CONTEMPORARY ORTHODONTICS

CONTEMPORARY ORTHODONTICS

WILLIAM R. PROFFIT, D.D.S., Ph.D.

Professor and Chairman, Department of Orthodontics,
School of Dentistry, University of North Carolina,
Chapel Hill, North Carolina

with

HENRY W. FIELDS, Jr., D.D.S., M.S., M.S.D.

and

James L. Ackerman
Paul M. Thomas
J.F. Camilla Tulloch

With **1400** *illustrations*

The C. V. Mosby Company

ST. LOUIS · TORONTO · LONDON   1986

MOSBY

A TRADITION OF PUBLISHING EXCELLENCE

Editor: Darlene Barela Warfel
Assistant editor: Donna Saya Sokolowski
Editing supervisor: Peggy Fagen
Manuscript editors: Jerie A. Jordan, Melissa Neves
Book design: Top Graphics
Cover design: Susan E. Lane
Production: Kathleen Teal, Jeanne Genz, Barbara Merritt

Printed in the United States of America

The C.V. Mosby Company
11830 Westline Industrial Drive, St. Louis, Missouri 63146

Library of Congress Cataloging-in-Publication Data

Proffit, William R.
    Contemporary orthodontics.

    Includes bibliographies and index.
    1. Orthodontics. I. Title. [DNLM: 1. Orthodontics—
methods.   WU 400 P964c]
RK521.P76 1986   617.6′43   85-21832
ISBN 0-8016-4084-9

GW/VH/VH 9 8 7 6 5 4 3 2 1   01/B/037

Contributors

HENRY W. FIELDS, Jr., D.D.S., M.S., M.S.D.

Associate Professor, Departments of Orthodontics and Pedodontics, School of Dentistry, University of North Carolina, Chapel Hill, North Carolina

JAMES L. ACKERMAN, D.D.S.

Private Practice, Bryn Mawr, Pennsylvania; formerly Professor and Chairman, Department of Orthodontics, University of Pennsylvania School of Dental Medicine, Philadelphia, Pennsylvania

PAUL M. THOMAS, D.D.S., M.S.

Assistant Professor, Departments of Orthodontics and Oral and Maxillofacial Surgery, School of Dentistry, University of North Carolina, Chapel Hill, North Carolina

J.F. CAMILLA TULLOCH, B.D.S., D.Orth.

Assistant Professor, Department of Orthodontics, School of Dentistry, University of North Carolina, Chapel Hill, North Carolina

Preface

Contemporary Orthodontics has two purposes: (1) to provide a comprehensive overview of orthodontics at the present time, in a format useful to practitioners at all levels, including specialty practice; and (2) to serve as an orthodontic text for students of dentistry, providing the information necessary for a basic understanding of orthodontics in a logical and comprehensible format.

The two purposes are not incompatible, and indeed the authors hope that all parts of the book will be interesting and accessible to readers with highly varied backgrounds. There is, however, a considerable spectrum of material, extending from a review of basic principles to a discussion of clinical procedures that commonly are considered beyond the scope of general dental practice. Given the differing needs of readers at varying levels, it is all but impossible to survey the present theory and practice of orthodontics without including some material that is beyond readers who are beginners in dentistry. Other material already forms the basic background of successful practitioners.

In its chapters on clinical treatment procedures, this text is written to provide a broad overview of treatment possibilities and the principles on which various treatment methods are based. An attempt is made to provide information about various possible treatment methods, with an emphasis on fixed appliance treatment with the edgewise appliance but without endorsement of specific techniques within the edgewise system or exclusion of other possible treatment approaches. The material on treatment techniques perhaps can be described best as a background against which graduate-level discussions of specific treatment techniques could begin. The attempt is to summarize the present state of the art at a level useful to specialists but comprehensible and interesting to nonspecialists who wish an understanding of the objectives, possibilities, and general approaches to orthodontic treatment.

The book is arranged so as to facilitate its use in a curriculum that follows the guidelines for predoctoral orthodontics developed by the American Association of Dental Schools in 1978. These guidelines, which are included in current accreditation standards, suggest that an appropriate curriculum should include instruction at four levels:

1. Basic growth and development
2. Applied growth and development, including diagnostic procedures
3. Biomechanics and basic orthodontic techniques
4. Clinical orthodontics, including adjunctive procedures for adults and treatment procedures of limited complexity for children

Material relating to these educational objectives in this text is found as follows:

Basic growth and development—Chapters 2, 3, 4

Applied growth and development and diagnostic procedures—Chapters 1, 6, 7

Biomechanics, basic orthodontic techniques, and simpler clinical procedures—Chapters 9-14, 19

In addition, to the extent that this was practical, material within each section and chapter is arranged in a sequence of increasing complexity, so that for example, concepts introduced in the early part of Chapter 4 are appropriately included in an introductory growth and development course, whereas material covered toward the end of that chapter often is reserved for an advanced-graduate level course. We hope that when the book is used as an orthodontic text, instructors will be able to easily identify and employ appropriate sections in conjunction with their preferred sequence and content of material.

Supplemental audiovisual materials to complement the sections of this text that normally are included in a predoctoral curriculum are available. These consist of a series of slide-tape sequences and video cassettes, along with teaching manuals. The instructional materials are grouped into four categories:

1. Basic growth and development: This is a complete self-instructional unit, including 8 video cassettes, 15 slide-tape sequences, a syllabus indicating the sequence and use of the instructional materials, and multiple-choice tests.
2. Applied growth and development: This also is a complete self-instructional unit, with 9 slide-tape sequences, 4 video cassettes, a syllabus, and test materials.
3. Biomechanics and laboratory technique: This consists of a laboratory manual and a series of video cassettes illustrating the fabrication and use of simple removable appliances and a fixed appliance technique for molar uprighting as an adjunctive orthodontic procedure.
4. Selected clinical topics: This includes a series of video cassettes on clinical procedures that often would be carried out outside the specialty practice of orthodontics.

Additional information about these audiovisual teaching materials can be obtained through direct contact with the Department of Orthodontics, UNC School of Dentistry, Chapel Hill, NC 27514.

The availability of color for the production of this book has been used in many line drawings in which color is used to enhance points requiring emphasis. A number of these drawings are modifications of illustrations by other authors, redrawn to take advantage of the availability of color. In all cases, these illustrations are used by permission and are acknowledged to the original source.

We would like to thank the staff of the UNC School of Dentistry Learning Resources Center, especially Warren McCollum, Tom Edwards, and Ramona Hutton-Howe, for art and photographic production; Nancy Arellano for secretarial and word processing support; Drs. Keith Black and Henry Zaytoun, Jr., for their assistance with organizing the illustrations for this volume; and our spouses and colleagues for their patience with this project.

Orthodontics has made tremendous strides in recent years, and it has been a pleasure to reflect on the extent of that progress during the preparation of this book. It also is gratifying to observe the increasing acceptance of orthodontic treatment in recent years and the continuing increase in the quality of treatment provided by well-trained and conscientious practitioners. We hope that this book contributes to continued progress in orthodontics.

William R. Proffit
Henry W. Fields, Jr.

Contents

THE ORTHODONTIC PROBLEM

Chapter 1

Malocclusion and Dentofacial Deformity in Contemporary Society

■ The Changing Goals of Orthodontic Treatment

Crowded, irregular, and protruding teeth have been a problem for some individuals since antiquity, and attempts to correct this disorder go back at least to 1000 BC. Primitive (and surprisingly well designed) orthodontic appliances have been found in both Greek and Etruscan materials. As dentistry developed in the eighteenth and nineteenth centuries, a number of devices for the "regulation" of the teeth were described by various authors and apparently used sporadically by the dentists of that era.

After 1850, the first texts that systematically described orthodontics appeared, the most notable being Norman Kingsley's *Oral Deformities*.[1] Kingsley (Fig. 1-1), who had a tremendous influence on American dentistry in the latter half of the nineteenth century, was among the first to use extraoral force to correct protruding teeth. He was also a pioneer in treatment of cleft palate and related problems.

Despite the contributions of Kingsley and his contemporaries, their emphasis in orthodontics remained the alignment of the teeth and the correction of facial proportions. Little attention was paid to the dental occlusion, and since it was common practice to remove teeth for many dental problems, extractions for crowding or malalignment were frequent. In an era when an intact dentition was a rarity, the details of occlusal relationships were considered unimportant.

In order to make good prosthetic replacement teeth, it was necessary to develop a concept of occlusion, and this occurred in the late 1800s. As the concepts of prosthetic occlusion developed and were refined, it was natural to extend this to the natural dentition. Edward H. Angle (Fig. 1-2), whose influence began to be felt about 1890, can be credited with much of the development of a concept of occlusion in the natural dentition. Angle's original interest was in prosthodontics, and he taught in that department in the dental schools at Pennsylvania and Minnesota in the 1880s. His increasing interest in occlusion in the natural definition and in the treatment necessary to obtain normal occlusion, led directly to his development of orthodontics as a specialty, with himself as the "father of modern orthodontics."

The publication of Angle's classification of malocclusion in the 1890s[2] was an important step in the development of orthodontics not only because it subdivided major types of malocclusion but also included the first clear and simple definition of normal occlusion in the natural dentition. Angle's postulate was that the upper first molars were the key to occlusion and that the upper and lower molars should be related so that the mesiobuccal cusp of the upper molar occludes in the buccal groove of the lower molar. If this

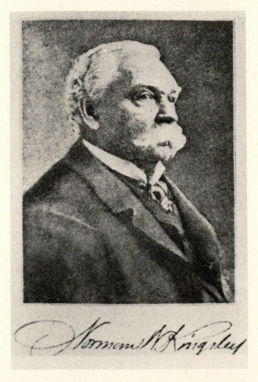

Fig. 1-1 ■ Norman Kingsley's self-portrait. Kingsley, who was a noted sculptor and artist as well as an influential dentist, also served as Dean of the School of Dentistry at New York University.

molar relationship existed and the teeth were arranged on a smoothly curving line of occlusion (Fig. 1-3), then normal occlusion would result. This statement, which nearly 100 years of experience have proved to be correct except when there are aberrations in the size of teeth, brilliantly simplified normal occlusion.

Angle then described three classes of malocclusion, based on the occlusal relationships of the first molars:

Class I   Normal relationship of the molars, but line of occlusion incorrect because of malposed teeth, rotations, or other causes

Class II   Lower molar distally positioned relative to upper molar, line of occlusion not specified

Class III   Lower molar mesially positioned relative to upper molar, line of occlusion not specified

Note that the Angle classification has four classes: normal occlusion, Class I malocclusion, Class II malocclusion, and Class III malocclusion (Fig. 1-4). Normal occlusion and Class I malocclusion share the same molar relationship, but differ in the arrangement of the teeth relative to the line of occlusion. The line of occlusion may or may not be correct in Class II and Class III.

With the establishment of a concept of normal occlusion and a classification scheme that incorporated the line of occlusion, by the early 1900s orthodontics was firmly established as the treatment of malocclusion, defined as any deviation from the ideal occlusal scheme described by Angle. Since precisely defined relationships required a full complement of teeth in both arches, maintaining an intact dentition became an important goal of orthodontic treatment. Angle and his followers strongly opposed extraction for orthodontic purposes. With the emphasis on dental occlusion that followed, however, less attention came to be paid to facial proportions and esthetics. Angle abandoned extraoral force because he found that it was not necessary to achieve proper occlusal relationships.

As time passed, it became clear that even an excellent occlusion was unsatisfactory if it was achieved at the expense of proper facial proportions. Not only were there esthetic problems, it often proved impossible to maintain an occlusal relationship achieved by prolonged use of heavy elastics to pull the teeth together as Angle and his followers had suggested. Extraction of teeth was reintroduced into orthodontics in the 1930s, to enhance facial esthetics and achieve better stability of the occlusal relationships.

Cephalometric radiography, which enabled orthodontists to measure the changes in tooth and jaw positions produced by growth and treatment, came into widespread use after World War II. These radiographs made it clear that many Class II and III malocclusions resulted from faulty jaw re-

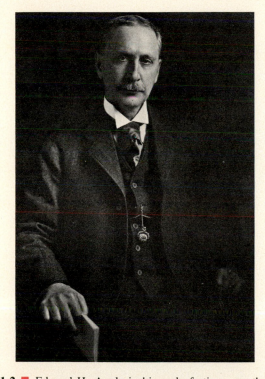

Fig. 1-2 ■ Edward H. Angle in his early forties, near the time that he estatablished himself as the first dental specialist. From 1905 to 1928, Angle operated proprietary orthodontic schools in St. Louis, New London, Connecticut, and Pasadena, California, in which many of the pioneer American orthodontists were trained.

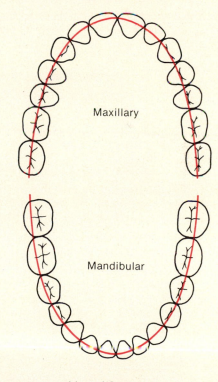

Maxillary

Mandibular

Line of Occlusion

Fig. 1-3 ■ The line of occlusion is a smooth (catenary) curve passing through the central fossa of each upper molar and across the cingulum of the upper canine and incisor teeth. The same line runs along the buccal cusps and incisal edges of the lower teeth, thus specifying the occlusal as well as interarch relationships once the molar position is established.

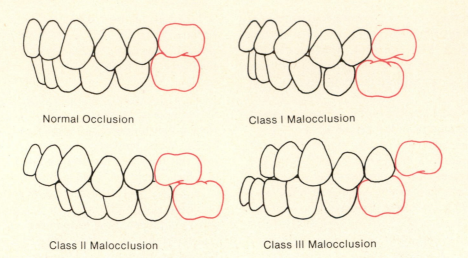

Normal Occlusion   Class I Malocclusion

Class II Malocclusion   Class III Malocclusion

Fig. 1-4 ■ Normal occlusion and malocclusion classes as specified by Angle. This classification was quickly and widely adopted early in the twentieth century. It is incorporated within all contemporary descriptive and classification schemes.

lationships, not just malposed teeth. By use of cephalometrics, it also was possible to see that jaw growth could be altered by orthodontic treatment. In Europe, the method of "functional jaw orthopedics" was developed to enhance growth changes, while in the United States, extraoral force came to be used for this purpose. At present, both functional and extraoral appliances are used internationally to control and modify growth and form.

The goal of modern orthodontics can be summed up as the creation of the best possible occlusal relationships, within the framework of acceptable facial esthetics and stability of the occlusal result (Figs. 1-5 to 1-7). The most recent definition of orthodontics, as adopted by the American Association of Orthodontists in 1981, includes these three goals within the definition following:

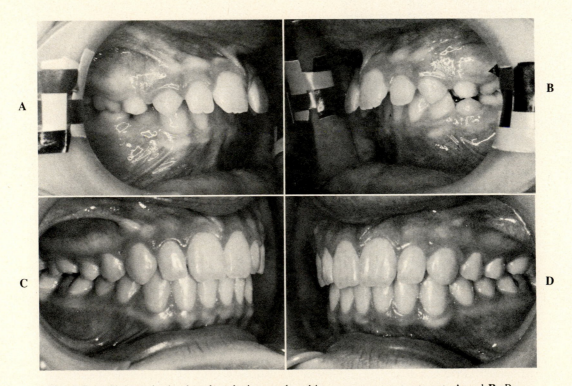

Fig. 1-5 ■ Changes in the dental occlusion produced by contemporary treatment. **A** and **B**, Pretreatment. **C** and **D**, Post-treatment. Two phases of treatment were used, first a functional appliance during the mixed dentition to influence jaw growth, then a fixed appliance to obtain excellent occlusal relationships.

Orthodontics (Dentofacial Orthopedics). The area of dentistry concerned with the supervision, guidance and correction of the growing and mature dentofacial structures, including those conditions that require movement of teeth or correction of malrelationships and malformations of related structures by the adjustment of relationships between and among teeth and facial bones by the application of forces and/or the stimulation and redirection of the functional forces within the craniofacial complex.

Major responsibilities of orthodontic practice include the diagnosis, prevention, interception and treatment of all forms of malocclusion of the teeth and associated alterations in their surrounding structures; the design, application and control of functional and corrective appliances; and the guidance of the dentition and its supporting structures to attain and maintain optimum relations in physiologic and esthetic harmony among facial and cranial structures.[3]

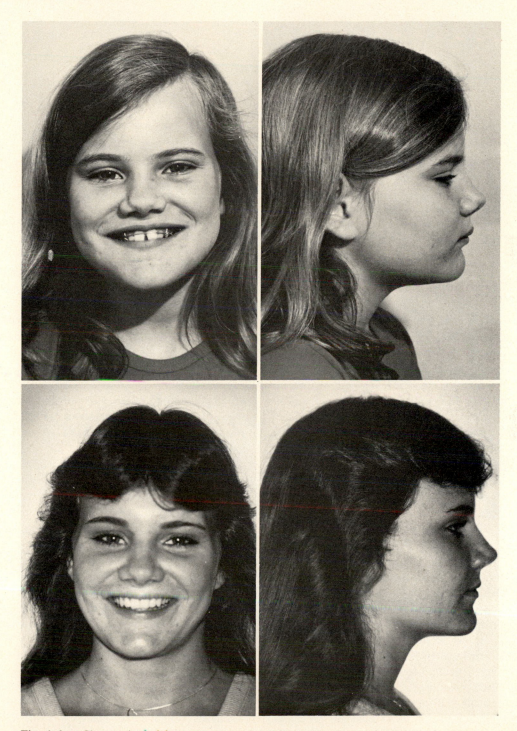

Fig. 1-6 ■ Changes in facial appearance produced by contemporary treatment (same patient as Fig. 1-5).

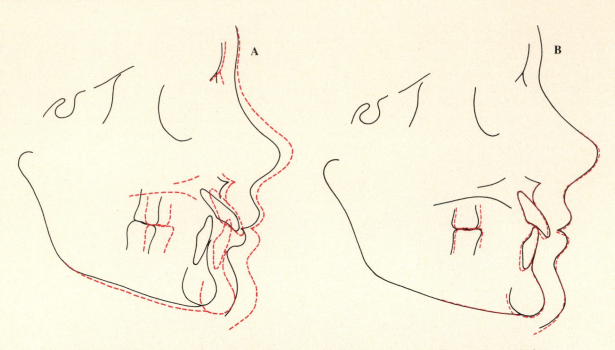

Fig. 1-7 ■ Superimposed cephalometric tracings, showing the skeletal and dental changes during treatment (same patient as Fig. 1-5). **A,** First phase of treatment (growth modification using functional appliance). **B,** Second phase of treatment (tooth positioning using complete fixed appliance).

■ *The Usual Orthodontic Problems: Epidemiology of Malocclusion*

What Angle defined as normal occlusion more properly should be considered the ideal normal, especially when the criteria are applied strictly. In fact, perfectly interdigitating teeth arranged along a perfectly regular line of occlusion are quite rare. For many years, epidemiologic studies of malocclusion suffered from considerable disagreement among the investigators about how much deviation from the ideal should be accepted within the bounds of normal. As a result, between 1930 and 1965 the prevalence of malocclusion in the United States was variously estimated as 35% to 95%.[4] These tremendous disparities were largely the result of the investigators' differing criteria for normal, not to population differences. Variations were also seen because the Angle classification is not a description of occlusal relationships sufficient for epidemiologic purposes.

Since 1960, a series of studies carried out by the U.S. Public Health Service (USPHS), the National Health Service in Britain, the World Health Organization, and other public health or university groups in most developed countries have provided a reasonably clear worldwide picture of the prevalence of various occlusal relationships or malrelationships. These studies of need and demand for orthodontic treatment have recently been reviewed.[5]

In the United States, two large scale surveys carried out by the Division of Health Statistics of the U.S. Public Health Service covered children ages 6 to 11 between 1963 and 1965, and youths ages 12 to 17 between 1969 and 1970. These surveys, published in the 1970s,[6,7] are by far the most thorough epidemiologic studies of occlusal relationships ever undertaken. Each was based on a sample of approximately 8,000 children or youths, selected to statistically represent the approximately 26 million individuals in the U.S. in those age ranges (excluding children living on Indian reservations).

To avoid judgment on how much was too much for a given characteristic, the data were tabulated by millimeters of deviation from ideal, allowing the user of the data to reach his own conclusions about admittedly controversial points. Data from these surveys are briefly discussed here and summarized in Tables 1 and 2.

The first point that the USPHS epidemiologic data makes clear is that the majority of American children and youths have a malocclusion of some type. In these studies, in addition to measurements of specific characteristics, Grainger's Treatment Priority Index (TPI)[8] was used to score the occlusion, providing an indicator of the overall severity of any occlusal problems. Approximately 25% had scores on the Treatment Priority Index of zero, indicating a near-ideal occlusion; the other 75% had some noticeable deviation from ideal occlusion. The percentage of youths age 12 to 17 with mild and moderate malocclusion was similar, but fewer in this age group had a zero score and considerably more had severe or very severe malocclusion (Table 1-1).

Since the Treatment Priority Index scores only occlusal characteristics, excluding skeletal and facial components, TPI scores do not necessarily coincide with the judgment clinicians would make, but they do indicate the relative proportions of children with increasingly severe malocclusion problems.

Table 1-1 ■ TPI Scores, U.S. children and youths

	Percent distribution			
	Age 6-11		Age 12-17	
TPI score	White	Black	White	Black
0 (near-ideal occlusion)	22.9	33.1	10.5	14.7
1-3 (mild malocclusion)	39.7	35.0	34.6	36.9
4-6 (moderate malocclusion)	23.7	15.0	25.7	21.0
>6 (severe or very severe)	13.7	16.9	29.2	27.4

Table 1-2 ■ Percent of U.S. children and youths with malocclusion types

	Age 6-11		Age 12-17	
	White	Black	White	Black
Crowding/malalignment problems				
Tooth displacement score 0 (ideal)	56.8	64.6	13.0	16.0
Tooth displacement score 1-5 (moderate)	38.9	32.6	43.6	49.5
Tooth displacement score >5 (severe)	4.3	2.6	43.4	34.5
Anteroposterior problems				
Overjet, 6 mm or more	17.3	13.5	15.3	11.8
Lower overjet, 1 mm or more	0.8	0.6	0.8	1.2
Vertical problems				
Open bite, 2 mm or more	1.4	9.6	1.2	10.1
Overbite, 6 mm or more	7.6	0.8	11.7	1.4
Transverse problems				
Lingual crossbite, 2 or more teeth	4.9	5.3	5.9	8.0
Buccal crossbite, 2 or more teeth	1.0	0.4	1.6	1.0

As might be expected, crowded malaligned teeth are the most common single contributor to malocclusion. About 40% of children and 85% of youths had some degree of malalignment within the dental arches, that is, a tooth displacement score other than zero (Table 1-2).

Excessive protrusion of maxillary incisors (overjet) was the second most common finding (Fig. 1-8). An overjet of 6 mm or more was found approximately 17% of children and 15% of youths. It is probable that many of these patients have a discrepancy in the size or position of the jaws, not just displacement of the teeth, but the survey provides no direct evidence on this point.

The other extreme in anteroposterior relationships, lower overjet with a Class III molar relationship, is uncommon in the U.S. population, occurring in less than 1% of all children and white youths, and just over 1% of black youths.

Vertical problems of anterior open bite versus excessive overbite (Fig. 1-9) are especially interesting because of the large racial differences in this characteristic. Just over 1% of white children, but nearly 10% of black, have 2 mm or more of anterior open bite. At the other end of the spectrum, 11.7% of white adolescents, but only 1.4% of blacks, have an overbite of 6 mm or more. This finding undoubtedly is related to different vertical facial proportions in the two groups, rather than to a different prevalence of habits or other causes (see Chapter 3 for a more detailed discussion.)

It is interesting to note that the number of children reported by their parents to suck their thumb every day or night is higher at all ages than the number of children with anterior open bite, indicating that even frequent thumb-sucking does not necessarily cause an open bite although a positive and significant correlation exists.

Problems in transverse dental relationships (posterior crossbites) (Fig. 1-10) are uncommon, occurring in about

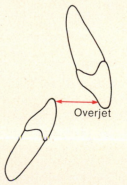

Fig. 1-8 ■ Overjet is defined as horizontal overlap of the incisors. Normally, the incisors are in contact, with the upper incisors ahead of the lower by only the thickness of the upper edges, i.e., 2 to 3 mm overjet is the normal relationship. If the lower incisors are in front of the upper incisors, the condition is called lower overjet, reverse overjet, or anterior crossbite.

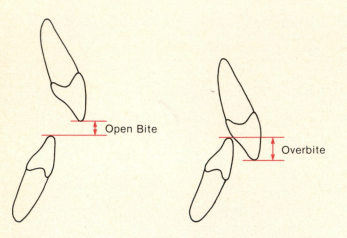

Fig. 1-9 ■ Overbite is defined as vertical overlap of the incisors. Normally, the lower incisal edges contact the lingual surface of the upper incisors at or above the cingulum, i.e., normally there is 1 to 2 mm overbite. In open bite, there is no vertical overlap, and the vertical separation is measured.

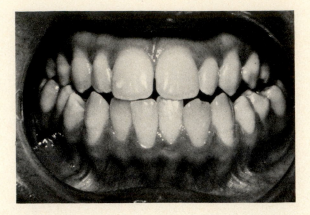

Fig. 1-10 ■ Posterior crossbite occurs when the line of occlusion is incorrect buccolingually. Usually, as in this child, the upper teeth are positioned lingually to the lower teeth. This is called lingual crossbite or just posterior crossbite. In buccal crossbite, which occurs rarely, if the upper teeth are too far buccally, there is no occlusal contact at all.

5% of children and 6% to 8% of youths, with minimal racial differences. When a transverse problem does exist, it is much more likely to be a relative narrowing of the maxillary arch (lingual crossbite) than buccal crossbite resulting from a relatively wide maxilla.

Although the Angle classification was not used in the USPHS survey—appropriately, since this classification scheme does not offer the necessary differentiation of vertical and transverse problems—it is interesting to calculate the percentage of individuals who would fall into Angle's four groups. From this approach, 25% at most have normal occlusion. Class I malocclusion (50% to 55%) is by far the largest single group; there are nearly but not quite as many Class II malocclusions (15% to 20%) as normal occlusion; Class III (1%) represents a very small proportion of the total.

■ *Need and Demand for Orthodontic Treatment*

■ Need for Treatment

Protruding, irregular, or maloccluded teeth can cause three types of problems for the patient: (1) psychosocial problems related to impaired dentofacial esthetics; (2) problems with oral function, including difficulties in jaw movement (muscle incoordination or pain), temporomandibular joint disturbances, and problems with mastication, swallowing, or speech; and (3) problems of accentuated periodontal disease or tooth decay related to malocclusion.

Psychosocial problems. A number of studies in recent years have confirmed what is intuitively obvious, that severe malocclusion can be a social handicap.[9,10] The usual caricature of an individual who is none too bright includes extremely protruding teeth. Several psychologic studies in recent years have confirmed that well aligned teeth and a pleasing smile carry positive status at all social levels, whereas irregular or protruding teeth carry negative status. Appearance can and does make a difference in teachers' expectations and therefore progress in school, in employability, and in competition for a mate and marriageability. Tests of the psychologic reactions of individuals to various dental conditions, carried out by showing photographs of various mouths to the individual whose response was being evaluated, show that cultural differences are smaller than might have been anticipated. A dental appearance pleasing to Americans is also judged pleasing in Australia and East Germany, whereas a dental appearance considered in the U.S. to carry with it some social handicap draws about the same response in these other cultural settings[11] (Fig. 1-11). There is no doubt that social responses conditioned by the appearance of the teeth can severely affect an individual's whole adaptation to life. This places the concept ''handicapping malocclusion'' in a larger and more important context. If the way you interact with other individuals is affected constantly by your teeth, your dental handicap is far from trivial.

It is interesting that psychic distress caused by disfiguring dental or facial conditions is not directly proportional to the anatomic severity of the problem. An individual who is grossly disfigured can anticipate a consistently negative response. An individual with an apparently less severe problem (for example, a protruding chin or irregular incisors) is sometimes treated differently because of this, but sometimes not. It seems to be easier to cope with a defect if other people's responses to it are consistent than if they are not. Unpredictable responses produce anxiety and can have strong deleterious effects.[12]

The impact of a physical defect on an individual also will be strongly influenced by that individual's self-esteem and

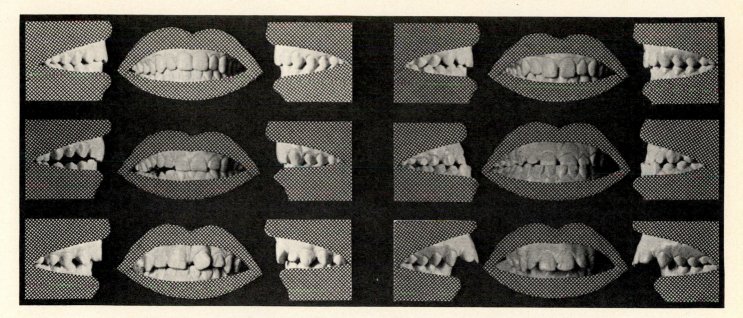

Fig. 1-11 ■ Examples of stimulus photographs used by Cons et al.[11] to study reactions to various dental conditions. A dental appearance like those in the bottom row carries negative social status; those in the top row are positive, and the middle row intermediate. Studies of this type have confirmed the impression that dental appearance affects social interactions.

Table 1-3 ■ Speech difficulties related to malocclusion

Speech sound	*Problem*	*Related malocclusion*
/s/, /z/ (sibilants)	Lisp	Anterior open bite, large gap between incisors
/t/, /d/ (linguoalveolar stops)	Diffulty in production	Irregular incisors, especially lingual position of maxillary incisors
/f/, /v/ (labiodental fricatives)	Distortion	Skeletal Class III
th, sh, ch (linguodental fricatives) (voiced or voiceless)	Distortion	Anterior open bite

the extent of his or her positive feelings about themselves. The result is that a degree of anatomic abnormality that is merely a condition of no great consequence to one individual can be a genuinely severe problem to another.

Oral function. A severe malocclusion may compromise all aspects of oral function. There may be difficulty in mastication if only a few teeth meet, and jaw discrepancies may force adaptive alterations in swallowing. It can be difficult or impossible to produce certain sounds in the presence of severe malocclusion (Table 1-3), and effective speech therapy may require some preliminary orthodontic treatment. Even less severe malocclusions tend to affect mastication, swallowing, and speech, not so much by making the function impossible as by requiring physiologic compensation for the anatomic deformity.

The relationship of malocclusion and adaptive function to the temporomandibular joint (TMJ) syndrome, manifested as pain in and around the temporomandibular joint, remains unclear and controversial. TMJ pain may result from pathologic changes within the temporomandibular joint, but more often is caused by muscle fatigue and spasm. Muscle pain almost always correlates with a history of posturing the mandible to an anterior or lateral position, or clenching or grinding the teeth as a response to stressful situations. The excessive muscle activity accompanying clenching or grinding may occur during the day or may be present during sleep.

Some dentists have suggested that even minor imperfections in the occlusion serve to trigger clenching and grinding activities. If this were true, it would indicate a real need for perfecting the occlusion in everyone, to avoid the possibility of developing facial muscle pain. Because the number of people with moderate degrees of malocclusion (50% to 75% of the population) far exceeds the number with TMJ problems (5% to 30%, depending on which symptoms are examined),[13,14] it seems unlikely that occlusal patterns alone are enough to cause hyperactivity of the oral musculature. Some individuals with poor occlusion have no problem with muscle pain when stressed, but do develop symptoms in other organ systems. Swedish data indicate that some types of malocclusion (Class III, anterior open bite, posterior crossbite, rotated/tipped teeth) correlate positively with TMJ problems, whereas other types of malocclusion do not.[15]

Since the postive correlations are not very large, it appears that malocclusion alone cannot explain the development of TMJ symptoms in most patients. On the other hand, if a patient does respond to stress by increased oral muscle activity, improper occlusal relationships of any type may make the problem more severe and harder to control. Therefore, malocclusion coupled with pain and spasm in the muscles of mastication may indicate a need for orthodontic treatment. If the problem is pathology within the joint itself, occlusal therapy is not a total answer but may be helpful in restoring proper internal relationships between the condyle and interarticular disk (see Chapter 19 for further details).

Relationship to dental disease. It seems obvious that malocclusion should contribute to both dental decay and periodontal disease by making it harder to care for the teeth properly. An individual's willingness and motivation determine his oral hygiene much more than how well the teeth are aligned, and presence or absence of dental plaque is the major determinant of the health of both the hard and soft tissues of the mouth. Studies of factors that influence tooth decay suggest that if individuals with malocclusion are more prone to tooth decay, the effect is small compared to hygiene status.[16]

It was once thought that trauma from occlusion played a significant role in the pathogenesis of periodontal disease. Studies in recent years reveal that how well the patient controls plaque is by far the strongest determinant of periodontal disease status, and the patient's occlusion in comparison plays a secondary role.[17] Occlusal trauma now receives much less emphasis as a primary etiologic factor for periodontal disease.

Two studies carried out in the late 1970s, in which a large number of patients were carefully examined 10 to 20 years after completion of orthodontic treatment, shed some light on the malocclusion–oral health relationship.[18,19] In both studies, comparison of the patients who underwent orthodontic treatment years ago with untreated individuals in the same age group showed similar periodontal status, despite the better functional occlusions of the orthodontically treated

group. There was only a tenuous link between untreated malocclusion and major periodontal disease later in life. No evidence of a beneficial effect of orthodontic treatment on future periodontal health was demonstrated, as would have been expected if untreated malocclusion had a major role in the etiology of periodontal problems.

It has been suggested that previous orthodontic treatment predisposes to later periodontal disease. The lack of association in these studies between occlusion and periodontal disease provided good news in this sense: there was no evidence that orthodontic treatment caused later periodontal problems. Patients with a history of orthodontic treatment appear to be more likely to seek later periodontal care than those who were not treated, and thus are over-represented among periodontal patients. This appears to be only another manifestation of the phenomenon that one segment of the population seeks dental treatment while another avoids it. Those who have had one type of dental treatment are more likely to seek another.

In summary, it appears that problems related to both esthetics and oral function can produce significant need for orthodontic treatment. The evidence is less clear that orthodontic treatment reduces the development of later dental disease.

■ Demand for Orthodontic Treatment

Demand for orthodontic treatment is indicated by the number of patients who actually make appointments and seek care. Need for treatment is more difficult to measure. This refers to the number of individuals who have an orthodontic problem and who would benefit from treatment. Not all patients with malocclusion, even those with extreme anatomic deviations from the normal, seek orthodontic treatment. Some do not recognize that they have a problem; others feel that they need treatment but cannot afford it or cannot obtain it. Data from the USPHS epidemiologic surveys[6,7] suggest that in typical American neighborhoods, about 35% of adolescents are perceived by parents and peers as needing orthodontic treatment. Dentists recommend treatment for another 20% (Table 1-4).

As might be expected, both the perceived need and demand vary with social and cultural conditions. More children in urban areas are thought (by parents and peers) to need treatment than children in rural areas, although the

Table 1-4 ■ Perceived need and demand for orthodontic treatment, United States, 1966-1970 (percent distribution)

| | Age 6-11 | | Age 12-17 | | | |
| | | | Boys | | Girls | |
	Boys	Girls	White	Black	White	Black
Parent/dentist perceived need	10.6	11.6	55.8		53.5	
Child/youth perceived need	—	—	17.6	20.3	18.3	21.5
Received treatment	2.4	2.6	9.6		11.8	
Perceived to need treatment, but not treated	—	—	10.9	9.3	13.3	9.7

prevalence of occlusal disharmony is similar. Dental and facial appearance is a major factor in the perception of need for treatment. Demand for orthodontic treatment is correlated with family income: all other factors being equal, the higher the income, the greater the demand for orthodontic treatment. This appears to reflect not only that higher income families can more easily afford orthodontic treatment but also that good facial appearance and avoidance of disfiguring dental conditions are associated with more prestigious social positions and occupations. The higher the aspirations for a child, the more likely the parent is to seek orthodontic treatment for him or her.

The effect of financial constraints on demand can be seen most clearly by the response to third-party payment plans. When third-party copayment is available, the number of individuals seeking orthodontic treatment rises considerably. Although reliable current data are not available, the number of children and youths who receive treatment has increased since the USPHS survey, perhaps to 15% to 20%. It is likely that demand for treatment will more closely approach the 35% level thought by the public to need treatment as orthodontic coinsurance becomes more widely available.

The number of adults seeking orthodontic treatment has increased rapidly since 1970. In the 1960s, 5% or less of all orthodontic patients were adults. By the mid-1980s, surveys of practitioners indicated that the figure was approaching 20%.[20] Many of these patients indicate that they wanted treatment earlier but did not receive it, often because their family could not afford it; now they can. Wearing braces as an adult is more socially acceptable than it was previously, though no one really knows why, and this too has made it easier for adults to seek treatment.

Orthodontics has become a more prominent part of den-

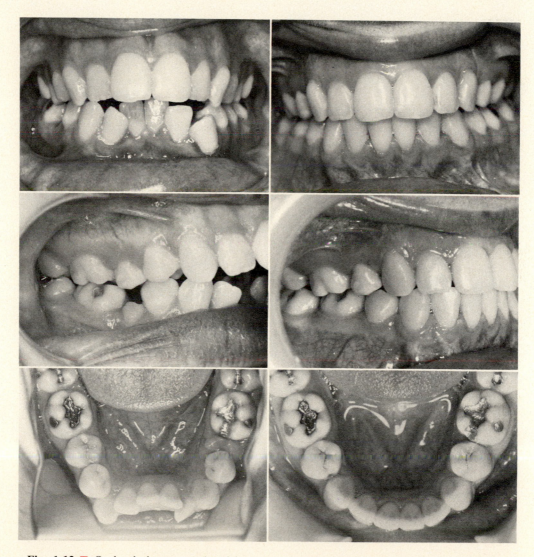

Fig. 1-12 ■ Occlusal changes produced in a nongrowing patient by contemporary orthodontic treatment (*Left column:* pre-treatment; *right column:* post-treatment). Note that first premolar teeth have been extracted to allow better lip contours and provide a more stable result.

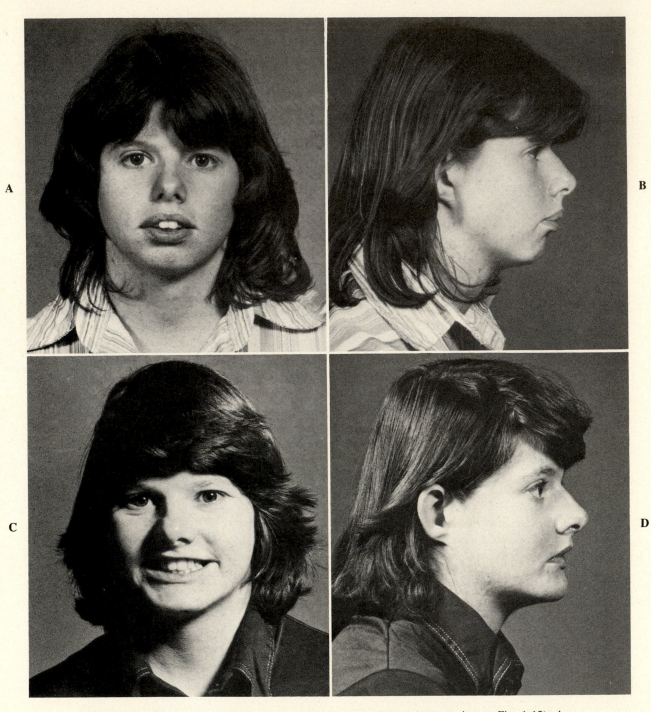

Fig. 1-13 ■ Facial changes produced by contemporary treatment (same patient as Fig. 1-12). **A** and **B,** Pre-treatment. **C** and **D,** Post-treatment. In this case, surgical repositioning of the upper jaw and chin was used to correct jaw relationships.

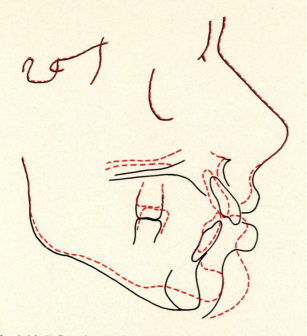

Fig. 1-14 ■ Superimposed cephalomatric tracings, showing skeletal and dental changes during treatment (same patient as Fig. 1-12).

tistry in recent years and this trend is likely to continue. The recent surveys of the long-term effects of orthodontic treatment reveal that the vast majority of individuals who had orthodontic treatment feel that they benefited from the treatment and are pleased with the result. Not all patients have the dramatic changes in dental and facial appearance shown in Fig. 1-12 to 1-14, but nearly all recognize an improvement in both dental condition and psychologic well-being.

■ *References*

1. Kingsley, N.W.: Treatise on oral deformities as a branch of mechanical surgery. New York, 1880, Appleton.
2. Angle, E.H.: Treatment of malocclusion of the teeth and fractures of the maxillae, Angle's system; ed. 6. Philadelphia, 1900, S.S. White Dental Manufacturing Co.
3. Hester, C.H., et al.: Glossary of dentofacial orthopedic terms. St. Louis, 1981, American Association of Orthodontists.
4. Zwemer, J.D., and Young, W.O.: Summary of studies on the prevalence of malocclusion. In Proffit, W.R., and Norton, L.A., editors: Education for orthodontics in general practice. Lexington, 1966, University of Kentucky, Department of Orthodontics.
5. McLain, J.B., and Proffit, W.R.: Oral health status in the United States: prevalence of malocclusion. J. Dent. Educ. **49:**386-396, 1985.
6. Kelly, J.E., Sanchez, M., and Van Kirk, L.E.: An assessment of the occlusion of teeth of children. Washington, D.C., 1973, National Center for Health Statistics, U.S. Public Health Service, DHEW Publication No. (HRA) 74-1612.
7. Kelly, J., and Harvey, C.: An assessment of the teeth of youths 12-17 years. Washington, D.C., 1977, National Center for Health Statistics, U.S. Public Health Service, DHEW Publication No. (HRA) 77-1644.
8. Grainger, R.M.: Orthodontic treatment priority index. Washington, D.C., 1967, National Center for Health Statistics, U.S. Public Health Service, PHS Publication No. 1000-Series 2, No. 25.
9. Morris, A.L. et al.: Seriously handicapping orthodontic conditions. Washington, D.C., 1977, National Academy of Sciences.
10. Jenny, J.: A social perspective on need and demand for orthodontic treatment. Int. Dent. J. **25:**248-256, 1975.
11. Cons, N.C., et al.: Perceptions of occlusal conditions in Australia, the German Democratic Republic, and the United States. Int. Dent. J. **33:**200-206, 1983.
12. Macgregor, F.C.: Social and psychological implications of dentofacial disfigurement. Angle Orthod. **40:**231-233, 1979.
13. Bush, F.M., et al.: Prevalence of mandibular dysfunction: subjective signs and symptoms. In Lundeen, H.C., and Gibbs, C.H., editors: Advances in Occlusion. Bristol, 1982, John Wright, pp. 106-118.
14. Rugh, J.I., and Solberg, W.K.: Oral health status in the United States: temporomandibular disorders. J. Dent. Educ. **49:**398-405, 1985.
15. Ingervall, B., Mohlin, B., and Thilander, B.: Prevalence of symptoms of functional disturbances of the masticatory system in Swedish men. J. Oral Rehab. **7:**185-197, 1980.
16. Bell, R.M., et al.: Treatment Effects in the National Preventive Dentistry Demonstration Program. Santa Monica, CA., 1984, Rand Corp.
17. Lindhe, J.: Trauma from occlusion. Dtsch. Zahnarztl. Z. **35:**680-684, 1980.
18. Sadowsky, C., and BeGole, E.A.: Long-term effects of orthodontic treatment on periodontal health. Am. J. Orthod. **80:**156-172, 1981.
19. Polson, L.A., et al.: Periodontal status after orthodontic treatment. International Association for Dental Research abstract, 1982.
20. Gottleib, E.L., and Vogel, D.S.: 1983 JCO Orthondontic Practice Study. J. Clin. Orthod. **18:**167-173, 1984.

THE DEVELOPMENT OF ORTHODONTIC PROBLEMS

Malocclusion and dentofacial deformity arise through variations in the normal developmental process, and so must be evaluated against a perspective of normal development. Because orthodontic treatment often involves manipulation of skeletal growth, clinical orthodontics requires an understanding not only of dental development but of more general concepts of physical growth.

This section begins in Chapter 2 with a discussion of basic concepts in physical growth and development. Information on physical growth and dental development at the various stages is then presented sequentially in Chapters 3 and 4, beginning with prenatal growth and extending into adult life where developmental changes continue at a slower pace. A brief discussion of psychologic development is included in Chapter 3, emphasizing emotional and cognitive development, and how the dentist can utilize this information to communicate with children and adolescents. The etiology of malocclusion and the special developmental problems of children with malocclusion and dentofacial deformity are considered in some detail in Chapter 5.

Chapter 2

Concepts of Physical Growth and Development

■ Growth: Pattern, Variability, and Timing

A thorough background in craniofacial growth and development is necessary for every dentist. Even for those who never work with children, it is difficult to comprehend conditions observed in adults without understanding the developmental processes that produced these problems. For those who do interact professionally with children—and almost every dentist does so at least occasionally—it is important to distinguish normal variation from the effects of abnormal or pathologic processes. Since dentists and orthodontists are heavily involved in the development of not just the dentition but the entire dentofacial complex, a conscientious practitioner may be able to manipulate facial growth for the benefit of the patient. Obviously, it is not possible to do so without a thorough understanding, not only of the pattern of normal growth but also of the mechanisms that underlie it.

The very terms *growth* and *development* can cause difficulties in understanding. Growth and development, though closely related, are not synonymous.

In conversational English, growth usually refers to an increase in size, but tends to be linked more to change than anything else. Only if growth meant change, after all, could someone seriously speak of a period of economic recession as one of "negative economic growth." Since some tissues grow rapidly and then shrink or disappear, a plot of physical growth versus time may include a negative phase. On the other hand, if growth is defined solely as a process of change, the term becomes almost meaningless. As a general

term, development connotes an increasing degree of organization, often with unfortunate consequences for the natural environment.

In this chapter, the term growth usually refers to an increase in size or number. Occasionally, however, the increase will be in neither size nor number, but in complexity. More often, the term development will be used to refer to an increase in complexity. Development carries an overtone of increasing specialization, so that one price of increased development is a loss of potential. Growth is largely an anatomic phenomenon, whereas development is physiologic.

In studies of growth and development, the concept of pattern is an important one. In a general sense, pattern (as in the pattern from which articles of clothing of different sizes are cut) reflects proportionality, usually of a complex set of proportions rather than just a single proportional relationship. Pattern in growth also represents proportionality, but in a still more complex way, because it refers not just to a set of proportional relationships at a point in time, but to the change in these proportional relationships over time. In other words, the physical arrangement of the body at any one time is a pattern of spatially proportioned parts. But there is a higher level pattern, the pattern of growth, which refers to the changes in these spatial proportions over time.

Fig. 2-1 illustrates the change in overall body proportions that occurs during normal growth and development. In fetal life, at about the third month of intrauterine development, the head takes up almost 50% of the total body length. At this stage, the cranium is large relative to the face and represents more than half the total head. In contrast, the limbs are still rudimentary and the trunk is underdeveloped. By the time of birth, the trunk and limbs have grown faster than the head and face, so that the proportion of the entire body devoted to the head has decreased to about 30%. The overall pattern of growth thereafter follows this course, with a progressive reduction of the relative size of the head to about 12% in the adult. At birth the legs represent about one-third of the total body length, while in the adult they represent about half. As Fig. 2-1 illustrates, there is more growth of the lower limbs than the upper during postnatal life. All of these changes, which are a part of the normal growth pattern, reflect the "cephalocaudal gradient of growth." This simply means that there is an axis of increased growth extending from the head toward the feet.

Another aspect of the normal growth pattern is that not

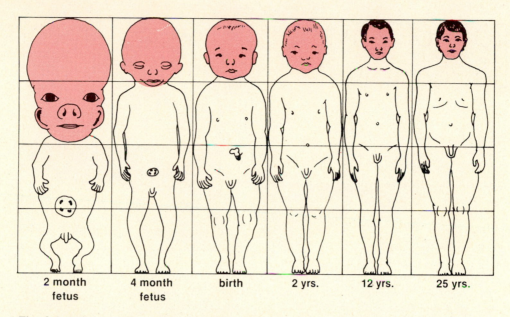

| 2 month fetus | 4 month fetus | birth | 2 yrs. | 12 yrs. | 25 yrs. |

Fig. 2-1 ■ Schematic representation of the changes in overall body proportions during normal growth and development. After the third month of fetal life, the proportion of total body size contributed by the head and face steadily declines. (Redrawn from Robbins, W.J., et al.: Growth. New Haven, 1928, Yale University Press.)

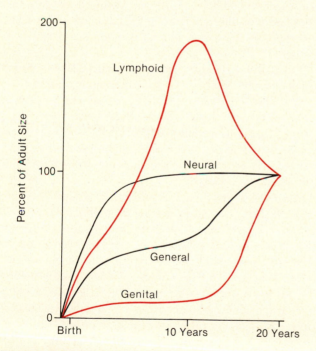

Fig. 2-2 ■ Scammon's curves for growth of the four major tissue systems of the body. As the graph indicates, growth of the neural tissues is nearly complete by 6 or 7 years of age. General body tissue, including muscle, bone, and viscera, show an S-shaped curve, with a definite slowing of the rate of growth during childhood and an acceleration at puberty. Lymphoid tissues proliferate far beyond the adult amount in late childhood, and then undergo involution at the same time that growth of the genital tissues accelerates rapidly. (From Scammon, R.E.: The measurement of the body in childhood. In Harris, J.A., editor: The measurement of Man. Minneapolis, 1930, University of Minnesota.)

all the tissue systems of the body grow at the same rate (Fig. 2-2). Obviously, the muscular and skeletal elements grow faster than the brain and central nervous system, as reflected in the relative decrease of head size. The overall pattern of growth is a reflection of the growth of the various tissues making up the whole organism. To put it differently, one reason for gradients of growth is that different tissue systems that grow at different rates are concentrated in various parts of the body.

Even within the head and face, the cephalocaudal growth gradient strongly affects proportions and leads to changes in proportion with growth (Fig. 2-3). When the skull of a newborn infant is compared proportionally to that of an adult, it is easy to see that the infant has a relatively much larger cranium and a much smaller face. This change in proportionality, with an emphasis on growth of the face relative to the cranium, is an important aspect of the pattern of facial growth. When the facial growth pattern is viewed against the perspective of the cephalocaudal gradient, it is not surprising that the mandible, being further away from the brain, tends to grow more than the maxilla, which is closer.

An important aspect of pattern is its predictability. Patterns repeat, whether in the organization of different colored tiles in the design of a floor or in skeletal proportions changing over time. The proportional relationships within a pattern can be specified mathematically, and the only difference between a growth pattern and a geometric one is the addition of a time dimension. Thinking about pattern in this way allows one to be more precise in defining what constitutes a change in pattern. Change, clearly, would denote an alteration in the predictable pattern of mathmatical relation-

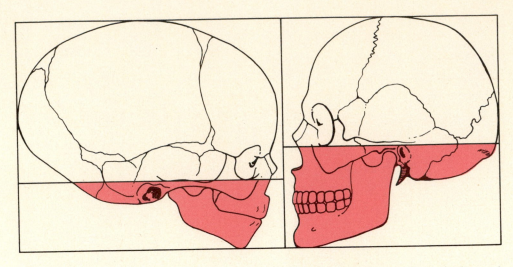

Fig. 2-3 ■ Changes in proportions of the head and face during growth. At birth, the face and jaws are relatively underdeveloped compared to their extent in the adult. As a result, there is much more growth of facial than cranial structures postnatally. (Redrawn from Lowery, G.H.: Growth and Development of Children, ed. 6. Chicago, 1973, Year Book Medical Publishers.)

ships. A change in growth pattern would indicate an alteration in the expected and predictable sequence of changes in proportions expected for that individual.

A second important concept in the study of growth and development is variability. Obviously, everyone is not alike, in the way that they grow as in everything else. It can be difficult, but clinically very important, to decide whether an individual is merely at the extreme of the normal variation or falls outside the normal range.

Rather than categorizing people as normal and abnormal, it is more useful to think in terms of deviations from the usual pattern and to express variability quantitatively. One way to do this is to evaluate a given child relative to peers on a standard growth chart (Fig. 2-4). Although charts of this type are commonly used for height and weight, the growth of any part of the body can be plotted in this way. The "normal variability," as derived from large-scale studies of groups of children, is shown by the solid lines on the graphs. An individual who stood exactly at the midpoint of the normal distribution would fall along the 50% line of the graph. One who was larger than 90% of the population would plot above the 90% line; one who was smaller than 10% of the population would plot below the 10% line.

These charts can be used in two ways to determine whether growth is normal or abnormal. First, the location of an individual relative to the group can be established. An individual who fell outside the range of 98% or 99% of the population certainly should receive special study before being accepted as just an extreme of the normal population. Second and perhaps more importantly, growth charts can be used to follow a child over time, to evaluate whether there is an unexpected change in growth pattern (Fig. 2-5). Pattern implies predictability. For the growth charts, this means that a child's growth should plot along the same percentile line at all ages. If the percentile position of an

individual relative to his or her peer group changes, especially if there is a marked change, the clinician should suspect some growth abnormality and should investigate further. Inevitably, there is a gray area at the extremes of normal variations, at which it is difficult to determine if growth is normal.

A final major concept in physical growth and development is that of timing. Variability in growth arises in several ways: from normal variation, from influences outside the normal experience (for example, serious illness), and from timing effects. Variation in timing arises because the same event happens for different individuals at different times—or, viewed differently, the biologic clocks of different individuals are set differently.

Variations in growth and development because of timing are particularly evident in human adolescence. Some children grow rapidly and mature early, completing their growth quickly and thereby appearing on the high side of developmental charts until their growth ceases and their contemporaries begin to catch up. Others grow and develop slowly, and so appear to be behind even though, given time, they will catch up with and even surpass children who once were larger. All children undergo a spurt of growth at adolescence, which can be seen more clearly by plotting change in height or weight (Fig. 2-6), but the growth spurt occurs at different times in different individuals.

Growth effects because of timing variation can be seen particularly clearly in girls, in whom the onset of menstruation, often referred to as menarche, gives an excellent indicator of the arrival of sexual maturity. Sexual maturation is accompanied by a spurt in growth. When the growth velocity curves for early, average, and late maturing girls are compared in Fig. 2-7, the marked differences in sizes between these girls during growth are apparent. At age 11, the early maturing girl is already past the peak of her ad-

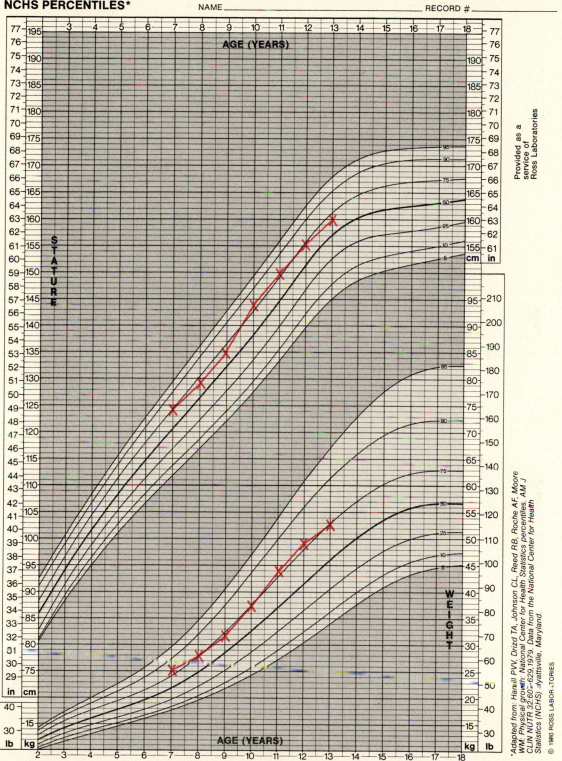

GIRLS: 2 TO 18 YEARS
PHYSICAL GROWTH
NCHS PERCENTILES*

Fig. 2-4 ■ Growth of a normal girl plotted on the female chart. Note that this girl remained at about the seventy-fifth percentile for height and weight over this entire period of observation. (Data from Hamill et al., National Center for Health Statistics, 1979; chart copyright Ross Laboratories, 1980.)

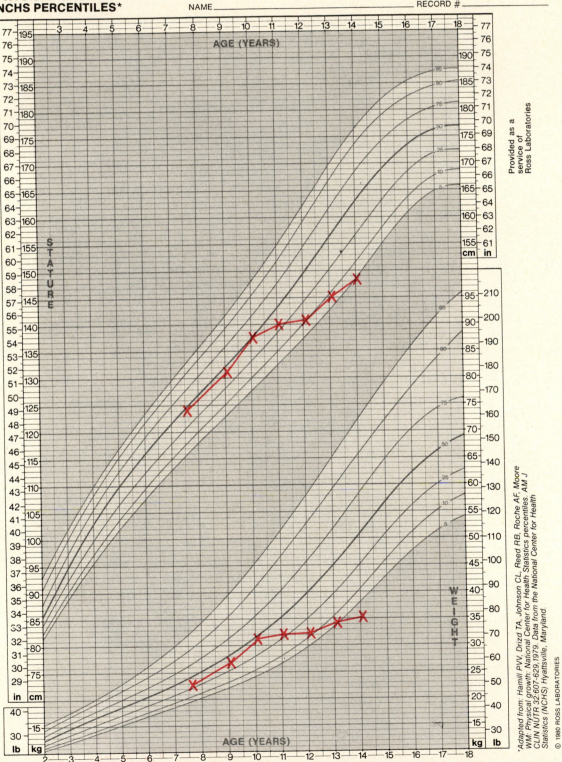

BOYS: 2 TO 18 YEARS
PHYSICAL GROWTH
NCHS PERCENTILES*

NAME _____   RECORD # _____

AGE (YEARS)

STATURE

WEIGHT

AGE (YEARS)

Provided as a
service of
Ross Laboratories

*Adapted from: Hamill PVV, Drizd TA, Johnson CL, Reed RB, Roche AF, Moore
WM: Physical growth: National Center for Health Statistics percentiles. AM J
CLIN NUTR 32:607-629,1979. Data from the National Center for Health
Statistics (NCHS) Hyattsville, Maryland.

© 1980 ROSS LABORATORIES

Fig. 2-5 ■ Growth of a boy, plotted on the male chart. Note the change in pattern between age 10 and 11, reflecting the impact of a serious illness on growth beginning at that time, with partial recovery after age 13 but a continuing effect on growth.

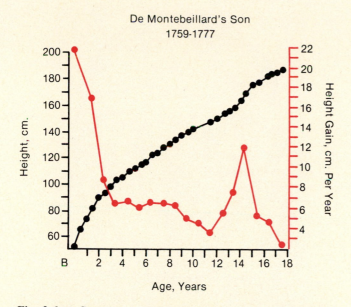

De Montebeillard's Son
1759-1777

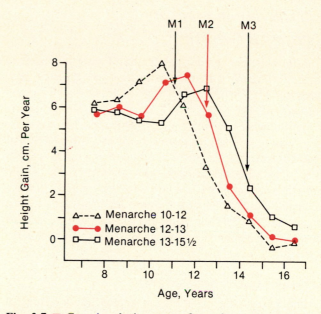

Fig. 2-6 ■ Growth can be plotted either in height and weight at any age (the black line here) or the amount of change in any given interval (the red line here, showing the same data as the black line). A curve like the black line is called a "distance curve," whereas the red line is a "velocity curve." Plotting velocity rather than distance makes it easier to see when accelerations and decelerations in the rate of growth occurred. These data are for the growth of one individual, the son of a French aristocrat in the late eighteenth century, whose growth followed the typical pattern. Note the acceleration of growth at adolescence, which occurred for this individual at about age 14. (Redrawn from Tanner, J.M.: Growth at Adolescence, ed. 2. Oxford, 1962, Blackwell Scientific Publications.)

Fig. 2-7 ■ Growth velocity curves for early, average, and late maturing girls. It is interesting to note that the earlier the adolescent growth spurt occurs, the more intense it appears to be. Obviously, at age 11 or 12, an early maturing girl would be considerably larger than one who matured late. In each case, the onset of menstruation (M1, M2, M3) came after the peak of growth velocity.

olescent growth spurt, whereas the late maturing girl has not even begun to grow rapidly. This sort of timing variation, which occurs in many ways other than that shown here, can be an important contributor to variability.

Because of time and variability, chronologic age often is not a good indicator of the individual's growth status. Although age is usually measured chronologically as the amount of time since birth or conception, it is also possible to measure age biologically, in terms of progress toward various developmental markers or stages. Timing variability can be reduced by using developmental age rather than chronologic age as an expression of an individual's growth status. For instance, if data for gain in height for girls are replotted, using the time of onset of menstruation as a reference time point (Fig. 2-8), it is apparent that girls who mature early, average, or late really follow a very similar growth pattern. This graph substitutes stage of sexual development for chronologic time, to produce a biologic time scale, and shows that the pattern is expressed at different times chronologically but not at different times physiologically. The effectiveness of biologic or developmental ages in reducing timing variability makes this approach very useful in evaluating a child's growth status.

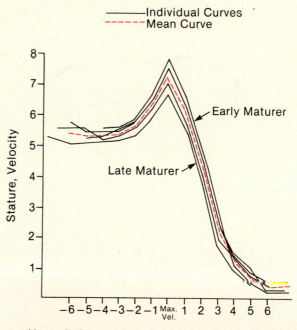

Fig. 2-8 ■ Velocity curves for four girls with quite different times of onset of menstruation, replotted using the onset of menstruation as a zero time point. It is apparent that the growth pattern in each case is quite similar, with almost all of the variation resulting from timing.

■ *Methods for Studying Physical Growth*

Before beginning the examination of growth data, it is important to have a reasonable idea of how the data were obtained. There are two basic approaches to studying physical growth. The first is based on techniques for measuring living animals (including humans), with the implication that the measurement itself does no harm and that the animal will be available for additional measurements at another time. The second approach uses experiments in which growth is manipulated in some way. This implies that the subject of the experiment will be available for study in some detail, and the detailed study may be destructive. For this reason, such experimental studies are restricted to subhuman species.

■ Measurement Approaches

The first of the measurement approaches for studying growth, with which the science of physical anthropology began, is craniometry, based on measurements of skulls found among human skeletal remains (Fig. 2-9). Craniometry was originally used to study the Neanderthal and Cro-Magnon peoples whose skulls were found in European caves in the eighteenth and nineteenth centuries. From such skeletal material, it has been possible to piece together a great deal of knowledge about extinct populations and to get some idea of their pattern of growth by comparing one skull to another. Craniometry has the advantage that rather precise measurements can be made on dry skulls; it has the important disadvantage for growth studies that, by necessity, all these growth data must be cross-sectional. Cross-sectional means that although different ages are represented in the population, the same individual can be measured at only one point in time.

It is also possible to measure skeletal dimensions on living individuals. In this technique, called anthropometry, various landmarks established in studies of dry skulls are measured in living individuals simply by using soft tissue points overlying these bony landmarks. For example, it is possible to measure the length of the cranium from a point at the bridge of the nose to a point at the greatest convexity of the rear of the skull. This measurement can be made on either a dried skull or a living individual, but results would be different because of the soft tissue thickness overlying both landmarks. Although the soft tissue introduces variation, anthropometry does make it possible to follow the growth of an individual directly, making the same measurements repeatedly at different times. This produces longitudinal data: repeated measures of the same individual.

The third measurement technique, cephalometric radiology, is of considerable importance not only in the study of growth but also in clinical evaluation of orthodontic patients. This approach can combine the advantages of craniometry and anthropometry. It allows a direct measurement of bony skeletal dimensions, since the bone can be seen

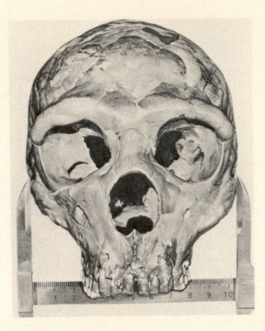

Fig. 2-9 ■ Craniometric studies are based on measurements between landmarks on dried skulls, typically those found in skeletal remains of earlier people. A classic craniometric measurement is the bizygomatic width, measured as shown here. Craniometry remains a valuable tool for the study of prehistoric populations.

through the soft tissue covering in a radiograph (Fig. 2-10), but it also allows the same individual to be followed over a period of time. The disadvantage of a cephalometric radiograph is that it produces a two-dimensional representation of a three-dimensional structure, and so even with precise head positioning, not all measurements are possible. To some extent, this can be overcome by taking more than one x-ray at different orientations and using triangulation to calculate oblique distances. The general pattern of craniofacial growth was known from craniometric and anthropometric studies before cephalometric radiography was invented, but much of the current picture of craniofacial growth is based on cephalometric studies.

Both anthropometric and cephalometric data can be expressed cross-sectionally rather than longitudinally. Obviously, it would be much easier and quicker to do a cross-sectional study, gathering data once for any individual and including subjects of different ages, rather than spending many years on a study in which the same individuals were measured repeatedly. For this reason, most studies are cross-sectional. When this approach is used, however, variability within the sample can conceal details of the growth pattern, particularly when there is no correction for timing variation (Fig. 2-11). Fluctuations in the growth curve that may occur for nearly every individual would be seen in a cross-sectional study only if they occurred at the same time for each person, which is unlikely. Longitudinal studies are efficient in the sense that a great deal of information can be gained from a relatively small number of subjects, fewer than would be needed in a cross-sectional study. In addition, the longitu-

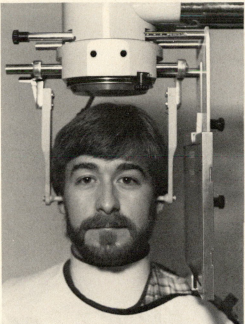

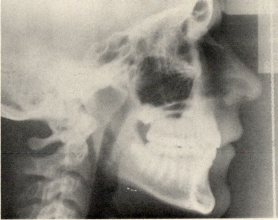

Fig. 2-10 ■ A cephalometric radiograph merits this name because of the use of a head positioning device to provide precise orientation of the head. This means that valid comparisons can be made between external and internal dimensions in members of the same population group, or that the same individual can be measured at two points in time, because the head orientation is reproducible.

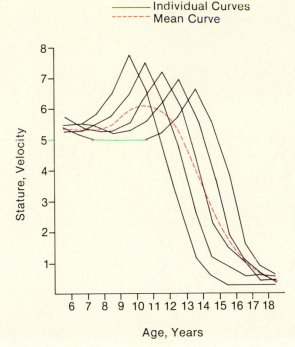

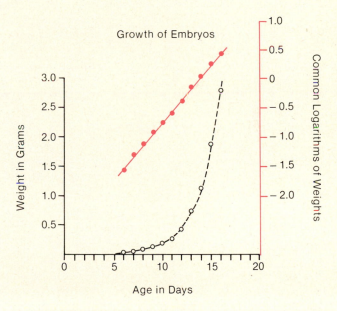

Fig. 2-11 ■ If growth velocity data for a group of individuals with a different timing of the adolescent growth spurt are plotted on a chronologic scale, it is apparent that the average curve is not an accurate representation of the pattern of growth for any particular individual. This smoothing of individual variation is a characteristic of cross-sectional data and a major limitation in use of the cross-sectional method for studies of growth. Only by following individuals through time in a longitudinal study is it possible to see the details of growth patterns.

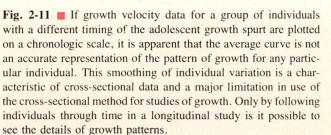

Fig. 2-12 ■ Data for the increase in weight of early embryos, with the raw data plotted in black and the same data plotted after logarithmic transformation in red. At this stage, the weight of the embryo increases dramatically but, as shown by the straight line after transformation, the rate of multiplication of individual cells remains fairly constant. When more cells are present, more divisions can occur, the weight increases faster. (From Lowery, G.H.: Growth and Development of Children, ed. 6. Chicago, 1973, Year Book Medical Publishers.)

dinal data highlight individual variations, particularly variations caused by timing effects.

Measurement data can be presented graphically in a number of different ways, and frequently it is possible to clarify growth changes by varying the method of display. For example, we have already seen that growth data can be presented by plotting the size attained as a function of age, which is called a "distance" curve (see Fig. 2-6) or as a "velocity" curve, showing not the total length by the increment added each year (see Fig. 6-8). Changes in the rate of growth are much more easily seen in the velocity curve than the distance curve.

Various other mathematical transformations can be used with growth data to make it easier to understand. For instance, the growth in weight of any embryo at an early stage follows a logarithmic or exponential curve, because the growth is based on division of cells; the more cells there are, the more cell divisions can occur. If the same data are plotted using the logarithm of the weight, a straight-line plot is attained (Fig. 2-12). This demonstrates that the rate of multiplication for cells in the embryo is remaining more or less constant. To correctly interpret data after mathematical transformation, it is important to understand how the data were transformed, but the approach is a powerful one in clarifying growth concepts.

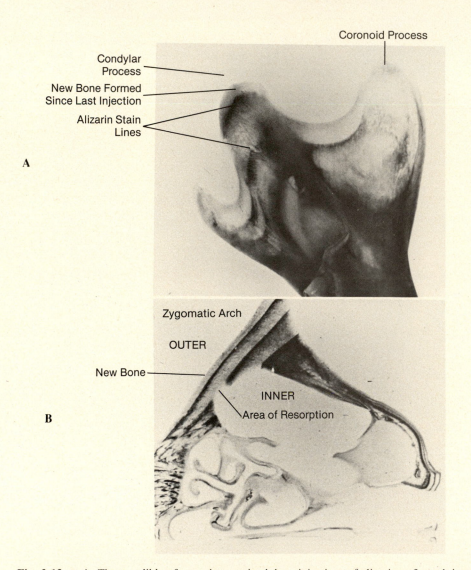

Fig. 2-13 ■ **A,** The mandible of a rat that received three injections of alizarin at 3-week intervals and was sacrificed 2 weeks after the last injection. Remodeling of the bone as it grows blurs some of the injection lines, but sequential lines in the condylar process can be seen clearly. **B,** Section through the zygomatic arch, from the same animal as in **A.** The zygomatic arch grows outward by apposition of bone on the outer surface and removal from the inner surface. The interruptions in the staining lines on the inner surface clearly show the areas where bone is being removed. What was the outer surface of the zygomatic arch at one point becomes the inner surface a relatively short time later, and then is removed.

■ Experimental Approaches

Much has been learned about skeletal growth using the technique called vital staining, in which dyes that stain mineralizing tissues (or occasionally, soft tissues) are injected into an animal. These dyes remain in the bones and teeth and can be detected later after sacrifice of the animal. This method was originated by the great English anatomist John Hunter in the eighteenth century. Hunter observed that the bones of pigs that occasionally were fed textile waste were often stained in an interesting way. He discovered that

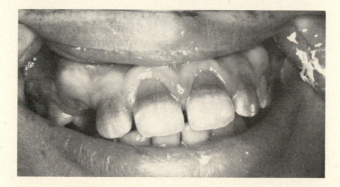

Fig. 2-14 ■ Tetracycline staining in the teeth of a boy who received large doses of tetracycline because of repeated upper respiratory infections in early childhood. From the location of the staining, it is apparent that tetracycline was not administered in infancy but was given in large doses beginning when the crowns of the central incisors were about half formed, or at approximately age 30 months.

the active agent was a dye called alizarin, which still is used for vital staining studies (Fig. 2-13). Alizarin reacts strongly with calcium at sites where bone calcification is occurring. Since these are the sites of active skeletal growth, the dye marks the locations at which active growth was occurring when it was injected. Bone remodels rapidly, and areas from which bone is being removed also can be identified by the fact that vital stained material has been removed from these locations.

Although studies using vital stains are not possible in humans, vital staining can occur. Many children born in the late 1950s and early 1960s who were given large quantities of the antibiotic tetracycline have permanently stained bones and teeth (Fig. 2-14). It was discovered too late that tetracycline is an excellent vital stain, which binds to calcium at growth sites in the same way as alizarin. The discoloration of incisor teeth that results from tetracycline given when the teeth are mineralizing has been an esthetic disaster for some individuals, and therefore tetracycline rarely is used for children.

With the development of radioactive tracers, it has become possible to use almost any radioactively labeled metabolite that becomes incorporated into the tissues as a sort of vital stain. The location, of course, must be detected by the weak radioactivity given off at the site where the material was incorporated. The gamma-emitting isotope ^{99m}Tc can be used to detect areas of rapid bone growth, but these images are more useful in diagnosis of localized growth problems (see Chapter 21) than for studies of growth patterns. For

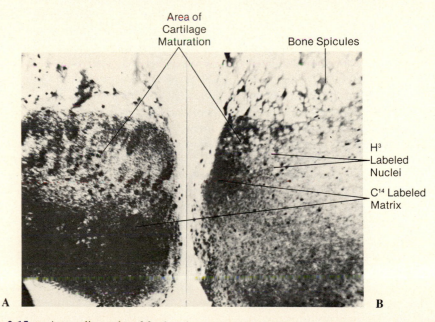

Fig. 2-15 ■ Autoradiographs of fetal rat bones growing in organ culture, with ^{14}C-proline and ^{3}H-thymidine incorporated in the culture medium. Thymidine is incorporated into DNA, which is replicated when a cell divides, so labeled nuclei are those of cells that underwent mitosis in culture. Because proline is a major constituent of collagen, cytoplasmic labeling indicates areas where proline was incorporated, primarily into extracellularly secreted collagen. **A,** Normal growth in this medium, with many labeled cells and heavy incorporation of proline. **B,** Decreased growth in a bone grown with a small amount of bacterial endotoxin added to the culture.

most studies of growth, radioactively labeled materials are detected by the technique of autoradiography, in which a film emulsion is placed over a thin section of tissue containing the isotope and then is exposed in the dark by the radiation. After the film is developed, the location of the radiation that indicates where growth is occurring, can be observed by looking at the tissue section through the film (Fig. 2-15).

Another experimental method, applicable to studies of humans, is implant radiography. In this technique, inert metal pins are placed in bones anywhere in the skeleton, including the face and jaws. These metal pins are well tolerated by the skeleton and become permanently incorporated into the bone without causing any problems (Fig. 2-16). If metallic implants are placed in the jaws, a considerable increase in the accuracy of a longitudinal cephalometric analysis of growth pattern can be achieved. This method of study, used extensively by Professor Bjork and coworkers at the Royal Dental College in Copenhagen, Denmark, has provided important new information about the growth pattern of the jaws.[1] The metal pins stay where they were placed within the bones in the absence of infection or inflammation, which is rarely a problem. Superimposing cephalometric radiographs on the implanted pins allows precise observation of both changes in the position of one bone relative to another, and changes in the external contours of individual bones. Before radiographic studies using implants, the extent of remodeling changes in the contours of the jaw bones was underestimated, and the rotational pattern of jaw growth described in Chapter 4 was not appreciated.

■ *The Nature of Skeletal Growth*

At the cellular level, there are only three possibilities for growth. The first is an increase in the size of individual cells, which is referred to as *hypertrophy.* The second possibility is an increase in the number of the cells, referred to as *hyperplasia.* The third is for the cells to *secrete extracellular material,* thus contributing to an increase in size independent of the number or size of the cells themselves.

In fact, all three of these processes occur in skeletal growth. Hyperplasia is a prominent feature of all forms of growth. Hypertrophy occurs in a number of special circumstances, but is a less important mechanism than hyperplasia in most instances. Although tissues throughout the body secrete extracellular material, this phenomenon is particularly important in the growth of the skeletal system, where extracellular material later mineralizes.

The fact that the extracellular material of the skeleton becomes mineralized leads to an important distinction between growth of the soft or nonmineralized tissues of the body and the hard or calcified tissues. Hard tissues are bones, teeth, and sometimes cartilages. Soft tissues are everything else. In most instances, cartilage, particularly the cartilages significantly involved in growth, behaves like soft tissue and should be thought of in that group, rather than as hard tissue.

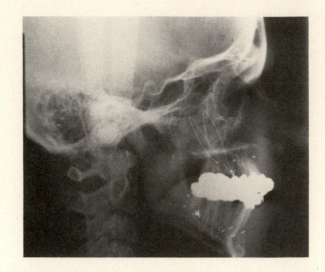

Fig. 2-16 ■ Cephalometric radiograph showing implants in a patient before surgery to reposition the jaws. The metallic implants appear as small white lines. Superimposing radiographs from before to after surgery on these implants allows a clear distinction between movements of the teeth and movements of the jaws.

Growth of soft tissues occurs by a combination of hyperplasia and hypertrophy. These processes go on everywhere within the tissues, and the result is what is called *interstitial growth,* which simply means that it occurs at all points within the tissue. Secretion of extracellular material can also accompany interstitial growth, but hyperplasia primarily and hypertrophy secondarily are its characteristics. Interstitial growth is characteristic of nearly all soft tissues and of uncalcified cartilage within the skeletal system.

In contrast, when mineralization takes place so that hard tissue is formed, interstitial growth becomes impossible. Hyperplasia, hypertrophy, and secretion of extracellular material all are still possible, but in mineralized tissues, these processes can occur only on the surface, not within the mineralized mass. Direct addition of new bone to the surface of existing bone can and does occur through the activity of cells in the periosteum, the soft tissue membrane that covers bone. Formation of new cells occurs in the periosteum, and extracellular material secreted there is mineralized and becomes new bone. This process is called *direct* or *surface apposition* of bone.

Interstitial growth is a prominent aspect of overall skeletal growth because a major portion of the skeletal system is originally modeled in cartilage. This includes the basal part of the skull as well as the trunk and limbs.

Fig. 2-17 shows the cartilaginous or chondrocranium at 8 and 12 weeks of intrauterine development. The height of cartilaginous skeletal development occurs during the third month of intrauterine life. A continuous plate of cartilage extends from the nasal capsule posteriorly all the way to the foramen magnum at the base of the skull. It must be kept in mind that cartilage is a nearly avascular tissue whose internal cells are supplied by diffusion through the outer layers. This means, of course, that the cartilage must be

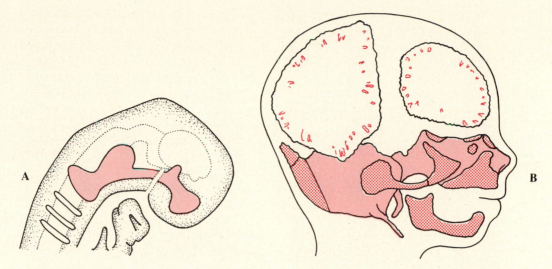

Fig. 2-17 ■ Development and maturation of the chondrocranium (cartilage: pink; bone: stippled red). **A,** Diagrammatic representation at about 8 weeks. Note that an essentially solid bar of cartilage extends from the nasal capsule anteriorly through to the occipital area posteriorly. **B,** Skeletal development at 12 weeks. Ossification centers have appeared in the midline cartilage structures, and in addition, intramembranous bone formation of the jaws and brain case has begun. From this point on, bone replaces cartilage of the original chondrocranium rapidly, so that only the small cartilaginous synchondroses connecting the bones of the cranial base remain.

thin. At early stages in development, the extremely small size of the embryo makes a chondroskeleton feasible, but with further growth, such an arrangement is no longer possible without an internal blood supply.

During the fourth month in utero, there is an ingrowth of blood vascular elements into various points of the chondrocranium (and the other parts of the early cartilaginous skeleton). These areas become centers of ossification, at which cartilage is transformed into bone, and islands of bone appear in the sea of surrounding cartilage (Fig. 2-17, *B*). The cartilage continues to grow rapidly but is replaced by bone with equal rapidity. The result is that the relative amount of bone increases rapidly and the relative (but not the absolute) amount of cartilage decreases. Eventually, the old chondrocranium is represented only by small areas of cartilage interposed between large sections of bone, which assume the characteristic form of the ethmoid, sphenoid, and basioccipital bones. Growth at these cartilaginous connections between the skeletal bones is similar to growth in the limbs.

In the long bones of the extremities, areas of ossification appear in the center of the bones and at the ends, ultimately producing a central shaft called the *diaphysis* and a bony cap on each end called the *epiphysis*. Between the epiphysis and diaphysis is a remaining area of uncalcified cartilage called the epiphyseal plate (Fig. 2-18). The epiphyseal plate cartilage of the long bones is a major center for their growth, and in fact this cartilage is responsible for almost all growth in length of these bones. The periosteum on the surface of the bones also plays an important role in adding to thickness and in reshaping the external contours.

Near the outer end of each epiphyseal plate is a zone of actively dividing cartilage cells. Some of these, pushed toward the diaphysis by proliferative activity beneath, undergo hypertrophy, secrete an extracellular matrix, and eventually degenerate as the matrix begins to mineralize and then is rapidly replaced by bone (Fig. 2-18). As long as the rate at which cartilage cells proliferate is equal to or greater than the rate at which they mature, growth will continue. Even-

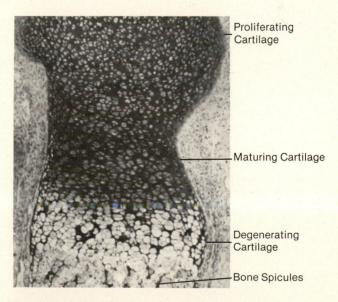

Proliferating Cartilage

Maturing Cartilage

Degenerating Cartilage

Bone Spicules

Fig. 2-18 ■ Endochondral ossification at an epiphyseal plate. Growth occurs by proliferation of cartilage, occurring here at the top. Maturing cartilage cells are displaced away from the area of proliferation, undergo hypertrophy, degenerate, and are replaced by spicules of bone, as seen in the bottom.

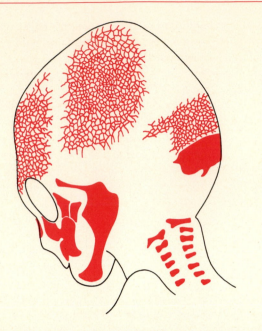

Fig. 2-19 ■ The bones of the skull of a 12-week-old fetus, drawn from a cleared alizarin-stained specimen. (Redrawn from Langman, J.: Medical Embryology, ed. 4. Baltimore, 1984, Williams & Wilkins.)

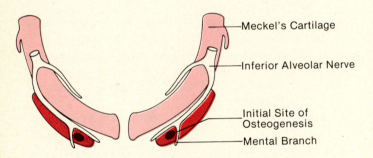

Meckel's Cartilage

Inferior Alveolar Nerve

Initial Site of Osteogenesis

Mental Branch

Fig. 2-20 ■ Diagrammatic representation of the relation of initial bone formation in the mandible to Meckel's cartilage and the inferior alveolar nerve. Bone formation begins just lateral to Meckel's cartilage and spreads posteriorly along it without any direct replacement of the cartilage by the newly forming bone of the mandible. (Redrawn from Ten Cate, A.R.: Oral Histology, St. Louis, 1985, The C.V. Mosby Co.)

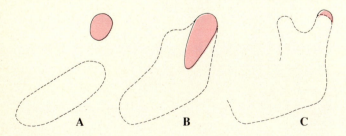

A   B   C

Fig. 2-21 ■ The condylar cartilage (pink) develops initially as a separate area of condensation from that of the body of the mandible, and only later is incorporated within it. **A,** Separate areas of mesenchymal condensation, at 8 weeks; **B,** fusion of the cartilage with the mandibular body, at 4 months; **C,** situation at birth (reduced in scale).

tually, however, toward the end of the normal growth period, the rate of maturation exceeds the rate of proliferation, the last of the cartilage is replaced by bone, and the epiphyseal plate disappears. At that point, the growth of the bone is complete, except for surface changes in thickness, which can be produced by the periosteum.

Not all bones of the adult skeleton were represented in the embryonic cartilaginous model, and it is possible for bone to form by secretion of bone matrix directly within connective tissues, without any intermediate formation of cartilage. Bone formation of this type is called *intramembranous bone formation*. This type of ossification occurs in the cranial vault and both jaws (Fig. 2-19).

Early in embryonic life, the mandible of higher animals develops in the same area as the cartilage of the first pharyngeal arch, Meckel's cartilage. It would seem that the mandible should be a bony replacement for this cartilage in the same way that the sphenoid bone beneath the brain replaces the cartilage in that area. In fact, development of the mandible begins as a condensation of mesenchyme just lateral to Meckel's cartilage and proceeds entirely as an intramembranous bone formation (Fig. 2-20). Meckel's cartilage disintegrates and largely disappears as the bony mandible develops. Remnants of this cartilage are transformed into a portion of two of the small bones that form the conductive ossicles of the middle ear, but not into a significant part of the mandible. Its perichondrium persists as the sphenomandibular ligament. The condylar cartilage develops initially as an independent secondary cartilage, which is separated by a considerable gap from the body of the mandible (Fig. 2-21). Early in fetal life, it fuses with the developing mandibular ramus.

The maxilla forms initially from a center of mesenchymal condensation in the maxillary process. This area is located on the lateral surface of the nasal capsule, the most anterior part of the chondrocranium, but although the growth cartilage contributes to lengthening of the head and anterior displacement of the maxilla, it does not contribute directly to formation of the maxillary bone. An accessory cartilage, the zygomatic or malar cartilage, which forms in the developing malar process, disappears and is totally replaced by bone well before birth, unlike the mandibular condylar cartilage, which persists.

Whatever the location for intramembranous bone formation, interstitial growth within the mineralized mass is impossible, and the bone must be formed entirely by apposition of new bone to free surfaces. Its shape can be changed through removal (resorption) of bone in one area and addition (apposition) of bone in another (see Fig. 2-13). This balance of apposition and resorption, with new bone being formed in some areas while old bone in removed in others, is an essential component of the growth process. *Remodeling* of this type is seen at the surfaces of bones that are growing primarily by endochondral replacement as well as in bones that formed directly within a connective tissue membrane.

■ *Types of Growth in the Craniofacial Complex*

To understand growth in any area of the body, it is necessary to understand: (1) the sites or location of growth, (2) the type of growth occurring at that location, and (3) the determinant or controlling factors in that growth.

For the following discussion of sites and types of growth, it is convenient to divide the craniofacial complex into four areas that grow rather differently: (1) the cranial vault, the bones that cover the upper and outer surface of the brain; (2) the cranial base, the bony floor under the brain, which also is the dividing line between the cranium and the face; (3) the nasomaxillary complex, the maxilla and the small bones associated with it; (4) the mandible. Determinants or controlling factors are discussed in the following section on theories of growth control.

■ Cranial Vault

The cranial vault is made up of a number of flat bones that are formed directly by intramembranous bone formation, without cartilaginous precursors. From the time that ossification begins at a number of centers that foreshadow the eventual anatomic bony units, the growth process is entirely the result of periosteal activity at the surfaces of the bones. Remodeling and growth occur primarily at the periosteum-lined contact areas between adjacent skull bones, the *skeletal sutures,* but periosteal activity also changes both the inner and outer surfaces of these plate-like bones.

At birth, the flat bones of the skull are rather widely separated by relatively loose connective tissues (Fig. 2-22). These open spaces, the fontanelles, allow a considerable amount of deformation of the skull at birth. As discussed in more detail in Chapter 3, this is important in allowing the relatively large head to pass through the birth canal.

After birth, apposition of bone along the edges of the fontanelles eliminates these open spaces fairly quickly, but the bones remain separated by a thin periosteum-lined suture for many years, eventually fusing in adult life.

Despite their small size, apposition of new bone at these sutures is the major mechanism for growth of the cranial vault. Although the majority of growth in the cranial vault occurs at the sutures, there is a tendency for bone to be removed from the inner surface of the cranial vault, while at the same time new bone is added on the exterior surface. This remodeling of the inner and outer surfaces allows for changes in contour during growth.

■ Cranial Base

In contrast to the cranial vault, the bones of the base of the skull (the cranial base) are formed initially in cartilage and are later transformed by endochondral ossification to bone. This is particularly true of the midline structures. As one moves laterally, growth at sutures and surface remodeling become more important, but the cranial base is essentially a midline structure. The situation is more complicated than in a long bone with its epiphyseal plates, however.

As indicated previously, centers of ossification appear early in embryonic life in the chondrocranium, indicating the eventual location of the basioccipital, sphenoid, and ethmoid bones that form the cranial base. As ossification proceeds, bands of cartilage called synchondroses remain between the centers of ossification (Fig. 2-23). These important growth sites are the synchondrosis between the sphenoid and occipital bones, or *sphenooccipital synchondrosis,* the *intersphenoid synchondrosis,* between two parts of the sphenoid bone, and the *sphenoethmoidal synchondrosis,* between the sphenoid and ethmoid bones. Histologically, a synchondrosis looks like a two-sided epiphyseal plate (Fig. 2-24). The area between the two bones consists of growing

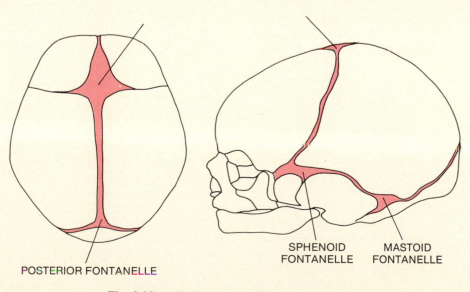

POSTERIOR FONTANELLE

SPHENOID FONTANELLE   MASTOID FONTANELLE

Fig. 2-22 ■ The fontanelles of the newborn skull.

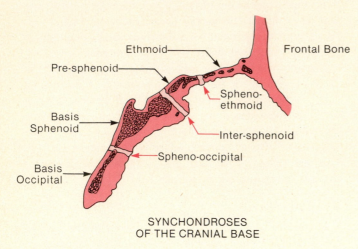

SYNCHONDROSES
OF THE CRANIAL BASE

Fig. 2-23 ■ Diagrammatic representation of the synchondroses of the cranial base, showing the location of these important growth sites.

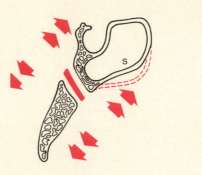
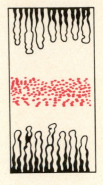

Fig. 2-24 ■ Diagrammatic representation of growth at the inter-sphenoid synchondrosis. A band of immature proliferating cartilage cells is located at the center of the synchondrosis, while a band of maturing cartilage cells extends in both directions away from the center, and endochondral ossification occurs at both margins. Growth at the synchondrosis lengthens this area of the cranial base. Even within the cranial base, bone remodeling on surfaces is also important—it is the mechanism by which the sphenoid sinus(es) enlarges, for instance.

cartilage. The synchondrosis has an area of cellular hyperplasia in the center, with bands of maturing cartilage cells extending in both directions that will eventually be replaced by bone.

A significant difference from the bones of the extremities is that immovable joints develop between the bones of the cranial base, in considerable contrast to the highly movable joints of the extremities. The cranial base is thus rather like a single long bone, except that there are multiple epiphyseal plate–like synchondroses. Immovable joints also occur between most of the other cranial and facial bones, the mandible being the only exception. The periosteum-lined sutures at other locations, containing no cartilage, are quite different from the cartilaginous synchondroses.

■ Maxilla (Nasomaxillary Complex)

The maxilla develops postnatally entirely by intramembranous ossification. Since there is no cartilage replacement, growth occurs in two ways: (1) by apposition of bone at the sutures that connect the maxilla to the cranium and cranial base and (2) by surface remodeling. In contrast to the cranial vault, however, surface changes in the maxilla are quite dramatic and as important as changes at the sutures.

The growth pattern of the face requires that it grow ''out from under the cranium,'' which means that the maxilla must move through growth a considerable distance downward and forward relative to the cranium and cranial base. As Fig. 2-25 illustrates, the sutures attaching the maxilla posteriorly and superiorly are ideally situated to allow its downward and forward repositioning. As the downward and forward movement occurs, the space that would otherwise open up at the sutures is filled in by proliferation of bone at these locations. The sutures remain the same width, and the various processes of the maxilla become longer. Bone apposition occurs on both sides of a suture, so the bones to which the maxilla is attached also become larger. Part of

the posterior border of the maxilla is a free surface in the tuberosity region. Bone is added at this surface, creating additional space into which the primary and then the permanent molar teeth successively erupt.

Interestingly, as the maxilla grows downward and forward, its front surfaces are remodeled, and bone is removed from most of the anterior surface. Note in Fig. 2-26 that almost the entire anterior surface of the maxilla is an area of resorption, not apposition. It might seem logical that if the anterior surface of the bone is moving downward and forward, this should be an area to which bone is added, not one from which it is removed. The correct concept, however, is that bone is removed from the anterior surface although the anterior surface is growing forward.

To understand this seeming paradox, it is necessary to comprehend that two quite different processes are going on simultaneously. The overall growth changes are the result of both a downward and forward translation of the maxilla and a simultaneous surface remodeling. The whole bony nasomaxillary complex is moving downward and forward relative to the cranium, being translated in space. Enlow,[2] whose careful anatomic studies of the facial skeleton underlie much of our present understanding, has illustrated this in cartoon form (Fig. 2-27). The maxilla is like the platform on wheels, being rolled forward, while at the same time its surface, represented by the wall in the cartoon, is being reduced on its anterior side and built up posteriorly, moving in space opposite to the direction of overall growth.

It is not necessarily true that remodeling changes oppose the direction of translation. Depending on the specific location, translation and remodeling may either oppose each other or produce an additive effect. The effect is additive, for instance, on the roof of the mouth. This area is carried downward and forward along with the rest of the maxilla, but at the same time bone is removed on the nasal side and

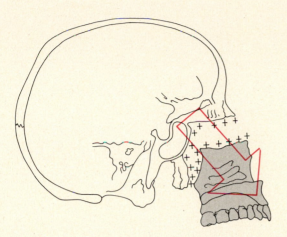

Fig. 2-25 ■ As growth of surrounding soft tissues translates the maxilla downward and forward, opening up space at its superior and posterior sutural attachments, new bone is added on both sides of the sutures. (Redrawn from Enlow, D.H.: Handbook of Facial Growth, ed. 2, Philadelphia, 1982, W.B. Saunders Co.)

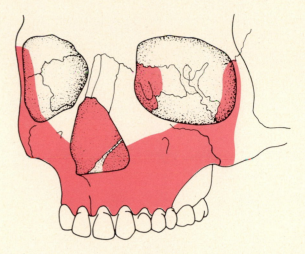

Fig. 2-26 ■ As the maxilla is carried downward and forward, its anterior surface tends to resorb. Resorption surfaces are shown here in pink. Only a small area around the anterior nasal spine is an exception. (Redrawn from Enlow, D.H.: Handbook of Facial Growth, ed. 2. Philadelphia, 1982, W.B. Saunders Co.)

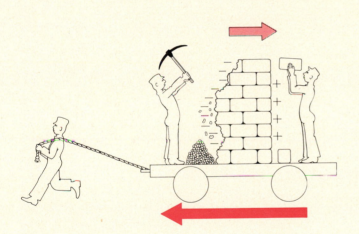

Fig. 2-27 ■ Surface remodeling of a bone in the opposite direction to that in which the bone is being translated by growth of adjacent structures creates a situation analagous to this cartoon, in which the wall is being rebuilt to move it backward at the same time the platform on which it is mounted is being moved forward. (Redrawn from Enlow, D.H.: Handbook of Facial Growth, ed. 2. Philadelphia, 1982, W.B. Saunders Co.)

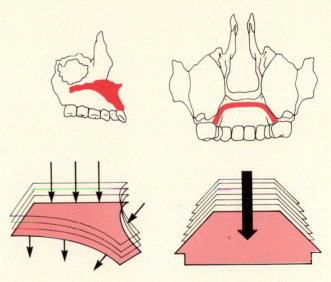

Fig. 2-28 ■ Remodeling of the palatal vault (which is also the floor of the nose) moves it in the same direction as it is being translated; bone is removed from the floor of the nose and added to the roof of the mouth. On the anterior surface, however, bone is removed, partially canceling the forward translation. As the vault moves downward, the same process of bone remodeling also widens it. (Redrawn from Enlow, D.H.: Handbook of Facial Growth, ed. 2. Philadelphia, 1982, W.B. Saunders Co.)

added on the oral side, thus creating an additional downward and forward movement of the palate (Fig. 2-28). Immediately adjacently, however, the anterior part of the alveolar process is a resorptive area, so removal of bone from the surface here tends to cancel some of the forward growth that otherwise would occur because of translation of the entire maxilla.

■ Mandible

In contrast to the maxilla both endochondral and periosteal activity are important in growth of the mandible. Cartilage covers the surface of the mandibular condyle at the temporomandibular joint. Although this cartilage is not like the cartilage at an epiphyseal plate or a synchondrosis, hyperplasia, hypertrophy, and endochondral replacement do

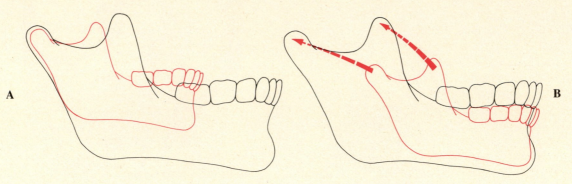

A   B

Fig. 2-29 ■ **A,** Growth of the mandible, as viewed from the perspective of a stable cranial base: the chin moves downward and forward; **B,** Mandibular growth, as viewed from the perspective of vital staining studies, which reveal minimal changes in the body and chin area, while there is exceptional growth and remodeling of the ramus, moving it posteriorly. The correct concept of mandibular growth is that the mandible is translated downward and forward and grows upward and backward in response to this translation, maintaining its contact with the skull.

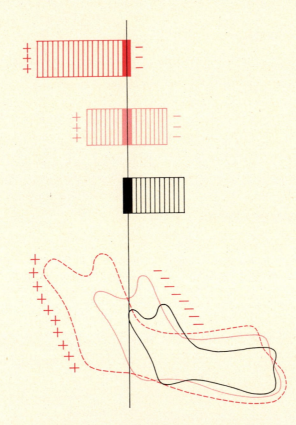

Fig. 2-30 ■ As the mandible grows in length, the ramus is extensively remodeled, so much so that bone at the tip of the condylar process at an early age can be found at the anterior surface of the ramus some years later. Given the extent of surface remodeling changes, it is an obvious error to emphasize endochondral bone formation at the condyle as the major mechanism for growth of the mandible. (Redrawn from Enlow, D.H.: Handbook of Facial Growth, ed. 2. Phaladelphia, 1982, W.B. Saunders Co.)

occur there. All other areas of the mandible are formed and grow by direct surface apposition and remodeling.

The overall pattern of growth of the mandible can be represented in two ways, as shown in Fig. 2-29. Depending on the frame of reference, both are correct. If the cranium is the reference area, the chin moves downward and forward. On the other hand, if data from vital staining experiments are examined, it becomes apparent that the principal sites of growth of the mandible are the posterior surface of the ramus and the condylar and coronoid processes. There is little change along the anterior part of the mandible. From this frame of reference, Fig. 2-29, *B,* is the correct representation.

As a growth site, the chin is almost inactive. It is translated downward and forward, as the actual growth occurs at the mandibular condyle and along the posterior surface of the ramus. The body of the mandible grows longer by periosteal apposition of bone on its posterior surface, while the ramus grows higher by endochondral replacement at the condyle accompanied by surface remodeling. Conceptually, it is correct to view the mandible as being translated downward and forward, while at the same time increasing in size by growing upward and backward. The translation occurs largely as the bone moves downward and forward along with the soft tissues in which it is embedded.

Nowhere is there a better example of remodeling resorption than in the backward movement of the ramus of the mandible. The mandible grows longer by apposition of new bone on the posterior surface of the ramus. At the same time, large quantities of bone are removed from the anterior surface of the ramus (Fig. 2-30). In essence, the body of the mandible grows longer as the ramus moves away from the chin, and this occurs by removal of bone from the anterior surface of the ramus and deposition of bone on the posterior surface. On first examination, one might expect a growth center somewhere underneath the teeth, so that the chin could grow forward away from the ramus. But that is not possible, since there is no cartilage and interstitial bone growth cannot occur. Instead, the ramus remodels. What was the posterior surface at one time becomes the center at a later date and eventually may become the anterior surface as remodeling proceeds.

In infancy, the ramus is located at about the spot where the primary first molar will erupt. Progressive posterior remodeling creates space for the second primary molar and then for the sequential eruption of the permanent molar teeth. More often than not, however, this growth ceases before enough space has been created for eruption of the third permanent molar, which becomes impacted in the ramus.

■ *Theories of Growth Control*

It is a truism that growth is strongly influenced by genetic factors, but it can also be significantly affected by the environment, in the form of nutritional status, degree of phys-

ical activity, health or illness, and a number of similar factors. Since a major part of the need for orthodontic treatment is created by disproportionate growth of the jaws, it is necessary to learn how skeletal growth is influenced and controlled to understand the etiology of malocclusion and dentofacial deformity. Great strides have been made in recent years in improving the understanding of growth control. Exactly what determines the growth of the jaws, however, remains unclear and continues to be subject of intensive research.

Three major theories in recent years have attempted to explain the determinants of craniofacial growth: (1) bone, like other tissues, is the primary determinant of its own growth; (2) cartilage is the primary determinant of skeletal growth, while bone responds secondarily and passively; and (3) the soft tissue matrix in which the skeletal elements are embedded is the primary determinant of growth, and both bone and cartilage are secondary followers.

The major difference in the theories is the location at which genetic control is expressed. The first theory implies that genetic control is expressed directly at the level of the bone, and therefore its locus should be the periosteum. The second or cartilage theory suggests that genetic control is expressed in the cartilage, while bone responds passively to being displaced. This indirect genetic control is called *epigenetic.* The third theory assumes that genetic control is mediated to a large extent outside the skeletal system and that growth of both bone and cartilage is controlled epigenetically, occurring only in response to a signal from other tissues.

It is apparent that the more indirectly growth is controlled, the greater the opportunity for environmental influences to affect it, and vice versa. Thus if the third theory were correct, considerably greater environmental influence could be expected than under the first theory. In contemporary thought, the truth is to be found in some synthesis of the second and third theories, while the first, though it was the dominant view as recently as the 1950s, has largely been discarded.

Distinguishing between a *site* of growth and a *center* of growth clarifies the differences between the theories of growth control. A site of growth is merely a location at which growth occurs, whereas a center is a location at which independent (genetically controlled) growth occurs. All centers of growth also are sites, but the reverse is not true. A major impetus to the theory that the tissues that form bone carry with them their own stimulus to do so came from the observation that the overall pattern of craniofacial growth is remarkably constant. The constancy of the growth pattern was interpreted to mean that the major sites of growth were also centers. Particularly, the sutures between the membranous bones of the cranium and jaws were considered growth centers, along with the sites of endochondral ossification in the cranial base and at the mandibular condyle. Growth, in this view, was the result of the expression at all these sites of a genetic program. The translation of the maxilla, there-

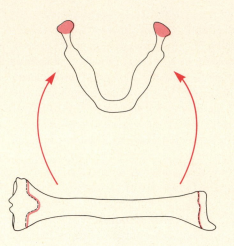

Fig. 2-31 ■ The mandible was once viewed conceptually as being analogous to a long bone that had been modified by (1) removal of the epiphysis, leaving the epiphyseal plates exposed, and (2) bending the shaft into a horseshoe shape. If this analogy were correct, of course, the cartilage at the distal ends of the bones should behave like true growth cartilage. Modern experiments indicate that, although the analogy is attractive, it is incorrect.

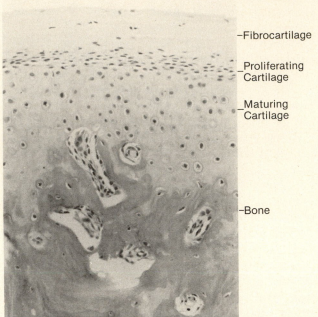

SURFACE OF CONDYLE

—Fibrocartilage

—Proliferating Cartilage

—Maturing Cartilage

—Bone

Fig. 2-32 ■ Endochondral ossification at the head of the mandibular condyle. A zone of proliferating cartilage is located just beneath the fibrocartilage on the articular surface, and endochondral ossification is occurring beneath this area. Compare the pattern of cellular activity to that of an epiphyseal plate (Fig. 2-18).

fore, was the result of pressure created by growth of the sutures, so that the bones were literally pushed apart.

If this theory were correct, growth at the sutures should occur largely independently of the environment, and it would not be possible to change the expression of growth at the sutures very much. While this was the dominant theory of growth, few attempts were made to modify facial growth because orthodontists "knew" that it could not be done.

It seems clear now that sutures, and the periosteal tissues more generally, are not primary determinants of craniofacial growth. Two lines of evidence lead to this conclusion. The first is that when an area of the suture between two facial bones is transplanted to another location (to a pouch in the abdomen, for instance), the tissue does not continue to grow. This indicates a lack of innate growth potential in the sutures. Second, it can be seen that growth at sutures will respond to outside influences under a number of circumstances. If cranial or facial bones are mechanically pulled apart at the sutures, new bone will fill in, and the bones will become larger than they would have been otherwise (Fig. 2-25). If a suture is compressed, growth at that site will be impeded. Thus sutures must be considered areas that react, not primary determinants. The sutures of the maxilla are sites of growth but are not growth centers.

The second major theory is that the determinant of craniofacial growth is growth of cartilages. The fact that, for many bones, cartilage does the growing while bone merely replaces it makes this theory attractive for the bones of the jaws. If cartilaginous growth were the primary influence, the cartilage at the condyle of the mandible could be considered as a pacemaker for growth of that bone, and the remodeling of the ramus and other surface changes could be viewed as secondary to the primary cartilaginous growth.

One way to visualize the mandible is by imagining that it is like the diaphysis of a long bone, bent into a horseshoe with the epiphyses removed, so that there is cartilage representing "half an epiphyseal plate" at the ends, which represent the mandibular condyles (Fig. 2-31). If this were the true situation, then indeed the cartilage at the mandibular condyle should act as a growth center, behaving basically like an epiphyseal growth cartilage (Fig. 2-32).

Growth of the maxilla is more difficult but not impossible to explain on a cartilage theory basis. Although there is no cartilage in the maxilla itself, there is cartilage in the nasal septum, and the nasomaxillary complex grows as a unit. Proponents of the cartilage theory hypothesize that the cartilaginous nasal septum serves as a pacemaker for other aspects of maxillary growth.[3] Note in Fig. 2-33 that the cartilage is located so that its growth could easily lead to a downward and forward translation of the maxilla. If the sutures of the maxilla served as reactive areas, as they seem to do, then they would respond to this translation by forming new bone when the sutures were pulled apart by forces from the growing cartilage. Although the amount of nasal septal cartilage reduces as growth continues, cartilage persists in this area throughout life, and the pacemaker role is certainly possible.

Two kinds of experiments have been carried out to test the idea that cartilage can serve as a true growth center. These involve an analysis of the results of transplanting

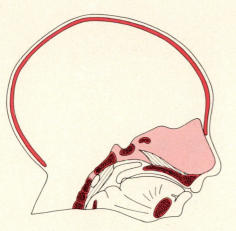

Fig. 2-33 ■ Diagrammatic representation of the chondrocranium at an early stage of development, showing the large amount of cartilage in the anterior region that eventually becomes the cartilaginous nasal septum.

cartilage and an evaluation of the effect on growth of removing cartilage at an early age.

Transplantation experiments demonstrate that not all skeletal cartilage acts the same when transplanted. If a piece of the epiphyseal plate of a long bone is transplanted, it will continue to grow in a new location or in culture, indicating that these cartilages do have innate growth potential. It seems likely that cartilage from the cranial base synchondroses behaves similarly. It is difficult to obtain cartilage from this area to transplant, particularly at an early age when the cartilage is actively growing under normal conditions, and so the data are scanty. Transplanting cartilage from the nasal septum gives equivocal results: sometimes it grows a bit, sometimes it does not. Cartilage from the mandibular condyle does not grow when transplanted.[4] Based on these results, it appears that epiphyseal cartilages and the cranial base synchondroses can act as independently growing centers, whereas the nasal septum has less independent growth potential and the mandibular condyle little or none. The condylar cartilage does not appear to be a growth center.

Experiments to test the effect of removing cartilages are also informative. The basic idea is that if removing a cartilaginous area stops or diminishes growth, perhaps it really was an important center for growth. The impact on a growing rabbit of having a segment of cartilaginous nasal septum removed is shown in Fig. 2-34. Obviously, extirpating the septum in the experimental rabbit caused a considerable deficit in growth of the midface.[5] It does not necessarily follow, however, that the entire effect on growth in such experiments results from loss of the cartilage. It can be argued that the surgery itself, and the accompanying interference with blood supply to the area, caused the growth changes rather than loss of cartilage.

There are few reported cases of early loss of the cartilaginous nasal septum in humans. One individual in whom

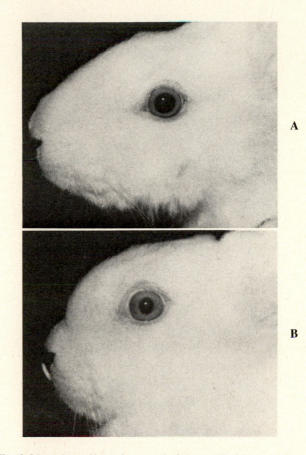

Fig. 2-34 ■ The effect of removal of the cartilaginous nasal septum on forward growth of the snout in the rabbit. **A,** Normal control; **B,** litter mate in whom cartilaginous nasal septum was removed soon after birth. The deficient forward growth of the nasomaxillary complex after this surgery is apparent. (From Sarnat, B.G.: In Factors Affecting the Growth of the Midface. Ann Arbor, 1976, University of Michigan Center for Human Growth and Development.)

the entire septum was removed at age 8 after an injury is shown in Fig. 2-35. It is apparent that a midface deficiency developed, but one cannot confidently attribute this to the loss of the cartilage. Nevertheless, the loss of growth in experimental animals when this cartilage is removed is great enough to lead most observers to conclude that the septal cartilage does have some innate growth potential, whose loss makes a difference in maxillary growth.

The neck of the mandibular condyle is a relatively fragile area. When the side of the jaw is struck sharply, the mandible often fractures just below the opposite condyle. When this happens, the condyle fragment is usually retracted well away from its previous location by the pull of the lateral pterygoid muscle (Fig. 2-36). The condyle literally has been removed when this occurs, and it resorbs over a period of time. Condylar fractures occur relatively frequently in children. If the condyle was an important growth center, one would expect to see severe growth impairment after such an injury at an early age. As recently as the 1960s it was

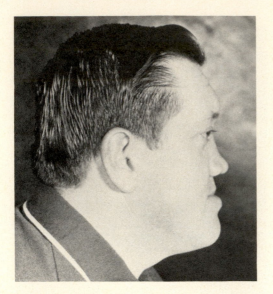

Fig. 2-35 ■ Profile view of man whose cartilaginous nasal septum was removed at age 8, after an injury. The obvious midface deficiency developed after the septum was removed.

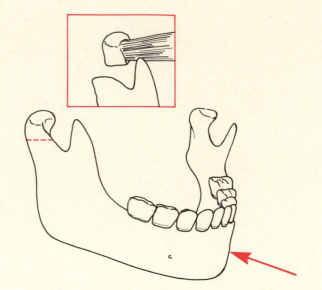

Fig. 2-36 ■ A blow to one side of the mandible may fracture the condylar process on the opposite side. When this happens, the pull of the lateral pterygoid muscle distracts the condylar fragment including all the cartilage, and it subsequently resorbs.

stated in standard texts that fracture of the mandibular condyle at an early age did invariably lead to severe growth disturbances.

Two excellent studies carried out in Scandinavia in the 1960s disproved this contention. Both Gilhuus-Moe[6] and Lund[7] demonstrated that after fractures of the mandibular condyle in a child, there was an excellent chance that the condylar process would regenerate to approximately its original size. In some children, there was actually an overgrowth on the side that had been fractured. In 15% to 20%, however, there was a reduction in growth after the injury. This growth reduction seems to relate to the amount of trauma to the soft tissues and resulting scarring in the area. The mechanism by which this occurs is discussed in the following section.

In experimental animals, after a fracture, all of the original bone and cartilage resorbs, and a new condyle regenerates directly from periosteum at the fracture site. Eventually, a new layer of cartilage forms at the condylar surface. Although there is no direct evidence that the cartilage layer itself regenerates in children after condylar fractures, it is likely that this occurs in humans also.

In short, neither transplanatation experiments nor experiments in which the condyle is removed lend any support to the idea that the cartilage of the mandibular condyle is an important center. It appears that the growth at the mandibular condyles is much more analogous to growth at the sutures of the maxilla, entirely reactive, than to growth at an epiphyseal plate.

If neither bone nor cartilage is the determinant for growth of the jaws, it would appear that the control would have to lie in the adjacent soft tissues. This point of view has been put formally in recent years by Moss, in his "functional matrix theory" of growth.[8] While granting the innate growth potential of cartilages of the long bones, his theory holds that neither the cartilage of the mandibular condyle nor the nasal septum cartilage is a determinant of jaw growth. Instead, he theorizes that growth of the face occurs as a response to functional needs and is mediated by the soft tissue in which the jaws are embedded. In this conceptual view, the soft tissues grow, and both bone and cartilage react.

The growth of the cranium illustrates this view of skeletal growth very well. There can be little question that the growth of the cranial vault is a direct response to the growth of the brain. Pressure exerted by the growing brain separates the cranial bones at the sutures, and new bone passively fills in at these sites so that the brain case fits the brain.

This phenomenon can be seen readily in humans in two experiments of nature (Fig. 2-37). First, when the brain is very small, the cranium is also very small, and the condition of microcephaly results. In this case, the size of the head is an accurate representation of the size of the brain. A second natural experiment is the condition called hydrocephaly. In this case, reabsorption of cerebrospinal fluid is impeded, the fluid accumulates, and intracranial pressure builds up. The increased intracranial pressure impedes development of the brain, so the hydrocephalic may have a small brain and be mentally retarded; but this condition also leads to an enormous growth of the cranial vault. Uncontrolled hydrocephaly may lead to a cranium two or three times its normal size, with enormously enlarged frontal, parietal, and occipital bones. This is perhaps the clearest example of a "functional matrix" in operation. Another excellent example is the relationship between the size of the eye and the size of the orbit. An enlarged eye or small eye will cause a corresponding change in the size of the orbital

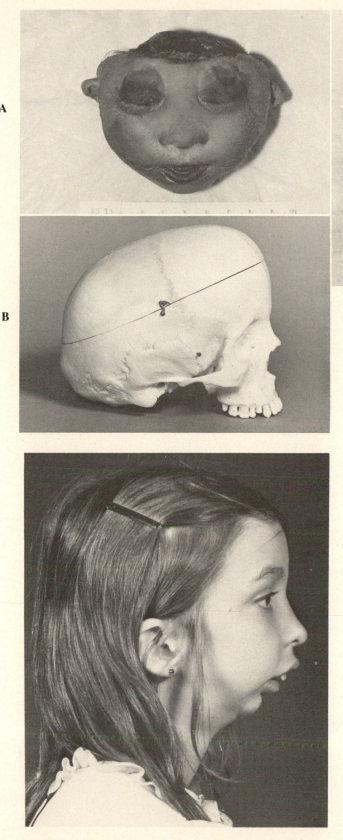

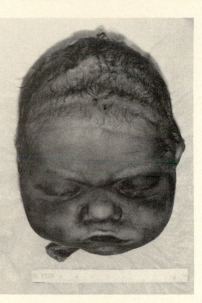

Fig. 2-37 ■ **A,** The brain case of an anencephalic full-term infant *(left);* in comparison with a facially-normal stillborn infant. Note the failure of the bony covering of the brain to develop in the absence of the brain. If the brain were very small, the brain case would also be small. **B,** The skull of a young child with hydrocephaly. Note the tremendous enlargement of the brain case in response to the increased intracranial pressure.

cavity. In this instance, the eye is the functional matrix.

Moss theorizes that the major determinant of growth of the maxilla and mandible is the enlargement of the nasal and oral cavities, which grow in response to functional needs. The theory does not make it clear how functional needs are transmitted to the tissues around the mouth and nose, but it does predict that the cartilages of the nasal septum and mandibular condyles are not important determinants of growth and that their loss would have little effect on growth if proper function could be obtained. From the view of this theory, however, absence of normal function would have wide-ranging effects.

We have already noted that in 75% to 80% of human children who suffer a condylar fracture, the resulting loss of the condyle does not impede mandibular growth. The condyle regenerates very nicely. What about the 20% to 25% of children in whom a growth deficit occurs after condylar fracture? Could some interference with function be the reason for the growth deficiency?

The answer seems to be a clear yes. It has been known for many years that mandibular growth is greatly impaired by an ankylosis (Fig. 2-38), defined as a fusion across the joint so that motion is prevented or extremely limited. Mandibular ankylosis can develop in a number of ways. For instance, one possible cause is a severe infection in the area of the temporomandibular joint, leading to destruction of tissues and ultimate scarring. Another cause, of course, is trauma, which can result in a growth deficiency if there is enough soft tissue injury to lead to severe scarring as the injury heals. It appears that the mechanical restriction caused

Fig. 2-38 ■ Profile view of a girl in whom a severe infection of the mastoid air cells involved the temporomandibular joints and led to ankylosis of the mandible. The resulting restriction of mandibular growth is apparent.

by scar tissue in the vicinity of the temporomandibular joint impedes translation of the mandible as the adjacent soft tissues grow, and that this is the reason for growth deficiency in some children after condylar fractures.

In summary, it appears that growth of the cranium occurs almost entirely in response to growth of the brain. Growth of the cranial base is primarily the result of endochondral growth and bony replacement at the synchondroses, which have independent growth potential. Growth of the maxilla and its associated structures occurs from a combination of growth at sutures and direct remodeling of the surfaces of the bone. The maxilla is translated downward and forward as the face grows, and new bone fills in at the sutures. The extent to which growth of cartilage of the nasal septum leads to translation of the maxilla remains unknown, but this cartilaginous growth does not seem vigorous enough to entirely account for the forward repositioning of the maxilla. Growth of the surrounding soft tissues seems to be important. Growth of the mandible occurs by both endochondral proliferation at the condyle and apposition and resorption of bone at surfaces. It seems clear that the mandible is translated in space by the growth of muscles and other adjacent soft tissues and that addition of new bone at the condyle is in response to the soft tissue changes.

■ *References*

1. Bjork, A.: The use of metallic implants in the study of facial growth in children: method and application. Am J. Phys. Anthropol. **29**:243-250, 1968.
2. Enlow, D.H.: Handbook of Facial Growth, ed 2. Philadelphia, 1982, W.B. Saunders.
3. Scott, J.H.: Dento-facial Development and Growth. Oxford, 1967, Pergamon Press.
4. Ronning, O.: Observations on the intracerebral transplantation of the mandibular condyle. Acta Odont. Scand. **24**:443-457, 1966.
5. Sarnat, B.G.: The postnatal maxillary nasal-orbital complex: Experimental surgery. In Factors Affecting the Growth of the Midface. Ann Arbor, 1976, University of Michigan Center for Human Growth and Development.
6. Gilhuus-Moe, O.: Fractures of the Mandibular Condyle in the Growth Period. Stockholm, 1969, Scandinavian University Books, Universitatsforlaget.
7. Lund, K.: Mandibular growth and remodelling process after mandibular fractures. Acta Odont. Scand. **32**(Suppl. 64), 1974.
8. Moss, M.L.: The functional matrix. In Kraus, B.S., and Riedel, R.A., editors: Vistas in Orthodontics. Philadelphia, 1962, Lea and Febiger.

Chapter 3

The Early Stages of Physical and Social Development

■ Prenatal Influences on Facial Development

A general understanding of the formation of the face, as presented in the standard embryology texts, is presumed in the discussion that follows. The focus here is on the events in prenatal development that are particularly pertinent to orthodontic problems later in life.

Some specific abnormalities in facial form and jaw relationships can be traced to very early stages. Since most structures of the face are ultimately derived from migrating neural crest cells[1] (Fig. 3-1), it is not surprising that interferences with this migration produce facial deformities. At the completion of the migration of the neural crest cells in the fourth week of human embryonic life, they form practically all of the loose mesenchymal tissue in the facial region, lying between the surface ectoderm and the underlying forebrain and eye. Most of the neural crest cells in the facial area later differentiate into skeletal and connective tissues, including the bones of the jaw and the teeth. Severe facial asymmetry in some patients (Fig. 3-2) may be related to unequal amounts of neural crest migration on the two sides, although it is difficult to be sure that this is the sole cause.

Diminished neural crest migration definitely has been implicated in Treacher Collins syndrome, also called mandibulofacial dysostosis. In this congenital syndrome, both the maxilla and mandible are underdeveloped as a result of a generalized lack of mesenchymal tissue (Fig. 3-3). Analogous problems in animals can be produced by drugs that

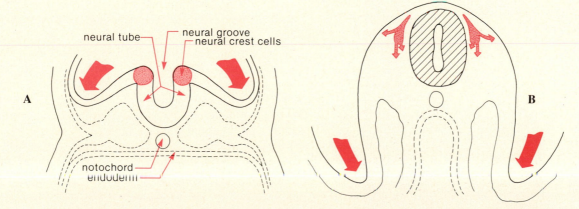

Fig. 3-1 ■ Diagrammatic lateral sections through embryos at 20 and 24 days, showing formation of the neural folds, neural groove, and neural crest. **A,** At 20 days, neural crest cells can be identified at the lips of the deepening neural groove, forerunner of the central nervous system. **B,** At 24 days, the neural crest cells (pink) have separated from the neural tube and are beginning their extensive migration beneath the surface ectoderm. The migration is so extensive, and the role of these neural crest cells so important in formation of structures of the head and face, they can almost be considered a fourth primary germ layer.

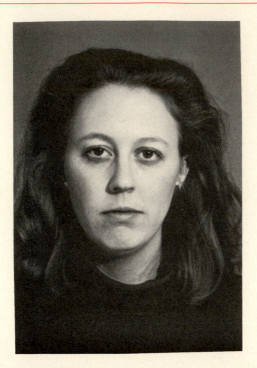

Fig. 3-2 ■ Severe facial asymmetry of this extent could have a number of embryologic causes, but it is likely that problems began at the stage of neural crest cell migration.

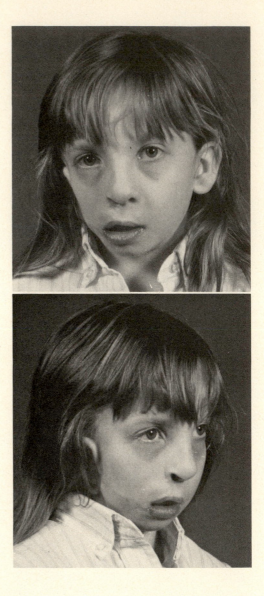

Fig. 3-3 ■ In the Treacher Collins syndrome, a generalized lack of mesenchymal tissue in the lateral part of the face is the major cause of the characteristic facial appearance.

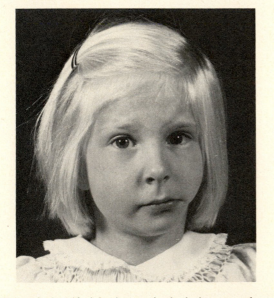

Fig. 3-4 ■ In hemifacial microsomia, both the external ear and the mandibular ramus are deficient or absent on the affected side.

decrease cell mobility.[2] The experiments suggest that the neural crest cells with the longest migration path, those taking a circuitous route to the lateral and lower areas of the face, are most affected, whereas those going to the central area tend to complete their migratory movement. This explains why midline defects including clefts rarely are part of the syndrome. Some degree of asymmetry may be present, but both sides are affected.

A second congenital defect with a somewhat later embryologic origin is hemifacial microsomia (Fig. 3-4). In this condition, the external ear is deformed and both the ramus of the mandible and associated soft tissues (muscle, fascia) are deficient or missing. Until the past decade, the embryologic origin of this condition was unknown. Poswillo's experimental work in animals indicates that defects resembling those of hemifacial microsomia can be produced by drugs that cause a hemorrhage from the stapedial artery[3]. At about 6 weeks after conception, this vessel, derived from the internal carotid artery, is replaced as the major supply

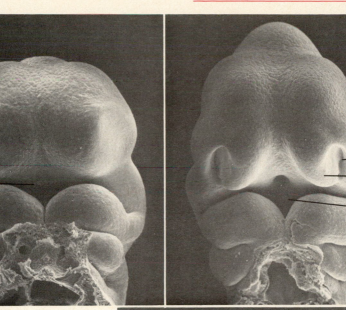
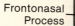
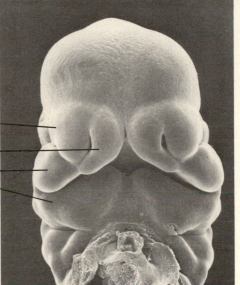

Fig. 3-5 ■ Scanning electron micrographs of mouse embryos (which are very similar to human embryos at this stage of development), showing the stages in facial development. **A,** Early formation of the face (about 24 days after conception in the human). Division of the first branchial arch into the maxillary and mandibular processes is just beginning. **B,** At a stage equivalent to about 31 days in the human, the medial and lateral nasal processes can be recognized alongside the nasal pit. **C,** Fusion of the median nasal, lateral nasal, and maxillary processes forms the upper lip, while fusion between the maxillary and mandibular processes establishes the width of the mouth opening. This stage is reached at about 36 days in the human. (Courtesy Dr. K. Sulik.)

to the facial region by the external carotid artery. If a hemorrhage occurs just as the two vessels coalesce, the result is a loss of tissue in the area where the ramus of the mandible and the structures of the external ear will form. These are the structures affected in hemifacial microsomia. Although there is no direct evidence that this same hemorrhage pattern causes hemifacial microsomia in humans, it seems likely that a similar mechanism is involved. Hemifacial micro-

somia is usually unilateral and rarely symmetric even if both sides are involved.

The most common congenital defect involving the face and jaws, second only to clubfoot in the entire spectrum of congenital deformities, is clefting of the lip, palate, or, less commonly, other facial structures. Exactly where clefts appear is determined by the locations at which fusion of the various facial processes failed to occur (Fig. 3-5, 3-6), and

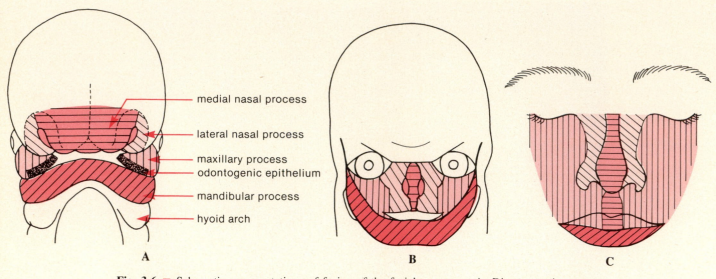

Fig. 3-6 ■ Schematic representations of fusion of the facial processes. **A,** Diagrammatic representation of structures at 31 days, when fusion is just beginning; **B,** relationships at 35 days, when the fusion process is well advanced; **C,** schematic representation of the contribution of the embryonic facial processes to the structures of the adult face. The medial nasal process contributes the central part of the nose and the philtrum of the lip. The lateral nasal process forms the outer parts of the nose, and the maxillary process forms the bulk of the upper lip and the cheeks. (**B** redrawn from TenCate, A.R.: Oral Histology, St. Louis, 1980, The C.V. Mosby Co.; **C** redrawn from Sulik, K.K.: Scan. Elect. Microscp., in press, 1985.)

this in turn is influenced by the time in embryologic life when there was some interference with development.

Clefting of the lip occurs because of a failure of fusion between the median nasal and lateral nasal processes. At least theoretically a midline cleft of the upper lip could develop because of a split within the median nasal process, but in fact this almost never occurs. Instead, clefts of the lip occur lateral to the midline on either or both sides (Fig. 3-7). Since the fusion of the median nasal processes creates not only the lip but the area of the alveolar ridge containing the central and lateral incisors, it is likely that a notch in

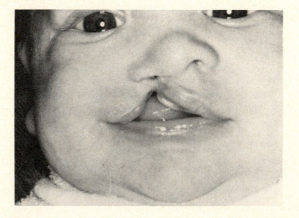

Fig. 3-7 ■ Unilateral cleft lip in an infant. Note that the cleft is not in the midline, but lateral to the midline. The cleft location indicates the separation between the lateral and medial nasal processes.

the alveolar process will accompany a cleft lip even if there is not clefting of the secondary palate.

Closure of the secondary palate by elevation of the palatal shelves (Fig. 3-8, and 3-9) follows that of the primary palate by nearly 2 weeks, which means that an interference with lip closure that still is present can affect the palate. About 60% of individuals with a cleft lip also have a palatal cleft[4] (Fig. 3-10). An isolated cleft of the secondary palate is the result of a problem that arose after lip closure was completed. Incomplete fusion of the secondary palate, which produces a notch in its posterior extent, indicates a very late-appearing interference with fusion.

The width of the mouth is determined by fusion of the maxillary and mandibular processes at their lateral extent, and so a failure of fusion in this area could produce an exceptionally wide mouth, or macrostomia. Failure of fusion between the maxillary and lateral processes could produce an obliquely directed cleft of the face. Other patterns of facial clefts are possible, based on the details of fusion. Fortunately, these conditions are rare.

One congenital craniofacial malformation seems to arise considerably later than the ones discussed so far, developing during the fetal period. This is Crouzon's syndrome, characterized by underdevelopment of the midface and eyes that seem to bulge from their sockets (Fig. 3-11).

It results from early closure of the sutures between the cranial and facial bones. From early in fetal life, normal cranial and facial development is dependent on growth adjustments at the sutures in response to growth of the brain and facial soft tissues. Early closure of a suture, called

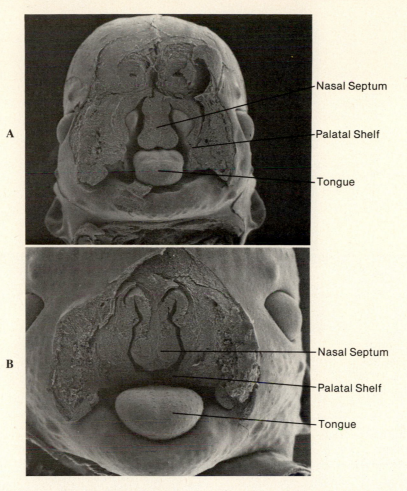

Fig. 3-8 ■ Scanning electron micrographs of mouse embryos sectioned in the frontal plane. **A,** Before elevation of the palatal shelves; **B,** immediately after depression of the tongue and elevation of the shelves. (Courtesy Dr. K. Sulik.)

synostosis, leads to characteristic distortions depending on the location of the early fusion. Crouzon's syndrome arises because of prenatal fusion of the superior and posterior sutures of the maxilla, along the wall of the orbit. The premature fusion frequently extends posteriorly into the cranium, producing distortions of the cranial vault as well. If fusion in the orbital area prevents the maxilla from translating downward and forward, the result must be severe underdevelopment of the middle third of the face. The characteristic protrusion of the eyes is largely an illusion—the eyes appear to bulge outward because the area beneath them is underdeveloped. There may be a component of true extrusion of the eyes, however, because when cranial sutures become synostosed, intracranial pressure increases.

Although the characteristic deformity is recognized at birth, the situation worsens as growth disturbances caused by the fused sutures continue postnatally. Surgery to release the sutures is necessary at an early age.

By the third trimester of intrauterine life, the human fetus weighs approximately 1000 grams and though far from ready for life outside the protective intrauterine environment, can often survive premature birth. Dental development, which begins in the third month, proceeds rapidly thereafter (Table 3-1). During the last 3 months, continued rapid growth results in a tripling of body mass to about 3000 grams.

Although the proportion of the total body mass represented by the head decreases from the fourth month of intrauterine life onward, at birth the head is still nearly half the total and represents the largest impediment to passage of the infant through the birth canal. Making the head longer and narrower obviously would facilitate birth, and this is accomplished by a literal distortion of the shape (Fig. 3-12). This change of shape is possible because at birth, relatively large uncalcified fontanelles persist between the flat bones of the brain case. As the head is compressed within the birth canal, the brain case (calvarium) can increase in length and decrease in width, assuming the desired tubular form and easing passage through the birth canal.

The relative lack of growth of the lower jaw prenatally also makes birth easier, since a prominent bony chin at the time of birth would be a considerable problem in passage

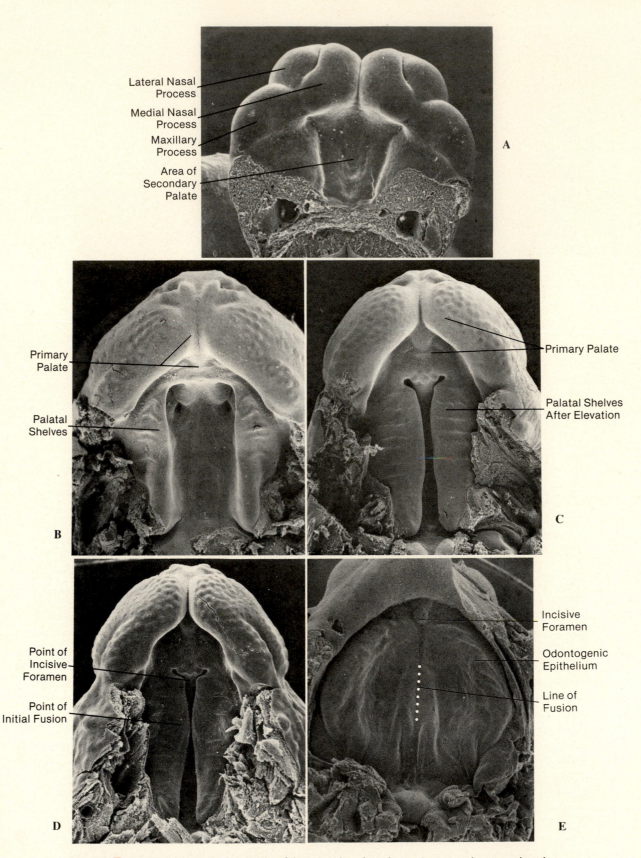

Fig. 3-9 ■ Scanning electron micrographs of the stages in palate closure (mouse embryos sectioned so that the lower jaw has been removed), analagous to the same stages in human embryos. **A,** At the completion of primary palate formation; **B,** before elevation of the palatal shelves, equivalent to Fig. 3-8, A; **C,** shelves during elevation; **D,** initial fusion of the shelves at a point about one-third of the way back along their length; **E,** secondary palate immediately after fusion. (Courtesy Dr. K. Sulik.)

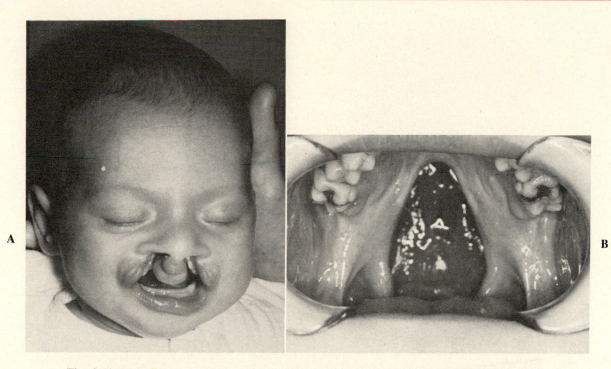

Fig. 3-10 ■ **A,** Bilateral cleft lip and palate in an infant. The separation of the premaxilla from the remainder of the maxilla is shown clearly; **B,** an unrepaired cleft of the secondary palate in a 12-year-old child. An isolated cleft of the palate can affect all of the secondary palate, as in this individual, or only the posterior portion of it.

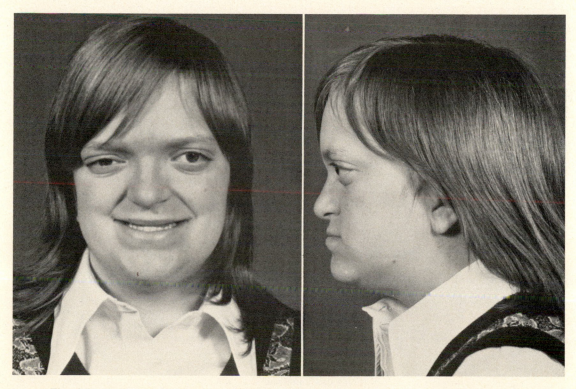

Fig. 3-11 ■ Typical facial appearance in Crouzon's syndrome of moderate severity. Note the deficiency of the midfacial structures, which usually is coupled with wide separation of the eyes (hypertelorism), as in this individual.

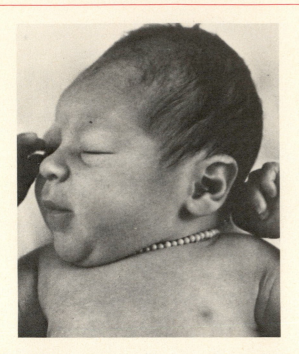

Fig. 3-12 ■ This photograph of a newborn infant clearly shows the head distortion accompanying passage through the birth canal. Note that the head has been squeezed into a more elliptical or tubular shape, a distortion made possible by the presence of the relatively large fontanelles. (Courtesy Mead Johnson Co.)

through the birth canal. Many a young dentist, acutely aware of the orthodontic problems that can arise later because of skeletal mandibular deficiency, has been shocked to discover how incredibly mandibular deficient his own newborn is and has required reassurance that this is a perfectly normal and indeed desirable phenomenon. Postnatally, the mandible grows more than the other facial structures and gradually catches up, producing the eventual adult proportions.

Despite the physical adaptations that facilitate it, birth is a traumatic process. In the best of circumstances, being thrust into the world requires a dramatic set of physiologic adaptations. For a short period, growth ceases and there may be a small decrease in weight during the first 7 to 10 days of life. Such an interruption in growth produces a physical effect in skeletal tissues that are forming at the time, because the orderly sequence of calcification is disturbed. The result is a noticeable line across both bones and teeth that are forming at the time. However, bones are not visible and are remodeled to such an extent that any lines caused by the growth arrest at birth would soon be covered over at any rate.

Teeth, on the other hand, are quite visible, and the extent of any growth disturbance related to birth can be seen in the enamel, which is not remodeled. Almost every child has a ''neonatal line'' across the surface of the primary teeth, its location varying from tooth to tooth depending on the

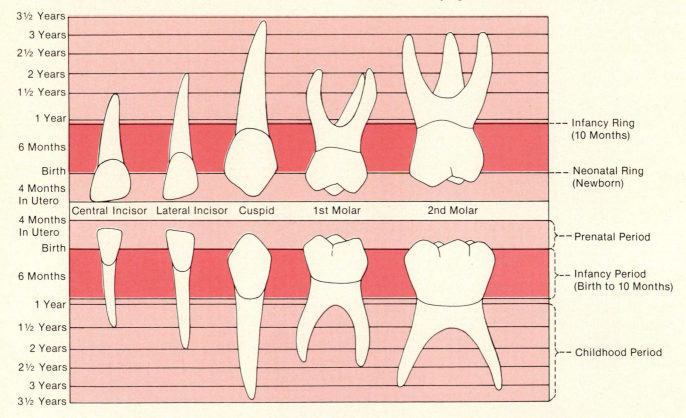

Fig. 3-13 ■ Primary teeth shown on a developmental scale that indicates the expected location of the neonatal line. From a chart of this type, the timing of illness or traumatic events that led to disturbances of enamel formation can be deduced from the location of enamel lines on various teeth.

stage of development at birth (Fig. 3-13). Under normal circumstances, the line can be seen only on close examination, but if the neonatal period was stormy, a prominent area of stained, distorted, or poorly calcified enamel can be observed.

Birth is not the only circumstance that can have this effect. As a general rule, it can be anticipated that growth disturbances lasting 1 to 2 weeks or more, such as the one that accompanies birth or a growth cessation caused by a febrile illness later, will leave a visible record in the enamel of teeth forming at the time. Permanent as well as primary teeth can be affected by illnesses during infancy and early childhood.

■ *Infancy and Early Childhood: The Primary Dentition Years*

■ Eruption of the Primary Teeth

At birth, neither the maxillary nor the mandibular alveolar process is well developed. Occasionally, a "natal tooth" is present, although the first primary teeth normally do not erupt until approximately 6 months of age. The natal tooth usually is a supernumerary one, formed by an aberration in the development of the dental lamina, but occasionally is merely a very early but otherwise normal central incisor. Because of the possibility that it is perfectly normal, such a natal tooth should not be extracted casually.

The timing and sequence of eruption of the primary teeth are shown in Table 3-1. The dates of eruption are relatively variable; up to 6 months of acceleration or delay is within the normal range. The eruption sequence, however, is usually preserved. One can expect that the mandibular central

incisors will erupt first, closely followed by the other incisors. After a 3 to 4 month interval, the mandibular and maxillary first molars erupt, followed in another 3 or 4 months by the maxillary and mandibular canines, which nearly fill the space between the lateral incisor and first molar. The primary dentition is usually completed at 24 to 30 months as the mandibular, then the maxillary second molars erupt.

Spacing is normal throughout the anterior part of the primary dentition, but is most noticeable in two locations called the primate spaces. (Most subhuman primates have these spaces throughout life, thus the name.) In the maxillary arch, the primate space is located between the lateral incisors and canines, whereas in the mandibular arch, the space is between the canines and first molars (Fig. 3-14). The primate spaces are normally present from the time the teeth erupt. Developmental spaces between the incisors are often present from the beginning, but become somewhat larger as the child grows and the alveolar processes expand. Generalized spacing of the primary teeth is a requirement for proper alignment of the permanent incisors.

■ Maturation of Oral Function

The principal physiologic functions of the oral cavity are respiration, swallowing, mastication, and speech. Although it may seem odd to list respiration as an oral function, since the major portal for respiration is the nose, respiratory needs are a primary determinant of posture of the mandible and tongue.

At birth, if the newborn infant is to survive, an airway must be established within a very few minutes and must be maintained thereafter. To open the airway, the mandible must be positioned downward and the tongue moved downward and forward away from the posterior pharyngeal wall (Fig. 3-15). This allows air to be moved through the nose

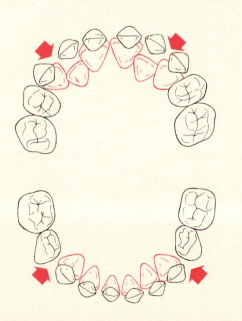

Fig. 3-14 ■ The crowns of the permanent incisors (red) lie lingual to the crowns of the primary incisors (black), particularly in the case of the maxillary laterals. Arrows point to the primate spaces.

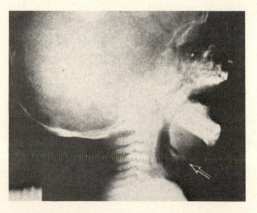

Fig. 3-15 ■ Radiograph of an infant immediately after birth, during the first breath of life. To breathe, the infant must position the mandible downward and the tongue forward to open up an airway and must maintain this posture thereafter. The arrow indicates the shadow of the tongue, and the open airway behind it is clearly visible. (From Bosma, J.F.: Am. J. Orthod. **49:**94-104, 1963.)

Table 3-1 ■ Chronology of tooth development

Tooth	Calcification begins		Crown completed		Eruption		Root completed	
	Max.	Mand.	Max.	Mand.	Max.	Mand.	Max.	Mand.
Primary								
Central	14 wk. in utero	14 wk. in utero	1½ mo.	2½ mo.	10 mo.	8 mo.	1½ yr.	1½ yr.
Lateral	16 wk. in utero	16 wk. in utero	2½ mo.	3 mo.	11 mo.	13 mo.	2 yr.	1½ yr.
Canine	17 wk.	17 wk. in utero	9 mo.	9 mo.	19 mo.	20 mo.	3¼	3¼ yr.
1st Molar	15 wk. in utero	15 wk. in utero	6 mo.	5½ mo.	16 mo.	16 mo.	2½ yr.	2¼ yr.
2nd Molar	19 wk. in utero	18 wk. in utero	11 mo.	10 mo.	29 mo.	27 mo.	3 yr.	3 yr.
Permanent								
Central	3 mo.	3 mo.	4½ yr.	3½ yr.	7¼ yr.	6¼ yr.	10½ yr.	9½ yr.
Lateral	11 mo.	3 mo.	5½ yr.	4 yr.	8¼ yr.	7½ hr.	11 yr.	10 yr.
Canine	4 mo.	4 mo.	6 yr.	5¾ yr.	11½ yr.	10½ yr.	13½ yr.	12¾ hr.
1st Premolar	20 mo.	22 mo.	7 yr.	6¾ yr.	10¼ yr.	10½ yr.	13½ yr.	13½ yr.
2nd Premolar	27 mo.	28 mo.	7¾ yr.	7½ yr.	11 yr.	11¼ yr.	14½ yr.	15 yr.
1st Molar	32 wk. in utero	32 wk. in utero	4¼ yr.	3¾ yr.	6¼ yr.	6 yr.	10½ yr.	10¾ yr.
2nd Molar	27 mo.	27 mo.	7¾ yr.	7½ yr.	12½ hr.	12 yr.	15¾ yr.	16 yr.
3rd Molar	8 yr.	9 yr.	14 yr.	14 yr.	20 yr.	20 yr.	22 yr.	22 yr.

and across the pharynx into the lungs. Newborn infants are obligatory nasal breathers and may not survive if the nasal passage is blocked at birth. Later, breathing through the mouth becomes physiologically possible. At all times during life, respiratory needs can alter the postural basis from which oral activities begin.

Respiratory movements are "practiced" in utero, although of course the lungs do not inflate at that time. Swallowing also occurs during the last months of fetal life, and it appears that swallowed amniotic fluid may be an important stimulus to activation of the infant's immune system.

Once an airway has been established, the newborn infant's next physiologic priority is to obtain milk and transfer it into the gastrointestinal system. This is accomplished by two maneuvers: suckling, not sucking with which it is frequently confused, and swallowing.

The milk ducts of lactating mammals are surrounded by smooth muscle, which contracts to force out the milk. To obtain milk, the infant does not have to suck it from the mother's breast and probably could not do so. Instead, the infant's role is to stimulate the smooth muscle to contract and squirt milk into his mouth. This is done by suckling, consisting of small nibbling movements of the lips. When the milk is squirted into the mouth, it is only necessary for the infant to groove the tongue and allow the milk to flow posteriorly into the pharynx and esophagus. The tongue, however, must be placed anteriorly in contact with the lower lip, so that milk is in fact deposited on the tongue.

This sequence of events defines an infantile swallow, which is characterized by active contractions of the musculature of the lips, a tongue tip brought forward into contact with the lower lip, and little activity of the posterior tongue or pharyngeal musculature. Tongue to lower lip apposition is so common in infants that this posture is usually adopted at rest, and it is frequently possible to gently move the infant's lip and note that the tongue tip moves with it, almost as if the two were glued together (Fig. 3-16).

As the infant matures, there is increasing activation of the elevator muscles of the mandible as the child swallows. As semisolid and eventually solid foods are added to the diet, it is necessary for the child to use the tongue in a more complex way to gather up a bolus, position it along the middle of the tongue, and transport it posteriorly. The chewing movements of a young child typically involve moving the mandible laterally as it opens, then bringing it back toward the midline and closing to bring the teeth into contact with the food. By the time the primary molars begin to

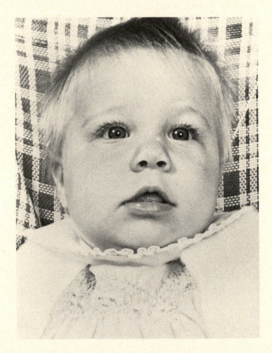

Fig. 3-16 ■ Characteristic placement of the tongue against the lower lip in an infant of a few months of age. At this stage of development, tongue contact with the lip is maintained most of the time.

erupt, this sort of juvenile chewing pattern is well established. By this time also, the more complex movements of the posterior part of the tongue have produced a definite transition beyond the infantile swallow.

Maturation of oral function can be characterized in general as following a gradient from anterior to posterior. At birth, the lips are relatively mature and capable of vigorous suckling activity, whereas more posterior structures are quite immature. As time passes, greater activity by the posterior parts of the tongue and more complex motions of the pharyngeal structures are required.

This principle of front to back maturation is particularly well illustrated by the acquisition of speech. The first speech sounds are the bilabial sounds /m/, /p/, and /b/—which is why an infant's first word is likely to be "mama" or "papa." Somewhat later, the tongue tip consonants like /t/ and /d/ appear. The sibilant /s/ and /z/ sounds, which require that the tongue tip be placed close to but not against the palate, come later still, and the last speech sound, /r/, which requires precise positioning of the posterior tongue, often is not acquired until age 4 or 5.

Nearly all modern infants engage in some sort of habitual non-nutritive sucking, sucking a thumb, finger, or a similarly shaped object. Some fetuses have been reported to suck their thumb in utero, and the vast majority of infants do so during the period from 6 months to 2 years or later. This practice is culturally determined to some extent, since children in primitive groups who are allowed ready access to the mother's breast for a long period of time rarely suck any other object.[5] It is probably true that if a child who is bottle-fed had constant access to the bottle, the habit of sucking on anything else would not develop.

After the eruption of the primary molars during the second year, drinking from a cup replaces drinking from a bottle or continued nursing at the mother's breast, and the number of children who engage in non-nutritive sucking diminishes. When sucking activity stops, a continued transition in the pattern of swallow leads to the acquisition of an adult pattern. This type of swallow is characterized by a cessation of lip activity, i.e., lips relaxed, the placement of the tongue tip against the alveolar process behind the upper incisors, and the posterior teeth brought into occlusion during swallowing. As long as sucking habits persists, however, there will not be a total transition to the adult swallow.

Surveys of American children indicate that at age , about 50% have achieved an adult swallow, while the remaining 50% are still somewhere in the transition.[6] After sucking habits are extinguished, a complete transition to the adult swallow may require some months. This is complicated, however, by the fact that an anterior open bite, which may well be present if a sucking habit has persisted for a long time, can delay the transition even further because of the physiologic need to seal the anterior space. The relationship of tongue position to malocclusion is discussed further in Chapter 5.

The chewing pattern of the adult is quite different from that of a typical child: an adult typically opens straight down, then moves the jaw laterally and brings the teeth into contact, whereas a child moves the jaw laterally on opening (Fig. 3-17). This transition in the chewing pattern appears to develop in conjunction with eruption of the permanent canines, at about age 12. Interestingly, adults who do not achieve normal function of the canine teeth because of a severe anterior open bite retain the juvenile chewing pattern.[7]

■ Physical Development in the Preschool Years

The general pattern of physical development after birth is a continuation of the pattern of the late fetal period: rapid growth continues, with a relatively steady increase in height and weight, although there is a continuing decline in the rate of growth as a percentage of the previous body size.

Three circumstances merit special attention:

1. *Premature birth (low birth weight).* Infants weighing less than 5 pounds at birth are at greater risk of problems in the immediate postnatal period. Since low birth weight is a reflection of premature birth, it is reasonable to establish the prognosis in terms of birth weight rather than estimated gestational age. Until recent years, children with birth weights below 4 pounds often did not survive, and even with the best current specialized neonatal services, the chances of extremely low birth weight infants (less than 3 pounds) are not good, though now many are saved.

If a premature infant survives the neonatal period, however, there is every reason to expect that growth will follow the normal pattern and that the child will gradually overcome the initial handicap (Fig. 3-18). Premature infants can be expected to be small throughout the first and into the second years of life. In many instances, by the third year of life

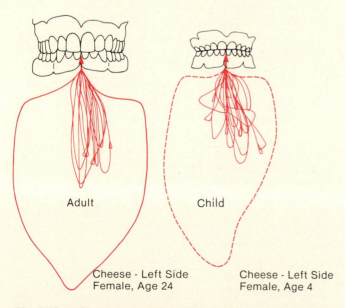

Adult   Child

Cheese - Left Side   Cheese - Left Side
Female, Age 24   Female, Age 4

Fig. 3-17 ■ Chewing movements of an adult contrasted to a child. (From Lundeen, H.C., and Gibbs, C.H.: Advances in Occlusion. Boston, 1982, John Wright's PSG, Inc.)

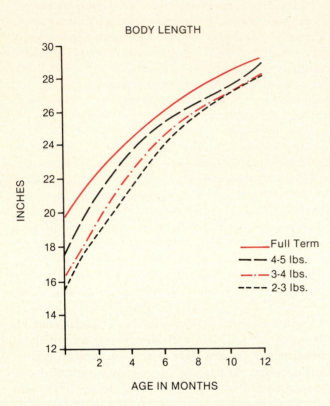

BODY LENGTH

Full Term
4-5 lbs.
3-4 lbs.
2-3 lbs.

INCHES

AGE IN MONTHS

Fig. 3-18 ■ Growth curves for premature compared to full-term infants. (From Lowery, G.H.: Growth and Development of Children, ed. 6. Chicago, 1973, Year Book Medical Publishers.)

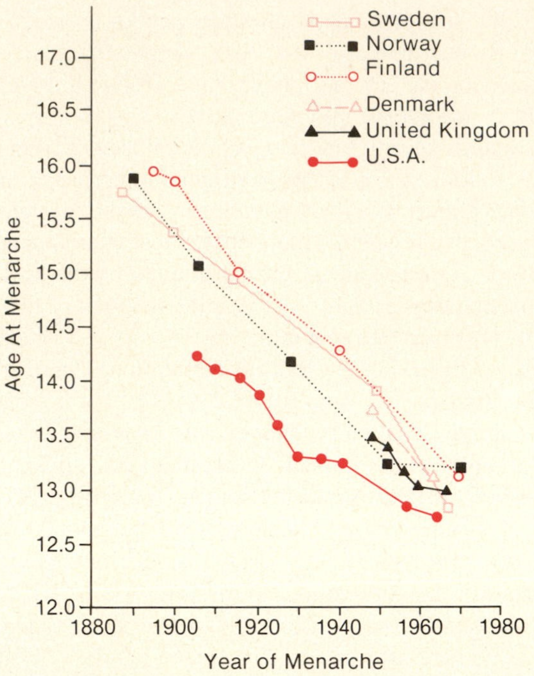

Sweden
Norway
Finland
Denmark
United Kingdom
U.S.A.

Age At Menarche

Year of Menarche

Fig. 3-19 ■ Age at menarche declined in both the United States and northern European countries in the first half of the twentieth century. On the average, children are now larger at any given age than in the early 1900s, and they also mature more quickly. This secular trend, however, seems to have leveled recently. (From Tanner, J.M.: Foetus into Man. Cambridge, Mass., 1978, Harvard University Press.)

premature and normal-term infants are indistinguishable in attainment of developmental milestones.[8]

2. *Chronic illness.* Skeletal growth is a process that can occur only when the other requirements of the individual have been met. For a normal child, perhaps 90% of the available energy must be "taken off the top" to meet the requirements for survival, leaving 10% for growth.

The impact of chronic illness is to alter this balance, leaving relatively less of the total energy requirement for growth. Children who are chronically ill typically fall behind their healthier peers, and if the chronic illness persists, the growth deficit is cumulative. An episode of acute illness leads to a temporary cessation of growth, but if the growth interruption is relatively brief, there will be no long-term effect. The more chronic the illness, the greater the cumulative impact. Obviously, the more severe the illness, the greater the impact at any given time.

3. *Nutritional status.* For growth to occur, there must be a nutritional supply in excess of the amount necessary for mere survival. Chronically inadequate nutrition, therefore, has an effect similar to chronic illness. On the other hand, once a level of nutritional adequacy has been achieved, additional nutritional intake is not a stimulus to more rapid growth. Adequate nutrition, in short, like reasonable overall health, is a necessary condition for normal growth but is not a stimulus to it.

An interesting phenomenon of the last 300 or 400 years, particularly the first half of the twentieth century, has been a generalized increase in size of most individuals. There has also been a lowering in the age of sexual maturation, so that children recently have grown faster and matured earlier than they did previously. Since 1900, in the United States the average height has increased 2 to 3 inches, and average age of girls at first menstruation has decreased by about a year[9] (Fig. 3-19). This "secular trend" toward more rapid growth and earlier maturation is undoubtedly related to better nutrition, which allows the faster weight gain that by itself can trigger earlier maturation.

Because a secular trend has been observed in populations whose nutritional status does not seem to have improved significantly, nutrition may not be the entire explanation. On the other hand, a deficiency in one or two essential nutritional components can serve to limit the rate of growth, even if the diet is generally adequate. Physical growth requires the formation of new protein, and it is likely that the amount of protein may have been a limiting factor for many populations in the past. A generally adequate diet that was low in trace minerals, vitamins, or other minor but important components may also have limited the rate of growth in the past, so that even a small change to supply previously deficient items may in some instances have allowed a considerable increment in growth.

■ *Social and Behavioral Development*

W.R. Proffit, J.M. George, and F.T. McIver

Physical growth can be considered the outcome of an interaction between genetically controlled cell proliferation and environmental influences that modify the genetic program. Similarly, behavior can be viewed as the result of an interaction between innate or instinctual behavioral patterns and behaviors learned after birth. In lower animals, it appears that the majority of behaviors are instinctive, although even they are capable of a degree of learned behavior. In humans, on the other hand, it is generally conceded that the great majority of behaviors are learned.

For this reason, it is less easy to construct stages of behavioral development in humans than stages of physical development. The higher proportion of learned behavior means that what might be considered environmental effects can greatly modify behavior. On the other hand, there are human instinctual behaviors, for example the sex drive, and in a sense, the outcome of behavior hinges on how the instinctual behavioral urges have been modified by learning. The older the individual, the more complex the behavioral pattern and the more important the learned overlay of behavior will be.

In this section, a brief overview of social, cognitive, and behavioral development is presented, greatly simplifying a complex subject and emphasizing the evaluation and management of children who will be receiving dental and orthodontic treatment. First, the process by which behavior can be learned is presented. Second, the structural substrate of behavior, which appears to relate both to the organization of the nervous system at various stages and to emotional components underlying the expression of behavior, will be reviewed.

■ Learning and the Development of Behavior

The basic mechanisms of learning appear to be essentially the same at all ages. As learning proceeds, more complex skills and behaviors appear, but it is difficult to define the process in distinct stages—a continuous flow model appears more appropriate. It is important to remember that this discussion is of the development of behavioral patterns, not the acquisition of knowledge or intellectual skills in the academic sense.

At present, psychologists generally consider that there are three distinct mechanisms by which behavioral responses are learned: (1) classical conditioning, (2) operant conditioning, and (3) observational learning.

Classical conditioning. Classical conditioning was first described by the Russian physiologist Ivan Pavlov, who discovered in the nineteenth century during his studies of reflexes that apparently unassociated stimuli could produce reflexive behavior. Pavlov's classic experiments involved the presentation of food to a hungry animal, along with some other stimulus, for example, the ringing of a bell. The sight and sound of food normally elicit salivation by a reflex

mechanism. If a bell is rung each time food is presented, the auditory stimulus of the ringing bell will become associated with the food presentation stimulus, and in a relatively short time, the ringing of a bell by itself will elicit salivation. Classical conditioning, then, operates by the simple process of association of one stimulus with another.

Classical conditioning occurs readily with young children, and can have a considerable impact on a young child's behavior on the first visit to a dental office. By the time a child is brought for the first visit to a dentist, even if that visit is at an early age, it is highly likely that he or she will have had many experiences with pediatricians and medical personnel. When a child experiences pain, the reflex reaction is crying and withdrawal. In Pavlovian terms, the infliction of pain is an unconditioned stimulus, but a number of aspects of the setting in which the pain occurs can come to be associated with this unconditioned stimulus.

For instance, it is unusual for a child to encounter people who are dressed entirely in white uniforms or long white coats. If the unconditioned stimulus of painful treatment comes to be associated with the conditioned stimulus of white coats (Fig. 3-20), a child may cry and withdraw immediately at the first sight of a white-coated dentist or dental assistant. In this case, the child has learned to associate the conditioned stimulus of pain and the unconditioned stimulus of a white-coated adult, and the mere sight of the white coat is enough to produce the reflex behavior initially associated with pain.

Associations of this type tend to become generalized. Painful and unpleasant experiences associated with medical treatment can become generalized to the atmosphere of a physician's office, so that the whole atmosphere of a waiting room, receptionist, and other waiting children may produce crying and withdrawal after several experiences in the physician's office, even before a white coat is sighted.

Because of this association, behavior management in the dentist's office is easier if the dental office looks as little like the typical pediatrician's office or hospital clinic as possible. In practices where the dentist and auxiliaries work with young children, they have found that it is helpful in reducing children's anxiety if their appearance is different from that associated with the physician. It also helps if they can make the child's first visit as different as possible from the previous visits to the physician. Treatment that might produce pain should be avoided if at all possible on the first visit to the dental office.

The association between a conditioned and an unconditioned stimulus is strengthened or reinforced every time they occur together (Fig. 3-21). Every time a child is taken to a hospital clinic where something painful is done, the association between pain and the general atmosphere of that clinic becomes stronger, as the child becomes more sure of his conclusion that bad things happen in such a place. Conversely, if the association between a conditioned and an unconditioned stimulus is not reinforced, the association between them will become less strong, and eventually the

CLASSICAL CONDITIONING

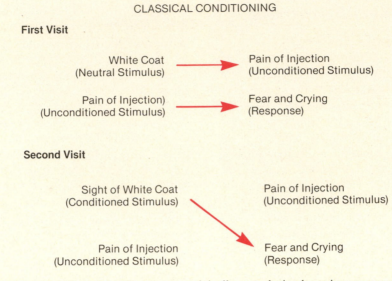

First Visit

White Coat (Neutral Stimulus) → Pain of Injection (Unconditioned Stimulus)

Pain of Injection) (Unconditioned Stimulus) → Fear and Crying (Response)

Second Visit

Sight of White Coat (Conditioned Stimulus)   Pain of Injection (Unconditioned Stimulus)

Pain of Injection (Unconditioned Stimulus) → Fear and Crying (Response)

Fig. 3-20 ■ Classical conditioning causes an originally neutral stimulus to become associated with one that leads to a specific reaction. If individuals in white coats are the ones who give painful injections that cause crying, the sight of an individual in a white coat soon may provoke an outburst of crying.

REINFORCEMENT

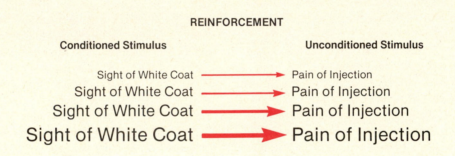

Conditioned Stimulus		Unconditioned Stimulus
Sight of White Coat	→	Pain of Injection
Sight of White Coat	→	Pain of Injection
Sight of White Coat	→	Pain of Injection
Sight of White Coat	→	Pain of Injection

Fig. 3-21 ■ Every time they occur, the association between a conditioned and unconditioned stimulus is strengthened. This process is called reinforcement.

conditioned response will no longer occur. This phenomenon is referred to as extinction of the conditioned behavior. Once a conditioned response has been established, it is necessary to reinforce it only occasionally to maintain it. If the conditioned association is one of white coats and doctors' offices with pain, it can take many visits without unpleasant experiences and pain to extinguish the associated crying and avoidance.

The opposite of generalization of a conditioned stimulus is discrimination. The conditioned association of white coats with pain can easily be generalized to any office setting. If a child is taken into other office settings that are somewhat different from the one where painful things happen, a dental office, for instance, where painful injections are not necessary, a discrimination between the two types of offices soon will develop and the generalized response to any office as a place where painful things occur will be extinguished.

Operant conditioning. Operant conditioning, which can be viewed conceptually as a significant extension of classical conditioning, has been emphasized by the preeminent behavioral theorist of recent years, B.F. Skinner. Skinner con-

tends that the most complex human behaviors can be explained by operant conditioning.[10] His theories, which downplay the role of the individual's conscious determination in favor of unconscious determined behavior, have met with much resistance but have been remarkably successful in explaining many aspects of social behavior far too complicated to be understood from the perspective of classical conditioning.

Since the theory of operant conditioning explains—or

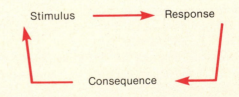

Stimulus → Response → Consequence →

Fig. 3-22 ■ Operant conditioning differs from classical conditioning in that the consequence of a behavior is considered a stimulus for future behavior. This means that the consequence of any particular response will affect the probability of that response occurring again in a similar situation.

	PROBABILITY OF RESPONSE INCREASES	PROBABILITY OF RESPONSE DECREASES
Pleasant Stimulus (S_1)	I S_1 Presented Positive Reinforcement or Reward	III S_1 Withdrawn Omission or Time-Out
Unpleasant Stimulus (S_2)	II S_2 Withdrawn Negative Reinforcement or Escape	IV S_2 Presented Punishment

Fig. 3-23 ■ The four basic types of operant conditioning.

attempts to explain—complex behavior, it is not surprising that the theory itself is more complex. Although it is not possible here to explore operant conditioning in any detail, a brief overview is presented as an aid in understanding the acquisition of behavior that older children are likely to demonstrate in the dentist's or orthodontist's office.

The basic principle of operant conditioning is that the consequence of a behavior is in itself a stimulus that can affect future behavior (Fig. 3-22). In other words, the consequence that follows a response will alter the probability of that response occurring again in a similar situation. In classical conditioning, a stimulus leads to a response; in operant conditioning, a response becomes a further stimulus. The general rule is that if the consequence of a certain response is pleasant or desirable, that response is more likely to be used again in the future; but if a particular response produces an unpleasant consequence, the probability that that response will be used in the future is diminished.

Skinner has described four basic types of operant conditioning, distinguished by the nature of the consequence (Fig. 3-23). The first of these is *positive reinforcement*. If a pleasant consequence follows a response, the response has been positively reinforced, and the behavior that led to this pleasant consequence becomes more likely in the future. For example, if a child is given a reward such as a toy for behaving well during her first dental visit, she is more likely to behave well during future dental visits; her behavior was positively reinforced.

A second type of operant conditioning, called *negative reinforcement,* involves the withdrawal of an unpleasant stimulus after a response. Like positive reinforcement, negative reinforcement increases the likelihood of a response in the future. In this context, the word negative is somewhat misleading. It merely refers to the fact that the response that is reinforced is a response that leads to the removal of an undesirable stimulus.

As an example, a child who views a visit to the hospital clinic as an unpleasant experience may throw a temper tantrum at the prospect of having to go there. If this behavior succeeds in allowing the child to escape the visit to the clinic, the behavior has been negatively reinforced and is more likely to occur the next time a visit to the clinic is proposed. The same can be true, of course, in the dentist's office. If behavior considered unacceptable by the dentist and his staff nevertheless succeeds in allowing the child to escape from dental treatment, that behavior has been negatively reinforced and is more likely to occur the next time the child is in the dental office. In dental practice, it is important to positively reinforce desired behavior, but it is equally important to avoid negatively reinforcing behavior not desired.

The other two types of operant conditioning decrease the likelihood of a response. The third type, called *omission,* involves removal of a pleasant stimulus after a particular response. For example, if a child who throws a temper tantrum has his favorite toy taken away for a short time as a consequence of this behavior, the probability of similar misbehavior is decreased.

The fourth type of operant conditioning, *punishment,* occurs when an unpleasant stimulus is presented after a response. This also decreases the probability that the behavior that prompted punishment will occur in the future. Punishment, like the other forms of operant conditioning, is effective at all ages, not just with children. For example, if the dentist with his new sports car receives a ticket for driving 50 miles per hour down a street marked for 35 miles per hour, he is likely to drive more slowly down that particular street in the future, particularly if he thinks that the same radar speed trap is still operating. Punishment, of course, has traditionally been used as a method of behavior modification in children, more so in some societies than others.

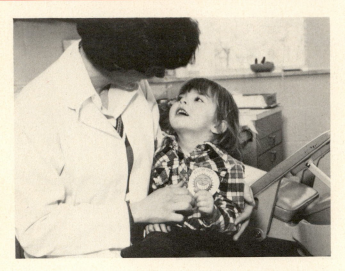

Fig. 3-24 ■ This 5-year-old is being positively reinforced by receiving a ''healthy teeth'' button after visiting his dentist. The same methods work well for older orthodontic patients, who enjoy receiving a button or t-shirt saying something like ''Braces are beautiful.''

In general, positive and negative reinforcement are the most suitable types of operant conditioning for use in the dental office, particularly for motivating orthodontic patients who must cooperate at home even more than in the dental office. Both types of reinforcement increase the likelihood of a particular behavior recurring, rather than attempting to suppress a behavior. Simply praising a child for desirable behavior produces positive reinforcement, and additional positive reinforcement can be achieved by presenting some tangible reward.

Older children are just as susceptible to positive reinforcement as younger ones. Adolescents in the orthodontic treatment age, for instance, can obtain positive reinforcement from a simple pin saying, ''World's Greatest Orthodontic Patient'' or something similar. A reward system, perhaps providing a t-shirt with some slogan as a prize for three consecutive appointments with good hygiene, is another simple example of positive reinforcement (Fig. 3-24).

Negative reinforcement, which also accentuates the probability of any given behavior, is more difficult to utilize as a behavioral management tool in the dental office. If a child is concerned about a procedure but behaves well and understands that the procedure has been shortened because of his good behavior, the desired behavior has been negatively reinforced. Orthodontic treatment is not an unpleasant experience, largely because pain develops well after the patient leaves the office and is not directly associated with the office. Negative reinforcement (''be good and we'll get this over with faster'') is less useful than in restorative dentistry.

The other two types of operant conditioning, omission and punishment, should be used sparingly and with caution in the dental office. Since a positive stimulus is removed in omission, the child may react with anger or frustration.

When punishment is used, both fear and anger sometimes result. In fact, punishment can lead to a classically conditioned fear response. Obviously, it is a good idea for the dentist and staff to avoid creating fear and anger in the child patient, and thus these two types of operant conditioning should be used cautiously.

One mild form of punishment that can be used with children is called ''voice control.'' Voice control involves speaking to the child in a firm voice to gain his (or her) attention, telling him that his present behavior is unacceptable, and directing him as to how he should behave. This technique should be used with care and the child should be immediately rewarded for an improvement in his behavior. It is most effective when a warm, caring relationship has been established between the dental team and the patient.

There is no doubt that operant conditioning can be used to modify behavior in individuals of any age, and that it forms the basis for many of the behavior patterns of life. Behavioral theorists believe that operant conditioning forms the pattern of essentially all behavior, not just the relatively superficial ones. Whether or not this is true, operant conditioning is a powerful tool for learning of behavior and an important influence throughout life.

Concepts of reinforcement as opposed to extinction, and generalization as opposed to discrimination, apply to operant conditioning as well as to classical conditioning. In operant conditioning, of course, the concepts apply to the situation in which a response leads to a particular consequence, not to the conditioned stimulus that directly controls the conditioned response. Positive or negative reinforcement becomes even more effective if repeated, although it is not necessary to provide a reward at every visit to the dental office to obtain positive reinforcement. Similarly, conditioning obtained through positive reinforcement can be extinguished if the desired behavior is now followed by omission, punishment, or simply a lack of further positive reinforcement.

Operant conditioning that occurs in one situation can also be generalized to similar situations. For example, a child who has been positively reinforced for good behavior in the pediatrician's office is likely to behave well on the first visit to a similarly equipped dentist's office because he or she will anticipate a reward at the dentist's also, based on an assessment of the similarity of the situation. A child who continues to be rewarded for good behavior in the pediatrician's office but does not receive similar rewards in the dentist's office, however, will learn to discriminate between the two situations and may eventually behave better for the pediatrician than for the dentist.

Observational learning (modeling). Another potent way that behavior is acquired is through imitation of behavior observed in a social context. This type of learning appears to be distinct from learning by either classical or operant conditioning. Acquisition of behavior through imitation of the behavior of others, of course, is entirely compatible with both classical and operant conditioning. Some theorists,

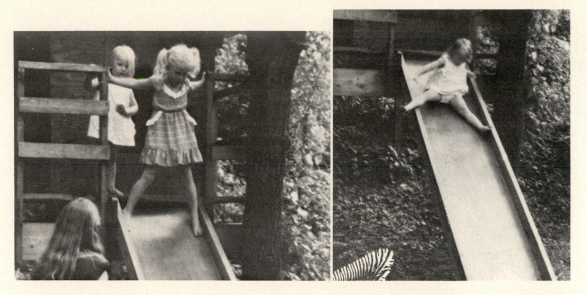

Fig. 3-25 ■ Observational learning: a child acquires a behavior by first observing it and then actually performing it, like this girl on her first visit to the playground slide.

notably A. Bandura,[11] emphasize the importance of learning by imitation in a social context, whereas others, especially Skinner and his followers,[12] argue that conditioning is more important although recognizing that learning by imitation can occur. It certainly seems that much of a child's behavior in a dental office can be learned from observing siblings, other children, or even parents.

There are two distinct stages in observational learning: *acquisition* of the behavior by observing it, and the actual *performance* of that behavior (Fig. 3-25). A child can observe many behaviors and thereby acquire the potential to perform them, without immediately demonstrating or performing that behavior. Children are capable of acquiring almost any behavior that they observe closely and which is not too complex for them to perform at their level of physical development. A child is exposed to a tremendous range of possible behaviors, most of which he acquires even though the behavior may not be expressed immediately or ever.

Whether a child will actually perform an acquired behavior depends on several factors. Important among these are the characteristics of the role model. If the model is liked or respected, the child is more likely to imitate him or her. For this reason, a parent or older sibling is often the object of imitation by the child. For children in the elementary and junior high school age groups, peers within their own age group, or individuals slightly older, are increasingly important role models, while the influence of parents and older siblings decreases. For adolescents, the peer group is the major source of role models.

Another important influence on whether a behavior is performed is the expected consequences of the behavior. If a child observes an older sibling refuse to obey his father's command and then sees punishment follow this refusal, he is less likely to defy the father on a future occasion, but he

probably still has acquired the behavior, and if he should become defiant, is likely to stage it in a similar way.

Observational learning can be an important tool in management of dental treatment. If a young child observes an older sibling undergoing dental treatment without complaint or uncooperative behavior, he or she is likely to imitate this behavior. If the older sibling is observed being rewarded, the younger child will also expect a reward for behaving well. Because the parent is an important role model for a young child, the mother's attitude toward dental treatment is likely to influence the child's approach.

Research has demonstrated that one of the best predictors of how anxious a child will be during dental treatment is how anxious the mother is. A mother who is calm and relaxed about the prospect of dental treatment teaches the child by observation that this is the appropriate approach to being treated, whereas an anxious and alarmed mother tends to elicit the same set of responses in her child (Fig. 3-26).

Observational learning can be used to advantage in the design of treatment areas. At one time, it was routine for dentists to provide small private cubicles in which all patients, children and adults, were treated. The modern trend, particularly in treatment of children and adolescents but to some extent with adults also, is to carry out dental treatment in open areas with several treatment stations.

Sitting in one dental chair watching the dentist work on someone else in an adjacent chair can provide a great deal of observational learning about what the experience will be like. Direct communication among patients, answering questions about exactly what happened, can add even further learning. Both children and adolescents do better, it appears, if they are treated in open clinics rather than in private cubicles, and observational learning plays an important part in this. The dentist hopes, of course, that what the patient

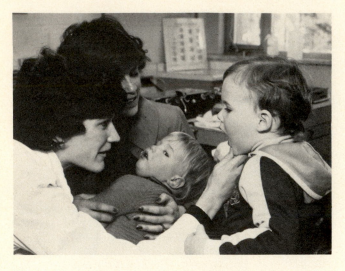

Fig. 3-26 ■ Observational learning from observing another child's treatment can help both an anxious child and his mother to respond positively to the treatment situation.

who is waiting for treatment observes is appropriate behavior on the part of the patient who is being treated, which will be the case in a well-managed clinical setting.

■ Stages of Emotional and Cognitive Development

Emotional development. In contrast to continuous learning by conditioning and observation, both emotional or personality development and cognitive or intellectual development seem to pass through relatively discrete stages. The contemporary description of emotional development is based on Sigmund Freud's psychoanalytic theory of personality development, but has been greatly extended by Erik Erikson.[13] Erikson's work, although connected to Freud's, represents a great departure from psychosexual stages as proposed by Freud. His ''eight ages of man'' illustrate a progression through a series of personality development stages. In Erikson's view, ''psychosocial development proceeds by critical steps—'critical' being a characteristic of turning points, of moments of decision between progress and regres-

sion, integration and retardation.''[13] In this view, each developmental stage represents a ''psychosocial crisis'' in which individuals are influenced by their social environment to develop more or less toward one extreme of the conflicting personality qualities dominant at that stage.

Although chronologic ages are associated with Erikson's developmental stages, as in physical development the chronologic age varies among individuals but the sequence of the developmental stages is constant. Rather differently from physical development, it is possible and indeed probable that qualities associated with earlier stages may be evident in later stages because of incomplete resolution of the earlier stages.

Erikson's stages of emotional development are as follows (Fig. 3-27):

1. *Development of basic trust (birth to 18 months).* In this initial stage of emotional development a basic trust—or lack of trust—in the environment is developed. Successful development of trust depends on a caring and consistent mother or mother-substitute, who meets both the physiologic and emotional needs of the infant. There are strongly held theories but no clear answers to exactly what constitutes proper mothering, but it is important that a strong bond develop between parent and child. This bond must be maintained to allow the child to develop basic trust in the world. In fact, physical growth can be significantly retarded unless the child's emotional needs are met by appropriate mothering.

The syndrome of ''maternal deprivation,'' in which a child receives inadequate maternal support, is well recognized though fortunately rare. Such infants fail to gain weight and are retarded in their physical as well as emotional growth (Fig. 3-28). The maternal deprivation must be extreme to produce a deficit in physical growth. Unstable mothering that produces no apparent physical effects can result in a lack of sense of basic trust. This may occur in children from broken families or who have lived in a series of foster homes.

The tight bond between parent and child at this early

ERIKSON'S "EIGHT AGES OF MAN"

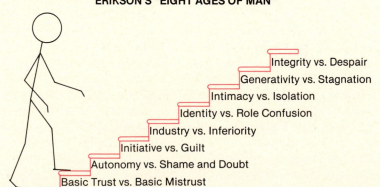

Integrity vs. Despair
Generativity vs. Stagnation
Intimacy vs. Isolation
Identity vs. Role Confusion
Industry vs. Inferiority
Initiative vs. Guilt
Autonomy vs. Shame and Doubt
Basic Trust vs. Basic Mistrust

Fig. 3-27 ■ Erikson's stages of emotional development: the sequence is more fixed than the time when each stage is reached. Some adults never reach the final steps on the developmental staircase.

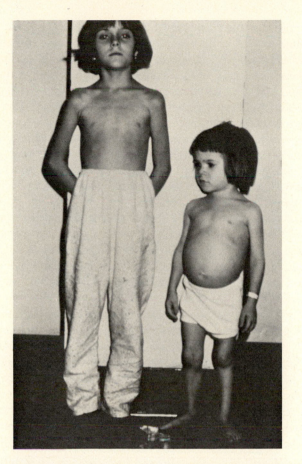

Fig. 3-28 ■ Both these girls are 7 years old. The one on the left is normal, whereas the one on the right had extreme emotional neglect from a mother who rejected her. The effect on physical growth in this "maternal deprivation syndrome" is obvious; fortunately, this condition is rare. The emotional response probably affects physical growth by altering hormone production, but the mechanism is not fully understood. (Courtesy Dr. F. Debusk.)

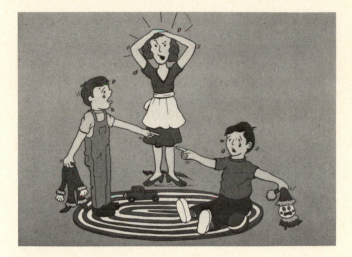

Fig. 3-29 ■ During the period in which children are developing autonomy, conflicts with siblings, peers, and parents can seem never-ending. Consistently enforced limits on behavior during this stage, often called the "terrible two's," are needed to allow the child to develop trust in a predictable environment.

stage of emotional development is reflected in a strong sense of "separation anxiety" in the child when separated from the parent. If it is necessary to provide dental treatment at an early age, it usually is preferable to do so with the parent present, and if possible, while the child is being held by one of the parents. At later ages, a child who never developed a sense of basic trust will have difficulty in entering into situations that require trust and confidence in another person. Such an individual is likely to be an extremely frightened and uncooperative patient who needs special effort to establish rapport and trust with the dentist and staff.

2. *Development of autonomy (18 months to 3 years).* Children around the age of 2 often are said to be undergoing the "terrible two's" because of their uncooperative and frequently obnoxious behavior. At this stage of emotional development, the child is moving away from the mother and developing a sense of individual identity or autonomy. Typically, the child struggles to exercise free choice in his life. He or she varies between being a little devil who says

no to every wish of the parents and insists on having his own way, and being a little angel who retreats to the parents in moments of dependence. The parents and other adults with whom the child reacts at this stage must protect him against the consequences of dangerous and unacceptable behavior, while providing opportunities to develop independent behavior. Consistently enforced limits on behavior at this time allow the child to further develop trust in a predictable environment (Fig. 3-29).

Failure to develop a proper sense of autonomy results in the development of doubts in the child's mind about his ability to stand alone, and this in turn produces doubts about others. Erikson defines the resulting state as one of shame, a feeling of having all one's shortcomings exposed. Autonomy in control of bodily functions is an important part of this stage, as the young child is toilet trained and taken out of diapers. At this stage (and later!), wetting one's pants produces a feeling of shame. This stage is considered as decisive in producing the personality characteristics of love as opposed to hate, cooperation as opposed to selfishness, and freedom of expression as opposed to self-consciousness.

To quote Erikson, "From a sense of self-control without a loss of self-esteem comes a lasting sense of good will and pride; from a sense of loss of self-control and foreign over-control come a lasting propensity for doubt and shame."[13]

A key toward obtaining cooperation with treatment from a child at this stage is to have the child think that whenever the dentist wants was his or her own choice, not something required by another person. For a 2-year-old seeking autonomy, it is all right to open your mouth if you want to, but almost psychologically unacceptable to do it if someone tells you to. One way around this is to offer the child reasonable choices whenever possible, for instance, either a green or a yellow napkin for the neck.

A child at this stage who finds the situation threatening is likely to retreat to mother and be unwilling to separate from her. Allowing the parent to be present during treatment may be needed.

3. *Development of initiative (3 to 6 years).* In this stage, the child continues to develop greater autonomy, but now adds to it planning and vigorous pursuit of various activities. The initiative is shown by physical activity and motion, extreme curiosity and questioning, and aggressive talking. A major task for parents and teachers at this stage is to channel the activity into manageable tasks, arranging things so that the child is able to succeed, and preventing him or her from undertaking tasks where success is not possible. At this stage, a child is inherently teachable. One part of initiative is the eager modeling of behavior on those whom he respects.

The opposite of initiative is guilt resulting from goals that are contemplated but not attained, from acts initiated but not completed, or from faults or acts rebuked by persons the child respects. In Erikson's view, the child's ultimate ability to initiate new ideas or activities depends on how well he or she is able at this stage to express new thoughts and do new things without being made to feel guilty about expressing a bad idea or failing to achieve what was expected.

For most children, the first visit to the dentist comes during this stage of initiative. Going to the dentist can be constructed as a new and challenging adventure in which the child can experience success. Success in coping with the anxiety of visiting the dentist can help develop greater independence and produce a sense of accomplishment. Poorly managed, of course, a dental visit can also contribute toward the guilt that accompanies failure. A child at this stage will be intensely curious about the dentist's office and eager to learn about the things found there. An exploratory visit with the mother present and with little treatment accomplished usually is important in getting the dental experience off to a good start. After the initial experience, a child at this stage can usually tolerate being separated from the mother for treatment and is likely to behave better in this arrangement, so that independence rather than dependence is reinforced.

4. *Mastery of skills (age 7 to 11 years).* At this stage, the child is working to acquire the academic and social skills that will allow him or her to compete in an environment where significant recognition is given to those who produce. At the same time, the child is learning the rules by which that world is organized. In Erikson's terms, the child acquires industriousness and begins the preparation for entrance into a competitive and working world. Competition with others within a reward system becomes a reality; at the same time, it becomes clear that some tasks can be accomplished only by cooperating with others. The influence of parents as role models decreases and the influence of the peer group increases.

The negative side of emotional and personality development at this stage can be the acquisition of a sense of inferiority. A child who begins to compete academically, socially, and physically is certain to find that others do some things better and that someone does nearly anything better. Somebody else gets put in the advanced section, is selected as leader of the group, or is chosen first for the team. Failure to measure up to the peer group on a broad scale predisposes toward personality characteristics of inadequacy, inferiority, and uselessness. Again, it is important for responsible adults to attempt to structure an environment that provides challenges, but challenges that have a reasonable chance of being met rather than guarantee failure.

By this stage, a child should already have experienced the first visit to the dentist, although a significant number will not have done so. Orthodontic treatment often begins during this stage of development. Children at this age are trying to learn the skills and rules that define success in any situation, and that includes the dental office. A key to behavioral management is clearly outlining for the child what is expected and positively reinforcing appropriate behavior.

Orthodontic treatment in this age group is likely to involve the faithful wearing of removable appliances (Fig. 3-30). Whether a child will do so is determined in large part by whether he or she understands what is needed to please the dentist and parents, whether the peer group is supportive, and whether the desired behavior is reinforced by the dentist.

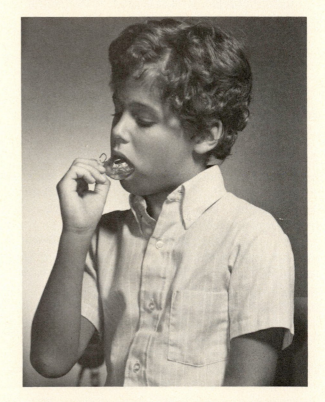

Fig. 3-30 ■ Instructions for a young child who will be wearing a removable orthodontic appliance must be explicit and concrete. Children at this stage cannot be motivated by abstract concepts, but are influenced by improved acceptance or status from their peer group.

Children at this stage still are not likely to be motivated by abstract concepts such as "If you wear this appliance your bite will be better." They can be motivated, however, by improved acceptance or status from the peer group. This means that emphasizing how the teeth will look better as the child cooperates is more likely to be a motivating factor than emphasizing a better occlusal relationship, which the peer group is not likely to notice.

5. *Development of personal identity (age 12 to 17 years).* Adolescence, a period of intense physical development, is also the stage in psychosocial development in which a unique personal identity is acquired. This sense of identity includes both a feeling of belonging to a larger group and a realization that one can exist outside the family. It is an extremely complex stage because of the many new opportunities that arise. Emerging sexuality complicates relationships with others. At the same time, physical ability changes, academic responsibilities increase, and career possibilities begin to be defined.

Establishing one's own identity requires a partial withdrawal from the family, and the peer group increases still further in importance because it offers a sense of continuity of existence in spite of drastic changes within the individual (Fig. 3-31). Members of the peer group become important role models, and the values and tastes of parents and other authority figures are likely to be rejected. At the same time, some separation from the peer group is necessary to establish one's own uniqueness and value. As adolescence progresses, an inability to separate from the group indicates some failure in identity development. This in turn can lead to a poor sense of direction for the future, confusion regarding one's place in society, and low self-esteem.

Most orthodontic treatment is carried out during the adolescent years, and behavioral management of adolescents

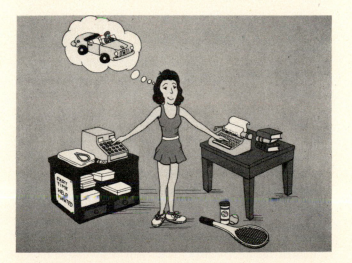

Fig. 3-31 ■ Adolescence is an extremely complex stage because of the many new opportunities and challenges thrust upon the teenager. Emerging sexuality, academic pressures, earning money, increased mobility, career aspirations, and recreational interests combine to produce stress and rewards.

can be extremely challenging. Since parental authority is being rejected, a poor psychologic situation is created by orthodontic treatment, if it is being carried out primarily because the parents want it, not the child. At this stage, orthodontic treatment should be instituted only if the patient wants it, not just to please the parents.

Motivation for seeking treatment can be defined as internal or external. External motivation is from pressure from others, as in orthodontic treatment "to get mother off my back." Internal motivation is provided by an individual's own desire for treatment to correct a defect that he perceives in himself, not some defect pointed to by authority figures whose values are being rejected anyway. Approval of the peer group is extremely important. At one time, there was a certain stigma attached to being the only one in the group so unfortunate as to have to wear braces. In some areas of the United States now, orthodontic treatment has become so common that there may be a loss of status attached to being one of the few in the group who is not receiving treatment, so that treatment may even be requested in order to remain "one of the crowd."

It is extremely important for an adolescent to actively desire the treatment as something being done *for,* not *to,* him or her. In this stage, abstract concepts can be grasped readily, but appeals to do something because of its impact on personal health are not likely to be heeded. The typical adolescent feels that health problems are concerns of somebody else, and this attitude covers everything from accidental death in reckless driving to development of decalcified areas on carelessly brushed teeth.

6. *Development of intimacy (young adult).* The adult stages of development begin with the attainment of intimate relationships with others. Successful development of intimacy depends on a willingness to compromise and even to sacrifice to maintain a relationship. Success leads to the establishment of affiliations and partnerships, both with a mate and with others of the same sex in working toward the attainment of career goals. Failure leads to isolation from others and is likely to be accompanied by strong prejudices and a set of attitudes that serve to keep others away rather than bringing them into closer contact.

A growing number of young adults are seeking orthodontic care. Often these individuals are seeking to correct a dental appearance they perceive as flawed. They may feel that a change in their appearance will facilitate attainment of intimate relationships. On the other hand, a "new look" resulting from orthodontic treatment may interfere with previously established relationships.

The factors that affect the development of an intimate relationship include all aspects of each person—appearance, personality, emotional qualities, intellect, and others. A significant change in any of these may be perceived by either partner as altering the relationship. Because of these potential problems, the potential psychologic impact of orthodontic treatment must be fully explained to and explored with the young adult patient before beginning therapy.

7. *Guidance of the next generation (adult).* A major responsibility of a mature adult is the establishment and guidance of the next generation. Becoming a successful and supportive parent is obviously a major part of this, but another aspect of the same responsibility is service to the group, community, and nation. The next generation is guided, in short, not only by nurturing and influencing one's own children but also by supporting the network of social services needed to ensure the next generation's success. The opposite personality characteristic in mature adults is stagnation, characterized by self-indulgence and self-centered behavior.

8. *Attainment of integrity (late adult).* The final stage in psychosocial development is the attainment of integrity. At this stage, the individual has adapted to the combination of gratification and disappointment that every adult experiences. The feeling of integrity is best summed up as a feeling that one has made the best of this life's situation and has made peace with it. The opposite characteristic is despair. This feeling is often expressed as disgust and unhappiness on a broad scale, frequently accompanied by a fear that death will occur before a life change that might lead to integrity can be accomplished.

Cognitive development. Cognitive development, the development of intellectual capabilities, also occurs in a series of relatively distinct stages. Like the other psychologic theories, the theory of cognitive development is strongly associated with one dominant individual, in this case the Swiss psychologist Jean Piaget. From the perspective of Piaget and his followers, the development of intelligence is another example of the widespread phenomenon of biologic adaptation. Every individual is born with the capacity to adjust or adapt to both the physical and sociocultural environments in which he or she must live.

In Piaget's view, adaptation occurs through two complementary processes, *assimilation* and *accommodation*.[14] From the beginning, a child incorporates or assimilates events within the environment into mental categories called cognitive structures. A cognitive structure in this sense is a classification for sensations and perceptions.

For example, a child who has just learned the word ''bird'' will tend to assimilate all flying objects into his idea of bird. When he sees a bee, he will probably say, ''Look, bird!'' However, for intelligence to develop, the child must also have the complementary process of accommodation. Accommodation occurs when the child changes his or her cognitive structure or mental category to better represent the environment. In the previous example, the child will be corrected by an adult or older child and will soon learn to distinguish between birds and bees. In other words, the child will accommodate to the event of seeing a bee, by creating a separate category of flying objects for bees.

Intelligence develops as an interplay between assimilation and accommodation. Each time the child in our example sees a flying object he or she will try to assimilate it into existing cognitive categories. If these categories do not

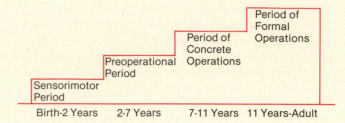

Fig. 3-32 ■ Cognitive development is divided into four major periods, as diagrammed here.

work, he or she will try to accommodate by creating new ones. However, the child's ability to adapt is limited by the current level of development. The notion that the child's ability to adapt is *age-related* is a crucial concept in Piaget's theory of development.

From the perspective of cognitive development theory, life can be divided into four major stages (Fig. 3-32): the *sensorimotor* period, extending from birth to 2 years of age; the *preoperational* period, from 2 to 7 years; the *concrete operational* period from about age 7 to puberty; and the period of *formal operations,* which runs from adolescence through adulthood. Like the other developmental stages, it is important to realize that the time frame is variable, especially for the later ones. Some adults never reach the last stage. The sequence of the stages, however, is fixed.

It appears that a child's way of thinking about and viewing the world is quite different at the different stages. A child simply does not think like an adult until the period of formal operations has been reached. Since a child's thought processes are quite different, one cannot expect a child to process and utilize information in the same way that an adult would. To communicate successfully with a child, it is necessary to understand his or her intellectual level and the way in which thought processes work at the various stages.

Considering the cognitive development stages in more detail:

1. *Sensorimotor period.* During the first 2 years of life, a child develops from a newborn infant who is almost totally dependent on reflex activities to an individual who can develop new behavior to cope with new situations. During this stage, the child develops rudimentary concepts of objects, including the idea that objects in the environment are permanent; they do not disappear when the child is not looking at them. Simple modes of thought that are the foundation of language develop during this time, but communication between a child at this stage and an adult is extremely limited because of the child's simple concepts and lack of language capabilities. At this stage, a child has little ability to interpret sensory data and a limited ability to project forward or backward in time.

2. *Preoperational period.* Because children above the age of 2 begin to use language in ways similar to adults, it appears that their thought processes are more like those of adults than is the case. During the preoperational stage, the

capacity develops to form mental symbols representing things and events not present, and children learn to use words to symbolize these absent objects. Because children's word symbolism is dictated by the external appearance or characteristics of an object, however, their use of words is different from adults'. To an adult, the word "coat" refers to a whole family of external garments that may be long or short, heavy or light, and so on. To a preoperational child, however, the word "coat" is initially associated with only the one he or she wears, and the garment that daddy wears would require another word.

A general feature of thought processes and language during the preoperational period is *egocentrism,* meaning that the child is incapable of assuming another person's point of view. At this stage, his own perspective is all that he can manage—assuming another's view is simply beyond his mental capabilities.

Still another characteristic of thought processes at this stage is *animism,* investing inanimate objects with life. Essentially everything is seen as being alive by a young child, and so stories that invest the most improbable objects with life are quite acceptable to children of this age. Animism can be used to the dental team's advantage by giving dental instruments and equipment life-like names and qualities. For example, the handpiece can be called "Whistling Willie" who is happy while he works at polishing the child's teeth.

At this stage, capabilities for logical reasoning are limited, and the child's thought processes are dominated by the immediate sensory impressions. This characteristic can be illustrated by asking the child to solve a liquid conservation problem. The child is first shown two equal size glasses with water in them. The child agrees that both contain the same amount of water. Then the contents of one glass are poured into a taller, narrower glass while the child watches. Now when asked which container has more water, the child will usually say that the tall one does. Her impressions are dominated by the greater height of the water in the tall glass.

For this reason, the dental staff should use immediate sensations rather than abstract reasoning in discussing concepts like prevention of dental problems with a child at this stage. Excellent oral hygiene is very important when an orthodontic appliance is present (a lingual arch to prevent drift of teeth, for instance). A preoperational child will have trouble understanding a chain of reasoning like the following: "Brushing and flossing remove food particles, which in turn prevents bacteria from forming acids, which cause tooth decay." He or she is much more likely to understand: "Brushing makes your teeth feel clean and smooth," and, "Toothpaste makes your mouth taste good," because these statements rely on things the child can taste or feel immediately.

A knowledge of these thought processes obviously can be used to improve communication with children of this age. A further example would be talking to a 4-year-old about how desirable it would be to stop thumb sucking. The dentist might have little problem in getting the child to accept the idea that "Mr. Thumb" was the problem and that the dentist and the child should form a partnership to control Mr. Thumb who wishes to get into the child's mouth. Animism, in other words, can apply even to parts of the child's own body, which seem to take on a life of their own in this view.

On the other hand, it would not be useful to point out to the child how proud his father would be if he stopped sucking his thumb, since the child would think his father's attitude was the same as the child's (egocentrism). Since the child's view of time is centered around the present, and he or she is dominated by how things look, feeel, taste, and sound now, there also is no point in talking to the 4-year-old about how much better his teeth will look in the future if he stops sucking his thumb. Telling him that the teeth will feel better now or talking about how bad his thumb tastes, however, may make an impact, since he can relate to that.

3. *Period of concrete operations.* As a child moves into this stage, typically after a year or so of preschool and first grade activity, an improved ability to reason emerges. He or she can use a limited number of logical processes, especially those involving objects that can be handled and manipulated, i.e., concrete objects. Thus, an 8-year-old could watch the water being poured from one glass to another, imagine the reverse of that process, and conclude that the amount of water remains the same no matter what size the container is. If a child in this stage is given a similar problem, however, stated only in words with no concrete objects to illustrate it, the child may fail to solve it. The child's thinking is still strongly tied to concrete situations, and the ability to reason on an abstract level is limited.

By this stage, the ability to see another point of view develops, while animism declines. Children in this period are much more like adults in the way they view the world but we must remain aware that they are still cognitively different from adults. Presenting ideas as abstract concepts rather than illustrating them with concrete objects can be a major barrier to communication. Instructions must be illustrated with concrete objects. "Now wear your retainer every night and be sure to keep it clean," is too abstract. More concrete directions would be: "This is your retainer. Put it in your mouth like this, and take it out like that. Put it in every evening right after dinner before you go to bed, and take it out before breakfast every morning. Brush it like this with an old toothbrush to keep it clean."

4. *Period of formal operations.* For most children, the ability to deal with abstract concepts and abstract reasoning develops by about age 11. At this stage, the child's thought process has become the same as an adult's, and the child is capable of understanding concepts like health, disease, and preventive treatment. At this stage, intellectually the child can and should be treated as an adult. It is as great a mistake to talk down to a child who has developed the ability to deal with abstract concepts, using the concrete approach

needed with an 8-year-old, as it is to assume that the 8-year-old can handle abstract ideas. Successful communication, in other words, requires a feel for the child's stage of intellectual development.

To be received, the dentist's message must be couched in the proper terms intellectually. It must also be acceptable psychologically, i.e., appropriately related to the child's stage of psychosocial development. An effective message must take into account the stages of development in learning theory. The adage "different strokes for different folks" applies strongly to children, whose variations in intellectual and psychosocial development affect the way they receive orthodontic treatment just as their differing stages of physical development do.

■ *References*

1. Johnston, M.C., and Listgarten, M.A.: The migration, interaction and early differentiation of orofacial tissues. In Slavkin, H.S., and Bavetta, L.A., editors: Developmental Aspects of Oral Biology. New York, 1972, Academic Press.
2. Poswillo, D.: The pathogenesis of the Treacher-Collins syndrome (mandibulofacial dysostosis). Br. J. Oral Surg. **13:**1-26, 1975.
3. Poswillo, D.: The pathogenesis of the first and second branchial arch syndrome. Oral Surg. **35:**302-328, 1973.
4. Cooper, H.K., et al., editor: Cleft Palate and Cleft Lip: A Team Approach to Clinical Management and Rehabilitation of the Patient. Philadelphia, 1979, W.B. Saunders Co.
5. Larsson, E.F., and Dahlin, K.G.: The prevalence of finger and dummy-sucking habits in European and primitive population groups. Am. J. Orthod., **87:**432-435, 1985.
6. Fletcher, S.G., Casteel, R.L., and Bradley, D.P.: Tongue-thrust swallow, speech articulation, and age. J. Speech Hear. Disord. **26:**201-214, 1961.
7. Lundeen, H.C., and Gibbs, C.H.: Advances in Occlusion. Boston, 1982, John Wright–PSG, Inc.
8. Lowery, G.H.: Growth and Development of Children, ed. 6. Chicago, 1973, Year-book Medical Publishers.
9. Tanner, J.M.: Earlier maturation in man. Sci. Am. **218:**28-35, 1968.
10. Skinner, B.F.: Science and Human Behavior. New York, 1953, Macmillan.
11. Bandura, A., and Walter, R.H.: Social Learning and Personality Development. New York, 1963, Holt, Rinehart & Winston.
12. Rachlin, H.: Introduction to Modern Behaviorism. San Francisco, 1970, W.H. Freeman.
13. Erikson, E.: Childhood and Society. New York, 1963, W.W. Norton.
14. Flavell, J.H.: The Developmental Psychology of Jean Piaget. New York, 1963, Van Nostrand Reinhold.

Chapter 4

The Later Stages of Development

■ Late Childhood: The Mixed Dentition Years

■ Eruption of the Permanent Teeth

The eruption of any tooth can be divided into several stages. The nature of eruption and its control before the emergence of the tooth into the mouth are somewhat different from eruption after emergence, and we will consider these major stages separately.

Preemergent eruption. During the period when the crown of a tooth is being formed, there is a very slow labial or buccal drift of the tooth follicle within the bone, but this follicular drift is not attributed to the eruption mechanism itself. In fact, the amount of change in the position of the tooth follicle is extremely small, so small that a follicle can be used as a natural marker in radiographic studies of growth, and is known to exist with certainty only because of vital staining experiments. Eruptive movement begins soon after the root begins to form. This supports the idea that metabolic activity within the periodontal ligament is a major part of, if not the only mechanism for, eruption.

Two processes are necessary for preemergent eruption. First, there must be resorption of bone and primary tooth roots overlying the crown of the erupting tooth; second, the eruption mechanism itself then must move the tooth in the direction where the path has been cleared (Fig. 4-1). Although the two mechanims normally operate in concert, in some circumstances they do not. Investigations of the results of a failure of bone resorption, or alternately, of a failure of the eruption mechanism when bone resorption is normal, have yielded considerable insight into the control of pre-emergent eruption.

Defective bone resorption occurs in a mutant species of mice, appropriately labeled *Ia,* for Incisors absent. In these animals, the deficient bone resorption means that the incisor teeth cannot erupt, and they never appear in the mouth. Failure of teeth to erupt because of a failure of bone resorption also occurs in humans, as for instance in the syndrome of cleidocranial dysplasia (Fig. 4-2). In children with this condition, not only is resorption of primary teeth and bone deficient but heavy fibrous gingiva and multiple supernumerary teeth also impede normal eruption. All of these serve to mechanically block the succedaneous teeth (those replacing primary teeth) from erupting.

It has been demonstrated experimentally in animals that the rate of bone resorption and the rate of tooth eruption are not controlled physiologically by the same mechanism. Cahill[2] showed, for instance, that if the tooth bud of a dog premolar was wired to the lower border of the mandible, the tooth would no longer erupt because of this mechanical obstruction, but resorption of overlying bone would proceed at the usual rate, resulting in a large cystic cavity overlying the ligated tooth bud.

On at least one occasion, the same experiment has inadvertently been done to a child, in whom a second molar was wired to the lower border of the mandible when a mandibular fracture was repaired (Fig. 4-3). The result was the same: bone resorption continued, but eruption of the tooth was prevented. In a rare but now well documented human syndrome called ''primary failure of eruption,'' affected posterior teeth fail to erupt, presumably because of a defect in the eruption mechanism (see Chapter 5). In these individuals, bone resorption apparently proceeds normally, but the involved teeth simply do not follow the path that has been cleared.

It appears, therefore, that resorption is the rate-limiting factor in preemergent eruption. Normally, the overlying bone and primary teeth resorb, and the eruption mechanism then moves the tooth into the space created by the resorption. Nevertheless, something about the erupting tooth (perhaps

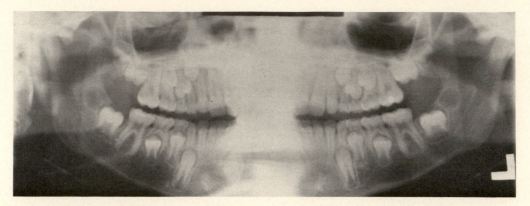

Fig. 4-1 ■ Panoramic radiograph of normal eruption in a 10-year-old boy. Note that the permanent teeth erupt as resorption of overlying primary teeth and bone occurs. Resorption must occur to make eruption possible.

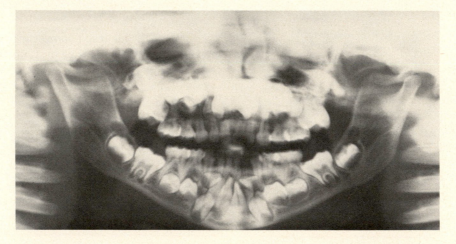

Fig. 4-2 ■ Panoramic radiograph of an 8-year-old-patient with cleidocranial dysplasia, showing the characteristic features of this condition. In cleidocranial dysplasia, the succedaneous teeth do not erupt because of abnormal resorption, and the eruption of nonsuccedaneous teeth is delayed by fibrotic gingiva. Supernumerary teeth often are also present, as in this patient, creating additional mechanical obstruction.

pressure within the follicle, or some chemical messenger) is the signal for bone resorption.

Despite many years of study, the precise mechanism through which the eruption force is generated remains unknown. Substances that interfere with the development of cross-links in maturing collagen interfere with eruption, which makes it tempting to theorize that cross-linking of maturing collagen in the periodontal ligament provides the eruptive force. From studies of root-resected and -transected rat incisors,[4] it seems clear that at least the major eruption mechanism (there may, after all, be more than one) is localized within the periodontal ligament.

Other possibilities for the eruption mechanism besides collagen maturation are localized variations in blood pressure or flow, forces derived from contraction of fibroblasts, and alterations in the extracellular ground substances of the periodontal ligament similar to those that occur in thixotropic gels (see Steedle and Proffit[5] for a review). A tooth will continue to erupt after its apical area has been removed,

so the proliferation of cells associated with lengthening of the root is not an essential part of the mechanism. Normally, the rate of eruption is such that the apical area remains at the same place while the crown moves occlusally, but if eruption is mechanically blocked, the proliferating apical area will move in the opposite direction, inducing resorption where it usually does not occur (Fig. 4-4). This often causes a distortion of root form.

Postemergent eruption. Once a tooth emerges into the mouth, it erupts rapidly until it approaches the occlusal level and is subjected to the forces of mastication. At that point, its eruption slows and then as it reaches the occlusal level of other teeth and is in complete function, all but halts. The stage of relatively rapid eruption from the time a tooth first penetrates the gingiva until it reaches the occlusal level is called the *postemergent spurt,* in contrast to the following phase of very slow eruption, termed the *juvenile occlusal equilibrium*.

There is no reason to believe that the eruption mechanism

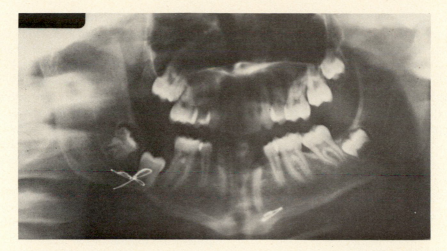

Fig. 4-3 ■ Panoramic radiograph from a 16-year-old patient whose lower jaw was broken at age 10. Neither the mandibular left canine nor the mandibular right second molar have erupted. The canine, in the line of a body fracture, has fused to the bone (traumatic ankylosis). A wire ligature in the area of the right ramus fracture has inadvertently pinned the right second molar, simulating Cahill's experiments in animals. Note that in this situation, bone resorption over the unerupted molar has continued, although eruptive movements of the tooth have not followed. (Courtesy Dr. Bruce King.)

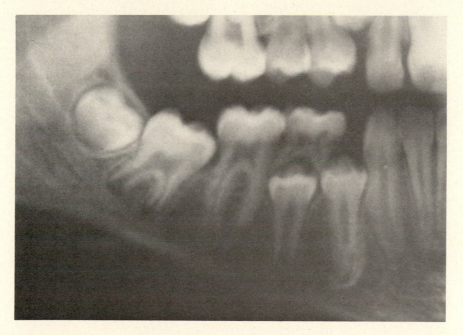

Fig. 4-4 ■ In this 14 year-old boy, normal resorption of the root of the second primary molar has not occurred, and eruption of the first premolar has been delayed by mechanical obstruction. Note the lengthening of the crypt of this tooth, with resorption at the apical area. Some distortion of root form is probably also occurring.

is any different after emergence than it was before, but the control mechanism certainly is different (Fig. 4-5). It seems obvious that as a tooth is subjected to biting forces that oppose eruption, the overall rate of eruption would be slowed, and in fact exactly this occurs. However, the way that forces applied to a tooth influence its rate of eruption remains unknown. Experiments with the erupting incisors of rodents indicate that there is a maximal rate achieved by a tooth when it is not subjected to any forces; when the tooth is in function, its eruption rate decreases by 40% to 60%.[6] In rodents, this impeded eruption rate equals the rate at which the tooth wears away.

In human teeth, tooth wear is not an important phenomenon, and after the teeth reach the occlusal level, eruption becomes almost imperceptibly slow although it definitely continues. During the juvenile equilibrium, teeth that are in function erupt at a rate that parallels the rate of vertical growth of the mandibular ramus (Fig. 4-6). As the mandible continues to grow, it moves away from the maxilla, creating a space into which the teeth erupt.

The amount of eruption necessary to compensate for jaw growth can best be appreciated by observing what happens

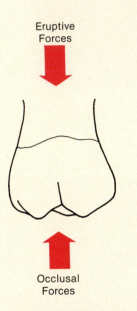

Eruptive
Forces

Occlusal
Forces

Fig. 4-5 ■ Diagrammatic representation of the equilibrium between forces promoting eruption and those opposing it, after a tooth has emerged into the oral cavity.

to a tooth that becomes ankylosed, i.e., fused to the alveolar bone. An ankylosed tooth appears to submerge over a period of time as the other teeth continue to erupt while it remains at the same vertical level (Fig. 4-7). The total eruption path of a first permanent molar is about 2.5 cm. Of that distance, nearly half is traversed after the tooth reaches the occlusal level and is in function. If a first molar becomes ankylosed at an early age, which fortunately is rare, it can "submerge" to such an extent that the tooth is covered over again by the gingiva as other teeth erupt and the alveolar process increases in height (Fig. 4-8).

Since the rate of eruption parallels the rate of jaw growth, it is not surprising that a pubertal spurt in eruption of the teeth accompanies the pubertal spurt in jaw growth. This pattern of eruption of the teeth in concert with growth of the jaws reinforces the concept that the rate of eruption is controlled by the forces opposing eruption, not those promoting it. After a tooth is in the mouth, the forces opposing eruption are those from chewing, and perhaps in addition, soft tissue pressures from lips, cheeks, or tongue contacting the teeth. Disturbances in the coordination between jaw growth and tooth eruption often contribute to the development of orthodontic problems.

When the pubertal growth spurt ends, a final phase in tooth eruption called the *adult occlusal equilibrium* is achieved. During adult life, teeth continue to erupt at an extremely slow rate. If its antagonist is lost at any age, a tooth can again erupt more rapidly, demonstrating that the eruption mechanism remains active and capable of producing significant tooth movement even late in life.

Wear of the teeth may become significant as the years

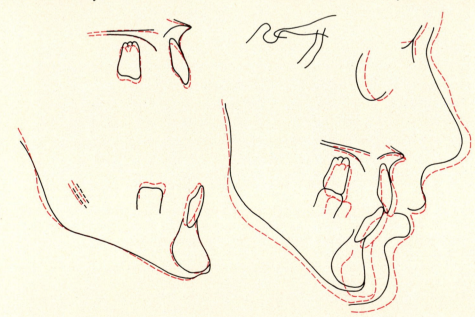

Fig. 4-6 ■ The amount of tooth eruption after the teeth have come into occlusion equals the vertical growth of the ramus, in a patient who is growing normally. Vertical growth increases the space between the jaws, and the maxillary and mandibular teeth normally divide this space equally. Note the equivalent eruption of the upper and lower molars in this patient between age 10 *(black)* and 14 *(red)*. This is a normal growth pattern.

pass. If wear is severe in adults, eruption may not compensate for the loss of tooth structure, so that the vertical dimension of the face is decreased. In most individuals, however, any wear of the teeth is compensated by additional eruption, so that face height remains constant or even increases slightly in the fourth, fifth, and sixth decades of life (see Maturation and Aging, in this chapter).

Eruption sequence and timing. The transition from the primary to the permanent dentition begins at about age 6 with the eruption of the first permanent molars, followed soon thereafter by the permanent incisors. The permanent teeth tend to erupt in groups, and it is less important to know the most common eruption sequence than to know the expected timing of these eruption stages. The stages are used in the calculation of dental age, which is particularly important during the mixed dentition years. Dental age is determined from three characteristics. The first is which teeth have erupted. The second and third, which are closely related, are the amount of resorption of the roots of primary teeth and the amount of development of permanent teeth.

The first stage of eruption of the permanent teeth is illustrated in Fig. 4-9. The most common eruption sequence is the eruption of the mandibular central incisor, closely followed by the mandibular first permanent molar and the maxillary first permanent molar. These teeth normally erupt at so nearly the same time, however, that it is quite within normal variation for the first molars to slightly precede the mandibular central incisors or vice versa. Usually, the man-

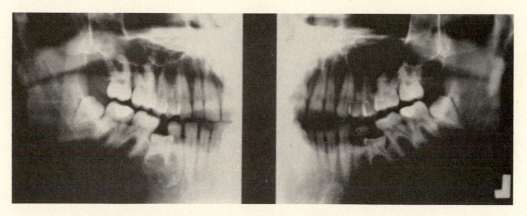

Fig. 4-7 ■ The mandibular second primary molars in this young adult, whose second premolars were congenitally missing, became ankylosed well before eruption of the other teeth was completed. Their apparent submergence is really because the other teeth have erupted past them. Note that the permanent first molars have tipped mesially over the submerged primary molars.

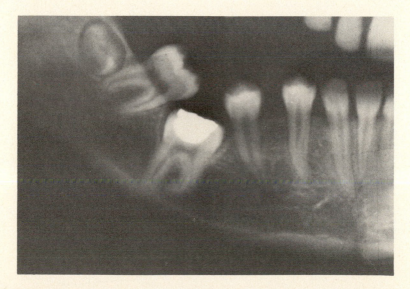

Fig. 4-8 ■ The first molar in this 15-year-old girl ceased erupting soon after its emergence into the mouth at age 6 or 7. At that time when the dentist placed an occlusal restoration, the tooth was apparently in or near occlusion. This dramatically illustrates the amount of eruption that must occur after the initial occlusal contact of first molars.

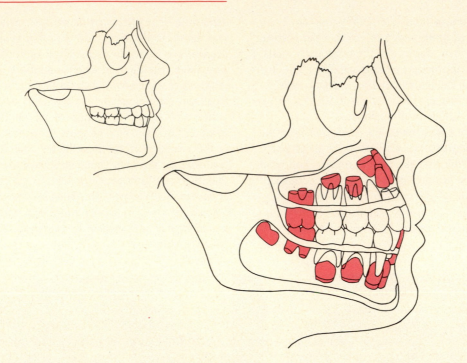

Fig. 4-9 ■ The first stage of eruption of the permanent teeth, at age 6, is characterized by the near-simultaneous eruption of the mandibular central incisors, the mandibular first molars, and the maxillary first molars.

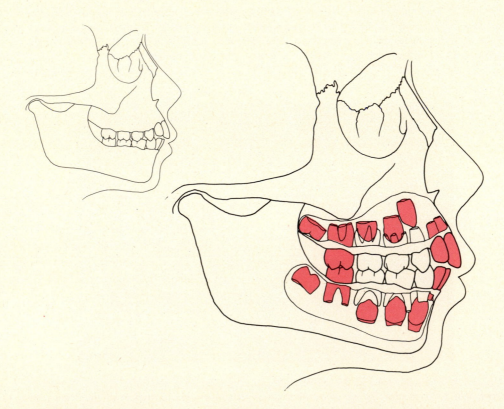

Fig. 4-10 ■ Dental age 8 is characterized by eruption of the maxillary lateral incisors.

dibular molar will precede the maxillary molar. The beginning eruption of this group of teeth characterizes dental age 6.

In the second stage of eruption at dental age 7, the maxillary central incisors and the mandibular lateral incisors erupt. The maxillary central incisor is usually a year behind the mandibular central incisor, but erupts simultaneously with the mandibular lateral incisor. At dental age 7, root formation of the maxillary lateral incisor is well advanced, but it is still about 1 year from eruption, while the canines and premolars are still in the stage of crown completion or just at the beginning of root formation.

Dental age 8 (Fig. 4-10) is characterized by the eruption of the maxillary lateral incisors. After this tooth comes into the arch, there is a delay of 2 to 3 years before any further permanent teeth appear.

Since no teeth are erupting at that time, dental ages 9 and 10 must be distinguished by the extent of resorption of the primary canines and premolars and the extent of root development of their permanent successors. At dental age 9, the primary canines, first molars, and second molars are present. Approximately one-third of the root of the mandibular canine and the mandibular first premolar is completed. Root development is just beginning, if it has started at all, on the mandibular second premolar (Fig. 4-11). In the maxillary arch, root development has begun on the first premolar but is just beginning, if it is present at all, on both the canine and the second premolar.

Dental age 10 is characterized by a greater amount of both root resorption of the primary canines and molars, and root development of their permanent successors. At dental age 10, approximately one-half of the roots of the mandibular canine and mandibular first premolar has been completed; nearly half the root of the upper first premolar is complete, and there is significant root development of the mandibular second premolar, maxillary canine, and maxillary second premolar.

Teeth usually emerge when three-fourths of their roots are completed.[7] Thus a signal of the impending eruption of a tooth that has not yet appeared is its root development approaching this level. The roots of the incisors were not complete, of course, when they first erupted. It takes about 2 to 3 years for roots to be completed after a tooth has erupted into occlusion.

Another indicator of dental age 10, therefore, would be completion of the roots of the mandibular incisor teeth and near completion of the roots of the maxillary laterals. By dental age 11, the roots of all incisors and first permanent molars should be well completed.

Dental age 11 (Fig. 4-12) is characterized by the eruption of another group of teeth: the mandibular canine, mandibular first premolar, and maxillary first premolar all erupt more

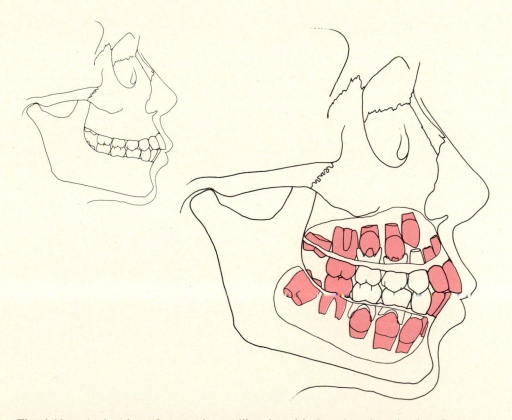

Fig. 4-11 ■ At dental age 9 years, the maxillary lateral incisors have been in place for a year, and root formation on other incisors and first molars is nearly complete. Root development of the maxillary canines and all second premolars is just beginning, while about one-third of the root of the mandibular canines and all first premolars have been completed.

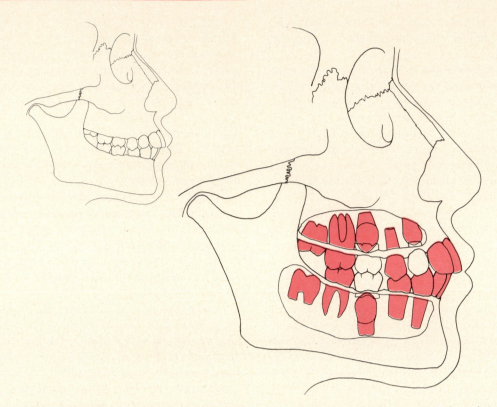

Fig. 4-12 ■ Dental age 11 is characterized by the more or less simultaneous eruption of the mandibular canines, mandibular first premolars, and maxillary first premolars.

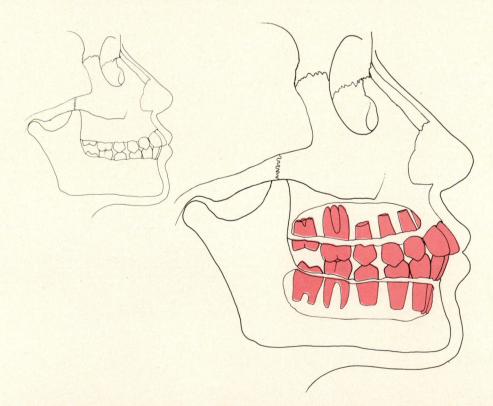

Fig. 4-13 ■ Dental age 12 years is characterized by eruption of the remaining succedaneous teeth (the maxillary canine and the maxillary and mandibular second premolars) and, typically a few months later, the maxillary and mandibular second molars.

or less simultaneously. In the mandibular arch, the odds slightly favor the eruption of the first premolar ahead of the canine, but the reverse sequence frequently occurs. In the maxillary arch, on the other hand, the first premolar erupts well ahead of either the canine or second premolar. At dental age 11, the only remaining primary teeth are the maxillary canine and second molar, and the mandibular second molar.

At dental age 12 (Fig. 4-13), the remaining succedaneous permanent teeth erupt. Succedaneous refers to permanent teeth that replace primary predecessors; thus a canine is a succedaneous tooth, whereas a first molar is not. In addition, at age 12 the second permanent molars in both arches are nearing eruption. Typically, the succedaneous teeth complete their eruption before the emergence of the second molars. Although mineralization often begins later, it is usually possible to note the early beginnings of the third molars by age 12.

Dental ages 13, 14, and 15 are characterized by the extent of completion of the roots of permanent teeth. By dental age 15 (Fig. 4-14), the third molar should be apparent on the radiographs, and the roots of all other permanent teeth should be complete.

Like all other developmental ages (discussed in more detail in paragraphs following), dental age correlates with chronologic age—but the correlation for dental age is one of the weakest. In other words, the teeth erupt with a con-siderable degree of variability from the chronologic age standards.[8] It remains true, however, that the teeth erupt in stages, as described here. A child who has precocious dental development might have the mandibular central incisors and first molars erupt at age 5 and could reach dental age 12 by chronologic age 10. A child with slow dental development might not reach dental age 12 until chronologic age 14, which is within the range of normal variation.

A change in the sequence of eruption is a much more reliable sign of a disturbance in normal development than a generalized delay or acceleration. The more a tooth deviates from its expected position in the sequence, the greater the likelihood of some sort of problem. For example, a delay in eruption of maxillary canines to age 14 is within normal variation if the second premolars are also delayed, but if the second premolars have erupted at age 12 and the canines have not, something is probably wrong.

Several reasonably normal variations in eruption sequence have clinical significance and should be recognized. These are: (1) eruption of second molars ahead of premolars in the mandibular arch, (2) eruption of canines ahead of premolars in the maxillary arch, and (3) asymmetries in eruption between the right and left sides.

Early eruption of the mandibular second molars can be unfortunate in a dental arch where room to accommodate the teeth is marginal. The eruption of the second molar

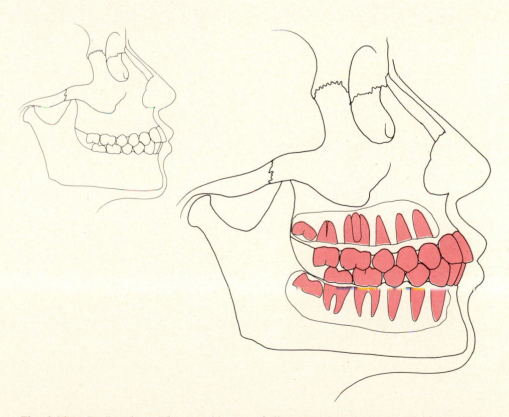

Fig. 4-14 ■ By dental age 15 years, the roots of all permanent teeth except the third molars are complete, and crown formation of third molars often has been completed.

before the second premolar tends to decrease the space for the second premolar and may lead to its being partially blocked out of the arch. Some dental intervention may be needed to get the second premolar into the arch when the mandibular second molar erupts early.

If the maxillary canines erupt at about the same time as the maxillary first premolar (remember that this is the normal eruption sequence of the lower arch but is abnormal in the upper), the maxillary canine will probably be forced labially. Labial positioning of maxillary canines often occurs when there is an overall lack of space in the arch, because this tooth is the last to erupt normally, but displacement of the canine can also be an unfortunate consequence of an eruption sequence abnormality.

An asymmetry in the rate of eruption on the two sides of the dental arch is a frequent enough variation to approach the bounds of normal. Usually when this happens, however, the patient has a lack of space to accommodate the erupting teeth and a different pattern of mechanical obstruction on one side compared to the other. As a general rule, if a permanent tooth on one side has erupted but its counterpart on the other has not, a radiograph should be taken to investigate the cause of the problem. Small variations from one side to the other may be normal, but large ones often indicate a problem.

■ Space Relationships in Replacement of the Incisors

If a dissected skull is examined, it can be seen that in both the maxillary and mandibular arches, the permanent incisor tooth buds lie lingual as well as apical to the primary incisors (Fig. 4-15). The result is a tendency for the mandibular permanent incisors to erupt somewhat lingually and in a slightly irregular position, even in children who have normal dental arches and normal spacing within the arches. In the maxillary arch, the lateral incisor is likely to be lingually positioned at the time of its emergence and to remain in that position if there is any crowding in the arch. The permanent canines are positioned to lie more nearly in line with the primary canines. If there are problems in eruption, these teeth can be displaced either lingually or labially, but usually they are displaced labially if there is not enough room to accommodate them within the arch.

The permanent incisor teeth are considerably larger than the primary incisors that they replace. For instance, the mandibular permanent central incisor is about 5.5 mm in width, whereas the primary central it replaces is about 3 mm in width. Because the other permanent incisors and canines are each 2 to 3 mm wider than their primary predecessors, spacing between the primary incisors is not only normal, it is critically important (Fig. 4-16). Otherwise, there will not be enough room for the permanent incisors when they erupt.

Spacing in the primary incisor region is normally distributed among all the incisors, not just in the "primate space" locations where permanent spaces exist in most

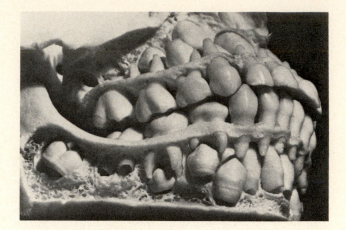

Fig. 4-15 ■ This photograph of the dissected skull of a child of approximately 6 years of age shows the relationship of the developing permanent tooth buds to the primary teeth. Note that the permanent incisors are positioned lingual to the roots of the primary incisors, while the canines are more labially placed. (From van der Linden, F.P.G.M., and Deuterloo, H.S.: Development of the Human Dentition: An Atlas. New York, 1976, Harper and Row.)

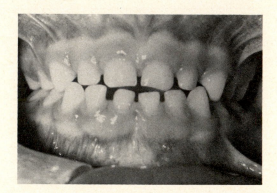

Fig. 4-16 ■ Spaces of this magnitude between the primary incisors are normal within the primary dentition and necessary for proper alignment of the permanent incisors when they erupt.

mammalian species. This arrangement of the primary incisor teeth with gaps between them may not be very pretty, but it is normal. All dentists sooner or later meet a mother like Janie's, who is very concerned that her child has crowded permanent incisors. Her frequent comment is, "But Janie had such beautiful baby teeth!" What the mother means is that Janie's primary incisors lacked the normal spacing. An adult appearing smile in a primary dentition child is an abnormal, not a normal finding—the spaces are very important for alignment of the permanent teeth.

Changes in the amount of space anterior to the canine teeth are shown graphically in Fig. 4-17. Note the excess space in the maxillary and mandibular arches before the permanent incisors begin to erupt. In the maxillary arch, the primate space is mesial to the canines and is included in the graph. In the mandibular arch, the primate space is distal to the canine, which adds nearly another millimeter

AVAILABLE SPACE · INCISOR SEGMENT

maxilla ——   mandible ——

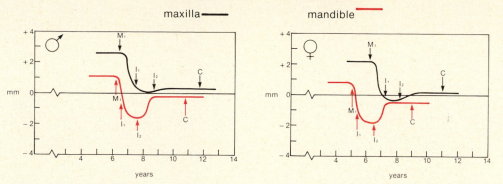

Fig. 4-17 ■ Graphic representation of the average amount of space available within the arches in boys (*(left)*) and girls *(right)*. The time of eruption of the first molar (M_1), central and lateral incisors (I_1 and I_2), and canines (c) are noted by arrows. Note that in the mandibular arch in both sexes, the amount of space for the mandibular incisors is negative for about 2 years after their eruption, meaning that a small amount of crowding in the mandibular arch at this time is normal. (From Moorrees, C.F.A., and Chadha, J.M.: Angle Orthod. **35:**12-22, 1965.)

to the total available space in the lower arch. The total amount of spacing in the two arches, therefore, is about the same. The primary molars normally have tight contacts, so there is no additional spacing posteriorly.

When the central incisors erupt, these teeth use up essentially all of the excess space found in the normal primary dentition. With the eruption of the lateral incisors, the space situation becomes tight in both arches. The maxillary arch, on the average, has just enough space to accommodate the permanent lateral incisors when they erupt. In the mandibular arch, however, when the lateral incisors erupt, there is on the average 1.6 mm less space available for the four mandibular incisors than would be required to perfectly align them (see Fig. 4-17). This difference between the amount of space needed for the incisors and the amount available for them is called the "incisor liability." Because of the incisor liability, a normal child will go through a transitory stage of mandibular incisor crowding at age 8 to 9 even if there will eventually be enough room to accommodate all the permanent teeth in good alignment (Fig. 4-18). In other words, a period when the mandibular incisors are slightly crowded is a normal developmental stage. Continued development of the arches improves the spacing situation, and by the time the canine teeth erupt, space is once again adequate.

Where did the extra space come from to align these mildly crowded lower incisors? Most jaw growth is in the posterior, and there is no mechanism by which the mandible can easily become longer in its anterior region. Rather than from jaw growth per se, the extra space comes from three sources[9] (Fig. 4-19):

1. A slight increase in the width of the dental arch across the canines. As growth continues, the teeth erupt not only upward but also slightly outward. This increase is small, about 2 mm on the average, but it does contribute to the resolution of early crowding of the incisors. More width is gained in the maxillary arch than in the mandibular, and more is gained by boys than by girls. For this reason, girls have a greater liability to incisor crowding, particularly mandibular incisor crowding.

2. Labial positioning of the permanent incisors relative to the primary incisors. The primary incisors tend to stand quite upright. As the permanent incisors replace them, these teeth lean slightly forward, which arranges them along the arc of a larger circle. Although this change is also small, it contributes 1 to 2 mm of additional space in the average child, and thus helps resolve crowding.

3. Repositioning of the canines in the mandibular arch. As the permanent incisors erupt, the canine teeth not only widen out slightly but move slightly back into the primate space. This contributes to the slight width increase already noted because the arch is wider posteriorly, and also provides an extra millimeter of space. Since the primate space in the maxillary arch is mesial to the canine, there is little

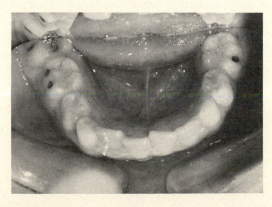

Fig. 4-18 ■ Mild irregularity of the mandibular incisors, of the magnitude pictured here, is normal at age 7 to 8, when the permanent incisors and first molars have erupted but the primary canines and molars are retained.

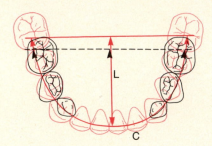

Fig. 4-19 ■ Tooth sizes and arch dimensions in the transition to the permanent dentition. The additional space to align mandibular incisors, after the period of mild normal crowding, is derived from three sources: (1) a slight increase in arch width across the canines, (2) slight labial positioning of the central and lateral incisors, and (3) a distal shift of the permanent canines when the primary first molars are exfoliated. The primary molars are significantly larger than the premolars that replace them, and the "leeway space" provided by this difference offers an excellent opportunity for natural or orthodontic adjustment of occlusal relationships at the end of the dental transition. Both arch length *(L)*, the distance from a line perpendicular to the mesial surface of the permanent first molars to the central incisors, and arch circumference *(C)* tend to decrease during the transition, i.e., some of the leeway space is used by mesial movement of the molars.

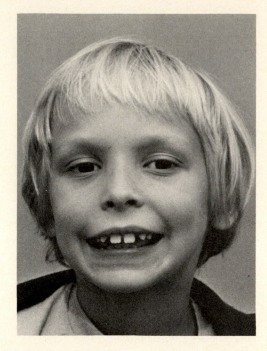

Fig. 4-20 ■ In some children, the maxillary incisors flare laterally and are widely spaced when they first erupt, a condition often called the "ugly duckling" stage. The spaced incisors tend to improve when the canines erupt, but this condition increases the possibility that the canines will become impacted.

opportunity for a similar change in the anteroposterior position of the maxillary canine.

It is important to note that all three of these changes occur without significant skeletal growth in the front of the jaws. The slight increases in arch dimension during normal development are not sufficient to overcome discrepancies of any magnitude, so crowding is likely to persist into the permanent dentition if it was severe initially. In fact, crowding of the incisors—the most common form of Angle's Class I malocclusion—is by far the most prevalent form of malocclusion.

The mandibular permanent central incisors are almost always in proximal contact from the time that they erupt. In the maxillary arch, however, there may continue to be a space between the maxillary central incisors, called a diastema in the permanent dentition, after the permanent teeth erupt. A central diastema tends to close as the lateral incisors erupt but may persist even after the lateral incisors have erupted, particularly if the primary canines have been lost or if the upper incisors are flared to the labial. This situation is another of the variations in the normal developmental pattern, which occurs frequently enough to be almost normal. Since the spaced upper incisors are not very esthetic, this is referred to as the "ugly duckling stage" of development (Fig. 4-20).

The spaces tend to close as the permanent canines erupt. The greater the amount of spacing, the less the likelihood that a maxillary central diastema will totally close on its

own. As a general guideline, a maxillary central diastema of 2 mm or less will probably close spontaneously, while total closure of a diastema initially greater than 2 mm is unlikely.[10]

■ Space Relationships in Replacement of Canines and Primary Molars

In contrast to the anterior teeth, the permanent premolars are smaller than the primary teeth they replace (Fig. 4-21). The mandibular primary second molar is on the average 2 mm larger than the second premolar, while in the maxillary arch, the primary second molar is 1.5 mm larger. The primary first molar is only slightly larger than the first premolar, but does contribute an extra 0.5 mm in the mandible. The result is that each side in the mandibular arch contains about 2.5 mm of what is called "leeway space," while in the maxillary arch, about 1.5 mm is available on the average.

When the second primary molars are lost, the first permanent molars move forward (mesially) relatively rapidly, using the leeway space. This decreases both arch length and arch circumference, which are related and frequently confused terms. The difference between them is illustrated in Fig. 4-19. Even if incisor crowding is present, the leeway space is normally used by mesial movement of the permanent molars. An opportunity for orthodontic treatment is created at this time, since crowding could be relieved by using the leeway space (see Chapter 13).

Occlusal relationships in the mixed dentition parallel

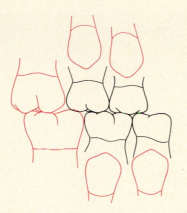

Fig. 4-21 ■ The size difference between the primary molars and permanent premolars, as would be observed in a panoramic radiograph.

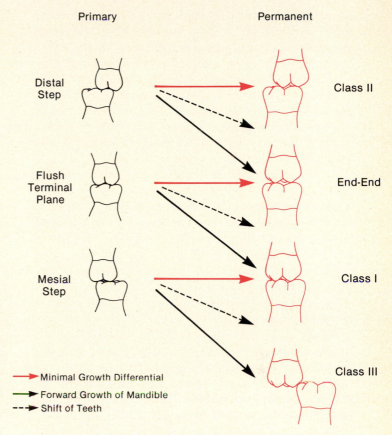

Fig. 4-22 ■ Occlusal relationships of the primary and permanent molars. The flush terminal plane relationship, shown in the middle left, is the normal relationship in the primary dentition. When the first permanent molars first erupt, their relationship is determined by that of the primary molars. The molar relationship tends to shift at the time the second primary molars are lost and the adolescent growth spurt occurs, as shown by the arrows. If leeway space is inadequate and there is no differential forward growth of the mandible, the change will be that shown in the red line. With available leeway space but without good growth, the change will be that shown by the dotted line. With good growth and a shift of the molars, the change shown by the solid black line can be expected. (Adapted from Moyers, R.E.: Handbook of Orthodontics, ed. 3. Chicago, 1973, Year Book Medical Publishers.)

those in the premanent dentition, but the descriptive terms are somewhat different. A normal relationship of the primary molar teeth is the *flush terminal plane* relationship illustrated in Fig. 4-22. The primary dentition equivalent of Angle's Class II is the *distal step*. A *mesial step* relationship corresponds to Angle's Class I. An equivalent of Class III is almost never seen in the primary dentition because of the normal pattern of craniofacial growth in which the mandible lags behind the maxilla.

At the time the primary second molars are lost, both the maxillary and mandibular molars tend to shift mesially into the leeway space, but the mandibular molar normally moves mesially more than its maxillary counterpart. This differential movement contributes to the normal transition from a flush terminal plane relationship in the mixed dentition to a Class I relationship in the permanent dentition.

Differential growth of the mandible relative to the maxilla is also an important contributor to the molar transition. As we have discussed, a characteristic of the growth pattern at this age is more growth of the mandible than the maxilla, so that a relatively deficient mandible gradually catches up. Conceptually, one can imagine that the upper and lower teeth are mounted on moving platforms, and that the platform on which the lower teeth are mounted moves a bit faster than the upper platform. This differential growth of the jaws carries the mandible slightly forward relative to the maxilla during the mixed dentition.

If a child has a flush terminal plane molar relationship early in the mixed dentition, about 3.5 mm of movement of the lower molar forward relative to the upper molar is required for a smooth transition to a Class I molar relationship in the permanent dentition. About half of this distance must be supplied by differential growth of the lower jaw, carrying the lower molar with it. The other half can be obtained from the leeway space, which allows greater mesial movement of the mandibular than the maxillary molar.

Only a modest change in molar relationship can be produced by this combination of differential growth of the jaws and differential forward movement of the lower molar. It must be kept in mind that the changes described here are those that happen to a child experiencing a normal growth pattern. There is no guarantee in any given individual that differential forward growth of the mandible will occur, nor that the leeway space will close in a way that moves the lower molar relatively forward.

The possibilities for the transition in molar relationship from the mixed to the early permanent dentition are summarized in Fig. 4-22. Note that the transition is usually accompanied by a one-half cusp (3 to 4 mm) relative forward movement of the lower molar, accomplished by a combination of differential growth and tooth movement. A child's initial distal step relationship may change during the transition to an end-to-end (one-half cusp Class II) relationship in the permanent dentition, but is not likely to be corrected all the way to Class I. It also is possible that the pattern of growth will not lead to greater prominence of the mandible, in which case the molar relationship in the permanent dentition probably will remain a full cusp Class II.

Similarly, a flush terminal plane relationship, which produces an end-to-end relationship of the permanent molars when they first erupt, can change to Class I in the permanent dentition, but can remain end-to-end in the permanent dentition if the growth pattern is not favorable.

Finally, a child who has experienced early mandibular growth may have a mesial step relationship in the primary molars, producing a Class I molar relationship at an early age. It is quite possible for this mesial step relationship to progress to a half-cusp Class III during the molar transition and proceed further to a full Class III relationship with continued mandibular growth. On the other hand, if differential mandibular growth no longer occurs, the mesial step relationship at an early age may simply become a Class I relationship later.

For any given child, the odds are that the normal growth pattern will prevail, and that there will be a one-half cusp transition in the molar relationship at the time the second primary molars are lost. It must be understood that although this is the most likely outcome, it is by no means the only one. The possibility that a distal step will become Class II malocclusion or that a flush terminal plane will become end-to-end is very real. Class III malocclusion is much less common than Class II, but a child who has a mesial step relationship at an early age is also at some risk of developing Class III malocclusion as time passes.

■ Assessment of Skeletal and Other Developmental Ages

As noted previously, dental development correlates reasonably well with chronologic age but occurs relatively independently. Of all the indicators of developmental age, dental age correlates least well with the other developmental indices. Physical growth status also varies from chronologic age in many children but does correlate well with skeletal age, which is determined by the relative level of maturation of the skeletal system. In planning orthodontic treatment it can be important to know how much skeletal growth remains, and so an evaluation of skeletal age is frequently needed.

An assessment of skeletal age must be based on the maturational status of markers within the skeletal system. Although a number of indicators could theoretically be used, the ossification of the bones of the hand and the wrist is normally the standard for skeletal development (Fig. 4-23). A radiograph of the hand and wrist provides a view of some 30 small bones, all of which have a predictable sequence of ossification. Although a view of no single bone is diagnostic, an assessment of the level of development of the bones in the wrist, hand, and fingers can give an accurate picture of a child's skeletal development status. To do this,

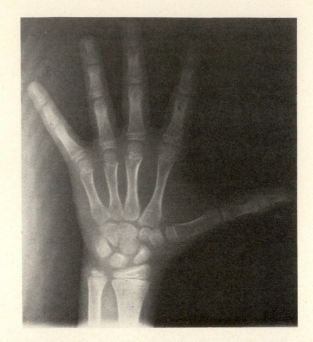

Fig. 4-23 ■ A radiograph of the hand and wrist can be used to assess skeletal age by comparing the degree of ossification of the wrist, hand, and finger bones to plates in a standard atlas of hand-wrist development.

a hand-wrist radiograph of the patient is simply compared with standard radiographic images in an atlas of the development of the hand and wrist.[11] The description is in exactly the same terms as a description of the status of the dentition: skeletal age 10 at chronologic age 12, for instance.

Developmental ages based on any of a large number of criteria can be established, if there is some scale against which a child's progress can be measured. For instance, one could measure a child's position on a scale of behavior, equating behavior of certain types as appropriate for 5-year-olds or 7-year-olds. In fact, behavioral age can be important in the dental treatment of children, since it is difficult to render satisfactory treatment if the child cannot be induced to behave appropriately and cooperate. The assessment of behavioral age is covered more completely in the section on social and behavioral development in Chapter 3.

The correlation between developmental ages of all types and chronologic age is quite good, as biologic correlations go (Fig. 4-24).[10] For most developmental indicators, the correlation coefficient between developmental status and chronologic age is about 0.8. The ability to predict one characteristic from another varies as the square of the correlation coefficient, so the probability that one could predict the developmental stage from knowing the chronologic age or vice versa is $(0.8)^2 = 0.64$. The correlation of dental age with chronologic age is not quite as good, about 0.7, which means that there is about a 50% chance of predicting the stage of dental development from the chronologic age.

It is interesting that the developmental ages correlate better among themselves than the developmental ages correlate with chronologic age.[12] Despite the caricature in our society

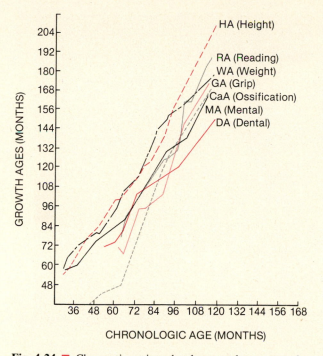

Fig. 4-24 ■ Changes in various developmental parameters for one normal child. Note that this child was advanced for his chronologic age in essentially all the parameters, and that all are reasonably well-correlated. For this individual, as for many children, dental age correlated less well with the group of developmental indicators than any of the others. (From Lowery, G.H.: Growth and Development of Children, ed. 6. Chicago, 1973, Year Book Medical Publishers.)

of the intellectually advanced but socially and physically retarded child, the chances are that a child who is advanced in one characteristic—skeletal age, for instance—is advanced in others as well. The mature looking and behaving 8-year-old is likely, in other words, also to have precocious development of the dentition. What will actually occur in any one individual is subject to the almost infinite variety of human variation, and the magnitude of the correlation coefficients must be kept in mind. Unfortunately for those dentists who want to examine only the teeth, the variations in dental development mean that it often is necessary to assess skeletal, behavioral, or other developmental ages in planning dental treatment.

■ *Adolescence: The Early Permanent Dentition Years*

Adolescence is a sexual phenomenon. It can be defined as the period of life when sexual maturity is attained. More specifically, it is the transitional period between the juvenile stage and adulthood, during which the secondary sexual characteristics appear, the adolescent growth spurt takes place, fertility is attained, and profound physiologic changes occur. All these developments are associated with the maturation of the sex organs and the accompanying surge in secretion of sex hormones.

This period is particularly important in dental and ortho-

dontic treatment, because the physical changes at adolescence significantly affect the face and dentition. Major events in dentofacial development that occur during adolescence include the exchange from the mixed to the permanent dentition, an acceleration in the overall rate of facial growth, and differential growth of the jaws.

■ Initiation of Adolescence

The first events of puberty occur in the brain, and the stimulus for their unfolding remains unknown. For whatever reason, perhaps in response to some type of internal clock, perhaps in response to a pattern of external stimuli not yet recognized, brain cells in the hypothalamus begin to secrete substances called releasing factors. Both the cells and their method of action are somewhat unusual. These neuroendocrine cells look like typical neurons, but they secrete materials in the cell body, which are carried by cytoplasmic transport down the axon toward a richly vascular area at the base of the hypothalamus near the pituitary gland (Fig. 4-25). The substances secreted by the nerve cells pass into capillaries in this vascular region and are carried by blood flow the short distance to the pituitary. It is unusual in the body for the venous return system to transport substances from one closely adjacent region to another, but here the special arrangement of the vessels seems made to order for this purpose. Accordingly, this special network of vessels, analogous to the venous supply to the liver but on a very much smaller scale, is called the pituitary portal system.

In the anterior pituitary gland, the hypothalamic releasing factors stimulate pituitary cells to produce several related but different hormones called pituitary gonadotrophins. Their function is to stimulate endocrine cells in the developing sex organs to produce sex hormones.

In the male, cells in the testes produce the male sex hormone testosterone, but other cells in the testes produce female sex hormones also. A different pituitary gonadotropin stimulates each of these cell types. Every individual has a mixture of male and female sex hormones, and it is a biologic fact as well as an everyday observation that there are feminine males and masculine females. Presumably this represents the balance of the competing male and female sex hormones.

In the female, the pituitary gonadotropins stimulate secretion of estrogen by the ovaries, and later progesterone by the same organ. In the female, male sex hormones are produced in the adrenal cortex, stimulated by still another pituitary hormone, and possibly some female hormones are produced in the male adrenal cortex.

Under the stimulation of the pituitary gonadotropins, sex hormones from the testes, ovary, and adrenal cortex are released into the bloodstream in quantities sufficient to cause development of secondary sexual characteristics and accelerated growth of the genitalia. The increasing level of the sex hormones also causes other physiologic changes, including the acceleration in general body growth and shrinkage of lymphoid tissues seen in the classic growth curves.

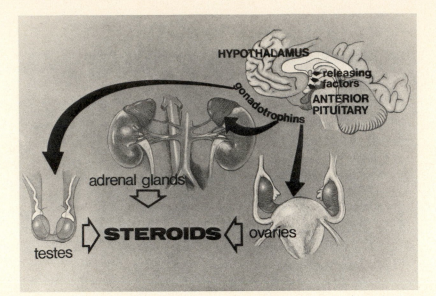

Fig. 4-25 ■ Diagrammatic representation of the cascade of endrocrine signals controlling sexual development. Releasing factors from the hypothalamus are carried via the pituitary portal circulation to the anterior pituitary gland, where they initiate the release of pituitary gonadotropic hormones. These in turn stimulate cells in the testes, ovaries, and adrenals, which secrete the steroid sex hormones.

Neural growth is unaffected by the events of adolescence, since it is essentially complete by age 6. The changes in the growth curves for the jaws, general body, lymphoid and genital tissues, however, can be considered the result of the hormonal changes that accompany sexual maturation (Fig. 4-26).

The system by which a few neurons in the hypothalamus ultimately control the level of circulating sex hormones may seem curiously complex. The principle, however, is one utilized in control systems throughout the body and also in modern technology. Each of the steps in the control process results in an amplification of the control signal, in a way analogous to the amplification of a small musical signal between the tape head and speakers of a stereo system. The amount of pituitary gonadotropin produced is 100 to 1000 times greater than the amount of gonadotropin releasing factors produced in the hypothalamus, and the amount of sex hormones produced is 1000 times greater than the amount of the pituitary hormones themselves. The system, then, is a three-stage amplifier. Rather than being a complex biologic curiosity, it is better viewed as a rational engineering design. A similar amplification of controlling signals from the brain is used, of course, in all body systems.

■ Timing of Puberty

There is a great deal of individual variation, but puberty and the adolescent growth spurt tend to occur nearly 2 years earlier on the average in girls than in boys[13] (Fig. 4-27). Why this occurs is not known, but the phenomenon has an important impact on the timing of orthodontic treatment, which must be done earlier in girls than in boys to take advantage of the adolescent growth spurt. Because of the

considerable individual variation, however, early maturing boys will reach puberty ahead of slow maturing girls, and it must be remembered that chronologic age has very little to do with where an individual stands developmentally. The stage of development of secondary sexual characteristics provides a physiologic calendar of adolescence that correlates with the individual's physical growth status. Not all the secondary sexual characteristics are readily visible, of course, but most can be evaluated in a normal fully clothed examination, such as would occur in a dental office.

Adolescence in girls can be divided into three stages, based on the extent of sexual development. The first stage, which occurs at about the beginning of the physical growth spurt, is the appearance of breast buds and early stages of the development of pubic hair. The peak velocity for physical growth occurs about 1 year after the initiation of stage one, and coincides with stage two of development of sexual characteristics (Fig. 4-27). At this time, there is noticeable breast development. Pubic hair is darker and more widespread, and hair appears in the armpits (axillary hair).

The third stage in girls occurs 1 to 1½ years after stage two and is marked by the onset of menstruation. By this time, the growth spurt is all but complete. At this stage, there is noticeable broadening of the hips with more adult fat distribution, and development of the breasts is complete.

The stages of sexual development in boys are more difficult to specifically define than in girls. Puberty begins later and extends over a longer period of time, about 5 years as compared to 3½ years for girls (Fig. 4-27). In boys, four stages in development can be correlated with the curve of general body growth at adolescence.

The initial sign of sexual maturation in boys usually is

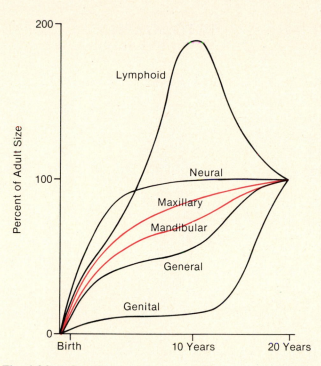

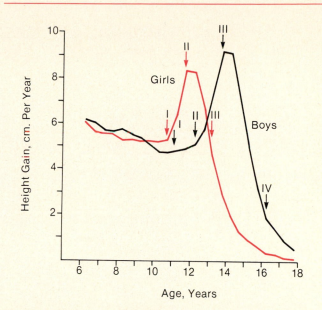

Fig. 4-26 ■ Growth curves for the maxilla and mandible shown against the background of Scammon's curves. Note that growth of the jaws is intermediate between the neural and general body curves, with the mandible following the general body curve more closely than the maxilla. The acceleration in general body growth at puberty, which affects the jaws, parallels the dramatic increase in development of the sexual organs. Lymphoid involution also occurs at this time.

Fig. 4-27 ■ Velocity curves for growth at adolescence, showing the difference in timing for girls and boys. Also indicated on the growth velocity curves are the corresponding stages in sexual development (see text). (From Tanner, J.M.: Growth at Adolescence, ed. 2. Oxford, 1962, Blackwell Scientific Publishers.)

the "fat spurt." The maturing boy gains weight and becomes almost chubby, with a somewhat feminine fat distribution. This probably occurs because estrogen production by the Leydig cells in the testes is stimulated before significant production of testosterone by the more abundant Sertoli cells. During this stage, boys may appear obese and somewhat awkward physically. At this time also, the scrotum begins to increase in size and may show some increase or change in pigmentation.

At stage two, about 1 year after stage one, the spurt in height is just beginning. At this stage, there is a redistribution and relative decrease in subcutaneous fat, pubic hair begins to appear, and growth of the penis begins.

The third stage occurs 8 to 12 months after stage two and coincides with the peak velocity in gain in height. At this time, axillary hair appears and facial hair appears on the upper lip only. A spurt in muscle growth also occurs, along with a continued decrease in subcutaneous fat and an obviously harder and more angular body form. Pubic hair distribution appears more adult, but has not yet spread to the medial of the thighs. The penis and scrotum are near adult size.

Stage four for boys, which occurs anywhere from 15 to 24 months after stage three, is difficult to pinpoint. At this time, the spurt of growth in height ends. There is facial hair

on the chin as well as the upper lip, adult distribution and color of pubic and axillary hair, and a further increase in muscular strength.

The timing of puberty makes an important difference in ultimate body size, in a way that may seem paradoxical at first: the earlier the onset of puberty, the smaller the adult size, and vice versa. Growth in height depends on endochondral bone growth at the epiphyseal plates of the long bones, and the impact of the sex hormones on endochondral bone growth is twofold. First, the sex hormones stimulate the cartilage to grow faster, and this produces the adolescent growth spurt. But the sex hormones also cause an increase in the rate of skeletal maturation, which for the long bones is the rate at which cartilage is transformed into bone. The acceleration in maturation is even greater than the acceleration in growth. Thus during the rapid growth at adolescence, the cartilage is used up faster than it is replaced. Toward the end of adolescence, the last of the cartilage is transformed into bone, and the epiphyseal plates close. At that point, of course, growth potential is lost and growth stops.

This early cessation of growth after early sexual maturation is particularly prominent in girls. It is responsible for much of the difference in adult size between men and women. Girls mature earlier on the average, and finish their growth much sooner. Boys are not bigger than girls until they grow for a longer time at adolescence. The difference arises because there is slow but steady growth before the growth spurt, and so when the growth spurt occurs, for those who mature late, it takes off from a higher plateau. The epiphyseal plates close more slowly in males than in females, and therefore the cutoff in growth that accompanies

ENDOMORPH
fatty tissues

MESOMORPH
musculature

ECTOMORPH
skin elements

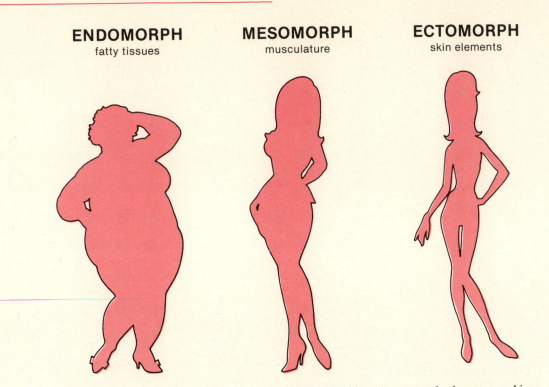

Fig. 4-28 ■ Caricatures of the body types described by Sheldon. As a general rule, ectomorphic individuals mature more slowly than mesomorphs and endomorphs.

the attainment of sexual maturity is also more complete in girls.

The timing of puberty seems to be affected by both genetic and environmental influences. There are early- and late-maturing families, and individuals in some racial and ethnic groups mature earlier than others. Body type also has an interesting effect on the timing of puberty and thereby the eventual height.

The anthropologist W.H. Sheldon classified body types by the relative predominance of tissues derived from the three primary germ layers[14] (Fig. 4-28). An individual who is slender, with relatively little muscle mass or body fat, is classified as an *ectomorph,* based on the predominance of skin and neural tissues derived from ectoderm. A highly muscular individual would be considered a *mesomorph,* and a short individual with little muscular development but large amounts of subcutaneous fat would be described as an *endomorph.*

Sheldon's body type classifications correlate with the timing of physical growth at adolescence: ectomorphs tend to mature later than mesomorphs or endomorphs, particularly the males in the group. Thus the ectomorph is likely to be considerably shorter than his mesomorphic friends in the junior high school years, at which time the mesomorphs but not the ectomorphs will have entered the adolescent growth spurt. By high school graduation, however, the relationships have reversed and at that point the ectomorphic individuals will be taller on the average than the mesomorphic ones, because their growth has continued for a longer time. Tall

adult males were often short compared to their peers at age 12, whereas the bigger boys then are often average sized adults.

In girls, it appears that the onset of menstruation requires the development of a certain amount of body fat, and endomorphic girls reach this level first. In ectomorphs, the onset of menstruation can be delayed until this level is reached. In fact, highly trained female athletes whose body fat levels are quite low may stop menstruating, apparently in response to the low body fat levels.

Seasonal and cultural factors also affect the overall rate of physical growth. All other factors being equal, growth tends to be faster in spring and summer than in fall and winter; city children tend to mature faster than rural ones. These effects are presumably mediated via the hypothalamus and affect the rate of secretion of gonadotropin-releasing factors.

The stages of adolescent development described here were correlated with growth in height. Fortunately, growth of the jaws usually correlates with the physiologic events of puberty in about the same way as growth in height (Fig. 4-29). There is an adolescent growth spurt in the length of the mandible, though not nearly as dramatic a spurt as that in body height, and a modest though discernible increase in growth at the sutures of the maxilla. The cephalocaudal gradient of growth, which is part of the normal pattern, is dramatically evident at puberty. More growth occurs in the lower extremity than in the upper, and within the face, more growth takes place in the lower jaw than in the upper. This produces an acceleration in mandibular growth relative to the maxilla and results in the differential jaw growth referred to previously. The maturing face becomes less convex as the mandible and chin become more prominent as a result of the differential jaw growth.

Although jaw growth follows the curve for general body growth, the correlation is not perfect. Longitudinal data from studies of craniofacial growth indicate that a significant number of individuals, especially among the girls, have a "juvenile acceleration" in jaw growth that occurs 1 to 2 years before the adolescent growth spurt[15] (Fig. 4-30). This juvenile acceleration can equal or even exceed the jaw growth that accompanies secondary sexual maturation. In boys, if a juvenile spurt occurs, it is nearly always less intense than the growth acceleration at puberty.

This tendency for a clinically useful acceleration in jaw growth to precede the adolescent spurt, particularly in girls, is a major reason for careful assessment of physiologic age in planning orthodontic treatment. If treatment is delayed too long, the opportunity to utilize the growth spurt is missed. In early-maturing girls, the adolescent growth spurt often precedes the final transition of the dentition, so that by the time the second premolars and second molars erupt, physical growth is all but complete. The presence of a juvenile growth spurt in girls accentuates this tendency for significant acceleration of jaw growth in the mixed dentition. If most girls are to receive orthodontic treatment while they are growing rapidly, the treatment must begin during the mixed dentition rather than after all succedaneous permanent teeth have erupted. In slow-maturing boys, on the other hand, the dentition can be relatively complete while a considerable amount of physical growth remains. In the timing of orthodontic treatment, clinicians have a tendency to treat girls too late and boys too soon, forgetting the considerable disparity in the rate of physiologic maturation.

■ *Growth Patterns in the Dentofacial Complex*

■ Dimensional Changes

Growth of the nasomaxillary complex. Growth of the nasomaxillary area is produced by two basic mechanisms: (1) passive displacement, created by growth in the cranial base that pushes the maxilla forward, and (2) active growth of the maxillary structures and the nose[16] (Fig. 4-31).

Passive displacement of the maxilla is a very important growth mechanism during the primary dentition years, but becomes less important as growth at the synchondroses of the cranial base slows markedly with the completion of neural growth at about age 7. Total forward movement of the maxilla and the amount resulting from forward displacement are shown in Table 4-1. Note that during the entire period between ages 7 to 15, about one-third of the total forward movement of the maxilla can be accounted for on the basis of passive displacement. The rest is the result of

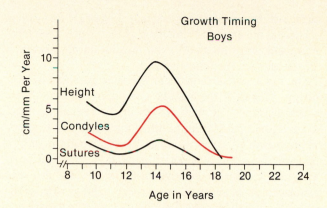

Fig. 4-29 ■ On the average, the spurt in growth of the jaws occurs at about the same time as the spurt in height, but it must be remembered that there is considerable individual variation. (From Woodside, D.G.: In Salzmann, J.A.: Orthodontics in Daily Practice. Philadelphia, 1974, J.B. Lippincott Co.)

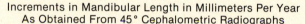

Increments in Mandibular Length in Millimeters Per Year As Obtained From 45° Cephalometric Radiographs

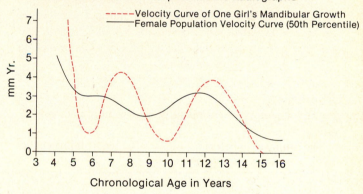

Fig. 4-30 ■ Longitudinal data for increase in length of the mandible in one girl, taken from the Burlington growth study in Canada, demonstrates an acceleration of growth at about 8 years of age (juvenile acceleration) equal in intensity to the pubertal acceleration between ages 11 and 14. Changes of this type in the pattern of growth for individuals tend to be smoothed out when cross-sectional or group average data are studied. (From Woodside, D.G.: In Salzmann, J.A.: Orthodontics in Daily Practice. Philadelphia, 1974, J.B. Lippincott Co.)

active growth of the maxillary sutures, in response to stimuli from the enveloping soft tissues (see Chapter 2).

The effect of surface remodeling must be considered when active growth of the maxilla is considered. Surface changes can either add to or subtract from growth in other areas, by surface apposition or resorption respectively. In fact, the maxilla grows downward and forward as bone is added in the tuberosity area posteriorly and at the posterior and superior sutures, but the anterior surfaces of the bone are resorbing at the same time (Fig. 4-32). For this reason, the distance that the body of the maxilla and the maxillary teeth are carried downward and forward during growth is greater by about 25% than the forward movement of the anterior surface of the maxilla. This tendency for surface remodeling to conceal the extent of relocation of the jaws is even more prominent when rotation of the maxilla during growth is considered (see the following sections).

The nasal structures undergo the same passive displacement as the rest of the maxilla. Growth of the nose occurs at a more rapid rate than growth of the rest of the face, however, particularly during the adolescent growth spurt. Nasal growth is produced in part by an increase in size of the cartilaginous nasal septum. In addition, proliferation of the lateral cartilages alters the shape of the nose and contributes to an increase in overall size. The growth of the nose is extremely variable, as a cursory examination of any group of people will confirm. Average increases in nasal dimensions of white Americans are illustrated in Table 4-2. Comparison with Table 4-1 shows that nasal dimensions increase at a rate about 25% greater than growth of the maxilla.

Mandibular growth. Growth of the mandible continues at a relatively steady rate before puberty. On the average, as Table 4-3 shows, ramus height increases 1 to 2 mm per year and body length increases 2 to 3 mm per year. These cross-sectional data tend to smooth out the juvenile and pubertal growth spurts, which (see previous discussion) do occur in growth of the mandible.

One feature of mandibular growth is an accentuation of the prominence of the chin. At one time, it was thought that this occurred primarily by addition of bone to the chin. It now is clear that, although small amounts of bone are added, the change in the contour of the chin itself occurs largely because the area just above the chin, between it and the base of the alveolar process, is a resorptive area. The increase in chin prominence with maturity results from a combination of forward translation of the chin as a part of the overall growth pattern of the mandible, and resorption above the chin that alters the bony contours.

An important source of variability in how much the chin grows forward is the extent of growth changes at the glenoid fossa. If the area of the temporal bone to which the mandible is attached moved forward relative to the cranial base during growth, this would translate the mandible forward in the same way that cranial base growth translates the maxilla for the mandible. However, this rarely happens.[17] More often, the attachment point moves straight down or posteriorly, thus subtracting from rather than augmenting the forward projection of the chin. In both the patients shown in Fig. 4-33, for instance, there was an approximately 7 mm increase in length of the mandible during orthodontic treatment around the time of puberty. In one of the patients, the

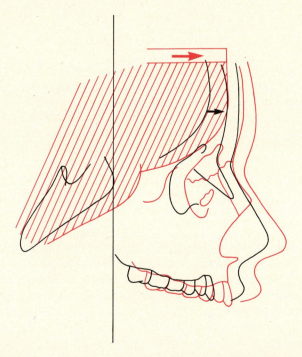

Fig. 4-31 ■ Diagrammatic representation of a major mechanism for growth of the maxilla: structures of the nasomaxillary complex are displaced forward as the cranial base lengthens and the anterior lobes of the brain grow in size. (Redrawn from Enlow, D.H.: Handbook of Facial Growth, ed. 2. Philadelphia, 1982, W.B. Saunders Co.)

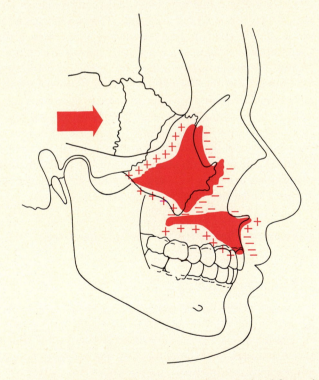

Fig. 4-32 ■ As the maxilla is translated downward and forward, bone is added at the sutures and in the tuberosity area posteriorly, but at the same time, surface remodeling removes bone from the anterior surfaces (except for a small area at the anterior nasal spine). For this reason, the amount of forward movement of anterior surfaces is less than the amount of displacement. In the roof of the mouth, however, surface remodeling adds bone, while bone is resorbed from the floor of the nose. The total downward movement of the palatal vault, therefore, is greater than the amount of displacement. (Redrawn from Enlow, D.H.: Handbook of Facial Growth, ed. 2. Philadelphia, 1982, W.B. Saunders Co.)

Table 4-1 ■ Maxillary length changes

	Total forward movement (mm) (basion-ANS increment)		Forward displacement (mm) (basion-PNS increment)	
Age	Male	Female	Male	Female
7	1.3	2.1	0.0	0.8
8	1.5	1.8	0.9	1.1
9	1.6	0.4	0.4	0.4
10	1.8	2.0	0.8	0.2
11	1.9	1.0	0.2	0.2
12	2.0	1.3	0.4	1.1
13	2.1	1.2	1.0	−0.1
14	1.1	1.5	0.3	0.1
15	1.2	1.1	0.4	0.8

Data from Riolo, M.L., et al.: An Atlas of Craniofacial Growth. Ann Arbor, 1974, University of Michigan, Center for Human Growth and Development.

Table 4-2 ■ Length and height of the nose

	Nose length (nasion to tip)		Vertical height of nose	
Age	Male	Female	Male	Female
6	43.3	41.1	36.0	34.2
9	47.7	45.2	40.1	37.0
12	51.7	50.2	43.5	41.1
15	54.9	54.4	46.6	44.3
18	60.2	57.8	49.0	46.1

Data from Subtelny, J.D.: Am. J. Orthod. **45:**481, 1959.

Table 4-3 ■ Mandibular length changes

	Body length increase (mm) (gonion-pogonion)		Ramus height increase (mm) (condylar-gonion)	
Age	Male	Female	Male	Female
7	2.8	1.7	0.8	1.2
8	1.7	2.5	1.4	1.4
9	1.9	1.1	1.5	0.3
10	2.0	2.5	1.2	0.7
11	2.2	1.7	1.8	0.9
12	1.3	0.8	1.4	2.2
13	2.0	1.8	2.2	0.5
14	2.5	1.1	2.2	1.7
15	1.6	1.1	1.1	2.3
16	2.3	1.0	3.4	1.6

Data from Riolo, M.L., et al.: An Atlas of Craniofacial Growth. Ann Arbor, 1974, University of Michigan, Center for Human Growth and Development.

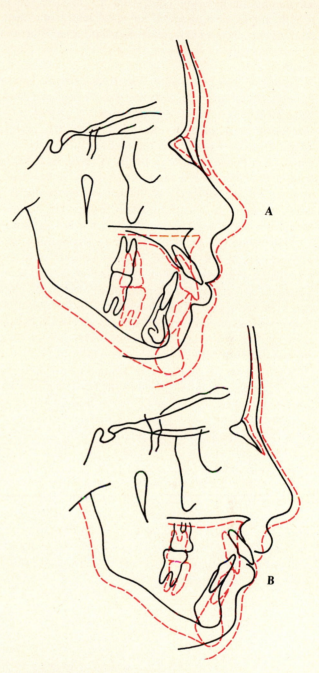

Fig. 4-33 ■ Cephalometric tracings of growth in two patients during the orthodontic correction of moderate Class II malocclusion (superimposed on sphenoethmoid triad in cranial base). **A,** Changes from age 11-10 to age 14-11. In this patient, approximately 7 mm of mandibular growth was expressed entirely as forward movement of the chin, while the area of the temporomandibular joint remained in the same anteroposterior position relative to the cranial base. **B,** Changes from age 11-8 to age 15-0. This patient also had approximately 7 mm of mandibular growth, but the TMJ area moved downward and backward relative to the cranial base, so that much of the growth was not expressed as forward movement of the chin. (Courtesy Dr. V. Kokich).

temporomandibular joint (TMJ) did not relocate during growth, and the chin projected forward 7 mm. In the other, the TMJ moved posteriorly, resulting in only a small forward projection of the chin despite the increase in mandibular length.

Timing of growth in width, length, and height. For the three planes of space in both the maxilla and mandible, there is a definite sequence in which growth is "completed," i.e., declines to the slow rate that characterizes normal adults. Growth in width is completed first, then growth in length, and finally growth in height. Growth in width of both jaws, including the width of the dental arches, tends to be completed before the adolescent growth spurt and is affected minimally if at all by adolescent growth changes. Intercanine width does not increase much if at all after age 12 (Fig. 4-34). There is a partial exception to this rule, however. As the jaws grow in length posteriorly, they also grow wider. For the maxilla, this affects primarily the width across the second, and if they are able to erupt, the third molars in the region of the tuberosity. For the mandible, both molar and bicondylar widths show small increases until the end of growth in length. Anterior width dimensions of the mandible stabilize earlier.

Growth in length of both jaws continues through the period of puberty. In girls, growth in length of the jaws has all but ceased by age 14 to 15 on the average (more accurately, by about 2 to 3 years after first menstruation). In boys, growth in length usually does not decline to the basal adult level until age 18 or so (about 4 years after attainment of sexual maturity).

Growth in vertical height of the jaws and face continues longer in both sexes than growth in length. Increases in facial height and concomitant eruption of teeth continue throughout life, but the decline to the adult level (which for vertical growth is surprisingly large—see the following section) often does not occur until age 17 or 18 in girls and in the early twenties in boys.

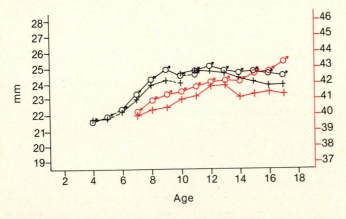

Fig. 4-34 ■ Average changes in mandibular canine and molar widths in both sexes during growth. Molar widths are shown in red, canine widths in black. (From Moyers, R.E., et al.: Standards of Human Occlusal Development. Ann Arbor, 1976, University of Michigan, Center for Human Growth and Development.)

■ Rotation of Jaws during Growth

Implant studies of jaw rotation. Until longitudinal studies of growth using metallic implants in the jaws were carried out in the 1960s, primarily by Bjork and coworkers in Copenhagen,[18] the extent to which both the maxilla and mandible rotate during growth was not appreciated. The reason is that rotation that occurs in the core of each jaw, called *internal rotation,* tends to be masked by surface changes and alterations in the rate of tooth eruption. The surface changes produce *external rotation.* Obviously, the overall change in the orientation of each jaw, as judged by the palatal plane and mandibular plane, results from a combination of internal and external rotation.

It is easier to visualize the internal and external rotation of the jaws by considering the mandible first. The core of the mandible is the bone that surrounds the inferior alveolar nerve. The rest of the mandible consists of its several functional processes (Fig. 4-35). These are the alveolar process (bone supporting the teeth and providing for mastication), the muscular processes (the bone to which the muscles of mastication attach), and the condylar process, the function in this case being the articulation of the jaw with the skull. If implants are placed in areas of stable bone away from the functional processes, it can be observed that in most individuals, the core of the mandible rotates during growth in a way that would tend to decrease the mandibular plane angle, i.e., up anteriorly and down posteriorly.

Bjork[19] distinguished two contributions to internal rotation (which he called total rotation) of the mandible: (1) matrix rotation, or rotation around the condyle, and (2) intramatrix rotation, or rotation centered within the body of the mandible (Fig. 4-36). By convention, the rotation of either jaw is considered "forward" and given a negative sign if there is more growth posteriorly than anteriorly. The rotation is "backward" and given a positive direction if it lengthens anterior dimensions more than posterior ones, bringing the chin downward and backward.

One of the features of internal rotation of the mandible is the variation between individuals, ranging up to 10 to 15 degrees. The pattern of vertical facial development, discussed in more detail later, is strongly related to the rotation of both jaws. For an average individual with normal vertical facial proportions, however, there is about −15 degrees of internal rotation from age 4 to adult life. Of this, about 25% results from matrix rotation and 75% from intramatrix rotation.

During the time that the core of the mandible rotates forward an average of 15 degrees, the mandibular plane angle, representing the orientation of the jaw to an outside observer, decreases only 2 to 4 degrees on the average. The reason that the internal rotation is not expressed in jaw orientation, of course, is that surface changes (external rotation) tend to compensate. This means that the posterior part of the lower border of the mandible must be an area of resorption, while the anterior aspect of the lower border is unchanged or undergoes slight apposition. Studies of surface changes reveal exactly this as the usual pattern of apposition and resorption (Fig. 4-37). On the average, then, there is about 15 degrees of internal, forward rotation and 11 to 12 degrees of external, backward rotation producing the 3 to 4 degree decrease in mandibular plane angle observed in the average individual during childhood and adolescence.

It is less easy to divide the maxilla into a core of bone and a series of functional processes. The alveolar process is certainly a functional process in the classic sense, but there are no areas of muscle attachment analogous to those of the mandible. The parts of the bone surrounding the air passages serve the function of respiration, and the form-function relationships involved are poorly understood. If implants are placed above the maxillary alveolar process, however, one can observe a core of the maxilla that un-

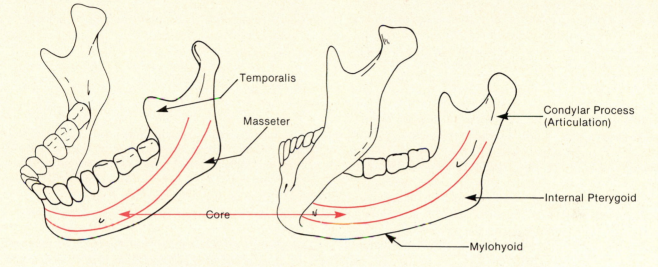

Fig. 4-35 ■ The mandible can be visualized as consisting of a core of bone surrounding the inferior alveolar neurovascular bundle, and a series of functional processes: the alveolar process, serving the function of mastication; the muscular processes, serving for muscle attachments; and the condylar process, serving to articulate the bone with the rest of the skull.

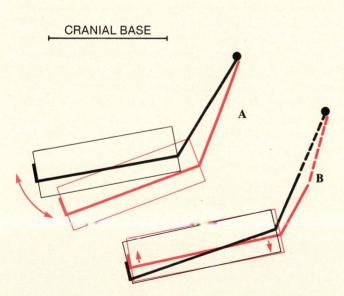

Fig. 4-36 ■ Internal rotation of the mandible, i.e., rotation of the core relative to the cranial base, has two components: **A**, rotation around the condyle, or matrix rotation; and **B**, rotations centered within the body of the mandible, or intramatrix rotation. (Redrawn from Bjork, A., and Skieller, V.: Eur. J. Orthod. **5:**1-46, 1983.)

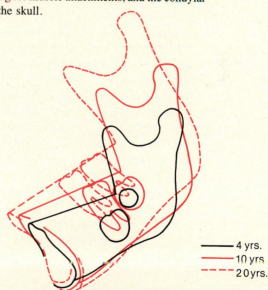

Fig. 4-37 ■ Superimposition on implants for an individual with a normal pattern of growth, showing surface changes in the mandible from age 4 to 20 years. For this patient there was −19 degrees internal rotation but only −3 degrees change in the mandibular plane angle. Note the dramatic remodeling in the area of the gonial angle, with a net resorption over this period of time. This surface remodeling or external rotation compensates for and conceals the extent of the internal rotation. (From Bjork, A., and Skieller, V.: Eur. J. Orthod. **5:**1-46, 1983.)

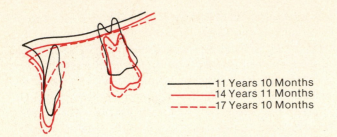

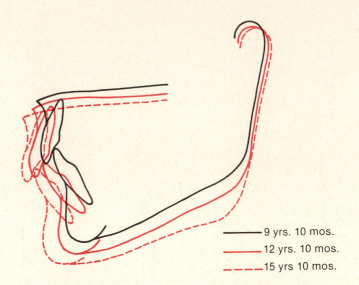

Fig. 4-38 ■ Superimposition on implants in the maxilla reveals that this patient experienced a small amount of backward internal rotation of the maxilla, i.e., down anteriorly. A small amount of forward rotation is the more usual pattern, but backward rotation occurs frequently. (From Bjork, A., and Skieller, V.: Am. J. Orthod. **62**:357, 1972.)

dergoes a small and variable degree of rotation, forward and backward (Fig. 4-38). This internal rotation is analogous to the intramatrix rotation of the mandible—matrix rotation, as defined for the mandible, is not possible for the maxilla.

At the same time that internal rotation of the maxilla is occurring, there also are varying degrees of resorption of bone on the nasal side and apposition of bone on the palatal side, in the anterior and posterior parts of the palate. Similar variations in the amount of eruption of the incisors and molars occur. These changes amount, of course, to an external rotation. For most patients, the external rotation is in the opposite direction to the internal rotation and is of the same magnitude, so that the two rotations cancel and the net change in jaw orientation (as evaluated by the palatal plane) is zero[22] (see Fig. 4-6).

Although the general pattern of internal rotation and external compensation described here occurs for the average individual, greater or lesser degrees of both internal rotation and external compensation are common. The result is moderate variation in jaw orientation, even in individuals with normal facial proportions. In addition, the rotational patterns of growth are quite different for individuals who have what are called the short face and long face types of vertical facial development.

Individuals of the short face type, who are characterized by short anterior face height, have excessive forward rotation of the mandible during growth, resulting from both an increase in the normal internal rotation and a decrease in external compensation. The result is a nearly horizontal palatal plane and mandibular morphology of the ''square jaw'' type, with a low mandibular plane angle and a square gonial angle (Fig. 4-39). A deep bite malocclusion and crowded incisors usually accompany this type of rotation (see following sections).

In long face individuals, who have excessive anterior face height, the palatal plane rotates down posteriorly, often creating a negative rather than the normal positive inclination to the true horizontal. The mandible shows an opposite, backward rotation, with an increase in the mandibular plane

Fig. 4-39 ■ Cranial base superimposition shows the characteristic pattern of forward jaw rotation in an individual developing in the ''short face'' pattern. The forward rotation flattens the mandibular plane and tends to increase overbite anteriorly. (From Bjork, A., and Skieller, V.: Am. J. Orthod. **62**:344, 1972.)

angle (Fig. 4-40). The mandibular changes result primarily from a lack of the normal forward internal rotation or even a backward internal rotation. The internal rotation, in turn, is primarily matrix rotation (centered at the condyle), not intramatrix rotation. This type of rotation is associated with anterior open bite malocclusion and mandibular deficiency (because the chin rotates back as well as down).

Backward rotation of the mandible also occurs in patients with abnormalities or pathologic changes affecting the temporomandibular joints. In these individuals, growth at the condyle is restricted. The interesting result in three cases documented by Bjork[19] was an intramatrix rotation centered in the body of the mandible, rather than the backward rotation at the condyle that dominated in individuals of the classic long face type. Jaw orientation changes in both the backward-rotating types, however, are similar, and the same types of malocclusions develop.

Interaction between jaw rotation and tooth eruption. As we have discussed, growth of the jaws creates a space into which the teeth erupt. The rotational pattern of jaw growth obviously influences the magnitude of tooth eruption. To a surprising extent, it can also influence the direction of eruption and the ultimate anteroposterior position of the incisor teeth.

The path of eruption of the maxillary teeth is downward and somewhat forward. In normal growth, the maxilla usually rotates a few degrees forward, but frequently rotates slightly backward. Forward rotation would tend to tip the incisors forward, increasing their prominence, while backward rotation directs the anterior teeth more posteriorly than would have been the case without the rotation, relatively uprighting them and decreasing their prominence.

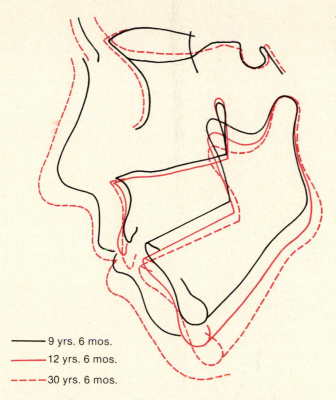

——— 9 yrs. 6 mos.

——— 12 yrs. 6 mos.

– – – 30 yrs. 6 mos.

Fig. 4-40 ■ The pattern of jaw rotation in an individual with the "long face" pattern of growth (cranial base superimposition). As the mandible rotates backward, anterior face height increases, there is a tendency toward anterior open bite, and the incisors are thrust forward relative to the mandible. (From Bjork, A., and Skieller, V.: Eur. J. Orthod. **5**:29, 1983.)

The eruption path of mandibular teeth is upward and somewhat forward. The normal internal rotation of the mandible carries the jaw upward in front. This rotation alters the eruption path of the incisors, tending to direct them more posteriorly than would otherwise have been the case (Fig. 4-41). Because the internal jaw rotation tends to upright the incisors, the molars migrate further mesially during growth than do the incisors, and this migration is reflected in the decrease in arch length that normally occurs (Fig. 4-42). Since the forward internal rotation of the mandible is greater than that of the maxilla, it is not surprising that the normal decrease in mandibular arch length is somewhat greater than the decrease in maxillary arch length.

Note that this explanation for the decrease in arch length that normally occurs in both jaws places relatively greater importance on lingual movement of the incisors and relatively less importance on the forward movement of molars than the traditional interpretation that emphasizes forward migration of the molar teeth. In fact, the same implant studies that revealed the internal jaw rotation also confirmed that changes in anteroposterior position of the incisor teeth are a major influence on arch length changes.

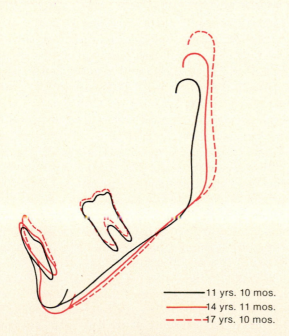

——— 11 yrs. 10 mos.

——— 14 yrs. 11 mos.

– – – 17 yrs. 10 mos.

Fig. 4-41 ■ Superimposition on mandibular implants shows the lingual positioning of the mandibular incisors relative to the mandible that often accompanies forward rotation during growth. (From Bjork, A., and Skieller, V.: Am. J. Orthod. **62**:357, 1972.)

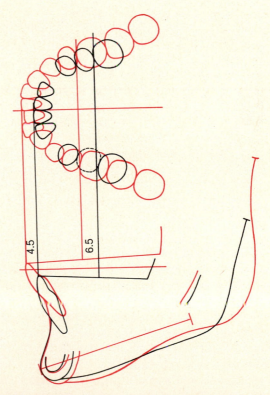

Fig. 4-42 ■ Superimposition on the mandible at ages 10 years 3 months (black) and 21 years 3 months (red) for this patient with a relatively small amount of internal rotation (-7.5 degrees) shows that the anterior and posterior teeth moved forward on the mandible, but the molars came forward more. (From Bjork, A., and Skieller, V.: Eur. J. Orthod. **5**:15, 1983.)

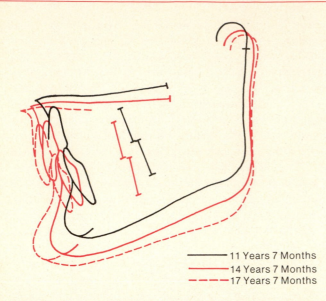

—— 11 Years 7 Months
—— 14 Years 7 Months
----- 17 Years 7 Months

Fig. 4-43 ■ Cranial base superimposition for a patient with the short face pattern of growth. As the mandible rotates upward and forward, the vertical overlap of the teeth tends to increase, creating a deep bite malocclusion. In addition, even though both the upper and lower teeth do move forward relative to cranial base, lingual displacement of incisors relative to the maxilla and mandible increases the tendency toward crowding. (From Bjork, A., and Skieller, V.: Am. J. Orthod. **62:**355, 1972.)

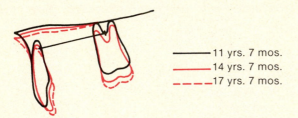

—— 11 yrs. 7 mos.
—— 14 yrs. 7 mos.
----- 17 yrs. 7 mos.

Fig. 4-44 ■ Superimposition on the maxilla reveals uprighting of the maxillary incisors in the short face growth pattern (same patient as Fig. 4-43). This decreases arch length and contributes to progressive crowding. (From Bjork, A., and Skieller, V.: Am. J. Orthod. **62:**355, 1972.)

Given this relationship between jaw rotation and incisor position, it is not surprising that both the vertical and anteroposterior positions of the incisors are affected in short face and long face individuals. When excessive rotation occurs in the short face type of development, the incisors tend to be carried into an overlapping position even if they erupt very little, hence the tendency for deep bite malocclusion in short face individuals (Fig. 4-43). The rotation also progressively uprights the incisors, displacing them lingually and causing a tendency toward crowding (Fig. 4-44). In the long face growth pattern, on the other hand, an anterior open bite will develop as anterior face height increases unless the incisors erupt for an extreme distance. The rotation of the jaws also carries the incisors forward, creating dental protrusion.

The interaction between tooth eruption and jaw rotation explains a number of previously puzzling aspects of tooth positioning in patients who have vertical facial disproportions. This topic is discussed from an etiologic perspective in Chapter 5 and is reviewed from the point of view of treatment planning in Chapter 8.

■ *Maturational and Aging Changes in the Dental Apparatus*

Maturational changes in the dentition affect the teeth and their supporting structures and the dental occlusion itself.

■ Changes in Teeth and Supporting Structures

At the time a permanent tooth erupts, the pulp chamber is relatively large. As time passes, additional dentin slowly deposits on the inside of the tooth, so that the pulp chamber gradually becomes smaller with increasing age (Fig. 4-45). This process continues relatively rapidly until the late teens, at which time the pulp chamber of a typical permanent tooth is about half the size that it was at the time of initial eruption. Because of the relatively large pulp chambers of young permanent teeth, complex restorative procedures are more likely to result in mechanical exposures in adolescents than in adults. Additional dentin continues to be produced at a slower rate throughout life, so that in old age, the pulp chambers of some permanent teeth are all but obliterated.

Maturation also brings about a tendency for a greater amount of the tooth to be exposed. At the time a permanent first molar erupts, the gingival attachment is high on the crown. Typically, the gingival attachment is still well above the cementoenamel junction when a tooth comes into full occlusion. The relative apical movement of the attachment that occurs thereafter in normal circumstances results more from vertical growth of the jaws and accompanying eruption of the teeth than from a downward migration of the gingival attachment. As we have noted previously in this chapter, vertical growth of the jaws and an increase in face height continue after transverse and anteroposterior growth has been completed. By the time the jaws all but stop growing vertically in the late teens, the gingival attachment is usually near the cementoenamel junction. In the absence of inflammation, mechanical abrasion, or pathologic changes, the gingival attachment should remain at about the same level almost indefinitely. In fact, however, most individuals experience some pathology of the gingiva or periodonteum as they age, and so further recession of the gingiva is common.

At one time, it was thought that "passive eruption" occurred, defined as an actual gingival migration of the attachment without any eruption of the tooth. It now appears that as long as the gingival tissues are entirely healthy, this sort of downward migration of the soft tissue attachment does not occur. What was once thought to be passive eruption during the teens is really active eruption, compensating for the vertical jaw growth still occurring at that time (Fig. 4-46).

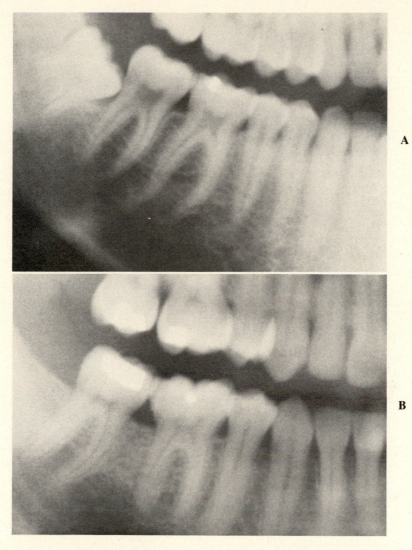

Fig. 4-45 ■ The size of the pulp chambers of permanent teeth decrease during adolescence, then continue to fill in more slowly for the rest of adult life. **A,** Age 17; **B,** age 26.

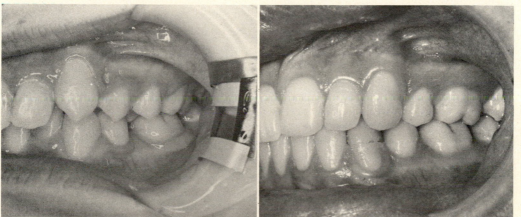

Fig. 4-46 ■ The increasing exposure of permanent teeth during adolescence was once thought to result from a downward migration of the attachment, but now is recognized to occur mostly in response to vertical growth. **A,** Age 13; **B,** age 18.

Both occlusal and interproximal wear, often to a severe degree, occurred in primitive people eating an extremely coarse diet. The elimination of most coarse particles from modern diets has also largely eliminated wear of this type. The observation of wear facets on the teeth of adults is now a reliable indicator of bruxism, not a natural consequence of mastication.

■ Changes in Alignment and Occlusion

Individuals in primitive societies who experienced wear of the teeth lost tooth substance interproximally as well as from the occlusal surfaces. The alveolar bone bends during heavy mastication, allowing the teeth to move slightly. (See Chapter 9 for more details.) When the teeth move back and forth relative to each other during mastication, abrasive particles can cause both interproximal and occlusal wear. The result in many primitive populations was a reduction in arch circumference of 5 to 10 mm or more after completion of the permanent dentition at adolescence (Fig. 4-47).

When this type of interproximal wear occurs, spaces do not open up between the posterior teeth, although some spacing may develop anteriorly. Instead, the permanent molars migrate mesially, keeping the contacts reasonably tight even as the contact points are worn off and the mesiodistal width of each tooth decreases.

In modern populations, there is a strong tendency for crowding of the mandibular incisor teeth to develop in the late teens and early twenties, no matter how well aligned the teeth were initially. Mild crowding of the lower incisors tends to develop if the teeth were initially well aligned, or initially mild crowding becomes worse. These changes appear as early as age 17 to 18 in some individuals and as late as the mid-twenties in others. Three major theories to account for this crowding have been proposed:

1. Lack of ''normal attrition'' in the modern diet.[20] As noted in Chapter 1, primitive populations tend to have a much smaller prevalence of malocclusion than do contemporary populations in developed countries. If a shortening of arch length and a mesial migration of the permanent molars is a natural phenomenon, it would seem reasonable that crowding would develop unless the amount of tooth structure was reduced during the final stages of growth. Raymond Begg, a pioneer Australian orthodontist, noted in his studies of the Australian aborigines that malocclusion is uncommon but that large amounts of interproximal and occlusal attrition occurred. Because of this, he advocated widespread extraction of premolar teeth in modern populations to provide the equivalent of the attrition he saw in aborigines. Unfortunately for this theory, when Australian aborigines change to a modern diet, as has happened to most of this group in the last 3 decades, occlusal and interproximal wear all but disappears, but late crowding rarely develops although periodontal disease does become a major problem. In other population groups, on the other hand, late crowding may develop even after premolars are extracted and arch length is reduced by modern orthodontic treatment.

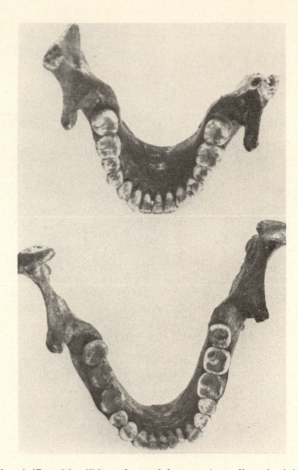

Fig. 4-47 ■ Mandibles of an adolescent Australian aboriginal *(top)* and an adult *(bottom)*, taken from prehistoric skeletal remains. Note the attrition of the teeth of the adult, resulting in interproximal as well as occlusal wear. Arch length in this population shortened by 1 cm or more after adolescence because of the extensive interproximal wear. (From Begg, P.R.: Am J. Orthod. **40**:298-312, 1954.)

Thus this theory, though superficially attractive, does not explain late crowding.

2. Pressure from third molars. Late crowding develops at about the time the third molars should erupt. In most individuals, these teeth are hopelessly impacted because the jaw length did not increase enough to accommodate them via backward remodeling of the ramus (Fig. 4-48). Erupting teeth produce pressure, and it has seemed entirely logical to many dentists that pressure from third molars with no room to erupt is the cause of late incisor crowding. Erupting teeth create a pressure of only 5 to 10 gm, however, and it is difficult to understand how that light a pressure at the posterior part of the dental arch could cause crowding in the anterior part. In fact, late crowding of lower incisors can develop in individuals whose lower third molars are congenitally missing. It seems, therefore, that pressure from third molars is not the explanation either.

3. Late mandibular growth. As a result of the cephalocaudal gradient of growth discussed in Chapter 2, the mandible can and does undergo more growth in the late teens

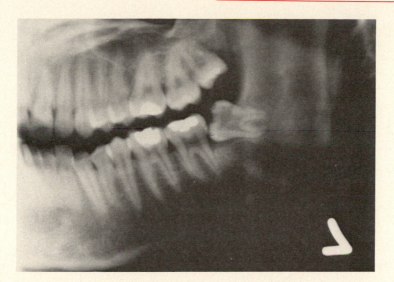

Fig. 4-48 ■ It seems reasonable that a horizontally impacted third molar would provide pressure against the dental arch, but it is highly unlikely that there is enough pressure from this source to cause the crowding of mandibular incisors that often develops in the late teens.

than the maxilla. Is it possible that late mandibular growth somehow causes late mandibular incisor crowding? If so, how? Bjork's implant studies[19] have provided an understanding of why late crowding occurs and how it indeed relates to the growth pattern of the jaw.

The position of the dentition relative to the maxilla and mandible is influenced by the pattern of growth of the jaws, a concept explored in some detail in previous sections. When the mandible grows forward relative to the maxilla, as it usually does in the late teens as well as earlier, the mandibular incisor teeth tend to be displaced lingually, particularly if any excessive rotation is also present.

In patients with a tight anterior occlusion before late differential mandibular growth occurs, the contact relationship of the lower incisors with the upper incisors must change if the mandible grows forward. In that circumstance, one of three events must occur: (1) the mandible is displaced distally, accompanied by a distortion of temporomandibular joint function and displacement of the articular disc; (2) the upper incisors flare forward, opening space between these teeth; or (3) the lower incisors displace distally and become crowded.

All three of these phenomena have been reported. The second response, flaring and spacing of the maxillary incisors, is the least common. Posterior displacement of the mandible accompanied by temporomandibular joint disturbances can definitely happen and may occasionally cause myofascial pain and dysfunction. However, distal displacement of the lower incisors, with concomitant crowding, is the most likely response.

It is not necessary for the incisors to be in occlusal contact for late crowding to develop. This also occurs commonly in individuals who have an anterior open bite and backward, not forward, rotation of the mandible (Fig. 4-42). In this situation, the rotation of the mandible carries the incisors forward and thrusts them against the lip. This creates light but lasting pressure by the lip, which tends to reposition the protruding incisors somewhat lingually, reducing arch length and causing crowding.

The current concept is that late incisor crowding develops as the mandibular incisors, and perhaps the entire mandibular dentition, move distally relative to the body of the mandible late in mandibular growth. This also sheds some light on the possible role of the third molars in determining whether crowding will occur, and how severe it will be. If space were available at the distal end of the mandibular arch, it might be possible for all the mandibular teeth to shift slightly distally, allowing the lower incisors to upright without becoming crowded. On the other hand, impacted third molars at the distal end of the lower arch would prevent the posterior teeth from shifting distally, and if differential mandibular growth occurred, their presence might guarantee that crowding would develop. In this case, the lower third molars could be the "last straw" in a chain of events that led to late incisor crowding. As noted previously, however, late incisor crowding does occur in individuals with no third molars at all, and so the presence of these teeth is not the critical variable. The extent of late mandibular growth is

■ Facial Growth in Adults

Until recently, although some anthropologists in the 1930s had reported small amounts of growth continuing into middle age, it was generally assumed that growth of the facial skeleton ceased in the late teens or early twenties. In the early 1980s, Behrents[21] succeeded in recalling over 100 individuals who never had orthodontic treatment but who had participated in the Bolton growth study in Cleveland in the 1930s and late 1940s, more than 40 years previously. While they were participants in the study, the growth of

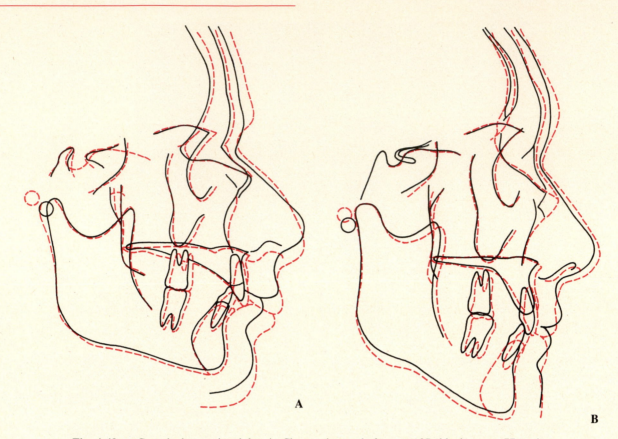

A

B

Fig. 4-49 ■ Growth changes in adults. **A,** Changes in a male from age 37 *(black)* to age 77 *(red)*. Note that both the maxilla and mandible grew forward, and the nose grew considerably. **B,** Growth changes in a woman between age 34 *(black)* and 83 *(red)*. Note that both jaws grew forward and somewhat downward, and that the nasal structure enlarged. (From Behrents, R.G.: A Treatise on the Continuum of Growth in the Aging Craniofacial Skeleton. Ann Arbor, 1984, Ph.D. Thesis, University of Michigan.)

these individuals had been carefully evaluated and recorded, by both measurements and serial cephalometric films. The magnification in the radiographs was known precisely, and it was possible to obtain new radiographs more than 4 decades later with known magnification, so that precise measurements of facial dimensions could be made.

The results were surprising but unequivocal: facial growth had continued during adult life (Fig. 4-49). There was an increase in essentially all of the facial dimensions, but both size and shape of the craniofacial complex altered with time. Vertical changes in adult life were more prominent than anteroposterior changes, whereas width changes were least evident, and so the alterations observed in the adult facial skeleton seem to be a continuation of the pattern seen during maturation. In a point of particular interest, an apparent deceleration of growth in females in the late teens was followed by a resumption of growth during the twenties. Although the magnitude of the adult growth changes, assessed on a millimeters per year basis, was quite small, the cumulative effect over decades was surprisingly large (Fig. 4-50).

The data also revealed that rotation of both jaws continued into adult life, in concert with the vertical changes and eruption of teeth. Because implants were not used in these patients, it was not possible to precisely differentiate internal from external rotation, but it seems likely that both internal rotation and surface changes did continue. In general, males showed a net rotation of the jaws in a forward direction, slightly decreasing the mandibular plane angle, whereas females had a tendency toward backward rotation, with an increase in the mandibular plane angle. In both groups, compensatory changes were noted in the dentition, so that occlusal relationships largely were maintained.

Both a history of orthodontic treatment and loss of multiple teeth had an impact on facial morphology in these adults and on the pattern of change. In a smaller group of patients who had orthodontic treatment many years previously, Behrents noted that the pattern of growth associated with the original malocclusion continued to express itself even in adult life. This finding is consistent with previous observations of growth in the late teens but also indicates how a gradual worsening of occlusal relationships could occur in

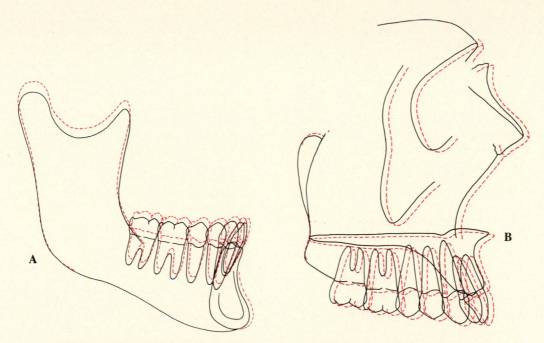

Fig. 4-50 ■ Growth changes in adults. **A,** Mean dimensional changes in the mandible for males in adult life. It is apparent that the pattern of juvenile and adolescent growth continues at a slower but ultimately significant rate. **B,** The mean positional changes in the maxilla during adult life, for both sexes combined. Note that the maxilla moves forward and slightly downward, continuing the previous pattern of growth. (From Behrents, R.G.: A Treatise on the Continuum of Growth in the Aging Craniofacial Skeleton. Ann Arbor, 1984, PhD. Thesis, University of Michigan.)

some patients long after the completion of orthodontic treatment. Loss of multiple teeth was associated with significant changes in vertical dimension.

As expected, changes in the facial soft tissue profile were greater than changes in the facial skeleton. The soft tissue changes involved an elongation of the nose (which often became significantly longer during adult life), flattening of the lips, and an augmentation of the chin.

In the light of Behrents' findings, it seems clear that the view of facial growth as a process that ends in the late teens or early twenties must be revised. It is correct, however, to view the growth process as one that declines to a basal level after the attainment of sexual maturity, and it is also correct to differentiate between growth in the three planes of space. Growth in width is not only the first to drop to adult levels, usually reaching essential completion by the onset of puberty, but the basal or adult level observed thereafter is quite low. Anteroposterior growth continues at a noticeable rate for a longer time, declining to basal levels only after puberty, with small but noticeable changes continuing throughout adult life. Vertical growth, which had previously been observed to continue well after puberty in both males and females, continues at a moderate level throughout adult life. Growth, in short, comes much closer to being a process that continues throughout life than most observers had suspected.

■ *References*

1. Darling, A.I., and Levers, B.G.: The pattern of eruption of some human teeth. Arch. Oral Biol. **20:**89-96, 1975.
2. Cahill, D.R.: The histology and rate of tooth eruption with and without temporary impaction in the dog. Anat. Rec. **166:**255-238, 1970.
3. Berkovitz, B.K.B., Migdalshia, A., and Solomon, M.: The effect of the lathyritic agent aminoacetonitrile on the unimpeded eruption rate in normal and root-resected rat lower incisors. Arch. Oral Biol. **17:**1755-1763, 1972.
4. Berkovitz, B.K.: The effect of root transection and partial root resection on the unimpeded eruption rate of the rat incisor. Arch. Oral Biol. **16:**1033-1043, 197.
5. Steedle, J.R., and Proffit, W.R.: The pattern and control of eruptive tooth movements. Am. J. Orthod. **87:**56-66, 1985.
6. Moxham, B.J.: Recording the eruption of the rabbit mandibular incisor using a device for continuously monitoring tooth movements. Arch. Oral Biol. **24:**889-899, 1980.
7. Gron, A.: Prediction of tooth emergence. J. Dent. Res. **41:**573-585, 1962.
8. Anderson, D.L., Thompson, G.W., and Popovich, F.: Interrelationship of dental maturity, skeletal maturity, height and weight from age 4 to 14 years. Growth **39:**453-462, 1975.
9. Moorrees, C.F.A., and Chadha, J.M.: Available space for the incisors during dental development—a growth study based on physiologic age. Angle Orthod. **35:**12-22, 1965.
10. Edwards, J.G.: The diastema, the frenum, the frenectomy. Am. J. Orthod. **71:**489-508, 1977.

11. Gruelich, W.W., and Pyle, S.I.: Radiographic Atlas of Skeletal Development of the Hand and Wrist. Palo Alto, CA., 1959, Stanford University Press.

12. Lowery, G.H.: Growth and Development of Children, ed. 6, Chicago, 1973, Year Book Publishers.

13. Tanner, J.M.: Growth at Adolescence, ed. 2, Springfield, IL., 1962, Charles C Thomas.

14. Sheldon, W.H.: The Varieties of Human Physique. New York, 1940, Harper Brothers.

15. Woodside, D.G.: Data from Burlington growth study. Cited in The activator. In Salzmann, J.A.: Orthodontics in Daily Practice. Philadelphia, 1974, J.B. Lippincott Co.

16. Enlow, D.H.: Handbook of Facial Growth, ed. 2, Philadelphia, 1982, W.B. Saunders Co.

17. Agronin, K.: Translation of the glenoid fossa: a cephalometric study during craniofacial development. Seattle, 1984, M.S.D. Thesis, University of Washington.

18. Bjork, A.: The use of metallic implants in the study of facial growth in children: method and application. Am. J. Phys. Anthropol. **29:**243-254, 1968.

19. Bjork, A., and Skieller, V.: Normal and abnormal growth of the mandible: a synthesis of longitudinal cephalometric implant studies over a period of 25 years. Eur. J. Orthod. **5:**1-46, 1983.

20. Begg, P.R.: Stone age man's dentition. Am. J. Orthod. **40:**298-312, 373-383, 462-475, 517-531, 1954.

21. Behrents, R.G.: A Treatise on the Continuum of Growth in the Aging Craniofacial Skeleton. Ann Arbor, 1984, Ph.D. Thesis, University of Michigan.

22. Bjork, A., and Skieller, V.: Postnatal growth and development of the maxillary complex. In McNamara, J.A., editor: Factors Affecting Growth of the Midface, Ann Arbor, 1976, University of Michigan Center for Human Growth and Development.

Chapter 5

The Etiology of Orthodontic Problems

Malocclusion and dentofacial deformity in most instances result not from some pathologic process, but from moderate distortions of normal development. In some patients, it is clear that an orthodontic problem is entirely the result of some environmental influence, as for example, mandibular deficiency secondary to a childhood fracture of the jaw. The etiology for a few other patients appears to be almost entirely genetic, as in the characteristic malocclusion that accompanies some rare genetic syndromes. The orthodontic problems of most patients, however, seem to arise from an interaction between environmental and innate influences.

The purpose of this chapter is to draw on the background of normal growth and development to illustrate possible and probable causes for orthodontic problems, and to place the etiology of malocclusion in perspective.

■ Possible Causes of Malocclusion

Malocclusion is presently so frequent that it occurs in a majority of the population—which does not mean that it is normal. Skeletal remains from northern European populations, whose descendents have the high rates of malocclusion discussed in Chapter 1, suggest that the present prevalence is several times greater than it was 1000 years ago. Crowding and malalignment of teeth within the arches (Class I malocclusion), the most common kind of malocclusion at present, was unusual until relatively recently[1] (but not unknown—see Fig. 5-1). Mild jaw discrepancies lead-ing to mild or moderate Class II and Class III malocclusion may have been fairly common in some primitive populations. Because the mandible tends to become separated from the rest of the skull when long-buried skeletal remains are unearthed, it is easier to be sure what has happened to alignment of teeth than to occlusal relationships. The skeletal remains suggest that all members of a group might tend toward a Class III, or less commonly, a Class II jaw relationship. Similar findings are noted in present population groups that have remained largely unaffected by modern development: crowding and malalignment of teeth are uncommon, but the majority of the group may have mild anteroposterior or transverse discrepancies, as in the tendency toward Class III found in South Pacific islanders[2] and buccal crossbite (X-occlusion) in Australian aborigines.[3]

Under primitive conditions, of course, excellent function of the jaws and teeth was an important predictor of the ability to survive and reproduce. A capable masticatory apparatus was essential to deal with uncooked or partially cooked meat and plant foods. Watching an Australian aboriginal using every muscle of the upper body to tear off a piece of kangaroo flesh from the barely cooked animal, for instance, makes one realize the decrease in demand on the masticatory apparatus that has accompanied civilization (Fig. 5-2). It seems that deviations from the present concept of ideal tooth interdigitation were more compatible than severe crowding and malalignment with the rigors of a primitive diet.

Although 1000 years is a long time relative to a single human life, it is a very short time from an evolutionary perspective. The fossil record documents evolutionary trends over many thousands of years that affect the present dentition, including a decrease in the size of individual teeth, a decrease in the number of the teeth, and a decrease in the size of the jaws. For example, there has been a steady reduction in the size of both anterior and posterior teeth over at least the last 50,000 years (Fig. 5-3). The number of teeth in the dentition of higher primates has been reduced compared to the usual mammalian pattern (Fig. 5-4). The third incisor and third premolar have disappeared, as has the fourth molar. At present, their frequent congenital absence indicates that the third molar, the second premolar, and the second incisor may be on their way out. In comparison to primitive peoples modern human beings have quite underdeveloped jaws.

It is easy to see that the progressive reduction in jaw size,

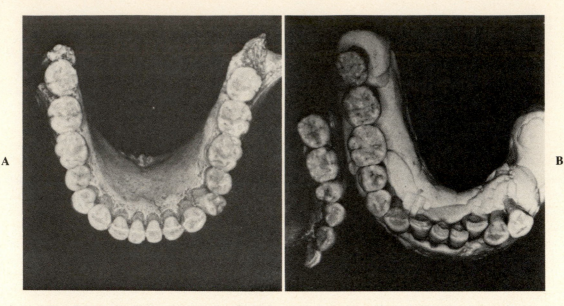

Fig. 5-1 ■ Mandibular dental arches from Neanderthal specimens from the Krapina cave in Yugoslavia, estimated to be approximately 100,000 years old. **A,** Note the excellent alignment in the specimen. **B,** Crowding and malalignment are seen in this specimen which had the largest teeth in this find of skeletal remains from approximately 80 individuals. (From Wolpoff, W.H.: Paleoanthropology. New York, 1980, Alfred A. Knopf.)

if not well matched to a decrease in tooth size and number, could lead to crowding and malalignment. It is less easy to see why such malalignment should have increased rather suddenly in recent years.

Cardiovascular disease and related health problems appear rapidly when a previously unaffected population group leaves agrarian life for the city and civilization. High blood pressure, heart disease, diabetes, and several other medical problems are so much more prevalent in developed than underdeveloped countries that they have been labeled "diseases of civilization." Dental problems including malocclusion are often included in the same category. The increase in malocclusion in modern times certainly parallels the development of modern civilization, but the parallel with stress-related diseases can be carried only so far.

There is some evidence that malocclusion increases within well-defined populations after a transition from rural villages to the city. Corruccini, for instance, reports a higher prevalence of crowding, posterior crossbite, and buccal segment discrepancy in urbanized compared to rural Punjabi youths of northern India.[4] The assessment is complicated by the fact that both dental caries and periodontal disease, which are rare on the primitive diet, do appear rapidly when the diet changes. The resulting dental pathology can make it difficult to establish what the occlusion might have been in the absence of early loss of teeth, gingivitis, and periodontal breakdown.

Corrucini argues that a higher prevalence of occlusal traits associated with malocclusion is found in a variety of circumstances having in common a greater contact with modern urban conditions and the modern soft diet[5]. His view is that the change in diet accompanying the development of contemporary civilization is an important cause of the increase in malocclusion. This implies that jaw size may have begun to decrease more rapidly in recent years because of a lack of functional stimulation of jaw growth. The mechanism by which that would happen is not obvious, and other possibilities are discussed in the following section.

Whatever the cause, malocclusion is an important problem in contemporary society. It is difficult to know the precise etiology of any specific malocclusion, but we do know in general what the possibilities are. In the remainder of this chapter, we will examine specific causes of malocclusion under three major headings: developmental, traumatic, and functional. The final section is devoted to considering the etiology of specific types of orthodontic problems, emphasizing the role of inherited dentofacial characteristics versus environmental factors as causes for malocclusion.

■ *Developmental Causes of Malocclusion*

■ Disturbances in Embryologic Development

Defects in embryologic development usually result in death of the embryo. As many as 20% of early pregnancies terminate because of lethal embryologic defects, often so early that the mother is not even aware that conception had occurred. Only a relatively small number of recognizable conditions that produce orthodontic problems are compatible with long-term survival. These conditions and their embryologic origin are discussed in Chapter 3.

A variety of causes for embryologic defects, ranging from

genetic disturbances to specific environmental insults, is known to exist. Chemical and other agents capable of producing embryologic defects if given at the critical time are called *teratogens*. Most drugs do not interfere with normal development or, at high doses, kill the embryo without producing defects, and therefore are not teratogenic. Teratogens typically cause specific defects if present at low levels but if given in higher doses, do have lethal effects. Teratogens known to produce orthodontic problems are listed in Table 5-1.

■ Disturbances of Dental Development

Disturbances of dental development may accompany major congenital defects, but more frequently occur as isolated findings that contribute to Class I malocclusion. Significant disturbances include:

Congenitally missing teeth. Congenital absence of teeth results from disturbances during the initial stages of formation of a tooth, initiation and proliferation. *Anodontia,* the total absence of teeth, is the extreme form. The term *oligodontia* refers to congenital absence of many but not all teeth, whereas the rarely used term *hypodontia* implies the absence of only a few teeth. Since the primary teeth give rise to the permanent tooth buds, there will be no permanent tooth if its primary predecessor was missing. It is possible,

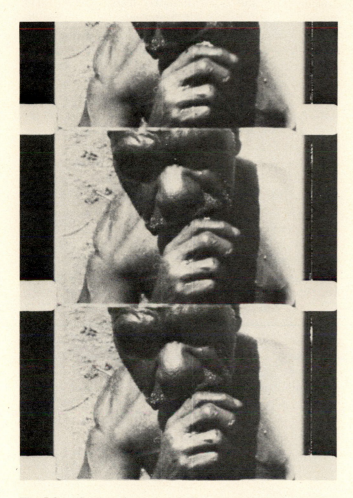

Fig. 5-2 ■ Sections from a movie film of an Australian aboriginal man eating a kangaroo prepared in the traditional fashion. Note the activity of muscles, not only in the facial region, but throughout the neck and shoulder girdle. (Courtesy M.J. Barrett.)

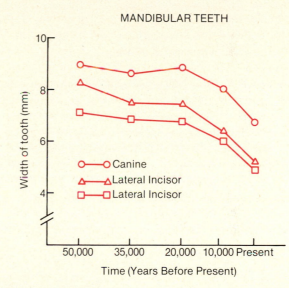

Fig. 5-3 ■ Graph showing the change in size of mandibular incisor and canine teeth over the past 50,000 years. (Plot of data from Wolpoff, W.H.: Paleoanthropology. New York, 1980, Alfred A. Knopf.)

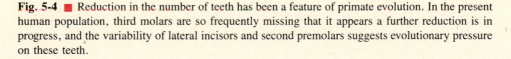

M-3	PM-4	C	I-3	Basic Mammalian
M-3	PM-3	C	I-2	Prosimian
M-3	PM-2	C	I-2	Higher Ape
M-3 (2)	PM-2	C	I-2	Man

Fig. 5-4 ■ Reduction in the number of teeth has been a feature of primate evolution. In the present human population, third molars are so frequently missing that it appears a further reduction is in progress, and the variability of lateral incisors and second premolars suggests evolutionary pressure on these teeth.

Table 5-1 ■ Teratogens affecting dentofacial development

Teratogens	Effect
Aminopterin	Anencephaly
Aspirin	Cleft lip and palate
Cigarette smoke (hypoxia)	Cleft lip and palate
Cytomegalovirus	Microcephaly, hydrocephaly, microphthalmia
Dilantin	Cleft lip and palate
Ethyl alcohol	Central mid-face discrepancy
6-Mercaptopurine	Cleft palate
13-cis Retinoic acid (Accutane)	Hemifacial microsomia, Treacher-Collins syndrome
Rubella virus	Microphthalmia, cataracts, deafness
Thalidomide	Hemifacial microsomia
Toxoplasma	Microcephaly, hydrocephaly, microphthalmia
X-radiation	Microcephaly
Valium	Cleft lip and palate
Vitamin D excess	Premature suture closure

however, for the primary teeth to be present and for all the permanent teeth to be absent. This would be referred to as anodontia of the permanent dentition.

Anodontia or oligodontia, the absence of all or most of the permanent teeth, is usually associated with an unusual but mild systemic abnormality, *ectodermal dysplasia* (Fig. 5-5). Individuals with ectodermal dysplasia have thin, sparse hair and an absence of sweat glands in addition to their characteristically missing teeth. Occasionally, oligodontia occurs in a patient with no apparent systemic problem or congenital syndrome. In these children, it appears as if there is a random pattern to the missing teeth.

Anodontia and oligodontia are rare, but hypodontia is a relatively common finding. As a general rule, if only one or a few teeth is missing, the absent tooth will be the most distal tooth of any given type. If a molar tooth is congenitally missing, it is almost always the third molar; if an incisor is missing, it is nearly always the lateral; if a premolar is missing, it almost always is the second rather than the first. Rarely is a canine the only missing tooth.

Malformed and supernumerary teeth. Abnormalities in tooth size and shape result from disturbances during the morphodifferentiation stage of development, perhaps with some carryover from the histodifferentiation stage. The most common abnormality is a variation in size, particularly of maxillary lateral incisors (Fig. 5-6) and second premolars.

About 5% of the total population have a significant "tooth size discrepancy" because of disproportionate sizes of the upper and lower teeth. Unless the teeth are matched for size, normal occlusion is impossible. As might be expected, the most variable teeth, the maxillary lateral incisors, are the major culprits. The diagnosis of tooth size discrepancy, discussed in Chapter 6, is based on comparison of the widths of teeth to published tables of expected tooth sizes.

Occasionally, tooth buds may fuse or geminate (partially split) during their development, resulting in a tooth with separate pulp chambers but joining of the dentin (Fig. 5-7). Cememtum is sometimes affected. The differentiation between gemination and fusion can be difficult, and is usually confirmed by counting the number of teeth in an area. If the other central and both lateral incisors are present, a bifurcated central incisor is the result of either gemination or, less probably, fusion with a supernumerary incisor. On the other hand, if the lateral incisor on the affected side is missing, the problem probably is fusion of the central and lateral incisor buds. Normal occlusion, of course, is all but impossible in the presence of geminated, fused, or otherwise malformed teeth.

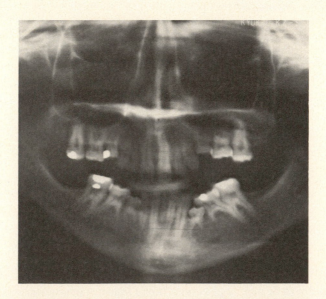

Fig. 5-5 ■ Panoramic radiograph of an individual with ectodermal dysplasia. The dental condition would be characterized as oligodontia, the absence of most of the permanent teeth. Ectodermal dysplasia is the most likely cause of this condition.

Supernumerary or extra teeth also result from disturbances during the initiation and proliferation stages of dental development. The most common supernumerary tooth appears in the maxillary midline and is called a mesiodens. Supernumerary lateral incisors also occur; extra premolars occasionally appear; a few patients have fourth as well as third molars. The presence of an extra tooth obviously has great potential to disrupt normal occlusal development (Fig. 5-8), and early intervention to remove it is usually required to obtain reasonable alignment and occlusal relationships. Many supernumerary teeth are most often seen in the congenital syndrome of cleidocranial dysplasia (see Fig. 4-2), which is characterized by missing clavicles (collar bones), multiple supernumerary and unerupted teeth, and failure of the succedaneous teeth to erupt (see further discussion following).

Interference with eruption. For a permanent tooth to erupt, the overlying bone as well as the primary tooth roots must resorb, and the tooth must make its way through the gingiva. Supernumerary teeth, sclerotic bone, and heavy fibrous gingiva can also interfere with eruption. All of these interferences are present in cleidocranial dysplasia. The multiple supernumerary teeth contribute an element of mechanical interference. More seriously, children with this condition have a defect in bone resorption, and the gingiva is quite heavy and fibrous[6]. If the eruption path can be cleared, the permanent teeth will erupt. To accomplish this, it is necessary not only to extract any supernumerary teeth that may be in the way but also to remove the bone overlying the permanent teeth and reflect the gingiva so that the teeth can break through into the mouth.

In patients with less severe problems, delays in eruption of permanent teeth contribute to malocclusion primarily because the other teeth drift to improper positions in the arch. In 10% to 15% of children, at least one primary molar becomes ankylosed (fused to the bone) before it finally resorbs and exfoliates. Although this delays eruption of its permanent successor, there is usually no lasting effect. Malocclusion develops only if the eruption delay is prolonged and drift of other teeth can occur.

Ectopic eruption. Occasionally, malposition of a permanent tooth bud can lead to eruption in the wrong place.

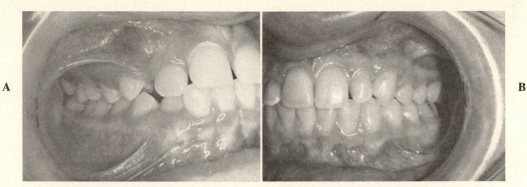

Fig. 5-6 ■ **A,** Anomalously large lateral incisors, leading to much more severe crowding in the maxillary than the mandibular arch. **B,** Normal-shaped but small lateral incisors. Maxillary lateral incisors show the greatest variation in size of all human teeth except third molars.

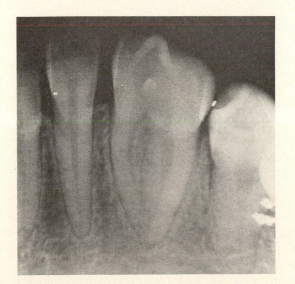

Fig. 5-7 ■ Fusion of a mandibular lateral incisor and canine.

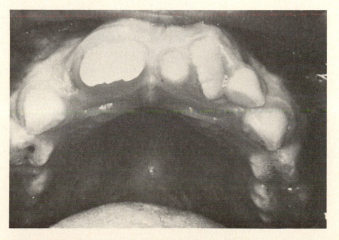

Fig. 5-8 ■ The most frequent orthodontic problem caused by a supernumerary tooth is an interference with eruption of a normal tooth, as seen here in the severe rotation of one central incisor because of the midline supernumerary tooth.

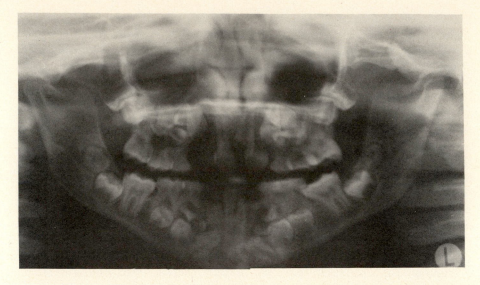

Fig. 5-9 ■ Panoramic film of an 9-year-old patient with cleidocranial dysplasia, 12 months after anterior supernumerary teeth and alveolar bone overlying the permanent incisors were removed. Note the eruption of the incisors when the mechanical obstruction is relieved (compare to Fig. 4-2, which is the same patient two years earlier). Also note the displacement of the mandibular canines and premolars by the supernumerary teeth in their area, which will have to be removed later.

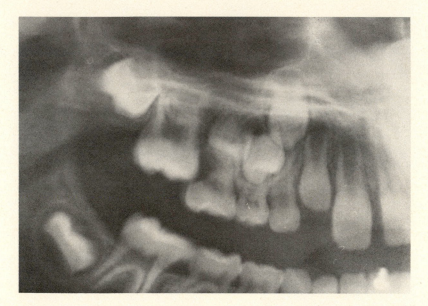

Fig. 5-10 ■ Ectopic eruption of the permanent maxillary first molar apparently results from mesial position or inclination of the tooth bud. This causes the eruptive path of the first molar to contact the root of the primary second molar. Delay in eruption of the first molar and root resorption of the second primary molar usually result, as shown here in an 8-year-old boy. Loss of space can cause crowding in the arch. Crowding of the permanent teeth is inevitable without treatment.

This condition is called *ectopic eruption*, and is most likely to occur in the eruption of maxillary first molars and incisors.[7,8]

If the eruption path of the maxillary first molar carries it too far mesially at an early stage, the permanent molar is unable to erupt, and the root of the second primary molar may be damaged (Fig. 5-10). The mesial position of the permanent molar means that the arch will be crowded unless the child receives treatment.

Ectopic eruption of mandibular lateral incisors, which occurs more frequently than first molars, may lead to transposition of the lateral incisor and canine.[9] A poor eruption direction of the canine, sometimes leading to impaction, is observed often but usually is due to the eruption path being altered by a lack of space. Sometimes, however, the bud is poorly positioned and the tooth erupts ectopically even when space is adequate, becoming transposed with a premolar, for instance (Fig. 5-11).

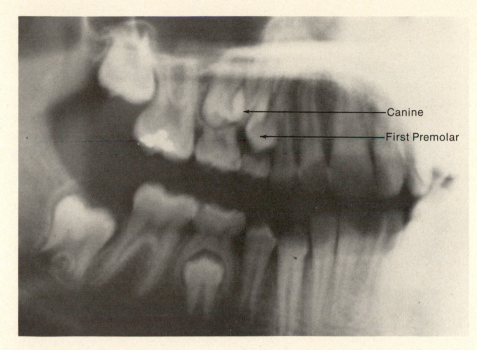

Fig. 5-11 ■ Ectopic eruption of the maxillary canine can lead to transposition of the canine and first premolar crowns.

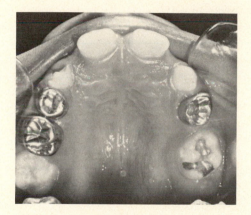

Fig. 5-12 ■ In this 8-year-old child, the space once occupied by the primary maxillary left second molar (on the right side in this mirror-image photograph) has almost totally closed as the permanent first molar drifted mesially.

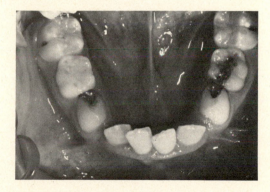

Fig. 5-13 ■ Premature loss of primary canines leads to closure of the space, not by mesial drift of the primary posterior teeth, but by distal drift of the permanent incisors.

■ Improper Guidance of Eruption

Early loss of primary teeth. When a unit within the dental arch is lost, the arch tends to contract and the space to close. At one time, this space closure was attributed entirely to mesial drift of posterior teeth, which in turn was confidently ascribed to forces from occlusion. The contemporary view is that mesial drift is a phenomenon of the permanent molars only. The major reason for mesial drift of the molars is the mesial inclination of the tooth, so that it erupts mesially as well as occlusally. Experimental data suggest that, rather than causing mesial drift, forces from occlusion actually retard it.[10] In other words, a permanent molar will drift mesially more rapidly in the absence of occlusal contacts than if they are present.

Mesial drift of the permanent first molar after a primary second molar is lost prematurely (Fig. 5-12) can significantly contribute to the development of crowding in the posterior part of the dental arch. This has been a significant cause of crowding and malalignment of premolars in the past. For this reason, maintenance of the space after a primary second molar has been lost is indicated (see Chapter 13).

When a primary first molar or canine is lost prematurely, there is also a tendency for the space to close. This occurs primarily by distal drift of incisors, not by mesial drift of posterior teeth (Fig. 5-13). The impetus for distal drift appears to have two sources: force from active contraction of transseptal fibers in the gingiva and pressures from the lips and cheeks.[11] The pull from transseptal fibers probably is the more consistent contributor to this space closure tendency, whereas lip pressure adds a variable component (see the following section on equilibrium below). If a primary canine or first molar is lost prematurely on only one side, the permanent teeth drift distally only on that side, leading to an asymmetry in the occlusion as well as a tendency toward crowding.

From this description, it is apparent that early loss of primary teeth can cause crowding and malalignment within the dental arches. Is this a major cause of Class I crowding problems? Perhaps the best indicator of the extent to which carious loss of primary teeth has caused crowding and malalignment in the past is the impact of fluoridation and other caries-preventive treatment on the prevalence of malocclusion. After some years of fluoridation, the prevalence of malocclusion may decrease in a typical U.S. community, but it is difficult to demonstrate a statistically significant change.[12] Crowding resulting from drift of permanent teeth, in other words, has not been the major cause of Class I malocclusion, which still affects almost half the population even when dental disease is under control. Even without fluoridation, it appears that only a small percentage of all crowding problems is caused by early loss of primary teeth, with the exact number obviously varying depending on the caries experience of any given population.

Functional shifts of the mandible. Functional shifts of the mandible while permanent teeth are erupting can produce both transverse and anteroposterior deviations in tooth position. (Possible effects on skeletal growth are discussed in the section of this chapter on functional influences.) Large displacements of teeth are unlikely, but this small displacement related to occlusal interferences can contribute to the development of both posterior and anterior crossbites.

Displaced teeth related to functional shifts are usually seen in two circumstances: posterior crossbite after prolonged thumbsucking, and anterior crossbite in mildly prognathic children. Prolonged sucking habits often produce a mildly narrowed maxillary arch and a tendency toward bilateral crossbite. Children with this condition usually shift the mandible to one side on closure to gain better function, which can guide permanent molars, or later, premolars into a crossbite relationship. If the sucking habit stops, the crossbite may persist until the maxillary arch is expanded (see Chapter 11).

A young child who has a tendency toward skeletal Class III malocclusion will have end-to-end contact of the primary incisors—a true anterior crossbite in the primary dentition is quite rare because mandibular growth lags behind maxillary growth. The primary incisors wear down rapidly, and an anterior shift of the mandible to escape occlusal interferences rarely occurs until the permanent incisors begin to erupt. A pattern of anterior displacement of the mandible may develop when the permanent incisors come into contact, however, producing an anterior crossbite from the shift. Because of its delayed arrival and lingual position, the maxillary lateral incisor is especially prone to being deflected

lingually rather than labially, and the chance that this will happen is obviously greater when there is a shift into anterior crossbite.

Malocclusion caused by improper eruption guidance from shifts of the mandible is uncommon. Although there is no doubt that it can and does occur, and that functional shifts are therefore a definite indication for treatment (see Chapter 11), improper eruption guidance accounts for only a small percentage of anterior or posterior crossbites.

■ *Problems Caused by Trauma*

■ Fetal Molding and Birth Injuries

Injuries apparent at birth fall into two major categories: (1) intrauterine molding and (2) trauma to the mandible during the birth process, particularly from the use of forceps in delivery.

Intrauterine molding. Occasionally, a limb of the fetus becomes pressed against another part of the body within the uterus, which can lead to distortion of rapidly growing areas. Strictly speaking, this is not a birth injury, but because the effects are noted at birth, it is considered in that category. The major impact of intrauterine molding on facial development results when an arm is positioned across the face, thereby restricting development of the maxilla (Fig. 5-14). As we have discussed, mandibular growth trails well behind maxillary growth before birth, and molding effects on the mandible are minimal. Although moderate to severe maxillary deficiency can result from intrauterine molding, this is quite a rare condition. There is good potential for catchup growth postnatally, and the intrauterine molding is unlikely to produce a severe long-term deformity.

Trauma to the mandible. Many deformity patterns now known to result from defects in embryologic development were once blamed on injuries during birth. Many parents, despite explanations from their doctors, will refer to their child's facial deformity as being caused by a birth injury even if the congenital syndrome pattern is evident. No matter what the parents say later, Treacher-Collins syndrome or Crouzon's syndrome obviously did not arise because of trauma during birth.

In some difficult births, however, the use of forceps to the head to assist in delivery might cause damage to the temporomandibular joint area. At least in theory, heavy pressure in the area of the temporomandibular joints could cause internal hemorrhage, loss of tissue, and a subsequent underdevelopment of the mandible. If the cartilage of the mandibular condyle were an important growth center, of course, the risk from damage to a presumably critical area would seem much greater. In light of the contemporary understanding that the condylar cartilage is not critical for proper growth of the mandible, it is not as easy to blame underdevelopment of the mandible on birth injuries.

It is interesting to note that although the use of forceps in deliveries has decreased considerably over the last 50 years, the prevalence of Class II malocclusion caused by

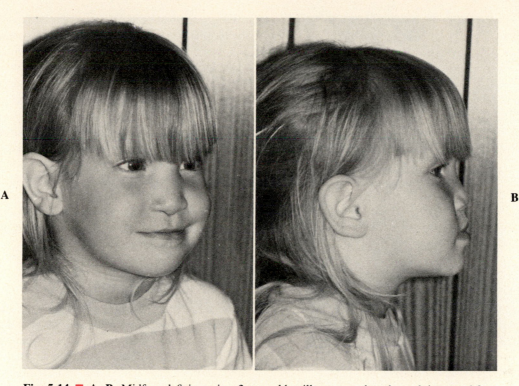

Fig. 5-14 ■ **A, B.** Midface deficiency in a 3-year-old, still apparent though much improved from the severe deficiency that was present at birth because of intrauterine molding.

mandibular deficiency has not decreased. In short, injury to the mandible during a traumatic delivery appears to be a rare and unusual cause of facial deformity. Children with deformities involving the mandible are much more likely to have a congenital syndrome.

■ Trauma to Teeth

Every child experiences a series of falls, and most manage to hit their teeth during their formative years. Occasionally, the impact is intense enough to knock out or severely displace a primary or permanent tooth. Dental trauma can lead to the development of malocclusion in three ways: (1) damage to permanent tooth buds from an injury to primary teeth, (2) drift of permanent teeth after premature loss of primary teeth, and (3) direct injury to permanent teeth.

Trauma to a primary tooth can displace the permanent tooth bud underlying it. There are two possible results. First, if the trauma occurs while the crown of the permanent tooth is forming, enamel formation will be disturbed, and there will be a defect in the crown of the permanent tooth.

Second, if the trauma occurs after the crown is complete, the crown may be displaced relative to the root. Root formation may stop, leaving a permanently shortened root. More frequently, however, root formation continues, but the remaining portion of the root then forms at an angle to the traumatically displaced crown (Fig. 5-15). This distortion of root form is called *dilaceration*, defined as a distorted root form. Dilaceration can occur from any distortion of the crown relative to the root, and so may result from mechan-

ical interference with eruption, but its usual cause, particularly in permanent incisor teeth, is trauma to primary teeth which also displaced the permanent buds.

If distortion of root position is severe enough, it is almost impossible for the crown to assume its proper position—that might require the root to extend out through the alveolar bone. For this reason, it may be necessary to extract a severely dilacerated tooth. Traumatically displaced tooth buds in children should be repositioned as early as possible, so that when root formation does resume, distortion of the root position will be minimized. This topic is discussed in more detail in Chapter 13.

Traumatic avulsion of primary incisors is unlikely to lead to significant drift of permanent teeth, but the child who knocks out her two front teeth at age 3 is more likely to have the permanent replacements finally erupt at age 9, 2 years late, than to have them erupt early. This occurs because of slow resorption of the overlying bone. The delay in itself, however, is unlikely to lead to malocclusion. The space tends to close if a permanent incisor is knocked out at an early age. It is rare for the space of a missing upper central incisor to close completely, but drift of the other permanent teeth may result in an unsightly space too small for a proper prosthetic replacement. Trauma is much more likely to affect anterior than posterior teeth, but if a posterior tooth is lost prematurely to trauma, the same patterns of drift will occur as if it had been lost to caries.

Permanent teeth are often displaced by trauma. If the tooth is knocked labially or lingually, the root of the tooth

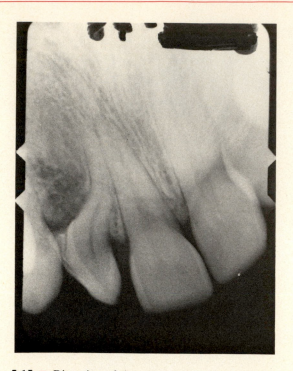

Fig. 5-15 ■ Distortion of the root (termed dilaceration) of this lateral incisor resulted from trauma at an earlier age that displaced the crown relative to the forming root.

is sometimes damaged, but there always is a fracture of the alveolar process. Immediately after the accident, an intact tooth can usually be moved back to its original position rapidly and easily, but after healing (which takes 2 to 3 weeks), months of orthodontic treatment may be needed to bring it back into the line of the arch. If the tooth is intruded traumatically, it may not re-erupt on its own. There is a significant chance of ankylosis, which will prevent, not only spontaneous re-eruption, but also later orthodontic treatment. In this situation also, immediate orthodontic treatment is preferred (see Chapter 13).

■ Childhood Fractures of the Jaw

The falls and impacts of childhood can fracture jaws just like other parts of the body. The condylar neck of the mandible is a particularly vulnerable area, and fractures of this area in childhood occur relatively frequently. Fortunately, the condylar process tends to regenerate well after early fractures (see Chapter 2). The best human data suggest that about 75% of children with early fractures of the mandibular condylar process have normal mandibular growth, and therefore do not develop a malocclusion because of this trauma that they would not have had in its absence.[13] Interestingly, the prognosis is better the earlier the condylar fracture occurs, perhaps because the growth potential is greater early in life.

From the number of children with later growth problems whose original fracture was not diagnosed, it appears that many early fractures of the condyle go completely unno-

ticed. It seems to be relatively common for a child to crash the bicycle, chip a tooth and fracture a condyle, cry a bit, and then continue to develop normally, complete with total regeneration of the condyle. Problems arise when there is enough scarring in the area to produce mechanical restrictions on displacement of the mandible during subsequent growth.

A survey of patients seen in the Dentofacial Clinic at the University of North Carolina indicates that about 5% of patients who need surgical correction of severe mandibular deficiency have this problem because of an early fracture of the jaw.[14] This suggests that childhood jaw fractures, though potentially a cause of severe orthodontic problems, do not make a large contribution to the total pool of patients with Class II malocclusion.

■ *Functional Influences*

A relationship between anatomic form and physiologic function is apparent in all animals. Over evolutionary time, adaptations in the jaws and dental apparatus are prominent in the fossil record. Form-function relationships at this level are controlled genetically and, though important for a general understanding of the human condition, have little to do with any individual's deviation from the current norm.

Form-function relationships during the lifetime of an individual may be significant in the etiology of malocclusion. Although the changes in body form are minimal, it is clear that an individual who does heavy physical work as an adolescent has both heavier and stronger muscles and a sturdier skeletal system than an individual who is sedentary. As noted in the introduction to this chapter, one theory for the modern increase in malocclusion is that jaws do not grow as much now because there is less functional demand from the soft modern diet. If the amount of function could affect the growth of the jaws in an individual, altered function could be a major cause of malocclusion. In addition, chewing exercises and other forms of physical therapy should be an important part of orthodontic treatment. On the other hand, if the pattern and amount of growth for any individual are largely controlled genetically, altering jaw function would have little if any impact, etiologically or therapeutically.

The pioneer orthodontists of 50 and 100 years ago were strong believers in function as a determinant of dental facial development. Practitioners of the mid-twentieth century, heavily influenced by the genetic discoveries during their professional lifetime, almost totally rejected the idea of functional influences on the jaws and dentition. At present, every shade of opinion on this subject has its vocal exponents, and the unsurprising result is that widely varying treatment methods are proposed. Because of the importance of the controversy in contemporary orthodontics, particular emphasis is placed here on evaluating the potential functional contributions to the etiology of malocclusion.

■ Equilibrium Theory and Development of the Dental Occlusion

Equilibrium theory, as applied in engineering, states that an object subjected to unequal forces will be accelerated and thereby will move to a different position in space (Fig. 5-16). It follows, therefore, that if any object is subjected to a set of forces but remains in the same position, those forces must be in balance or equilibrium. From this perspective, the dentition is obviously in equilibrium, since the teeth are subjected to a variety of forces, but do not move to a new location under usual circumstances. Even when teeth are moving, the movements are so slow that a static equilibrium can be presumed to exist at any instant in time.

The effectiveness of orthodontic treatment is itself a demonstration that forces on the dentition are normally in equilibrium. If a tooth is subjected to a continuous force from an orthodontic appliance, it does move. From an engineering point of view, the force applied by the orthodontist has altered the previous equilibrium, resulting in tooth movement. Although the dentition is subjected to very heavy forces during function, small additional forces, if they are maintained for a long enough time, can upset the equilibrium and lead to tooth movement. The nature of the forces necessary for tooth movement is discussed in detail in Chapter 9.

Equilibrium considerations also apply to the skeleton, including the facial skeleton. Skeletal alterations in response to functional demand occur under ordinary circumstances and are magnified under unusual experimental situations. As discussed in Chapter 2, the bony processes to which muscles attach are especially influenced by the muscles and the location of the attachments. The form of the mandible, because it is largely dictated by the shape of its functional processes, is particularly prone to alteration. Size changes in the skeleton in response to function are limited to the muscular processes of the bones, but the density of the skeleton as a whole increases when heavy work is done and decreases in its absence.

Equilibrium effects on the dentition. Equilibrium effects on the dentition can be understood best by observing the effect of various types of pressures. Although one might think that force multiplied by duration would explain the effects, this is not the case. The duration of a force, because of the biologic response, is more important than its magnitude.

When heavy masticatory forces are applied to the teeth, the fluid-filled periodontal ligament acts as a shock absorber, stabilizing the tooth for an instant while alveolar bone bends and the tooth is displaced for a short distance along with the bone. If the heavy pressure is maintained for more than a few seconds, increasingly severe pain is felt, and so the biting force is related quickly. This type of heavy intermittent pressure has no impact on the long-term position of a tooth (see Chapter 9 for more detail). A number of pathologic responses to heavy intermittent occlusal contacts on a

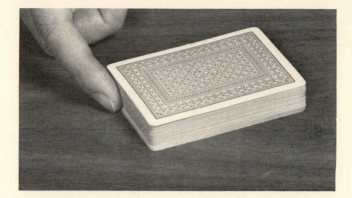

Fig. 5-16 ■ If you push lightly against a deck of cards on a table top, the cards do not move initially because there is an equilibrium between the force applied by your finger and frictional resistance. When the force of the finger exceeds the friction, however, the cards must move. Tooth movement occurs only when the equilibrium against the dentition is unbalanced.

tooth may occur, including increased mobility and pain, but as long as the periodontal apparatus is intact, forces from occlusion are rarely prolonged enough to move the tooth to a new position in which the occlusal trauma is lessened.

A second possible contributor to the equilibrium that governs tooth position is pressure from the lips, cheeks, and tongue. The pressures are much lighter than those from masticatory function, but are also much greater in duration. Experiments suggest that even very light forces are successful in moving teeth, if the force is of long enough duration.[15] The duration threshold seems to be approximately 6 hours in humans. Since the light pressures from lips, cheeks, and tongue at rest are maintained most of the time, tooth position should be affected by these soft tissue pressures.

It is easy to demonstrate that this is indeed the case. For example, if an injury to the soft tissue of the lip results in scarring and contracture, the incisors in this vicinity will be moved lingually as the lip tightens against them (Fig. 5-17). On the other hand, if restraining pressure by the lip or cheek is removed, the teeth move outward in response to unopposed pressure from the tongue (Fig. 5-18). An enlargement of the tongue from a tumor or other source will result in labial displacement of the teeth even though the lips and cheeks are intact, because the equilibrium is altered (Fig. 5-19).

These observations make it plain that, in contrast to forces from mastication, light sustained pressures from lips, cheeks, and tongue at rest are important determinants of tooth position. It seems unlikely, however, that the intermittent short-duration pressures created when the tongue and lips contact the teeth during swallowing or speaking would have any significant impact on tooth position.[16] As with masticatory forces, the pressure magnitudes would be great enough to move a tooth, but the duration is inadequate (Table 5-2).

Another possible contributor to the equilibrium could be pressures from external sources, of which various habits and orthodontic appliances would be most prominent. As an example, an orthodontic appliance that created light pressure on the inside of the dental arch might be used to expand the teeth laterally and anteriorly, creating enough space to bring all teeth into alignment. After a certain amount of arch expansion, cheek and lip pressure begins to increase. One could expect that as long as the appliance remained in place, even though it no longer exerted any active force, it would serve as a retainer to counter these increased forces. When the appliance was removed, however, the equilibrium would again be unbalanced, and the teeth would collapse lingually until a new position of balance was reached.

Whether a habit can serve in the same way as an orthodontic appliance to reposition teeth has been the subject of controversy since at least the first century AD, when Celsus recommended that a child with a crooked tooth be instructed to apply finger pressure against it so that it would be moved to its proper position. From our present understanding of equilibrium, we would expect that this would work, *if* the child kept the finger pressure against the tooth for 6 hours or more per day.

The same reasoning can be applied to other habits: if a habit like thumbsucking created pressure against the teeth for more than the threshold duration (6 hours or more per day), it certainly could move teeth (Fig. 5-20). On the other hand, if the habit had a shorter duration, even if the pressures were heavy, little or no effect would be expected. Whether a behavior pattern is essential or nonessential, innate or learned, its effect on the position of the teeth is determined not by the force that it applies to the teeth, but by how long that force is sustained.

Another possible contributor to the dental equilibrium is the periodontal fiber system, both in the gingival tissues and

Table 5-2 ■ Possible equilibrium influences: magnitude and duration of force against the teeth during function

Possible equilibrium influence	Force magnitude	Force duration
Tooth contacts		
Mastication	Very heavy	Very short
Swallowing	Light	Very short
Soft tissue pressures of lip, cheek and tongue		
Swallowing	Moderate	Short
Speaking	Light	Very short
Resting	Very light	Long
External pressures		
Habits	Moderate	Variable
Orthodontics	Moderate	Variable
Intrinsic pressures		
PDL fibers	Light	Long
Gingival fibers	Variable	Long

within the periodontal ligament. We have already noted that if a tooth is lost, the space tends to close, in part because of force created by the trans-septal fibers in the gingiva. The importance of this force has been demonstrated experimentally in monkeys by extracting a tooth and then making repeated incisions in the gingiva so that the trans-septal fiber network is disrupted and cannot reestablish continuity. Space closure is almost completely abolished under these circumstances.[17]

The same gingival fiber network stretches elastically dur-

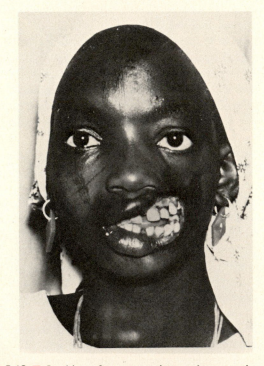

Fig. 5-18 ■ In this unfortunate patient, a large portion of the cheek has been lost because of a tropical infection. The outward splaying of the teeth when the restraining force of the cheek is lost illustrates the effect of a change in equilibrium. (From Moss, J.P., and Picton, D.C.A.: Arch. Oral Biol. **12:**1313-1320, 1967.)

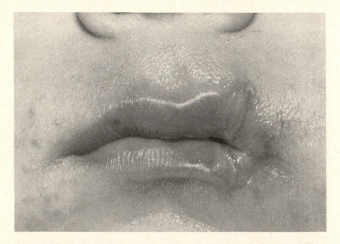

Fig. 5-17 ■ Scarring of the corner of the mouth in this child is related to a burn suffered at an early age from biting an electrical cord. From equilibrium theory, one would expect a distortion in the form of the dental arch in the region of the contracting scar, and exactly this occurs.

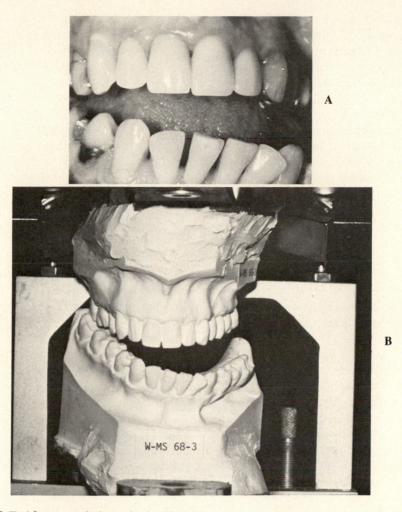

Fig. 5-19 ■ After a paralytic stroke in this patient, the side of the tongue rested against the mandibular left posterior teeth. **A,** Intraoral view; **B,** casts mounted on an articulator. The extreme displacement of teeth in this adult resulted from the increased tongue pressure, altering the equilibrium. (Courtesy Dr. T. Wallen).

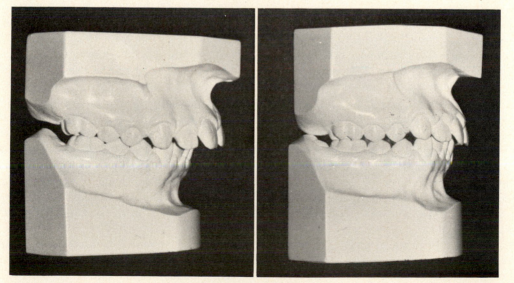

Fig. 5-20 ■ Dental casts from 11-year-old identical twins, one of whom (**A**) continued to suck her thumb several hours per day while the other (**B**) stopped at age 6. Displacement of the anterior teeth and narrowing of the arch in the thumbsucker are obvious. (Courtesy Dr. T. Wallen).

ing orthodontic treatment and tends to pull the teeth back toward their original position.[18] Clinical experience has shown that, after orthodontic treatment, it is often wise to make gingival incisions that sever the stretched trans-septal fibers, and then allow them to heal with the teeth properly aligned, to eliminate this force (see Chapter 17). In the absence of a space created by extraction or orthodontic tooth movement, however, the gingival fibers network apparently has minimal effects on the dental equilibrium.

Exactly how the eruption mechanism works is still not completely understood, but it seems clear now that the eruptive force is generated within the periodontal ligament. This force is large enough and sustained enough to move a tooth. It seems likely that the same metabolic activity can and does produce forces that serve as a part of ''active stabilization'' for teeth, directly contributing to the equilibrium. The extent to which this occurs in teeth that are not erupting is not known. It is known, however, that the eruption mechanism remains at least potentially active throughout life, since a tooth can begin to erupt again many years after eruptive movements have apparently ceased, if its antagonist is extracted. Thus there is at least the potential for metabolic activity in the periodontal ligament to affect equilibrium.

Consideration of eruptive forces leads to a final aspect of the dental equilibrium: the effect of forces against the teeth must be considered, not only in the antero-posterior and transverse planes of space that relate to the position of a tooth within the arch, but also vertically in relation to how much or how little a tooth erupts. The vertical position of any tooth, of course, is determined by the equilibrium between the forces that produce eruption and those that oppose it. Forces from mastication are the primary ones opposing eruption, but lighter, more sustained forces from soft tissues such as the tongue interposed between the teeth probably are more important, just as they are for the horizontal equilibrium.

As we will discuss more fully, it appears that malocclusions related to function are characterized more by vertical malposition of teeth, as in anterior open bite, than by malalignment or horizontal jaw discrepancies. The vertical equilibrium, in short, is an important part of the total equilibrium picture.[19]

Equilibrium effects on jaw size and shape. The jaws can be thought of as consisting of a core of bone to which functional processes are attached. The functional processes of bones will be altered if the function is lost or changed. For example, the bone of the alveolar process exists only to support the teeth. If a tooth fails to erupt, alveolar bone never forms in that area, and if a tooth is extracted, the alveolus resorbs after the extraction until finally the alveolar ridge completely atrophies. When one of a pair of opposing teeth is extracted, the other usually begins to erupt again, and even as bone is resorbing in one jaw where the tooth was lost, new alveolar bone forms in the other as the erupting tooth brings bone with it. The position of the tooth, not the functional loads on it, determines the shape of the alveolar ridge.

The same is true for the muscular processes: the location of the muscle attachments is more important in determining bone shape than mechanical loading or degree of activity. Growth of the muscle, however, determines the position of the attachment, and so muscle growth can produce a change in shape of the jaw, particularly at the angle of the mandible (see Chapter 3 for examples). The extent of muscular activity has little or no impact on morphology, but is reflected in the density of the bone. Powerful biting forces translate not into a mandible with significantly altered morphology, but into greater density as observed on x-ray films.

If the condylar processes of the mandible can be considered functional processes, as apparently they can, the intriguing possibility is raised that altering the position of the mandible might alter mandibular growth. The idea that holding the mandible forward or pressing it backward would change its growth has been accepted, rejected, and partially accepted again during the past century. Obviously, this theory has important implication for the etiology of malocclusion. If a child positions his mandible forward on closure because of interferences with the incisor teeth or because the tongue is large, will this stimulate the mandible to grow larger and ultimately produce a Class III malocclusion? Would allowing a young child to sleep on the stomach, so that the weight of the head rested on the chin, cause underdevelopment of the mandible and a Class II malocclusion?

The effect of force duration is not as clear for equilibrium effects on the jaws as for the teeth. It appears, however, that the same principle applies: the magnitude of force is less important than its duration. Positioning the jaw forward only when the teeth are brought into occlusion means that most of the time, when the mandible is in its rest position, there is no protrusion. We would expect no effects on a functional process from repeated intermittent force because of the short total duration, and the condylar process seems to respond in accordance with this principle. Neither experimental nor clinical evidence suggests that mandibular growth is any different because of occlusal interferences (though it should be kept in mind that tooth eruption, and thereby the final position of the teeth, can be altered).

If the mandible is protruded at all times, as might well be the case if the tongue is large, the duration threshold should be surpassed, and growth effects might be observed. It does appear that individuals with a large tongue have a well-developed mandible. A change in tongue morphology, as from thyroid deficiency, may contribute to excessive growth of the mandible to some people (Fig. 5-21). This is unlikely to be a major cause of mandibular prognathism.

Although it was widely believed 50 years ago that pressures against the mandible from various habits, particularly sleeping on the stomach, interfered with growth and caused Class II malocclusion, little or no evidence supports this contention. Growth of the soft tissue matrix that moves the mandible forward and creates a space between the condyle and the temporal fossa is the normal mechanism by which growth occurs, but inhibition of mandibular growth by pres-

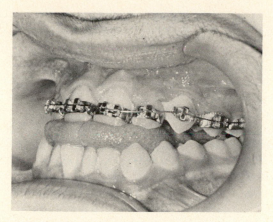

Fig. 5-21 ■ A large tongue, as in this patient with a history of thyroid deficiency from infancy onward, may contribute to the development of mandibular prognathism by causing the mandible to be positioned forward at all times.

sure is not a feature of normal development and is much harder to achieve, if indeed it is possible at all.

From the perspective of equilibrium theory, then, we can conclude that intermittent pressures or forces have little if any effect on either the position of the teeth or the size and shape of the jaws. Density of bone in the alveolar process and throughout the basal areas of the jaws should differ as a function of masticatory forces, but shape should not. Neither masticatory forces nor soft tissue pressures during swallowing and speaking should have any major influence on tooth position.

Major equilibrium influences for the teeth should be the light but long-lasting pressures from tongue, lips, and cheeks at rest. In addition, significant equilibrium effects should be expected from the elasticity of gingival fibers and from metabolic activity within the periodontal ligament (see Table 5-2). These equilibrium influences would affect the vertical as well as horizontal position of the teeth and could have a profound effect on how much tooth eruption occurred as well as where a tooth was positioned within the dental arch. The major equilibrium influences on the jaws should be positional changes affecting the functional processes, including the condylar process.

In the remainder of this section, functional patterns and habits that might produce malocclusion are examined as potential etiologic agents from the perspective of equilibrium theory.

■ Functional Influences on Dentofacial Development

Sucking and other habits. Although almost all normal children engage in non-nutritive sucking, prolonged sucking habits can lead to malocclusion. As a general rule, sucking habits during the primary dentition years have little if any long-term effect. If these habits persist beyond the time that the permanent teeth begin to erupt, however, malocclusion characterized by flared and spaced maxillary incisors, lingually positioned lower incisors, anterior open bite, and a

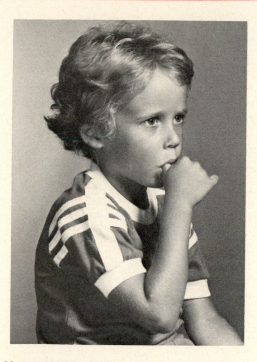

Fig. 5-22 ■ A child sucking his thumb usually places it as shown here, causing pressure that pushes the lower incisors lingually and the upper incisors labially. In addition, the jaw is positioned downward, providing additional opportunity for posterior teeth to erupt, and cheek pressure is increased while the tongue is lowered vertically away from the maxillary posterior teeth, altering the equilibrium that controls width dimensions. If the thumb is placed asymmetrically, the symmetry of the arch may be affected.

narrow upper arch is the likely result. The characteristic malocclusion associated with sucking arises from a combination of direct pressure on the teeth and an alteration in the pattern of resting cheek and lip pressures.

When a child places a thumb or finger between the teeth, it is usually positioned at an angle so that it presses lingually against the lower incisors and labially against the upper incisors (Fig. 5-22). This direct pressure is presumably responsible for the displacement of the incisors. There can be considerable variation in which teeth are affected and how much, depending on which teeth are contacted. How much the teeth are displaced should correlate better with the number of hours per day of sucking than with the magnitude of the pressure. Children who suck vigorously but intermittently may not displace the incisors much if at all, whereas others who produce 6 hours or more of pressure, particularly those who sleep with a thumb or finger between the teeth all night, can cause a significant malocclusion.

The anterior open bite associated with thumbsucking arises by a combination of interference with normal eruption of incisors and excessive eruption of posterior teeth. When a thumb or finger is placed between the anterior teeth, the mandible must be positioned downward to accommodate it. The interposed thumb directly impedes incisor eruption. At the same time, the separation of the jaws alters the vertical equilibrium on the posterior teeth, and as a result, there is more eruption of posterior teeth than might otherwise have occurred. Because of the geometry of the jaws, 1 mm of elongation posteriorly opens the bite about 2 mm anteriorly, so this can be a powerful contributor to the development of anterior open bite (Fig. 5-23).

Although negative pressure is created within the mouth during sucking, there is no reason to believe that this is responsible for the constriction of the maxillary arch that usually accompanies sucking habits. Instead, it seems reasonably clear that the maxillary arch fails to develop in width because of an alteration in the balance between cheek and tongue pressures. If the thumb is placed between the teeth, the tongue must be lowered, which decreases pressure by the tongue against the lingual of upper posterior teeth. At the same time, cheek pressure against these teeth is increased as the buccinator muscle contracts during sucking (Fig. 5-24). Cheek pressures are greatest at the corners of the mouth, and this probably explains why the maxillary arch tends to become V-shaped, with more constriction across the canines than the molars.

Sucking habits can be a powerful contributor to malocclusion, but sucking by itself does not create a severe malocclusion unless a long-duration habit persists well into the mixed dentition years. Mild displacement of the primary incisor teeth is often noted in 3- or 4-year-old children, but if sucking stops at this stage, normal lip and cheek pressures soon restore the teeth to their usual position. If the habit persists after the permanent incisors begin to erupt, orthodontic treatment may be necessary to overcome the resulting tooth displacements. The constricted maxillary arch is the aspect of the malocclusion least likely to correct spontaneously. In many children, if the maxillary arch is expanded transversely, both the incisor protrusion and anterior open bite will improve spontaneously (see Chapter 13). There is no point in beginning orthodontic therapy, of course, until the habit has stopped.

Many other habits have been indicted as causes of malocclusion. As noted previously, a "sleeping habit" in which the weight of the head rested on the chin once was thought to be a major cause of Class II malocclusion. Facial asymmetries have been attributed to always sleeping on one side of the face or even to "leaning habits," as when an inattentive child leans the side of his face against one hand to doze without falling out of the classroom chair.

Contemporary research makes it plain that it is not nearly as easy to distort the basic form of the facial skeleton as these views implied. Sucking habits often exceed the time threshold necessary to produce an effect on the teeth, but even prolonged sucking has little impact on the underlying form of the jaws. On close analysis most other habits have such a short duration that dental effects, much less skeletal effects, are unlikely.

Tongue thrusting. Much attention has been paid at various times to the tongue and tongue habits as possible etiologic factors in malocclusion. The possible deleterious effects of "tongue thrust swallowing" (Fig. 5-25), defined as placement of the tongue tip forward between the incisors during swallowing, received particular emphasis in the 1950s and 1960s.

Laboratory studies indicate that individuals who place the tongue tip forward usually do not have more tongue force against the teeth than those who keep the tongue tip back; in fact, tongue pressure may be lower.[20] The term "tongue thrust" is therefore something of a misnomer, since it implies that the tongue is forcefully thrust forward. Swallowing is not a learned behavior, but is integrated and controlled physiologically at subconscious levels, so whatever the pattern of swallow, it cannot be considered a habit in the usual sense. It is true, however, that individuals with an anterior open bite malocclusion place their tongue between the anterior teeth when they swallow while those who have a

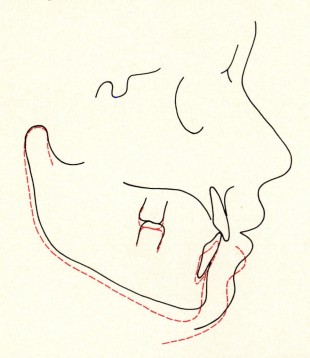

Fig. 5-23 ■ Cepalometric tracing showing the effects of posterior eruption on the extent of anterior opening. The only difference between the red and black tracings is that the first molars have been elongated 2 mm in the red one. Note that the result is 4 mm of separation of the incisors, because of the geometry of the jaw.

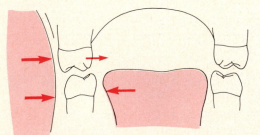

Fig. 5-24 ■ Diagrammatic representation of soft tissue pressures in the molar region in a child with a sucking habit. As the tongue is lowered and the cheeks contract during sucking, the pressure balance against the upper teeth is altered, and the upper but not the lower molars are displaced lingually.

normal incisor relationship usually do not, and it is tempting to blame the open bite problem on this pattern of tongue activity.

Maturation of oral activities including swallowing has been discussed in some detail in Chapter 3. The mature or adult swallow pattern appears in some normal children as early as age 3, but is not present in the majority until about age 6 and is never achieved in 10% to 15% of a typical population.[21] The infantile swallow is characterized by placement of the tongue between the gum ridges, in contact with the lower lip. Tongue thrust swallowing in older patients superficially resembles the infantile swallow, and sometimes children or adults who place the tongue between the anterior teeth are spoken of as having a retained infantile swallow. This is clearly incorrect. Only brain damaged children retain a truly infantile swallow in which the posterior part of the tongue has little or no role.

Since coordinated movements of the posterior tongue and elevation of the mandible tend to develop before protrusion of the tongue tip between the incisor teeth disappears, what is called ''tongue thrusting'' in young children is often a normal transitional stage in swallowing. During the transition from an infantile to a mature swallow, a child can be expected to pass through a stage in which the swallow is characterized by muscular activity to bring the lips together, separation of the posterior teeth, and forward protrusion of the tongue between the teeth. This is also a description of the classic tongue thrust swallow. A delay in the normal swallow transition can be expected when a child has a sucking habit.

When there is an anterior open bite, as often occurs from sucking habits, it is more difficult to seal off the front of the mouth during swallowing to prevent food or liquids from escaping. Bringing the lips together and placing the tongue between the separated anterior teeth is a successful maneu-ver to form an anterior seal, closing off the front of the mouth. When there is an open bite, in other words. a tongue thrust swallow is a necessary physiologic adaptation. Nearly every patient with an open bite also has a tongue thrust swallow. The reverse is not true—a tongue thrust swallow is often present in children with good anterior occlusion. After a sucking habit stops, the anterior open bite tends to close spontaneously, but the position of the tongue between the anterior teeth persists for a while as the open bite closes. Until the open bite disappears, an anterior seal by the tongue tip remains necessary.

The modern viewpoint is, in short, that the presence of an anterior open bite conditions a child (or adult) to place the tongue between the anterior teeth as a necessary physiologic adaptation. Anterior tongue placement, therefore, should be considered the result of anterior open bite, not its cause. It follows, of course, that therapy to alter the way a child swallows in unwarranted. If the tongue tip position during swallow is an adaptation to the position of the teeth rather than the other way around, correcting the tooth position by orthodontic treatment should cause a change in swallow pattern, and this usually happens.

This is not to say that the tongue has no etiologic role in the development of open bite malocclusion. From equilibrium theory, light but sustained pressures by the tongue against the teeth would be expected to have significant effects, and it is easy to demonstrate that such effects occur. Tongue thrust swallowing simply has too short a duration to have an impact on tooth position. Pressure by the tongue against the teeth during a typical swallow lasts for approximately 1 second. A typical individual swallows about 800 times per day while awake, but has only a few swallows per hour while asleep. The total per day, therefore, is usually under 1000. One thousand seconds of pressure, of course, totals only a few minutes, not nearly enough to affect the equilibrium.

On the other hand, if a patient with a tongue thrust swallow also has a forward resting posture of the tongue, the change in the pattern of resting pressures might affect tooth position, vertically or horizontally. Tongue tip protrusion during swallowing is sometimes associated with an alteration in tongue posture. If the position from which tongue movements start is different from normal, so that the pattern of resting pressures is different, there is likely to be an effect on the teeth, whereas if the postural position is normal, the tongue thrust swallow has no clinical significance.

Perhaps this point can best be put in perspective by comparing the number of children who have an anterior open bite malocclusion with the number of children of the same age reported to have a tongue thrust swallow. As Fig. 5-26 shows, at every age above 6, the number of children reported to have a tongue thrust swallow is about 10 times greater than the number reported to have an anterior open bite. Thus, there is no reason to believe that a tongue thrust swallow always implies an altered rest position and will lead to malocclusion. The odds are approximately 10 to 1 that

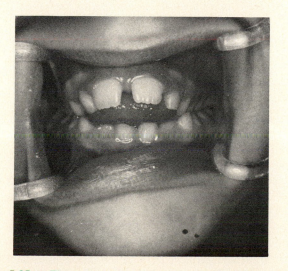

Fig. 5-25 ■ The typical appearance of a ''tongue thrust swallow,'' with the tongue tip between the incisors protruding forward to put in contact with the elevated lower lip.

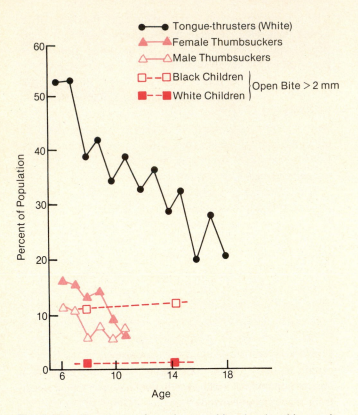

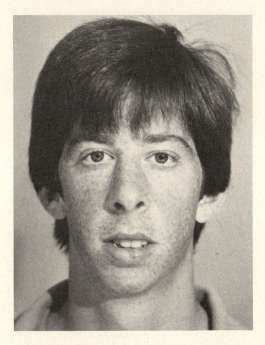

Fig. 5-26 ■ Prevalence of anterior open bite, thumbsucking, and tongue thrust swallowing as a function of age. Open bite occurs much more frequently in blacks than in whites. Note that the prevalence of anterior open bite at any age is only a small fraction of the prevalence of tongue thrust swallowing and is also less than the prevalence of thumbsucking. (Data from Fletcher, S.G., et al.: J. Speech Hear. Disord. **26**:201-208, 1961, Kelly, J.E., et al.: DHEW Pub. No. [HRA] 77-144, 1977.)

Fig. 5-27 ■ The classic ''adenoid facies,'' consisting of narrow width dimensions, protruding teeth, and lips separated at rest, has often been attributed to mouth breathing. Since it is perfectly possible to breathe through the nose with the lips separated, simply by creating an oral seal posteriorly with the soft palate, the facial appearance is not diagnostic of the respiratory mode. On careful study, many of these patients are found not to be obligatory mouth breathers.

this is not the case for any given child. In a child who has an open bite, tongue posture may be a factor, but the swallow itself is not.

Mouth breathing. Mouth breathing has also been in and out of vogue as a possible etiologic factor for malocclusion. Because respiratory needs are the primary determinant of the posture of the jaws and tongue (and of the head itself, to a lesser extent), it seems entirely reasonable that mouth breathing could cause different head, jaw, and tongue posture, which would then alter the equilibrium and affect both jaw growth and tooth position.

All humans are primarily nasal breathers, but everyone breathes through the mouth under certain physiologic conditions, the most prominent being an increased need for air during exercise. For the average individual, there is a transition to partial oral breathing when ventilatory exchange rates above 35 to 40 liters per minute are reached.[22] At maximum effort, 60 to 80 liters of air per minute are needed, about half of which is obtained through the mouth.

During resting conditions, greater effort is required to breathe through the nose than through the mouth—the tortuous nasal passages introduce an element of resistance to

airflow as they perform their function of warming and humidifying the inspired air. The increased work for nasal respiration is physiologically acceptable up to a point. If the nose is partially obstructed, the work increases, and at a certain level of resistance to nasal airflow, the individual switches to mouth breathing. This crossover point varies among individuals, but is usually reached at resistance levels of about 3.5 to 4.0 cm H_2O/liter/minute.[23]

The nasal inflammation accompanying a common cold occasionally converts all of us to mouth breathing by this mechanism. Chronic respiratory obstruction can be produced by prolonged inflammation of the nasal mucosa associated with allergies or chronic infection. It can also be produced by mechanical obstruction anywhere within the nasal passages. Since the pharyngeal tonsils or adenoids normally are large in children, partial obstruction from this source may contribute to mouth breathing in children. Individuals who have had chronic nasal obstruction may continue to breathe partially through the mouth even after the obstruction has been relieved. In this sense, mouth breathing can sometimes be considered a habit.

To breathe through the mouth, one must open up and

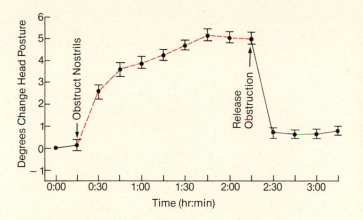

Fig. 5-28 ■ Data from an experiment with dental students, showing the immediate change in head posture when the nostrils are totally blocked: the head tips back about 5 degrees, increasing the separation of the jaws. When the obstruction is relieved, head posture returns to its original position. (From Vig, P.S., et al.[23]: Am. J. Orthod. **77**:258-268, 1980.)

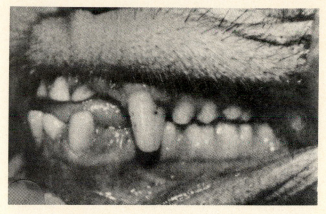

Fig. 5-29 ■ Malocclusion in a monkey who underwent several months of total nasal obstruction during growth. Note the mandibular prognathism, the most common response in this series of experiments. (From Harvold, E.P., et al.: Am. J. Orthod. **79**:359-372, 1981.)

maintain an oral airway. Three changes in posture are needed to accomplish this: lowering the mandible, positioning the tongue downward and forward, and extending (tipping back) the head. Like any other functional cause of malocclusion, mouth breathing would be expected to produce malocclusion, if indeed it did so, by its effects on equilibrium. These postural changes could affect vertical and horizontal positions of the teeth and perhaps could influence the growth of the jaws to a lesser extent.

The type of malocclusion most often associated with mouth breathing is called ''skeletal open bite'' or the ''long face syndrome.'' Diagnostic criteria are discussed in detail in Chapter 6. Briefly, in this condition, there is a downward and backward rotation of the mandible during growth (illustrated in Chapter 4). This is accompanied by excessive eruption of the posterior teeth, a tendency toward maxillary constriction, excessive overjet, and an anterior open bite. The association has been noted for many years: the descriptive term ''adenoid facies'' has appeared in the English literature for at least a century, probably longer (Fig. 5-27). At first glance, this distortion of normal growth appears to be exactly what should result from the postural adaptations if they persisted over a long period of time. Fortunately or unfortunately, the relationship between mouth breathing, altered posture, and the development of malocclusion is not so clearcut. Recent experimental studies with monkeys and human patients have only partially clarified the situation.

Experiments with human subjects have shown that a change in posture does accompany nasal obstruction.[24] For instance, when the nose is completely blocked, there is an immediate change of about 5 degrees in the craniovertebral angle (Fig. 5-28). The jaws move apart, as much by elevation of the maxilla because the head tips back, as by depression of the mandible. In the experiments, when the nasal obstruction is removed, the original posture immediately returns. This physiologic response occurs to the same extent, however, in individuals who already have some nasal obstruction, which indicates that it may not totally result from respiratory demands.

Experiments with growing monkeys show that totally obstructing the nostrils for a prolonged period in this species does lead to the development of malocclusion, but not of the type commonly associated with mouth breathing in humans.[25] Instead, the monkeys tend to develop some degree of mandibular prognathism, although their response shows considerable variety (Fig. 5-29). Placing a block in the roof of a monkey's mouth, which forces a downward position of the tongue and mandible, also produces a variety of malocclusions. It seems clear that altered posture is the mechanism by which growth changes were produced. The variety of responses in the monkeys suggests that the type of malocclusion is determined by the individual animal's pattern of adaptation.

In evaluating these experiments, it must be kept in mind that mouth breathing of any extent is completely unnatural for monkeys, who will die if the nasal passages are obstructed abruptly. To carry out the experiments, it was necessary to gradually obstruct their noses, giving the animals a chance to learn how to survive as mouth breathers. Total nasal obstruction is also extremely rare in humans, for whom partial obstruction is the potentially important etiologic agent.

A major problem in studying the effect of mouth breathing in humans is knowing what the pattern of respiration really is at any given time. How can you tell who is a mouth breather? How much do you have to breathe through your mouth to be classified a mouth breather? Human observers tend to equate lip separation at rest with mouth breathing (Fig. 5-27), but this is simply not correct. It is perfectly possible for an individual to breathe through the nose while the lips are apart. To do this, it is only necessary to seal off the mouth by placing the tongue against the palate. Since some lip separation at rest (lip incompetence) is normal in children, many children who appear to be mouth breathers may not be.

Simple clinical tests for mouth breathing can also be misleading. The highly vascular nasal mucosa undergoes cycles of engorgement with blood and shrinkage. The cycles alternate between the two nostrils: when one is clear, the other is at least slightly obstructed. For this reason, clinical tests to determine whether the patient can breathe freely through both nostrils nearly always show negative results. One partially obstructed nostril should not be interpreted as a problem with normal nasal breathing.

Instrumentation that simultaneously measures the nasal and oral airflow is required to accurately establish the percentage of nasal compared to oral respiration.[26] It seems obvious that a certain percentage of oral respiration, maintained for a certain percentage of the time, should be the definition of significant mouth breathing. The necessary measurements are just beginning to be made. At this point,

the information to define what mouth breathing really is, or what percentage of mouth breathing makes a difference, is simply not available. Total nasal obstruction is so rare in humans that knowing that this condition may create a malocclusion is of little value. It is partial, not total, mouth breathing that must be evaluated as an etiologic agent.

The best present data for the effects of partial nasal obstruction are based on Linder-Aronson's studies of Swedish children who underwent adenoidectomy. It seems reasonable to presume that a child who requires adenoidectomy for medical purposes does have some degree of nasal obstruction, although this condition was not evaluated directly. The Swedish data show that children in the adenoidectomy group had a significantly longer anterior face height than control children (Fig. 5-30). They also had a tendency toward maxillary constriction and more upright incisors.[27] Furthermore, when children in the adenoidectomy group were followed after their treatment, they tended to return toward the mean of the control group, though the differences persisted[28] (Fig. 5-31). Although the differences were statistically significant, they were not large. Face height on the average was about 3 mm greater in the adenoidectomy group. Earlier English workers indicated that the percentage of children with various malocclusions was about the same in a group being seen in an ear, nose, and throat clinic as in controls without respiratory problems.[29]

Another line of evidence allowing some evaluation of the relationship of mouth breathing to the long-face pattern of dentofacial deformity comes from examination of older patients needing surgical-orthondontic treatment. In a group with severe long-face problems studied at North Carolina, approximately one-third had increased nasal resistance, while two-thirds fell into the normal range[30] (Fig. 5-32).

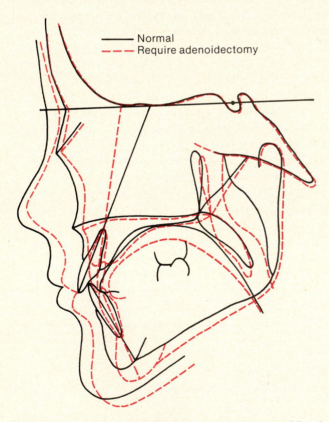

Fig. 5-30 ■ Average cephalometric tracings for a group of Swedish children requiring adenoidectomy for medical purposes, compared to a group of normal controls. The adenoidectomy group had statistically significantly greater anterior face height and steeper mandibular plane angles than the controls, but the differences were quantitatively not large. (From Linder-Aronson, S.: Acta Otolaryngol. Scand. [Supp. 265], 1970.)

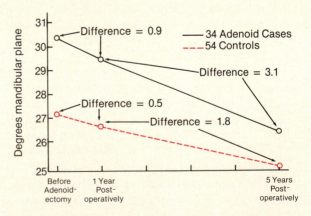

Fig. 5-31 ■ Comparison of mandibular plane angles in a group of postadenoidectomy children compared to normal controls. Note that the differences existing at the time of adenoidectomy decreased in size but did not totally disappear. (From Linder-Aronson, S.: In Cook, J.T., editor: Transactions of the Third International Orthodontic Congress. St. Louis, 1975, The C.V. Mosby Co.)

This finding does not, of course, provide any evidence on the actual mode of breathing, since these patients with normal resistance may have been breathing through the mouth even though there was nothing to keep them from breathing through the nose. There was nothing to indicate, however, that the majority of these patients had nasal obstruction. It appears that the long face pattern of deformity does occur in patients who have no problems with nasal respiration.

It simply will not be possible to unravel the relationship between mouth breathing and malocclusion until careful studies using the new instruments to quantify the nasal/oral respiratory ratio can be carried out. The postural changes associated with a degree of nasal obstruction can alter the equilibrium, and this change could either predispose an individual to malocclusion or accentuate an existing tendency. Posturing the mandible downward allows excessive eruption of posterior teeth, and low tongue posture changes the balance of labial and lingual forces on the upper teeth in a way that tends to constrict the upper arch.

It is thus easy to understand Linder-Aronson's results of changes in face height and arch width in the Swedish group and relate them to equilibrium disturbances, but it is important to note the small magnitude of the change. The alterations in posture associated with partial nasal obstruction are not great enough by themselves to create a major deformity. Mouth breathing, in short, can undoubtedly contribute to the development of orthodontic problems but partial nasal obstruction is difficult to indict as a major etiologic agent.

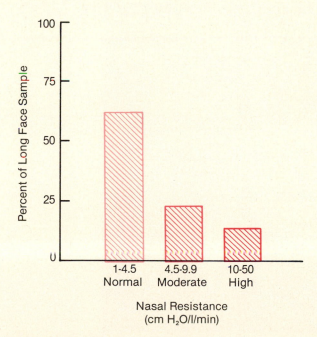

Fig. 5-32 ■ Nasal resistance values in a group of adult long face patients who were evaluated for possible orthognathic surgery. About two-thirds of this group had normal nasal resistance, while one-third had elevated values, some extremely so. (From Turvey, T.A., et al.: Am. J. Orthod. **85**:109-114, 1984.)

■ *Etiology in Contemporary Perspective*

■ Environment versus Heredity as Etiologic Factors

Part of the philosophy of the early orthodontists was their belief in the perfectability of man. Edward Angle and his contemporaries, influenced by the romanticized view of primitive peoples commonly held 100 years ago, took it for granted that malocclusion was a disease of civilization and blamed it on improper function of the jaws under the "degenerate" modern conditions. Classical (Mendelian) genetics developed rapidly in the first part of the twentieth century, and a different view of malocclusion gradually replaced the earlier one. This was that malocclusion is primarily the result of inherited dentofacial proportions, which may be altered somewhat by developmental variations, trauma, or altered function, but which are basically established at conception. A strong influence of inheritance on facial features is obvious at a glance—it is easy to recognize familial tendencies in the tilt of the nose, the shape of the jaw, and the look of the smile.

It is also apparent that certain types of malocclusion run in families. The Hapsburg jaw, the prognathic mandible of the German royal family, is the best known example, but dentists see repeated instances of similar malocclusions in parents and their offspring. The pertinent question for the etiology of malocclusion is not whether there are inherited influences on the jaws and teeth, because obviously there are, but whether malocclusion is often caused by inherited characteristics.

Malocclusion could be produced by inherited characteristics in two major possible ways. The first would be an inherited disporportion between the size of the teeth and the size of the jaws, which would produce crowding or spacing. The second possibility would be an inherited disproportion between size or shape of the upper and lower jaws, which would cause improper occlusal relationships. The more independently these characteristics are determined, the more likely that disproportions could be inherited. In that circumstance, a child could inherit large teeth but a small jaw, for instance, or a large upper jaw and a small lower one. Conversely, if dentofacial characteristics tended to be linked, an inherited mismatch of this type would be unlikely.

Primitive human populations in which malocclusion is less frequent than in modern groups are characterized by genetic isolation and uniformity. If everyone in a group carries the same genetic information for tooth size and jaw size, there would be no possibility of a child inheriting discordant characteristics. In the absence of processed food, one would expect strong selection pressure for traits that produced good masticatory function. Genes that introduced disturbances into the masticatory system would tend to be eliminated from the population (unless they conferred some other advantage). The result should be exactly what is seen in primitive populations: individuals in whom tooth size–

jaw size discrepancies are infrequent, and groups in which everyone tends to have the same jaw relationship. Different human groups have developed impressive variations in facial proportions and jaw relationships. What happens, then, when there is outbreeding between originally distinct human population groups?

One of the characteristics of civilization is the collection of large groups of people into urban centers, where the opportunities for mating outside one's own small population group are greatly magnified. If an inherited disproportion of the functional components of the face and jaws were possible, one would predict that modern urban populations would have a high prevalence of malocclusion and a great variety of orthodontic problems. The United States, reflecting its role as a ''genetic melting pot,'' should have one of the world's highest rates of malocclusion—which it does. From the perspective of the 1930s and 1940s, with the new knowledge of genetics, it would be tempting to conclude that the great increase in outbreeding that occurred as human populations grew and became more mobile, is the major explanation for the increase in malocclusion in recent years.

This view of malocclusion as primarily a genetic problem was greatly strengthened by breeding experiments with animals carried out in the 1930s. By far the most influential individual in this regard was Professor Stockard, who methodically cross-bred dogs and recorded the interesting effects on body structure.[31] Present-day dogs, of course, come in a tremendous variety of breeds and sizes. What would happen if one crossed a Boston terrier with a collie? Might the offspring have the collie's long, pointed lower jaw and the terrier's diminutive upper jaw? Could unusual crowding or spacing result because the teeth of one breed were combined in the offspring with the jaw of the other? Stockard's experiments indicated that dramatic malocclusions did occur in his cross-bred dogs, more from jaw discrepancies than from tooth size–jaw size imbalances (Fig. 5-33). These experiments seemed to confirm that independent inheritance of facial characteristics could be a major cause of malocclusion and that the rapid increase in malocclusion accompanying urbanization was probably the result of increased outbreeding.

The classic dog experiments, it turns out, are misleading because many breeds of small dogs carry the gene for achondroplasia. Animals or humans affected by this condition have deficient growth of cartilage. The result is extremely short extremities and an underdeveloped midface. The dachshund is the classic achondroplastic dog, but most terriers and bulldogs also carry this gene. Achrondroplasia is an autosomal dominant trait. Like many dominant genes, the gene for achondroplasia sometimes has only partial penetrance, meaning simply that the trait will be expressed more dramatically in some individuals than in others. It appears that most of the unusual malocclusions produced in Stockard's breeding experiments can be explained, not on

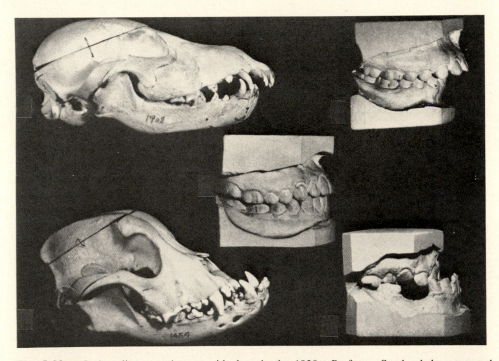

Fig. 5-33 ■ In breeding experiments with dogs in the 1930s, Professor Stockard demonstrated that severe malocclusions could be developed by crossing morphologically different breeds. His analogy to human malocclusion was a powerful influence in the rejection of the prevailing belief of the 1920s that improper jaw function caused malocclusion. (From Stockard, C.R., and Johnson, A.L.: Genetic and Endocrinic Basis for Differences in Form and Behavior. Philadelphia, 1941, The Wistar Institute of Anatomy and Biology, pp. 149-205.)

the basis of inherited jaw size, but by the extent to which achondroplasia was expressed in that animal.

Achondroplasia is rare in humans, but it does occur, and it produces the expected changes (Fig. 5-34). In addition to short limbs, the cranial base does not lengthen normally because of the deficient growth at the synchondroses, the maxilla is not translated forward to the normal extent, and a relative midface deficiency occurs. In a number of rela-

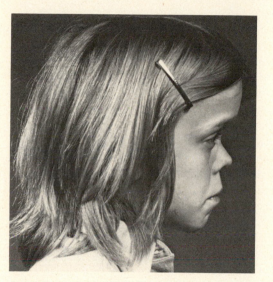

Fig. 5-34 ■ Characteristic facial appearance in an individual with achondroplasia. Note the deficient midface, particularly at the bridge of the nose. This results from decreased growth of cartilage in the cranial base, with a resulting lack of forward translation of the maxilla.

tively rare genetic syndromes like achondroplasia, influences on the form of the face, jaws, and teeth can be discerned, but those cause only a very small percentage of orthodontic problems.

A careful examination of the results of outbreeding in human populations also casts doubt on the hypothesis that independently inherited tooth and jaw characteristics are a major cause of malocclusion. The best data are probably from investigations carried out in Hawaii by Chung et al.[32] Before its discovery by the European explorers of the eighteenth century, Hawaii had a homogeneous Polynesian population. These people have large stature, broad and well developed jaws, and an unusual and distinctive form of the lower jaw, the "rocker jaw" (Fig. 5-35). Large scale migration to the islands by northern European and Chinese and Japanese groups has resulted in an exceptionally heterogeneous modern population. Tooth size, jaw size, and jaw proportions are rather different for the Polynesian, Oriental, and European contributors to the Hawaiian melting pot. If tooth and jaw characteristics were inherited independently, a high prevalence of severe malocclusion would be expected in this population.

In fact, the prevalence and type of malocclusion in the current Hawaiian population, though greater than the prevalence of malocclusion in the original populations, does not support this concept. The effects of interracial crosses appear to be more additive than multiplicative. For example, about 10% of the Chinese who migrated to Hawaii had Class III malocclusion, while about 10% of the Polynesians had crowded teeth. The offspring of this cross seem to have about a 10% prevalence of each characteristic, but there is

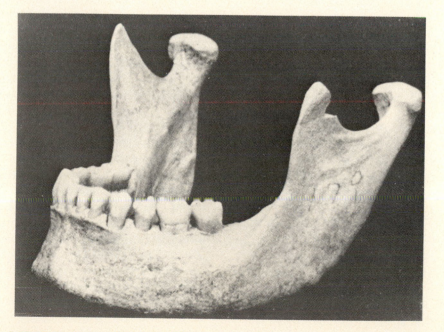

Fig. 5-35 ■ The characteristic form of the mandible in Polynesians has a smoothly curved gonial angle, hence the descriptive term "rocker jaw." (From Marshall, D.S., and Snow, C.E.: Am. J. Phys. Anthropol. **14:**405-427, 1956.)

no evidence of dramatic facial deformities like those seen in the cross-bred dogs. If malocclusion or a tendency to malocclusion is inherited, in other words, it is clear that the mechanism is not the independent inheritance of discrete morphologic characteristics like tooth and jaw sizes.

Studies of variations in twins allow an estimation of the heritability (role of genetic factors in total variability) of craniofacial structures. A basic assumption of twin research is that identical or monozygotic twins occur because of the early division of a fertilized egg, so each individual has the same chromosal DNA and the two are genetically identical. Differences between these individuals then should be solely the result of environmental influences. Twins also occur when two eggs are released at the same time and fertilized by different spermatozoa. These dizygotic or fraternal twins are not more similar than ordinary siblings except that they have shared the same intrauterine environment.

By comparing identical twins, fraternal twins, and ordinary siblings, an estimate of the effect of heredity in relation to the effect of the environment can be calculated. Lundstrom,[33] summarizing a number of research investigations of this type, concludes that about 40% of the dental and facial variations that lead to malocclusion can be attributed to hereditary factors. Corrucini[34] argues that the true figure is much lower.

In short, contemporary research has refuted the simplistic picture of malocclusion as resulting from independent inheritance of dental and facial characteristics, but has not yet clarified the precise role of heredity as an etiologic agent for malocclusion. The earlier concepts that jaw function is related to the development of malocclusion have been revived and strengthened, both by the evidence against simple inheritance and by a more optimistic view of the extent to which the human skeleton can be altered.

On the other hand, research findings consistently have shown that there are no simple explanations for malocclusion in terms of oral function. Mouth breathing, tongue thrusting, soft diet, sleeping posture—none can be regarded as the sole or even the major reason for most malocclusions. Conclusions about the etiology of orthodontic problems are difficult, especially since they may have arisen because of several interacting factors. The following discussion is an attempt to synthesize present knowledge into a contemporary overview and is offered in full awareness that the facts do not yet allow definite conclusions.

■ Etiologic Possibilities for Specific Types of Malocclusion

Crowding of the teeth, the most common type of malocclusion at present, undoubtedly is related in part to the continuing reduction in jaw and tooth size in human evolutionary development. It seems unlikely that there are genes for dental occlusion, ideal or otherwise, but genetic influences are obviously an important background for the development of the masticatory system. Increased outbreeding can explain at least part of the increase in crowding in recent centuries. The additive effects on malocclusion seen in the Hawaiian studies indicate how outbreeding could lead to an increased prevalence of malocclusion even if independent inheritance of dentofacial characteristics did not occur.

Environmental factors must have played some role, however, and it is not clear what these are. There is no theoretical explanation of how a coarser diet and more powerful jaw function could significantly alter the dimensions of the dental arches. Perhaps the relatively recent alterations in diet, which without question have reduced the functional demands on the jaws, have accelerated the trend toward reduction in jaw size that was already occurring.

The judgment that inherited characteristics contribute to crowding is an important one in planning orthodontic therapy, for it implies that a significant number of patients will continue to require extractions to provide space for aligning the remaining teeth. Physical therapy to make the dental apparatus grow larger seems an unlikely alternative. In the era when all malocclusion was attributed to a degenerate environment, extraction of teeth was never recommended. At the height of enthusiam for inherited characteristics as determinants of malocclusion, the majority of patients were treated with extractions. In contemporary perspective, the truth—and the extraction percentage—is somewhere in between.

Other types of Class I (nonskeletal) problems—crossbites, individual tooth malalignments—appear to arise from an interaction between the initial position of tooth buds and the pressure environment that guides eruption of the teeth. Forces from the lips, cheek, tongue, fingers, or other objects can influence tooth position, both vertically and horizontally, if the pressures are maintained for a long enough time. A small increment of continuous pressure can be quite effective in displacing teeth. Any individual tooth or all teeth in a section of the arch can be displaced buccally or lingually, or caused to erupt more or less than might otherwise have been the case. Minor problems, especially nonskeletal crossbites, often are caused primarily by alterations in function. Major problems usually have an additional genetic or developmental component.

Skeletal orthodontic problems, those resulting from malpositions or malformations of the jaws rather than just from irregularity of the teeth, can arise from a number of causes. Inherited patterns, defects in embryologic development, trauma, and functional influences can and apparently do contribute. Specific genetic syndromes or congenital defects involving the jaws are rare, as are malocclusions caused primarily by trauma. The fact that ideal occlusion does not necessarily occur in primitive populations suggests that variations from our ideal occlusal scheme are quite compatible with normal function. Perhaps greater variations in the jaws are tolerated now, with the change in diet, than were once compatible with long-term survival and reproductive success.

It seems reasonable to view the majority of moderate skeletal malocclusions as being the result of an inherited pattern which, although it is not consonant with our concept of ideal occlusion, is compatible with acceptable function. Fifteen to 20% of the contemporary U.S. and northern European population have a Class II malocclusion, and it is likely that most are inherited. There is little reason to believe that any significant number of Class II malocclusions result from functional causes and only a few are from some specific interference with growth—which is not to say that functional alterations in equilibrium cannot accentuate these problems when they appear. The more severe skeletal discrepancies probably fall into this category of inherited tendencies made worse by environmental effects.

Class III problems could arise because of mandibular posture, since constant distraction of the mandibular condyle from the fossa may be a stimulus to growth. Functional mandibular shifts affect only tooth position, but constant posturing because of respiratory needs, tongue size, or pharyngeal dimensions may affect the size of the jaw. There is a definite familial and racial tendency to mandibular prognathism,[35] and in the final analysis, it may not matter whether the inherited tendency is for a large mandible primarily, or for a large tongue or other characteristics that lead secondarily to a large mandible. It certainly appears that like Class II, the majority of Class III problems are related to inherited jaw proportions.

Altered function has traditionally been associated with vertical growth problems, especially anterior open bite. A child with an anterior open bite of moderate severity should be presumed to have a sucking habit until proved otherwise. Open bite may also be related to tongue posture, although not to tongue activity during swallowing. The postural changes dictated by partial nasal obstruction may also play a role. Excessive eruption of posterior teeth predisposes any individual to anterior open bite, and downward posturing of the mandible and tongue can allow excessive posterior eruption. However, vertical jaw proportions are inherited just as are anteroposterior proportions. Anterior open bite is much more common in blacks than whites, whereas deep bite is much more common in whites, and it seems reasonably clear that this reflects a different inherent facial morphology rather than environmental influences. Perhaps posture and the associated equilibrium effects interact with inherited jaw proportions to produce open bite or deep bite in some individuals.

A final word on etiology: whatever the malocclusion, it is nearly always stable after growth has been completed. If an orthodontic problem is corrected in adult life, which can be difficult because so much of treatment depends on growth, a surprising amount of change is also stable. The etiologic agents, in other words, are usually no longer present when growth is completed. Malocclusion, after all, is a developmental problem.

■ *References*

1. Wolpoff, W.H.: Paleoanthropology. New York, 1980, Alfred A. Knopf.
2. Baume, L.J.: Uniform methods for the epidemiologic assessment of malocclusion. Am J. Orthod. **66:**251-272, 1974.
3. Campbell, T.D., and Barrett, M.J.: Dental observations on Australian aborigines. Aust. Dent. J. **57:**1-6, 1953.
4. Corrucini, R.S., et al.: Epidemiological survey of occlusion in North India. Br. J. Orthod. **10:**44-47, 1983.
5. Corrucini, R.S.: An epidemiologic transition in dental occlusion in world populations. Am. J. Orthod. **86:**419-426, 1984.
6. Smylski, P.T., Woodside, D.G., and Harnett, B.E.: Surgical and orthodontic treatment of cleidocranial dysostosis. Int. J. Oral Surg. **3:**380-385, 1974.
7. O'Meara, W.F.: Ectopic eruption patterns in selected permanent teeth. J. Dent. Res. **41:**607-616, 1962.
8. Bjorklin, K., and Kurol, J.: Ectopic eruption of the maxillary first permanent molar: etiologic factors. Am. J. Orthod. **84:**147-155, 1983.
9. Shapira, Y., and Kuftinec, M.M.: The ectopically erupted mandibular lateral incisor. Am. J. Orthod. **82:**426-429, 1982.
10. Moss, J.P., and Picton, D.C.A.: Experimental mesial drift in adult monkeys *(Macaca irus)*. Arch. Oral Biol.**12:**1313-1320, 1967.
11. Moss, J.P.: The soft tissue environment of teeth and jaws: an experimental and clinical study. Part I. Br. J. Orthod. **7:**107-137, 1980.
12. Blayney, J.R., and Hill, I.N.: Fluorine and dental caries. J. Am. Dent. Assoc. **74:**233-302, 1967.
13. Lund, K.: Mandibular growth and remodelling process after mandibular fractures. Acta Odont. Scand. **32**(Suppl. 64): 1974.
14. Proffit, W.R., Vig, K.W.L., and Turvey, T.A.: Early fracture of the mandibular condyles: frequently an unsuspected cause of growth disturbances. Am. J. Orthod. **78:**1-24, 1980.
15. Weinstein, S., et al.: On an equilibrium theory of tooth position. Angle Orthod. **33:**1-26, 1963.
16. Proffit, W.R.: Equilibrium theory revisited. Angle Orthod. **48:**175-186, 1978.
17. Picton, D.C.A., and Moss, J.P.: The part played by the transseptal fibre system in experimental approximal drift of the cheek teeth of monkeys *(Macaca irus)*. Arch. Oral Biol. **18:**669-680, 1973.
18. Reitan, K.: Tissue rearrangement during retention of orthodontically rotated teeth. Angle Orthod. **29:**105-113, 1959.
19. Steedle, J.R., and Proffit, W.R.: The pattern and control of eruptive tooth movements. Am. J. Orthod. **87:**56-66, 1985.
20. Proffit, W.R.: Lingual pressure patterns in the transition from tongue thrust to adult swallowing. Arch. Oral Biol. **17:**555-563, 1972.
21. Proffit, W.R., and Mason, R.M.: Myofunctional therapy for tongue-thrusting: background and recommendations. J. Am. Dent. Assoc. **90:**403-411, 1975.
22. Niinimaa, V., et al.: Oronasal distribution of respiratory airflow. Respir. Physiol. **43:**69-75, 1981.
23. Watson, R.M., Warren, D.W., and Fischer, N.D.: Nasal resistance, skeletal classification, and mouth breathing in orthodontic patients. Am. J. Orthod. **54:**367-379, 1968.

24. Vig, P.S., Showfety, K.J., and Phillips, C.: Experimental manipulation of head posture. Am. J. Orthod. **77:**258-268, 1980.

25. Harvold, E.P., et al.: Primate experiments on oral respiration. Am. J. Orthod. **79:**359-372, 1981.

26. Warren, D.W.: A quantitative technique for assessing nasal airway impairment. Am. J. Orthod. **86:**306-314, 1984.

27. Linder-Aronson, S.: Adenoids: their effect on mode of breathing and nasal airflow and their relationship to characteristics of the facial skeleton and dentition. Acta Otolaryngol. Scand. (Suppl. 265), 1970.

28. Linder-Aronson, S.: Effects of adenoidectomy on the dentition and facial skeleton over a period of five years. In Cook, J.T., editor: Transactions of the Third International Orthodontic Congress. St. Louis, 1975, The C.V. Mosby Co.

29. Leech, H.L.: A clinical analysis of orofacial morphology and behavior of 500 patients attending an upper respiratory research clinic. Dent. Practitioner **9:**57-68, 1958.

30. Turvey, T.A., Hall, D.J., and Warren, D.W.: Alterations in nasal airway resistance following superior repositioning of the maxilla. Am. J. Orthod. **85:**109-114, 1984.

31. Stockard, C.R., and Johnson, A.L.: Genetic and Endocrinic Basis for Differences in Form and Behavior. Philadelphia, 1941, The Wistar Institute of Anatomy and Biology, pp. 149-205.

32. Chung, C.S., et al.: Genetic and epidemiologic studies of oral characteristics in Hawaii's schoolchildren. II. Malocclusion. Am. J. Human Genet. **23:**471-495, 1971.

33. Lundstrom, A.: Nature vs. nurture in dentofacial variation. Eur. J. Orthod. **6:**77-91, 1984.

34. Corrucini, R.S., and Potter, R.H.Y.: Genetic analysis of occlusal variation in twins. Am. J. Orthod. **78:**140-154, 1980.

35. Litton, S.F., Ackerman, L.V., Isaacson, R.J., and Shapiro, B.: A genetic study of Class III malocclusion. Am. J. Orthod. **58:**565-577, 1970.

DIAGNOSIS AND TREATMENT PLANNING

Diagnosis in orthodontics, as in other disciplines of dentistry and medicine, requires two steps: the collection of an adequate database of information about the patient, and the distillation from that database of a comprehensive but clearly stated list of the patient's problems. The process of orthodontic diagnosis and treatment planning lends itself well to the problem-oriented approach, and an adaptation of problem-oriented diagnosis and treatment planning will be presented here. In this approach, the diagnosis and treatment planning can be reduced to a series of logical steps (see also the figure below):

1. Development of an adequate diagnostic database
2. Formulation of a problem list from the database
3. Arrangement of the items on the orthodontic problem list in priority order, so that the most important problem receives highest priority for treatment
4. Consideration of possible solutions to each problem, with each problem evaluated for the moment as if it were the only problem that the patient had
5. Evaluation of the interaction among possible solutions to the individual problems
6. Synthesis of an optimal treatment plan, calculated to maximize benefit to the patient and minimize risks, costs, and complexity

The key to accurate diagnosis is this process of clearly separating the elements of the problem into a discrete list. Then the task of treatment planning is to synthesize the often disparate solutions to these specific problems into a unified overall treatment strategy.

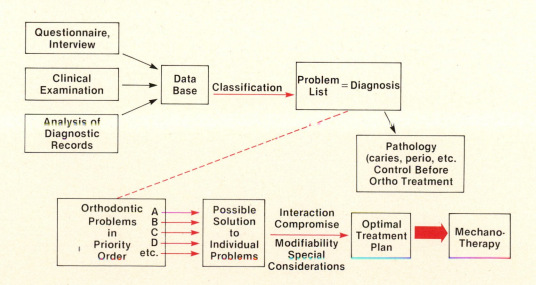

It is often said that the health professions are both science and art. This sequence of steps in the diagnosis and treatment planning process makes it easier to differentiate the science and art portions. In the development of a database and formulation of a problem list, the goal is *truth,* the goal of scientific inquiry. At this stage, there is no room for opinion or judgment; instead, a totally factual appraisal of the situation is required. On the other hand, the goal of the process that begins with setting priorities on the problem list and proceeds through the remaining steps is not scientific truth but *wisdom,* the plan that a wise and prudent clinician would follow to maximize benefit for the patient. Judgment by the clinician is required as problems are placed in priority order and as alternate treatment procedures are evaluated. Wise treatment choices, of course, are facilitated if no significant points have been overlooked previously.

Diagnosis, which we define here as the acquisition of a database and development of a problem list, is a scientific procedure. Treatment planning, on the other hand, has more elements of an art form. In Chapter 6, the focus is on the database–problem list stage. Chapters 7 and 8 discuss the more subjective treatment planning process.

Orthodontic Diagnosis: The Development of a Problem List

■ The Problem-Oriented Approach

In diagnosis, whether in orthodontics or other areas of dentistry or medicine, it is important not to concentrate so closely on one aspect of the patient's overall condition that other significant problems are overlooked. In a medical context, if a patient has an acute infection, it nevertheless will be important to detect that he is also suffering from diabetes. In an orthodontic context, it is an inaccurate diagnosis to characterize the dental occlusion while overlooking a jaw discrepancy, developmental syndrome, periodontal problem, or systemic disease. The natural bias of any specialist (and one does not have to be a dental specialist to already take a very specialized point of view) is to characterize problems in terms of his own special interest. Diagnosis, in short, should be comprehensive, not focused only on a single aspect of what in many instances can be a complex situation. Orthodontic diagnosis should proceed only after a broad overview of the patient's situation has been achieved.

The problem-oriented approach to diagnosis and treatment planning has been widely advocated in medicine and dentistry as a way to overcome the tendency to concentrate on only one part of a patient's problem. Weed's pioneering work in medical diagnosis[1] has been followed by numerous applications to dentistry and orthodontics. The essence of the problem-oriented approach is the development of a comprehensive database of pertinent information, so that no problems will be overlooked. From that database, the list of problems that is the diagnosis is abstracted.

For orthodontic purposes, the database may be thought of as being derived from three major sources: (1) information from questioning the patient, (2) information from clinical examination of the patient, and (3) information from evaluation of diagnostic records, including dental casts, radiographs, and photographs. Since all possible diagnostic records will not be obtained for all patients, some judgment must be used at an early stage in determining what information is essential and what is not. The steps in assembling an adequate database, including a discussion of which diagnostic records are needed, are presented below in sequence.

■ Questionnaire/Interview Information

The first step in the interview process should be to establish the patient's chief complaint, usually by a direct question to the patient. Further information should be sought in three major areas: (1) medical and dental history, (2) physical growth status, and (3) motivation, expectations, and other social-behavioral factors.

■ Medical and Dental History

Orthodontic problems are almost always the culmination of a developmental process, not the result of pathology. Nevertheless, a careful medical and dental history is needed for orthodontic patients both to provide a proper background for understanding the patient's overall situation and to evaluate specific orthodontically related concerns. The outline of a medical and dental history is presented in Fig. 6-1. Several of the questions included in the tables are annotated to explain their implications for an orthodontic patient. Ad-

MEDICAL/DENTAL HISTORY (CHILD/ADOLESCENT)

Name: _____   Date of birth: _____

Parent's name: _____

Address: _____

Yes   No   Has your child:

___ ___   1. Seen a physician for routine physical examination?

              Date of last physical examination _____

              Results _____

___ ___   2. Been immunized? Date of last immunization: _____

___ ___   3. Ever had a health problem? If yes, explain: _____

              _____

___ ___   4. Ever been under the care of a physician? If yes, explain: _____

              _____

___ ___   5. Ever been treated in an emergency room? Why? _____

___ ___   6. Ever been treated in a hospital? Why? _____

___ ___   7. Ever been allergic to anything? What? _____

___ ___   8. Ever taken any medicine? What? _____

___ ___   9. Had any unfavorable reactions to medicine? _____

___ ___ 10. Ever had any emotional, mental, or nervous disorders? If yes, explain:

              _____

___ ___ 11. Does your child presently take any daily medication? What? _____

         12. Please check if your child has had any of the following:

              a___ Heart disease   i___ Cleft lip/palate

              b___ Rheumatic fever   j___ Arthritis

              c___ Bleeding problems   k___ Kidney problems

              d___ Anemia   l___ Speech/hearing problems

              e___ Hepatitis   m___ Epilepsy/convulsions

              f___ Diabetes   n___ Tonsils removed

              g___ Asthma   o___ Adenoids removed

              h___ Liver problems   p___ Contact lenses

              ___ Any other physical/mental problems

              Comments: _____

___ ___ 13. Has any member of your immediate family had problems with any of the

              above? What? _____

Fig. 6-1 ■ Form for obtaining medical/dental history for young orthodontic patients. A separate but similar form is needed for older patients. Annotated comments, explaining why some of the questions are asked, are placed immediately below the form and are keyed by number to the question to which they refer.

MEDICAL/DENTAL HISTORY cont'd

Yes No

14. Do you consider your child to be (check one):

___ Advanced learner   ___ Progressing normally   ___ Slow learner

__ __ 15. Were there any problems at birth? What? _____

__ __ 16. Has your child had any recent rapid growth? How much? _____

17. Parents: Ht. _____ Wt. _____

Ht. _____ Wt. _____

Older brothers and sisters: Ht. _____ Sex ____ Age ____

Ht. _____ Sex ____ Age ____

Ht. _____ Sex ____ Age ____

__ __ 18. Females: Has menstruation begun? If yes, when? _____

__ __ Pregnant?

__ __ 19. Has your child ever been to a dentist? If yes, date of last examination:

_____ Date of last x-ray films: _____

__ __ 20. Has your child ever sucked his/her finger or thumb?

__ __ 21. Has your child inherited any family facial or dental characteristics?

If yes, explain: _____

__ __ 22. Do you give your child any form of fluoride?

23. Please check if your child has had problems with any of the following:

a___ Cavities   e___ Teeth sensitive to hot/cold

b___ Toothaches   f___ Teeth sensitive to sweets

c___ Teeth bumped   g___ Gum infection

d___ Color of teeth   h___ Other dental problems

Comments: _____

_____

24. What is your main concern in seeking this appointment? _____

_____

25. Child's physician: _____

Family dentist: _____

26. Child's school: _____ Grade in school: ____

27. Whom may we thank for referring you? _____

_____   _____

Signature of person completing this form   Relationship

Continued.

Fig. 6-1, cont'd ■ For legend see opposite page.

ANNOTATIONS ON SELECTED QUESTIONS

2. In the instance of oral facial trauma the DPT status is critical to establish the child's need for protection. Soft tissue injury is increased with appliances in place.

5. This helps establish a history of trauma.

10. This helps establish the patient's social emotional status.

12. (a and b) These patients need SBE coverage during banding and debanding procedures.

   (f) Tissue response may be altered especially in the presence of appliances.

   (i) Cleft lip/palate patients require altered treatment plans.

   (j) Arthritis has been related to TM joint problems and growth disturbances of the mandible.

   (n and o) This may detail previous treatment aimed at airway problems.

   (p) Certain antisialagogies may be contraindicated in patients who wear contact lenses.

16-18. These questions help establish growth status.

19. Reduction in unnecessary radiation is critical to the highest quality care. Many practitioners will request films as part of the examination procedures. Those patients seeking second opinions have already had some records obtained.

20. Habits may explain dental anomalies in question.

21. Familial tendency is indicated in some skeletal patterns and missing teeth have a documented genetic component.

23. (a) Dental trauma may have implications during tooth movement due to the increased possibility of root resorption.

   (g) Orthodontic treatment in the face of periodontal disease either acute or chronic is contraindicated until the disease stage is either controlled or reversed.

24. The chief complaint is critical to determine why the patient is seeking care. This should be foremost in the planning of treatment.

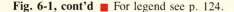

Fig. 6-1, cont'd ■ For legend see p. 124.

ditional comments on specific situations appear in the following paragraphs.

Trauma to teeth or jaws may be a factor in the etiology of some orthodontic problems. It has become apparent in recent years that early fractures of the condylar neck of the mandible occur more frequently than was previously thought (see Chapter 5). Although most children with condylar fractures recover uneventfully, a growth deficit related to an old condylar injury should be considered in the evaluation of a patient with facial asymmetry (Fig. 6-2). A mandibular fracture may be overlooked in the aftermath of an accident that caused widespread trauma. Although old fractures have particular significance, trauma to the teeth may also affect the development of the occlusion and should not be overlooked in the history.

It is important to note whether the patient is on long-term medication of any type, and if so, for what purpose. This may reveal systemic disease or metabolic problems that the patient did not report in any other way. Chronic medical problems in adults or children do not contraindicate orthodontic treatment, if the medical problem is under control,

but special precautions may be necessary if orthodontic treatment is to be carried out. For example, orthodontic treatment would be possible in a patient with controlled diabetes but would require especially careful monitoring, since the periodontal breakdown to which these individuals are susceptible might be accentuated by orthodontic forces (see Chapter 8).

Another common chronic problem for children and adolescents is a history of rheumatic fever or cardiac anomalies. In such a child, antibiotic coverage is required before any manipulation (fitting orthodontic bands, for instance) that would cause gingival bleeding. If these precautions are not observed, subacute bacterial endocarditis, which may be life-threatening, can occur. Finally, chronic medical problems can lead to alterations in the growth status of patients (see Chapter 4).

■ Physical Growth Evaluation

A second major area that should be explored by questions to the patient or parents is the individual's physical growth status. For normal youths who are approaching puberty,

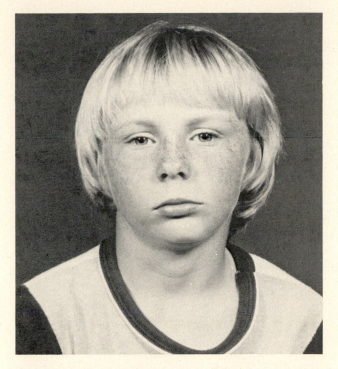

Fig. 6-2 ■ Facial asymmetry developed in this boy after fracture of the left mandibular condylar process at age 5, because scarring in the fracture area prevented normal translation of the mandible on that side during growth (see Chapter 2). Trauma is a frequent cause of asymmetry of this type.

questions about how rapidly the child has grown recently, whether clothes sizes have changed, whether there are signs of sexual maturation, and when sexual maturation occurred in older siblings usually provide the necessary information. In many instances, height-weight records and the child's progress on standard growth charts can be obtained from the pediatrician. Valuable information can also be obtained from clinical examination. Occasionally, a more precise assessment of skeletal maturation is needed, and a radiograph of the wrist to assess the patient's stage of bone ossification can be helpful (see the section on diagnostic records in this chapter).

One of the frustrations in evaluating growth status is that this assessment is most difficult for the very patients who need it most, those at the extremes of the normal range. Individuals with mandibular prognathism tend to have both more and longer-lasting mandibular growth, making it hard to establish when growth has stopped. This is important because if growth continues after an operation to reposition the mandible, the problem will recur. At the other extreme, some patients with deficient jaw growth have little or no change after an early puberty. Serial cephalometric radiographs offer the most accurate way to determine whether growth has stopped or is continuing.

■ Social and Behavioral Evaluation

Social and behavioral evaluation should explore several related areas: the patient's motivation for treatment, what

he or she expects as a result of treatment, and how cooperative or uncooperative the patient is likely to be.

Motivation for seeking treatment can be classified as external or internal. External motivation is that supplied by pressure from another individual, as with a reluctant child who is being brought for orthodontic treatment by a determined mother, or with an older patient who is seeking alignment of incisor teeth because her boyfriend (or his girlfriend) wants the teeth to look better. Internal motivation, on the other hand, comes from within the individual and is based on his or her own assessment of the situation and desire for treatment.

The distinction is vitally important in adults: internal motivation correlates strongly with patient satisfaction after treatment, whereas external motivation often produces unhappy and dissatisfied patients. Since children tend to do many things because a dominant adult requires it, true internal motivation may be rare in a child, but even in a young patient, cooperation is likely to be much better if the child genuinely wants treatment for himself or herself, rather than just putting up with it to please a parent. The child or adult who feels that the treatment is being done *for* him will be a much more receptive patient than one who views the treatment as something being done *to* him. Often it is necessary to follow up the question, ''Why are you seeking treatment?'' to establish what the motivation really is.

What the patient expects from treatment is very much related to the type of motivation and should be explored carefully with adults, especially those with primarily cosmetic problems. If the incisor teeth are irregular, and it turns out that the young adult expects his or her social adjustment problems to be solved after the dentist has aligned the teeth, the patient may be a poor risk for orthodontic treatment. It is one thing to undertake to correct a diastema between the maxillary incisors to improve the patient's appearance and dental function, and something else to do this so the patient will now experience greater social or job success. If the social problems continue after treatment, as is quite likely, the orthodontic treatment may become a focus for resentment.

Cooperation is more likely to be a problem with a child than an adult. Two factors are important in determining this: (1) the extent to which the child sees the treatment as a benefit, as opposed to something else he or she is required to undergo; (2) the degree of parental control. A resentful and rebellious adolescent, particularly one with ineffective parents, can become a real problem in treatment.

■ *Clinical Evaluation*

Patients seek orthodontic treatment for two major purposes: improvement of dental and facial esthetics, and correction of problems with occlusal and jaw function. Both are important. Both should be assessed during the clinical examination and evaluated further when additional diagnostic records are available. The goals of the orthodontic clinical examination are to document and evaluate facial,

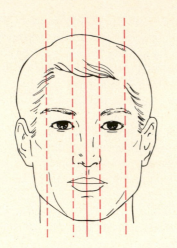

Fig. 6-3 ■ Facial symmetry in the frontal plane.

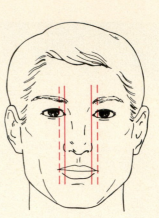

Fig. 6-4 ■ For ideal proportions from the frontal view, the width of the base of the nose should be approximately the same as the interinnercanthal distance (solid line), while the width of the mouth should approximate the distance between the irises (dotted line).

occlusal, and functional characteristics, and to decide which diagnostic records are required.

■ Evaluation of Facial Esthetics

Esthetic judgments are notoriously and unavoidably subjective. Although no real objectivity can be brought to esthetic judgment, it can be helpful to recast the purpose of this part of the clinical evaluation as an evaluation of facial proportions, not esthetics per se. Disproportionate and asymmetric facial features are a major contributor to facial esthetic problems. An appropriate goal for orthodontic treatment is to improve facial harmony by correcting disproportions.

Frontal view. From the front, the face should be examined for bilateral symmetry (Fig. 6-3), size proportions of midline to lateral structures (Fig. 6-4), and vertical pro-

portionality (Fig. 6-5, *A*). A small degree of bilateral facial asymmetry exists in essentially all normal individuals. This can be revealed most readily by comparing the real full face photograph with composites consisting of two right or two left sides (Fig. 6-6). This "normal asymmetry," which usually results from a small size difference between the two sides, should be distinguished from a chin or nose that deviates to one side. Similarly, mild deviations in vertical proportions often occur, but should be distinguished from disproportionate shortness or length of the middle or lower thirds of the face.

Another important point for the full face examination is the relationship of the dental midline of each arch to the skeletal midline of that jaw, i.e., the lower incisor midline related to the midline of the mandible, and the upper incisor midline related to the midline of the maxilla. Dental casts

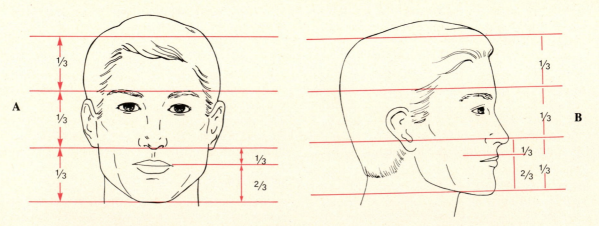

Fig. 6-5 ■ **A,** Vertical facial proportions in the frontal view: the vertical height of the midface, from the supraorbital ridges to the base of the nose, should equal the height of the lower face. **B,** Profile view. Within the lower face, the mouth should be about one-third of the way between the base of the nose and the chin.

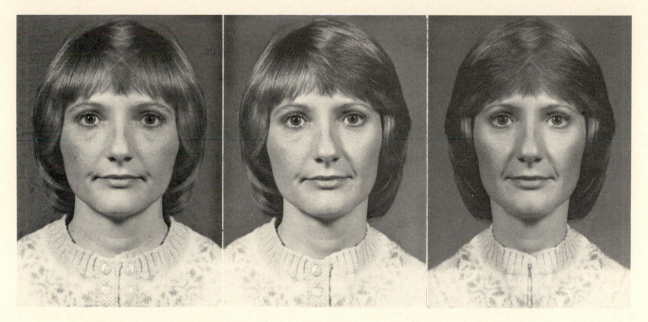

Fig. 6-6 ■ Composite photographs to indicate normal facial asymmetry. The true photograph is in the center. On the right is a composite of the two right sides, while on the left is a composite of the two left sides. This technique dramatically illustrates the difference in the two sides, which occurs normally.

will record the relationship of the midlines to each other if the casts are trimmed to represent the occlusion, but provide no information about the dental-skeletal midlines. For this reason, it is critical that the midline relationship be recorded during the clinical examination.

Finally, in a step particularly important for children around the age of puberty when most orthodontic treatment is carried out, the patient's developmental age should be assessed. Everyone becomes a more or less accurate judge of other people's ages—we expect to come within a year or two simply by observing the other person's facial appearance. Occasionally, we are fooled, as when we say that a 12-year-old girl looks 15, or a 15-year-old boy looks 12. With adolescents, the judgment is one of relatively physical maturity. This is valuable information when orthodontic treatment is contemplated because the stage of physical maturity correlates well with how much jaw growth remains. Before sexual maturity, continuing growth can be expected; after sexual maturity, much less growth is available.

The attainment of recognizable secondary sexual characteristics for girls and boys is discussed in Chapter 4. The degree of the development of these characteristics is much more important than chronologic age in determining how much growth remains.

Profile view. The object of the full face examination is to detect gross asymmetry or disproportion. Analysis of profile relationships must be carried out in greater depth, since skeletal proportions revealed in this view affect both anteroposterior and vertical tooth relationships in addition to facial esthetics. A careful examination of the profile yields the same information, though in less detail, as that obtained

from analysis of lateral cephalometric radiographs. For diagnostic purposes, particularly for separation of patients with more severe problems from those with good or reasonably good facial proportions, careful clinical evaluation of facial proportions is adequate. For this reason, the technique of facial form analysis has sometimes been called the "poor man's cephalometric analysis."[2] This is a vital diagnostic technique for all dentists and is one that must be mastered by all those who will see patients for primary care in dentistry, not just by orthodontists.

There are three goals of lateral facial form analysis, approached in three clear and distinct steps. These are:

1. Establishing whether the jaws are proportionately positioned in the anteroposterior plane of space. This step requires that the patient be placed in natural head position, either sitting upright or standing but not reclining in a dental chair, and looking at a distant object. With the head in this position, it can be noted whether the face is approximately vertical, or whether it slopes either anteriorly (anterior divergence) or posteriorly (posterior divergence) (Fig. 6-7). This divergence of the face (the term was coined by the eminent orthodontist-anthropologist Milo Hellman[3]) is influenced by the patient's background. Within reasonable limits, a divergent face is not necessarily disproportionate. American Indians and Orientals, for example, tend to have an anteriorly divergent face, while whites of Mediterranean ancestry tend to have a posteriorly divergent face.

Profile convexity or concavity reveals jaw disproportions. This is detected by viewing the relationship between two lines, one dropped from the bridge of the nose to the base of upper lip, a second extending from that point downward

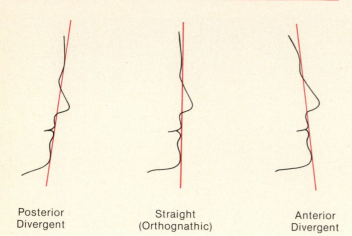

Posterior
Divergent

Straight
(Orthognathic)

Anterior
Divergent

Fig. 6-7 ■ Divergence of the face is defined as an anterior or posterior inclination of the lower face relative to the forehead. Anterior or posterior divergence can be compatible with good facial esthetics and proportions, and in fact a degree of facial divergence is a racial and ethnic characteristic.

to the chin (Fig. 6-8). These line segments should form a nearly straight line. An angle between them indicates either profile convexity (upper jaw prominent relative to chin) or profile concavity (upper jaw behind chin). A convex profile, therefore, indicates a skeletal Class II jaw relationship, whereas a concave profile indicates a skeletal Class III. A straight profile line, regardless of whether the face is divergent, does not indicate a problem.

2. Evaluation of lip protrusion, and thereby the extent of incisor protrusion. This step is done by relating the lips to a true vertical line passing through the concavity at the base of the upper lip (soft tissue point A) and through the similar concavity between the lower lip and chin (soft tissue point B) (Fig. 6-9). The lip should lie along or only slightly in front of this line. If the lip is significantly forward from this line, it can be judged to be protrusive; if the lip falls behind the line, it is retrusive.

This evaluation should be carried out with the patient's lips relaxed. It is also important to note the extent to which the lips are separated when they are relaxed and whether the patient must strain to bring the lips together (Fig. 6-10). When the lips are protrusive and separated at rest by more than 3 to 4 mm, it can be concluded that the lip protrusion results from protrusion of the incisors, and that both lip function and facial esthetics would improve if the protruding teeth were retracted. If the lips are protrusive but close over the teeth without strain, on the other hand, retraction of the incisor teeth will result in minimal changes in lip prominence.

Like facial divergence, lip protrusion is strongly influenced by racial and ethnic characteristics. Whites of northern European backgrounds have relatively thin lips and minimal lip prominence. Whites of southern European and middle eastern origin normally have more lip prominence than their northern cousins. Greater degrees of lip prominence normally occur in Orientals, and in blacks. This difference simply means that a degree of lip prominence normal for many whites would be considered retrusive for many Orientals or blacks, while a degree of lip prominence normal for blacks would be protrusive for most whites.

Detecting protrusion of incisors (which is relatively common) or retrusion of incisors (which is rare) is important

A   B   C

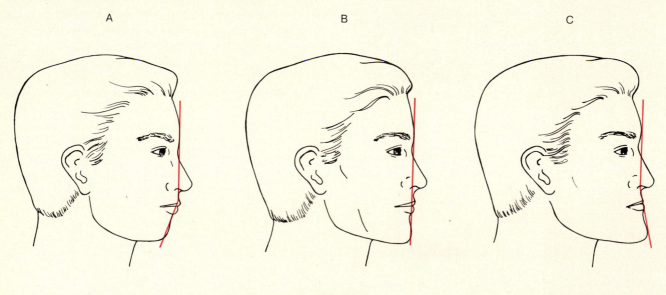

Convex

Straight

Concave

Fig. 6-8 ■ Profile convexity or concavity results from a disproportion in the size of the jaws, but does not by itself indicate which jaw is at fault. A convex facial profile indicates a Class II jaw relationship, which can result from either a maxilla that projects too far forward or a mandible too far back (as shown in *A*). A concave profile indicates a Class III relationship, which can result from either a maxilla that is too far back or a mandible that protrudes forward, as shown in *C*.

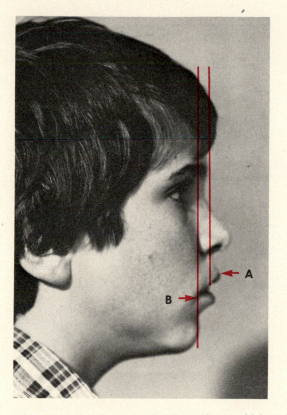

Fig. 6-9 ■ Excessive lip protrusion in a 10-year-old boy. Lip protrusion is evaluated by observing the distance that each lip projects forward from a true vertical line through the concavity at its base, i.e., a different reference line is used for each lip, as shown here.

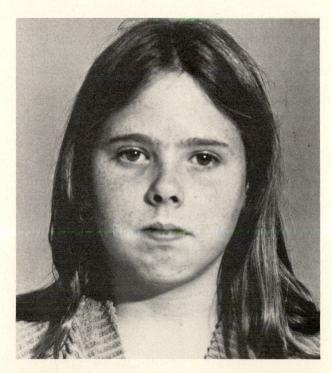

Fig. 6-10 ■ Lip strain, as the girl pulls her lips over her protruding teeth.

because of the effect of this on space within the dental arches. If the incisors protrude, they align themselves on the arc of a larger circle as they lean forward, whereas if the incisors are retrusive, less space is available to accommodate the canines and premolars (Fig. 6-11). In the extreme case, incisor protrusion in what might have been a patient with severe crowding can produce ideal alignment of the dental arches, at the expense of lips that protrude and are difficult to bring into function over the protruding incisor teeth. This condition can be termed bimaxillary dentoalveolar protrusion, meaning simply that in both jaws the teeth protrude (Fig. 6-12). The condition is often referred to as just bimaxillary protrusion, a simpler term but a misnomer since it is not the jaws but the teeth that protrude.

3. Evaluation of vertical facial proportions and mandibular plane angle. Vertical proportions were already observed during the full face examination, but sometimes can be seen more clearly in profile. Division of the face into vertical thirds is shown in Fig. 6-5. The inclination of the mandibular plane to a true horizontal line is visualized readily by placing a finger or mirror handle along the lower border (Fig. 6-13). A steep mandibular plane angle correlates with long anterior facial vertical dimensions and anterior open bite malocclusion, while a flat mandibular plane angle correlates with short anterior facial height and deep bite malocclusion. There is also an interaction between face height and the anteroposterior position of the mandible: all other things being equal, a long face predisposes the patient to Class II malocclusion, a short face to Class III. This is discussed in the section on cephalometric analysis later.

Facial form analysis carried out this way takes only a couple of minutes, but provides information that simply is not present from dental radiographs and casts. Such an evaluation by the primary care practitioner is an essential part of the evaluation of every prospective orthodontic patient.

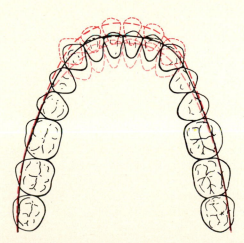

Fig. 6-11 ■ If the incisors flare forward, they can align themselves along the arc of a larger circle, which provides more space to accommodate the teeth and alleviates crowding. Conversely, if the incisors move lingually, this decreases the amount of space.

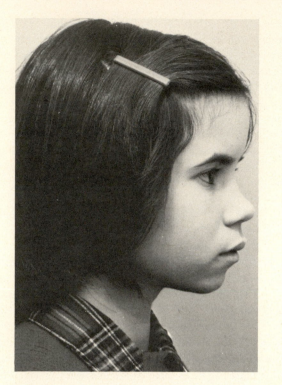

Fig. 6-12 ■ Bimaxillary dentoalveolar protrusion in a young girl. The severe dental and lip protrusion is accompanied by equally severe lip strain to bring the lips into closure.

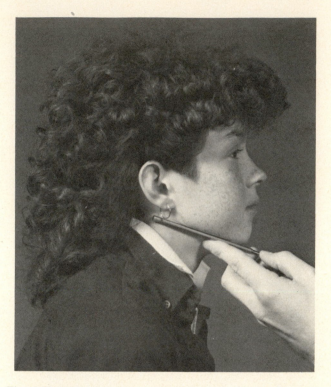

Fig. 6-13 ■ The mandibular plane angle can be visualized clinically by placing a mirror handle or other instrument along the border of the mandible. For this patient, the mandibular plane angle is normal, neither inclined too steeply nor too flatly.

■ Evaluation of Oral Health

The health of oral hard and soft tissues must be assessed for potential orthodontic patients as for any other. It is important that any dental caries or pulpal pathology be treated before orthodontic therapy. A thorough periodontal evaluation is an important part of the orthodontic examination. Potential or actual mucogingival problems are of special interest. Inadequate attached gingiva around crowded incisors indicates the possibility of tissue dehiscence developing when the teeth are aligned, especially with nonextraction (arch expansion) treatment (Fig. 6-14). The interaction between periodontic and orthodontic treatment for both children and adults is discussed in Chapter 8.

■ Evaluation of Jaw and Occlusal Function

Palpation of the temporomandibular joints (TMJ) should be a routine part of any dental examination, and it is important to note any signs of TMJ problems such as joint pain, noise, or limitation of opening. For orthodontic purposes, any lateral or anterior shifts of the mandible on closure are of special interest. Because the articular eminence is not well developed in children, it can be quite difficult to find the sort of positive "centric relation" position that can be determined in adults. Nevertheless, it is important to note whether the mandible shifts laterally or anteriorly when a child closes.

A child with an apparent unilateral crossbite usually has a bilateral narrowing of the maxillary arch, with a shift to

the unilateral crossbite. It is vitally important to verify this, or to rule out a shift and confirm a true unilateral crossbite, during the clinical examination. Similarly, many children and adults with a skeletal Class II relationship and an underlying skeletal Class II jaw relationship will position the mandible forward in a "Sunday bite," making the occlusion look better than it really is. Sometimes an apparent Class III relationship results from a forward shift to escape incisor interferences in what is really an end-to-end relationship (Fig. 6-15). These patients are said to have pseudo–Class III malocclusion.

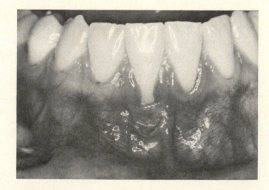

Fig. 6-14 ■ Dehiscence of soft tissue around a lower incisor after orthodontic alignment of the previously irregular teeth. This is likely to occur when there is inadequate attached gingiva. A free gingival graft or other periodontal therapy is indicated before orthodontic treatment.

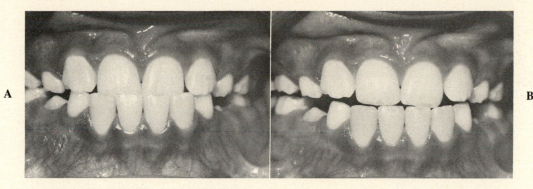

Fig. 6-15 ■ The anterior crossbite in this 10-year-old child **(A)** results largely from an anterior shift of the mandible because of incisor interferences **(B).** This shift into anterior crossbite is often referred to as a pseudo–Class III relationship because it frequently is not a reflection of a true Class III jaw relationship.

Occlusal interferences with functional mandibular movements, though of interest, are less important than they would be if treatment to alter the occlusion were not being contemplated. Balancing interferences, presence or absence of canine protection in lateral excursions, and other such factors should be noted in the clinical examination. These take on greater significance if they are still present when the occlusal changes produced by orthodontic treatment are nearing completion.

■ Which Diagnostic Records Are Needed?

Diagnostic records for orthodontic purposes fall into three major categories: (1) records for evaluation of the teeth and oral structures, (2) records for evaluation of the occlusion, and (3) records for evaluation of facial and jaw proportions.

Records for intraoral evaluation. After clinical evaluation of the health and status of oral structures, records demonstrating any hard or soft tissue lesions, and appropriate charting of the periodontal condition, are needed. A major purpose of intraoral photographs, which should be obtained routinely for patients receiving complex orthodontic treatment, is to document the initial condition of the hard and soft tissues.

A panoramic intraoral radiograph is valuable for orthodontic evaluation at any age. The panoramic film has a significant advantage over a series of intraoral radiographs in that it yields a broader view and thus is more likely to show any pathologic lesions and supernumerary or impacted teeth. It also gives a view of the mandibular condyles, which can be helpful, both in its own right and as a screening film to determine if other temporomandibular joint radiographs are needed.

The panoramic film should be supplemented with periapical and bitewing radiographs only as required for the individual patient. For an adult with periodontal disease, a full series of individual radiographs is often required in addition to the panoramic film. For children and adolescents, bitewing radiographs may be needed to evaluate interproximal caries; periapical views of incisors are indicated if there

is evidence or suspicion of root resorption. Periapical views should be taken of any suspicious areas in the panoramic film. The principle is that periapical films to supplement the panoramic radiograph are ordered only if there is a specific indication for doing so. It is no longer appropriate to routinely obtain a full intraoral series of films for every orthodontic patient.

Radiographs of the temporomandibular joint should be reserved for patients who have symptoms of dysfunction of that joint or who may have anomalies of the condyle that are not seen clearly on the panoramic film. Routine transcranial or laminagraphic TMJ films simply are not needed. Laminagraphic films taken to evaluate the position of the condyle relative to the fossa look more precise than they really are and must be interpreted cautiously. The problem is that the condyle is more than 1 cm wide mediolaterally, and a laminagraphic view of the medial area can give a different impression of condylar position than a cut through the lateral pole in the same individual.

Records for occlusal evaluation. Evaluation of the occlusion requires that impressions be made for dental casts and that the occlusion be recorded so that the casts can be articulated. Impressions for orthodontic evaluation differ from other impressions in that maximum displacement of soft tissues, created by maximum extension of the impression, is desired. The inclination of the teeth, not just the location of the crown, is important. If the impression is not well extended, important diagnostic information may be missing.

At the minimum, a wax bite of the patient's usual interdigitation (centric occlusion) should be made, and a check should be made to be sure that this does not differ significantly from the retruded position. An anterior shift of 1 to 2 mm from the retruded position is of little consequence, but lateral shifts or anterior shifts of greater magnitude should be noted carefully and a wax bite in an approximate centric relation position should be made for these patients. After the casts are poured, the wax bite is used to trim them so that when the casts are placed on their back, the teeth are in proper occlusion.

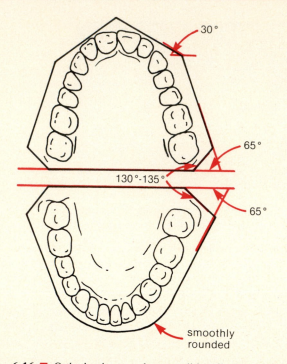

30°

65°

130°-135°

65°

smoothly
rounded

Fig. 6-16 ■ Orthodontic casts have traditionally been trimmed with symmetric bases. The backs are trimmed perpendicular to the midsagittal line, most easily visualized as the midpalatal raphe for most patients. The angles shown for the casts are suggested values; symmetry is more important than the precise angulation.

Dental casts for orthodontic purposes are usually trimmed so that the bases assume a symmetric shape (Fig. 6-16) and then are polished. There are two reasons for doing this: (1) If the casts are trimmed so that there is a symmetric base oriented to the midlline of the palate, it is much easier to detect asymmetry within the dental arches. Viewing the dentition against a symmetric backdrop provided by the base, in other words, makes it easier to analyze arch form. (2) Neatly trimmed and polished models are more acceptable for presentation to the patient, as will be necessary during any consultation about orthodontic treatment.

Knowing the position of the condyles is obviously important for orthodontic diagnostic purposes. Whether it is necessary or even desirable to mount casts on an articulator so that the functional occlusal paths before orthodontic treatment are recorded, is a matter of continuing debate. The current consensus is that for adolescent or preadolescent patients, i.e., those who have not completed their growth, there is little point in an articulator mounting. In young patients, the anatomy of the temporomandibular joint is less well developed, so that condylar guidance is much less prominent than in adults. Current research makes it clear that the form of the joint reflects function during growth. Thus, until mature canine function is reached and the chewing pattern changes from that of the child to the normal adult, completion of the articular eminence and the medial contours of the joint should not be expected (see Chapter 3). In addition, the relationships between the dentition and

the joint that are recorded in articulator mountings change rapidly while skeletal growth is continuing and tend to be only of historic interest after orthodontic treatment.

The situation is different for individuals whose growth is complete or largely complete. In adults, articulator-mounted casts should be obtained if symptoms of the TMJ syndrome (clicking, limitation of motion, pain) are present or if there is evidence of significant discrepancies between the occlusal and retruded mandibular positions. Lateral shifts of any magnitude would be considered significant. Only forward shifts of more than 2 or 3 mm would require an articulator mounting. An articulator mounting may also be needed for some surgical treatment planning (see Chapter 21).

Records for evaluation of facial proportions. For any orthodontic patient, facial and jaw proportions, not just dental occlusal relationships, must be evaluated. This can be done by a careful clinical evaluation of the patient's face, with a recording of positive findings, or by cephalometric radiographs if indicated.

The technique of facial form analysis, presented in detail previously, provides a record of facial proportions in the form of judgments about profile relationships. Facial photographs document these findings and should be taken when comprehensive orthodontic treatment is planned. A minimum of three views is needed: full face with lips relaxed, full face smiling, and profile with lips relaxed. Additional full face views with the lips together, and a three-quarter smiling view, are desirable but optional. Patients with asymmetry problems should have photographs of both profiles.

If orthodontic treatment for an individual who has significant facial asymmetry is contemplated, a frontal (posteroanterior, not anteroposterior) cephalometric film is indicated (but routine PA cephalometric films are not recommended). If there are significant anteroposterior or vertical jaw discrepancies, a lateral cephalometric radiograph is needed. Like all radiographic records, cephalometric films should be taken only when they are indicated. Comprehensive orthodontic treatment almost always requires a lateral cephalometric film. It is irresponsible to undertake growth modification treatment in a child without a pretreatment cephalometric film. For treatment of minor problems in children, or for adjunctive treatment procedures in adults, cephalometric radiographs are not usually required.

Minimal diagnostic records for any orthodontic patient consist of dental casts trimmed to represent the occlusal relationship, a panoramic radiograph or a series of periapical radiographs, and data from facial form analysis. A lateral cephalometric film is needed for all patients except those with minor or adjunctive treatment needs.

■ *Analysis of Diagnostic Records*

Comments on the analysis of intraoral radiographs appear in the previous section on clinical evaluation, as does information about intraoral and facial clinical findings that

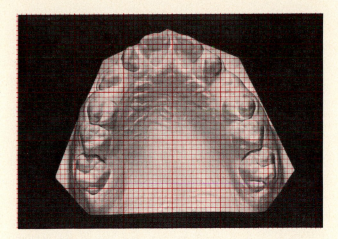

Fig. 6-17 ■ Placing a transparent ruled grid over the dental cast, so that the grid axis is on the midline, makes it easier to spot asymmetries in arch form (wider on the patient's left than right, in this example) and in tooth position (molars drifted forward on the right).

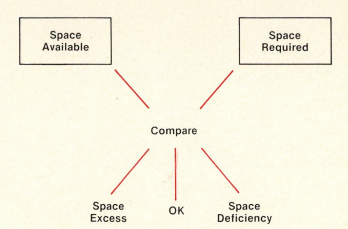

Fig. 6-18 ■ A comparison of space available versus space required establishes whether a deficiency of space within the arch will ultimately lead to crowding, whether the correct amount of room is available to accommodate the teeth, or whether excess space will result in gaps between the teeth.

were recorded photographically. In this section, the focus is on evaluation of space and symmetry within the dental arches by dental cast analysis and on dentofacial relationships as related by cephalometric analysis. Cephalometric analysis is not required for all patients but is needed for those with severe problems. Cast analysis is required for all potential orthodontic patients, whether problems are moderate or severe.

■ Cast Analysis: Symmetry and Space

Symmetry. An asymmetric position of an entire arch should have been detected already in the facial/esthetic examination. An asymmetry of arch form usually accompanies this finding, but may also be present even if the face looks symmetric. A transparent ruled grid placed over the upper dental arch and oriented to the midpalatal raphe can make it easier to see a distortion of arch form (Fig. 6-17).

The ruled grid also helps in seeing where drift of teeth has occurred. Asymmetry within the dental arch, but with symmetric arch form, usually results either from lateral drift of incisors or from drift of posterior teeth unilaterally. Lateral drift of incisors occurs frequently in patients with severe crowding, particularly if a primary canine was lost prematurely on one side. This often results in one permanent canine being blocked out of the arch while the other canine is nearly in its normal position, with all the incisors shifted laterally. Drift of posterior teeth is usually caused by early loss of a primary molar, but sometimes develops even when primary teeth were exfoliated on a normal schedule.

Alignment (crowding): space analysis. Since malalignment of the teeth usually results from lack of space and therefore is best considered as a reflection of crowding, this analysis is primarily one of space within the arches. Analysis of crowding or spacing (space analysis) requires a comparison between the amount of *space available* for the alignment of the teeth and the amount of *space required* to align them properly (Fig. 6-18).

The first step in space analysis is the calculation of space available. This is accomplished by measuring arch perimeter from one first molar to the other, over the contact points of posterior teeth and incisal edge of anteriors.

There are two basic ways to accomplish this: (1) by dividing the dental arch into segments that can be measured as straight line approximations of the arch (Fig. 6-19), or (2) by contouring a piece of wire to the line of occlusion, and then straightening out the wire for measurement. The first method is preferred because of its greater reliability.

The second step is to calculate the amount of space required for alignment of the teeth. This is done by measuring the mesiodistal width of each tooth from contact point to contact point, and then summing the widths of the individual teeth (Fig. 6-20). If the sum of the widths of the permanent teeth is greater than the amount of space available (arch

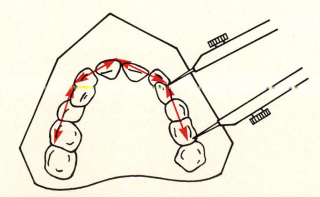

Fig. 6-19 ■ Space available can be measured most easily by dividing the dental arch into 4 straight line segments as shown. Each segment is measured individually with a sharp-pointed measuring instrument.

Table 6-1 ■ Moyers prediction values (75% level)

Total Mandibular-*Incisor Width*		*19.5*	*20.0*	*20.5*	*21.0*	*21.5*	*22.0*	*22.5*
Predicted width of	Maxilla	20.6	20.9	21.2	21.3	21.8	22.0	22.3
canine and premolars	Mandible	20.1	20.4	20.7	21.0	21.3	21.6	21.9

From Moyers, R.E.: Handbook of Orthodontics, ed.3, Chicago, 1973, Yearbook Medical Publishers, Inc.

perimeter deficiency), crowding must occur. If available space is larger (excess space), gaps will appear between some teeth.

Since it is usually a mixed dentition child for whom space analysis is carried out, it is often necessary to estimate the size of the unerupted permanent teeth to calculate the space required. There are three basic approaches for doing this:

1. Measurement of the teeth on radiographs. This requires an undistorted radiographic image, which is more easily achieved with individual periapical than with panoramic films. Even with individual films, it is often difficult to obtain an undistorted view of the canines, and this inevitably reduces the accuracy. With any type of radiograph, it is necessary to compensate for enlargement of the radiographic image. This can be done by measuring an object that can be seen both in the radiograph and on the casts, usually a primary molar tooth (Fig. 6-21). A simple proportional relationship can then be set up:

$$\frac{\text{True width of primary molar}}{\text{Apparent width of primary molar}} =$$

$$\frac{\text{True width of unerupted premolar}}{\text{Apparent width of unerupted premolar}}$$

Accuracy is fair to good, depending on the quality of the radiographs and their position in the arch. The technique can be used in maxillary and mandibular arches for all ethnic groups.

2. Estimation from proportionality tables. There is a reasonably good correlation between the size of the erupted permanent incisors and the unerupted canines and premo-

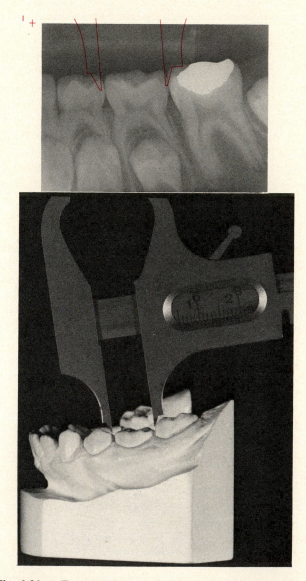

Fig. 6-21 ■ To correct for magnification in films, the same object is measured on the cast and on the film, which will yield the percentage of magnification. This ratio is used to correct for magnification on unerupted teeth.

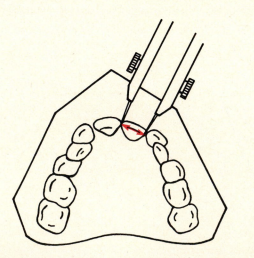

Fig. 6-20 ■ Space required is the sum of the mesiodistal width of each individual tooth, measured from contact point to contact point.

23.0	23.5	24.0	24.5	25.0	25.5	26.0	26.5	27.0	27.5	28.0	28.5	29.0
22.6	22.9	23.1	23.4	23.7	24.0	24.2	24.5	24.8	25.0	25.3	25.6	25.9
22.2	22.5	22.8	23.1	23.4	23.7	24.0	24.3	24.6	24.8	25.1	25.4	25.7

lars. These data have been tabulated for white American children by Moyers[3] (Table 6-1). To utilize the Moyers prediction tables, the mesiodistal width of the *lower* incisors is measured and this number is used to predict the size of *both* the lower and upper unerupted canines and premolars. The size of the lower incisors correlates better with the size of the upper canines and premolars than does the size of the upper incisors, because upper lateral incisors are extremely variable teeth. Accuracy with this method is fairly good for the northern European white children on whose data it is based, despite a tendency to overestimate the size of unerupted teeth. No radiographs are required, and it can be used for the upper or lower arch.

Tanaka and Johnston[4] have developed another way to use the width of the lower incisors to predict the size of unerupted canines and premolars (Table 6-2). The method has good accuracy despite a small bias toward overestimating the unerupted tooth sizes. It requires neither radiographs nor reference tables (once the method is memorized), which makes it very convenient.

3. Combination of radiographic and prediction table methods. Since the major problem with using radiographic images comes in evaluating the canine teeth, it would seem reasonable to use the size of permanent incisors measured from the dental casts and the size of unerupted premolars measured from the films, to predict the size of unerupted canines. This approach, developed by Hixon and Oldfather,[5] has been revised and improved by Staley and Kerber.[6] Their graph (Fig. 6-22) allows canine width to be read directly from the sum of incisor and premolar widths. This method can be used only for the mandibular arch and, of course, requires periapical radiographs. For white children, it is quite accurate.

Which of these methods is best for an individual patient will depend on the circumstances. The prediction tables work surprisingly well when applied to the population group from which they were developed. The Moyers, Tanaka-Johnston, and Staley-Kerber predictions are all based on data from white school children of northern European descent. If the patient fits this population group, the Staley-Kerber method will give the best prediction, followed by the Tanaka-Johnston and Moyers approaches. These methods are superior to measurement from radiographs. On the other hand, if the patient does not fit the population group, as a black or Oriental would not, direct measurement from the radiographs is the best approach. Obvious anomalies in tooth size or form seen in the radiographs contraindicate the use of tables for any patient.

The estimate of space available, obtained by measuring the arch perimeter, may not accurately represent the true situation after growth. It is assumed in space analysis that arch form will not change, there will be no increase in arch perimeter from growth, and no other unexpected changes will occur, so that arch perimeter will remain unchanged as the child develops. On the average, this is true, but changes do occur for some children, resulting in a chance of significant error in the prediction of space available. The assumptions are not valid at all for children with skeletal jaw discrepancies. Space analysis should be done only for children with good facial proportions—the results are inaccurate and misleading for the others.

The anteroposterior position of the incisors must also be considered in interpreting the space analysis result. There is an interaction between crowding and protrusion: if the incisors are positioned lingually, this accentuates any crowding; but if the incisors protrude, the potential crowding will be at least partially alleviated. One should keep in mind that crowding and protrusion are really different aspects of the same phenomenon, i.e., if there is not enough room to properly align the teeth, some combination of crowding and protrusion may occur. For this reason, information about how much the incisors protrude must be available from clinical examination to evaluate the results of space analysis. This information comes from facial form analysis or from cephalometric analysis if available.

A comtemporary form for space analysis is shown in Fig. 6-23. Note that the result from facial form analysis is required to use this form.

Table 6-2 ■ Tanaka and Johnston prediction values

| One half of the mesiodistal width of the four lower incisors | + 10.5 mm = | estimated width of mandibular canine and premolars in one quadrant |
| | + 11.0 mm = | estimated width of maxillary canine and premolars in one quadrant |

From Tanaka, M.M., and Johnston, L.E. J. Am. Dent. Assoc. **88**:798, 1974.

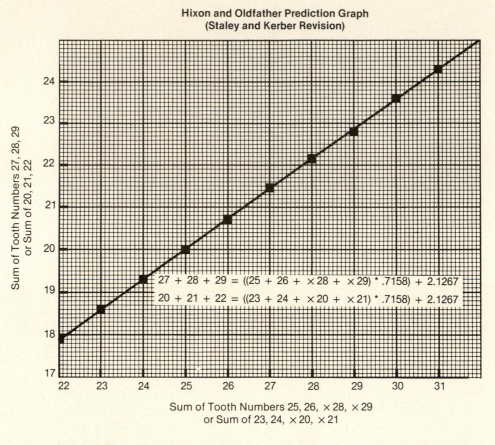

**Hixon and Oldfather Prediction Graph
(Staley and Kerber Revision)**

Sum of Tooth Numbers 27, 28, 29
or Sum of 20, 21, 22 (y-axis)

$27 + 28 + 29 = ((25 + 26 + \times 28 + \times 29) * .7158) + 2.1267$
$20 + 21 + 22 = ((23 + 24 + \times 20 + \times 21) * .7158) + 2.1267$

Sum of Tooth Numbers 25, 26, × 28, × 29
or Sum of 23, 24, × 20, × 21

Standard Error of Estimate = 0.44 mm

Fig. 6-22 ■ Graph showing relationship between size of lower incisors measured from cast plus lower first and second premolars measured from radiographs (*x*-axis) and size of canine plus premolars (*y*-axis). (From Staley, R.N., and Kerber, R.E.: Am. J. Orthod. **78:**296-302, 1980.)

Tooth size analysis. For good occlusion, the teeth must be proportional in size. If large upper teeth are combined with small lower teeth, as in a denture setup with mismatched sizes, there is no way to achieve ideal occlusion. Although the natural teeth match very well in most individuals, approximately 5% of the population have some degree of disproportion among the sizes of individual teeth, defined as tooth size discrepancy. When this occurs, an anomaly in the size of the upper lateral incisors is the most common cause, but variation in premolars or other teeth may be present. Occasionally, all the upper teeth will be too large or too small to fit properly with the lowers.

Tooth size analysis, sometimes called Bolton analysis after its developer,[7] is carried out by measuring the mesiodistal width of each permanent tooth. A standard table (Fig. 6-24) is then used to compare the summed widths of the maxillary to the mandibular anterior teeth and the total width of all upper to lower teeth (excluding second and third molars). A quick check for anterior tooth size discrepancy can be done by comparing the size of upper and lower lateral incisors. Unless the upper laterals are larger, a discrepancy almost surely exists. A discrepancy of less than 1.5 mm is rarely significant, but larger discrepancies create treatment problems and must be included in the orthodontic problem list.

■ Cephalometric Analysis

The introduction of radiographic cephalometrics in 1934 by Hofrath in Germany and Broadbent in the United States provided both a research and a clinical tool for the study of malocclusion and underlying skeletal disproportions (Fig. 6-25). The original purpose of cephalometrics was research on growth patterns in the craniofacial complex. The concepts of normal development presented in Chapters 2 and 3 were largely derived from such cephalometric studies.

It soon became clear that cephalometric films could be used to evaluate dentofacial proportions and clarify the anatomic basis for a malocclusion. Any malocclusion is the result of an interaction between jaw position and dental compensation or adaptation. It is possible to have normal occlusion in spite of an underlying jaw discrepancy through the mechanism of dental compensation, or to have a significant dental malocclusion within a normal skeletal pattern. Still another possibility is additive rather than compensatory dental and skeletal deviations, so that a combination of moderate jaw discrepancy and moderate dental

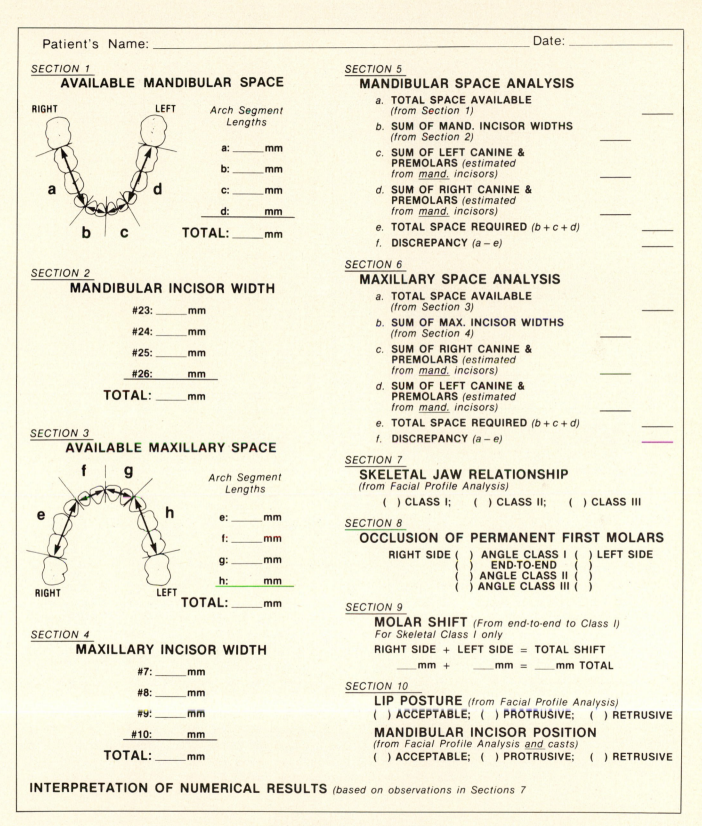

Patient's Name: _____ Date: _____

SECTION 1
AVAILABLE MANDIBULAR SPACE

RIGHT   LEFT

Arch Segment Lengths

a: _____ mm

b: _____ mm

c: _____ mm

d: _____ mm

TOTAL: _____ mm

SECTION 2
MANDIBULAR INCISOR WIDTH

#23: _____ mm

#24: _____ mm

#25: _____ mm

#26: _____ mm

TOTAL: _____ mm

SECTION 3
AVAILABLE MAXILLARY SPACE

Arch Segment Lengths

e: _____ mm

f: _____ mm

g: _____ mm

h: _____ mm

RIGHT   LEFT

TOTAL: _____ mm

SECTION 4
MAXILLARY INCISOR WIDTH

#7: _____ mm

#8: _____ mm

#9: _____ mm

#10: _____ mm

TOTAL: _____ mm

SECTION 5
MANDIBULAR SPACE ANALYSIS

a. TOTAL SPACE AVAILABLE
(from Section 1) _____

b. SUM OF MAND. INCISOR WIDTHS
(from Section 2) _____

c. SUM OF LEFT CANINE &
PREMOLARS *(estimated
from mand. incisors)* _____

d. SUM OF RIGHT CANINE &
PREMOLARS *(estimated
from mand. incisors)* _____

e. TOTAL SPACE REQUIRED *(b + c + d)* _____

f. DISCREPANCY *(a – e)* _____

SECTION 6
MAXILLARY SPACE ANALYSIS

a. TOTAL SPACE AVAILABLE
(from Section 3) _____

b. SUM OF MAX. INCISOR WIDTHS
(from Section 4) _____

c. SUM OF RIGHT CANINE &
PREMOLARS *(estimated
from mand. incisors)* _____

d. SUM OF LEFT CANINE &
PREMOLARS *(estimated
from mand. incisors)* _____

e. TOTAL SPACE REQUIRED *(b + c + d)* _____

f. DISCREPANCY *(a – e)* _____

SECTION 7
SKELETAL JAW RELATIONSHIP
(from Facial Profile Analysis)

( ) CLASS I;   ( ) CLASS II;   ( ) CLASS III

SECTION 8
OCCLUSION OF PERMANENT FIRST MOLARS

RIGHT SIDE ( ) ANGLE CLASS I ( ) LEFT SIDE
( ) END-TO-END ( )
( ) ANGLE CLASS II ( )
( ) ANGLE CLASS III ( )

SECTION 9
MOLAR SHIFT *(From end-to-end to Class I)*
For Skeletal Class I only

RIGHT SIDE + LEFT SIDE = TOTAL SHIFT

_____ mm + _____ mm = _____ mm TOTAL

SECTION 10
LIP POSTURE *(from Facial Profile Analysis)*
( ) ACCEPTABLE; ( ) PROTRUSIVE; ( ) RETRUSIVE

MANDIBULAR INCISOR POSITION
(from Facial Profile Analysis and casts)
( ) ACCEPTABLE; ( ) PROTRUSIVE; ( ) RETRUSIVE

INTERPRETATION OF NUMERICAL RESULTS *(based on observations in Sections 7*

Fig. 6-23 ■ Space analysis form.

BOLTON ANALYSIS

Maxillary Anterior Excess

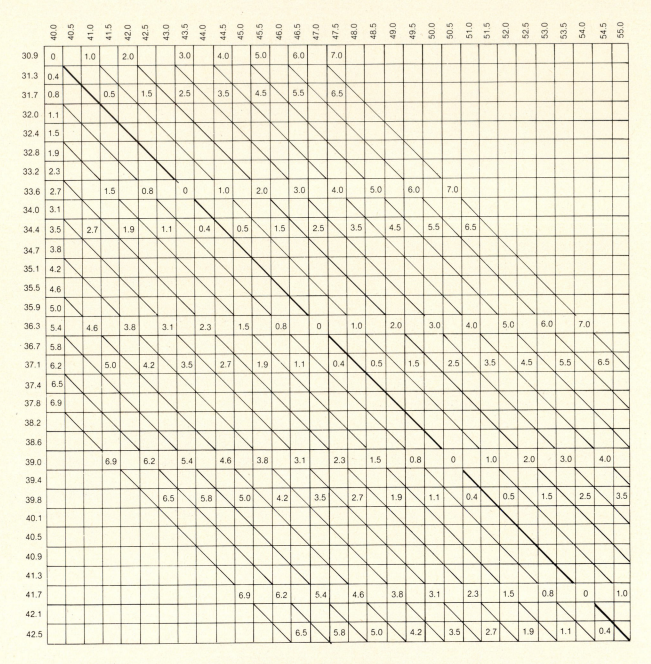

Mandibular Anterior Excess

Fig. 6-24 ■ Tables for calculating tooth-size discrepancy. **A,** Table for anterior relationships. The width of the mandibular incisors is indicated on the vertical axis, and the width of the maxillary incisors on the horizontal axis. The magnitude of discrepancy and whether it is relative mandibular or maxillary excess are indicated by the intersection of the lines (courtesy Dr. Robert Little).

BOLTON ANALYSIS

Maxillary Overall Excess

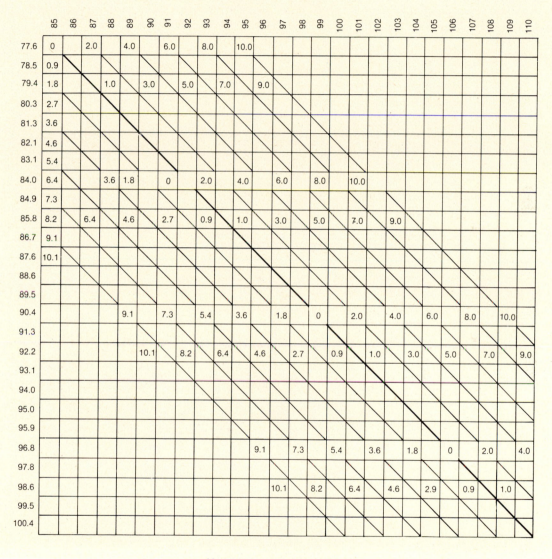

Mandibular Overall Excess

Fig. 6-24, cont'd ■ **B,** Similar table for overall tooth relationships.

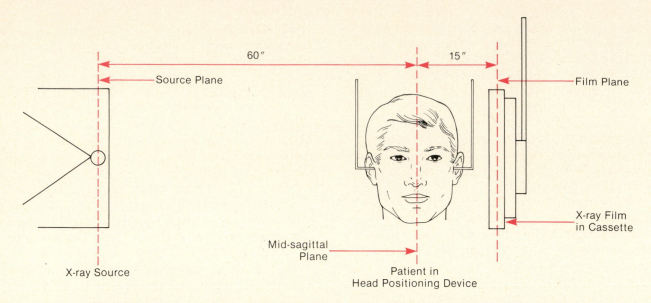

Fig. 6-25 ■ Diagrammatic representation of the American standard cephalometric arrangement. By convention, the distance from the x-ray source to the subject's midsagittal plane is 5 feet. The distance from the midsagittal plane to the cassette can vary in many machines, but must be the same for each patient every time.

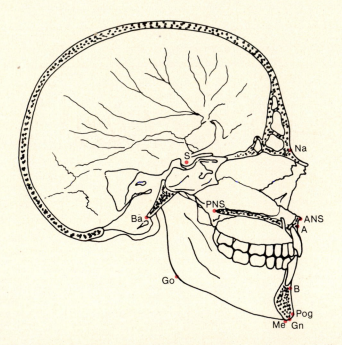

Fig. 6-26 ■ Definitions of cephalometric landmarks (as seen in a dissected skull): *Point A*, the innermost point on the contour of the premaxilla between anterior nasal spine and the incisor tooth. *ANS* (anterior nasal spine), the tip of the anterior nasal spine (sometimes modified as the point on the upper or lower contour of the spine where it is 3 mm thick: see Harvold analysis). *Point B*, the innermost point on the contour of the mandible between the incisor tooth and the bony chin; *Ba* (basion), the lowest point on the anterior margin of foramen magnum, at the base of the clivus; *Gn* (gnathion); the center of the inferior contour of the chin; *Go* (gonion), the center of the inferior contour of the mandibular angle; *Me* (menton), the most inferior point on the mandibular symphysis, i.e., the bottom of the chin; *Na* (nasion), the anterior point of the intersection between the nasal and frontal bones; *PNS* (posterior nasal spine), the tip of the posterior spine of the palatine bone, at the junction of the hard and soft palates; *Pog* (pogonion), the most anterior point on the contour of the chin.

displacement adds up to a severe malocclusion. Two apparently similar malocclusions as evaluated from the dental casts may turn out to be quite different when evaluated more completely, using cephalometric analysis to reveal differences in dentofacial proportions.

Cephalometric analysis is commonly carried out, not on the radiograph itself, but on a tracing that emphasizes the relationship of selected points. In essence, a tracing is used to reduce the amount of information on the film to a manageable level. The common cephalometric landmarks and a typical tracing are shown in Figs. 6-26 and 6-27. Cephalometric landmarks can be represented as a series of points whose coordinates are specified, making it possible to handle cephalometric data in a computer-compatible format.

Another way that radiographic cephalometrics is a useful clinical tool is in the study of changes brought about by orthodontic treatment. Serial cephalometric radiographs taken at intervals before, during, and after treatment can be superimposed to study changes in jaw and tooth positions retrospectively (Fig. 6-28). The observed changes result from a combination of growth and treatment (except in nongrowing adults), and with our present knowledge, it is difficult to determine which were caused by treatment.

Still another use for cephalometrics is to estimate growth changes that should occur for a patient, predicting future facial growth. If predicted growth changes are combined with a forecast of treatment changes, the result is an architectural plan or blueprint of orthodontic treatment called a visualized treatment objective (VTO). Preparation of a VTO can be very helpful in planning treatment for patients with complex problems and is mandatory in the development of a surgical-orthodontic treatment plan (see Chapter 21).

For diagnostic purposes, the major use of radiographic cephalometrics is in characterizing the patient's dental and

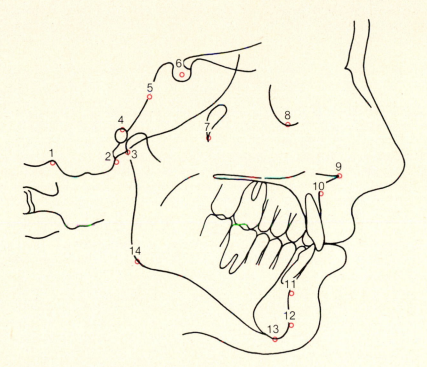

Fig. 6-27 ■ Definitions of cephalometric landmarks (as seen in a lateral cephalometric tracing): *1. Bo* (Bolton point), the highest point in the upward curvature of the retrocondylar fossa of the occipital bone; *2. Ba* (basion), the lowest point on the anterior margin of the foramen magnum, at the base of the clivus; *3. Ar* (articulare), the point of intersection between the shadow of the zygomatic arch and the posterior border of the mandibular ramus; *4. Po* (porion), the midpoint of the upper contour of the external auditory canal (anatomic porion); or, the midpoint of the upper contour of the metal ear rod of the cephalometer (machine porion); *5. SO* (sphenooccipital sychondrosis), the junction between the occipital and basisphenoid bones (if wide, the upper margin); *6. S* (sella), the midpoint of the cavity of sella turcica; *7. Ptm* (pterygomaxillary fissure), the point at the base of the fissure where the anterior and posterior walls meet; *8. Or* (orbitale), the lowest point on the inferior margin of the orbit; *9. ANS* (anterior nasal spine), the tip of the anterior nasal spine (sometimes modified as the point on the upper or lower contour of the spine where it is 3 mm thick; see Harvold analysis); *10. Point A,* the innermost point on the contour of the premaxilla between anterior nasal spine and the incisor tooth; *11. Point B,* the innermost point on the contour of the mandible between the incisor tooth and the bony chin; *12. Pog* (pogonion), the most anterior point on the contour of the chin; *13. Me* (menton), the most inferior point on the mandibular symphysis, i.e., the bottom of the chin.

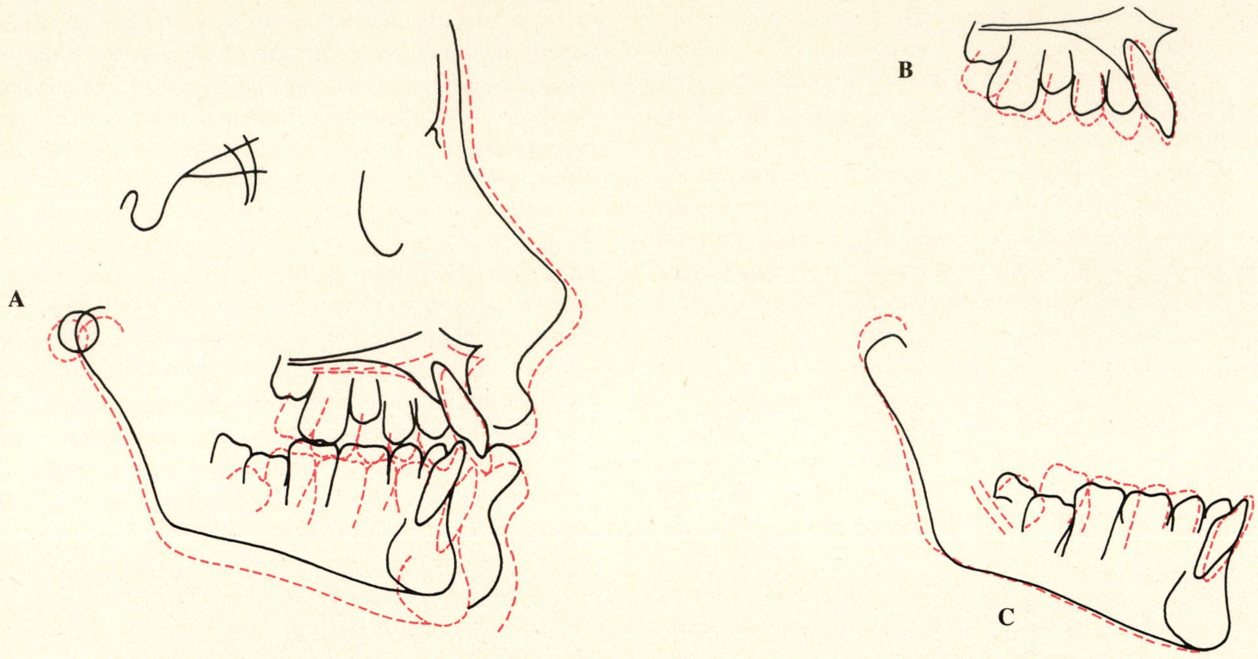

Fig. 6-28 ■ The three major cephalometric superimpositions showing tracings of the same individual at an earlier (black) and later (red) time. **A,** Superimposition on the anterior cranial base along the SN line. This superimposition shows the overall pattern of changes in the face, which result from a combination of growth and orthodontic treatment in children receiving orthodontic therapy. Note in this patient that the lower jaw grew downward and forward, while the upper jaw moved straight down. This allowed the correction of the patient's Class II malocclusion. **B,** Superimposition on the maxilla. This view shows changes of the maxillary teeth relative to the maxilla. In this patient's case, minimal changes occurred, the most notable being a forward movement of the upper first molar when the second primary molar was lost. **C,** Superimposition on the mandible, specifically on the inner surface of the mandibular symphysis and the outline of the mandibular canal and unerupted third molar crypts. This superimposition shows both changes of the mandible and changes of the mandibular teeth relative to the mandible. Note that the mandibular ramus increased in length posteriorly, while the condyle grew upward and backward. As would be expected, the mandibular molar teeth moved forward as the transition from the mixed to the early permanent dentition occurred.

skeletal relationships. In this section, we will focus on the use of cephalometric analysis to compare a patient to his or her peers, using population standards. The use of cephalometrics to estimate the magnitude and direction of future growth, and techniques for developing visualized treatment objectives combining growth prediction and estimated orthodontic treatment effects, are covered in Chapter 8.

Development of cephalometric analysis. To use cephalometrics to compare an individual to his or her population group, average values for various measurements must be established by studying a sample of individuals of the same sex, race, and age. This type of cephalometric analysis was first popularized after World War II in the form of the Downs analysis, developed at the University of Illinois and based on skeletal and facial proportions of 25 untreated adolescent whites selected because of their ideal dental occlusions.[8]

From the very beginning, the issue of how to establish the normal reference standards was difficult. It seems obvious that patients with severe cranial disproportions should be excluded from a normal sample. Since normal occlusion

is not the usual finding in a randomly selected population group, one must make a further choice in establishing the reference group, either excluding only obviously deformed individuals while including most malocclusions, or excluding essentially all those with malocclusion to obtain an ideal sample. In the beginning, the latter approach was chosen. Comparisons were made only with patients with excellent occlusion and facial proportions, as in the 25 individuals chosen for the Downs standards. Perhaps the extreme of selectivity in establishing a reference standard was exemplified by Steiner, whose original ideal measurements were reputedly based on one Hollywood starlet. Although the story is apocryphal, if it is true, Dr. Steiner had a very good eye, because recalculation of his original values based on much larger samples produced only minor changes.

The standards developed for the Downs analysis are still useful, but have largely been replaced by newer standards based on less rigidly selected groups. A major database for contemporary analysis is the Michigan growth study, carried out in Ann Arbor and involving a typical group of children

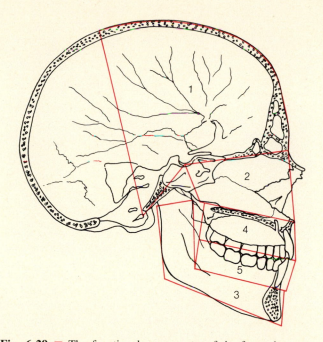

Fig. 6-29 ■ The functional components of the face, shown superimposed on the anatomic drawing. The cranium and cranial base *(1)*, the skeletal maxilla and nasomaxillary complex *(2)*, and the skeletal mandible *(3)* are parts of the face that exist whether or not there is a dentition. The maxillary teeth and alveolar process *(4)* and the mandibular teeth and alveolar process *(5)* are independent functional units, which can be displaced relative to the supporting bone of the maxilla and mandible, respectively. The goal of cephalometric analysis is to establish the relationship of these functional components in both the anteroposterior and vertical planes of space.

including mild and moderate malocclusions.[9] Other major sources are the Burlington (Ontario) growth study,[10] the Bolton study in Cleveland,[11] and several smaller growth studies, along with numerous specific samples collected in university projects to develop standards for specific racial and ethnic groups.

It can be helpful to conceptualize the goal of cephalometric analysis as evaluating the relationships, both horizontally and vertically, of the five major functional components of the face (Fig. 6-29): the cranium and cranial base, the skeletal maxilla (described as the portions of the maxilla that would remain if there were no teeth and alveolar processes), the skeletal mandible (similarly defined), the maxillary dentition, and the mandibular dentition. In this sense, any cephalometric analysis is a set of measurements designed to yield a description of the relationships between these functional units, so that the relationships and their patterns can be described accurately.

There are two basic ways to approach this goal. One is the approach chosen originally in the Downs analysis and followed by most workers in the field since that time. This is the use of selected measurements to establish the appropriate comparisons. Three measurement techniques have been suggested. The first of these utilizes linear measurements of the distance between two points on the cephalometric film or, more commonly, on a tracing of the film. These distances can be compared directly or in the form of proportions. The second method utilizes the angles formed between lines drawn on the radiograph or tracing. This has the advantage that one does not have to use ratios or make corrections for size differences between individuals. The third measurement technique is an arcial-type analysis, in which a series of arcs is utilized to evaluate the location of anatomic structures. It is possible to combine all three types of measurement within a single analytic method (demonstrated in the contemporary analyses below).

The other basic approach is to express the normative data graphically rather than as a series of measurements and to compare the patient's dentofacial form directly with an ideal normal via a template. In the early years of cephalometric analysis, it was recognized that representing the norm in graphic form might make it easier to recognize a pattern of relationships. The "Moorrees mesh" advocated in the early 1960s presented the patient's disproportions as the distortion of a grid,[12] but was not widely accepted because the normative relationships were not clearly established. In recent years, direct comparison of patients to templates has been advocated as a method of analysis.[13,14]

In the sections following, the contemporary measurement approaches are discussed first, and then the template methods are presented.

Measurement analysis

Choice of a horizontal reference line. In any technique for cephalometric analysis, it is necessary to establish a reference area or reference line. The same problem was faced in the early anthropometric and craniometric studies of the nineteenth century. By the late 1800s, skeletal remains of human beings had been found at many locations and were under extensive study. An international congress of anatomists and physical anthropologists was held at Frankfort in Germany in 1882, with the choice of a horizontal reference line for orientation of skulls an important item for the agenda. At the conference, the Frankfort plane, extending from the upper rim of the external auditory meatus (porion) to the inferior border of the orbital rim (orbitale), was adopted as the best representation of the natural orientation of the skull (Fig. 6-30). This Frankfort plane was employed for orientation of the patient from the beginning of cephalometrics and remains commonly used for analysis.

In cephalometric use, however, the Frankfort plane suffers from two difficulties. The first is that both its anterior and posterior landmarks, particularly porion, can be difficult to locate reliably on a cephalometric film. A radiopaque marker is placed on the rod that extends into the external auditory meatus as part of the cephalometric head positioning device, and the location of this marker, referred to as "machine porion" is often used to locate porion. The shadow of the auditory canal can be seen on cephalometric films, usually located slightly above and posterior to machine porion. The upper edge of this canal can also be used to

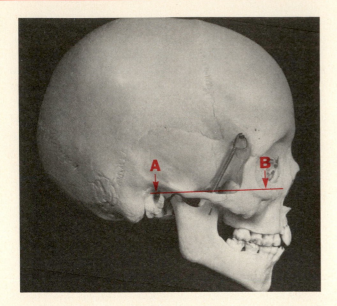

Fig. 6-30 ■ The Frankfort plane as originally described for orientation of dried skulls. This plane extends from the upper border of the external auditory canal *(A)* (porion) anteriorly to the upper border of the lower orbital rim (orbitale) *(B)*.

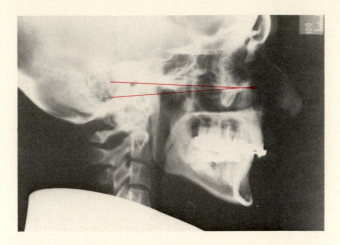

Fig. 6-31 ■ Using "machine porion," the upper surface of the ear rod of the cephalometric headholder, can give a different Frankfort plane than using "anatomic porion," the upper surface of the shadow of the auditory canal. Both porion and orbitale, the landmarks for the Frankfort plane, are difficult to locate accurately on cephalometric films, making Frankfort a relatively unreliable reference for cephalometric analysis.

establish "anatomic porion," which gives a slightly different Frankfort plane (Fig. 6-31).

An alternative horizontal reference line, easily and reliably detected on cephalometric films, is the line from sella turcica (S) to the junction between the nasal and frontal bones (N). In the average individual, the SN plane is oriented at 6 to 8 degrees to the Frankfort plane. Another way to obtain a Frankfort line is simply to draw it at 7 degrees to SN, but although this increases reliability and reproducibility, it decreases accuracy.

Finally, it is possible to use a "true horizontal" line, established physiologically rather than anatomically, as the horizontal reference plane. The Frankfort plane was originally adopted, in fact, as the best anatomic estimator of natural head position. This approach requires that cephalometric radiographs be taken with the patient in natural head position i.e., with the patient holding his head level. This position is obtained when relaxed individuals look at a distant object or into their own eyes in a mirror. As the anatomists of a century ago deduced, for most patients the true horizontal line closely approximates the Frankfort plane. Some patients, however, show significant differences. Similarly, a line at 7 degrees to SN is usually a good approximation to both Frankfort and the true horizontal, but there are individual differences of plus or minus 10 degrees in this relationship. The natural head position can be reproduced within 1 or 2 degrees.[25]

In contemporary usage, cephalometric films should be taken in the natural head position, so that the physiologic true horizontal plane is established. The inclination of SN to the true horizontal plane (or to the Frankfort plane if true horizontal plane is not known) should always be noted, and if the inclination of SN differs significantly from 6 degrees, measurements based on SN should be corrected by this difference.

Steiner analysis. The Steiner analysis, developed and promoted by Cecil Steiner in the 1950s,[15] can be considered the first of the modern cephalometric analyses for two reasons: it displayed measurements in a way that emphasized not just the individual measurements but their interrelationship into a pattern, and it offered specific guides for use of cephalometric measurements in treatment planning. The analysis remains widely used today.

In the Steiner analysis, the first measurement is the angle SNA, which is designed to evaluate the anteroposterior position of the maxilla relative to the anterior cranial base (Fig. 6-32). The "norm" for SNA is 82 ± 2 degrees. Thus, if a patient's SNA were greater than 84 degrees, this would be interpreted as maxillary protrusion, while SNA values of less than 80 degrees would be interpreted as maxillary retrusion. This interpretation is valid only if the SN plane is normally inclined to the true horizontal and the position of N is normal. Similarly, the angle SNB is used to evaluate the anteroposterior position of the mandible, for which the norm is 78 ± 2 degrees. The difference between SNA and SNB, the ANB angle, indicates the magnitude of the skeletal jaw discrepancy. What is important is not so much which jaw is at fault as the magnitude of the discrepancy that must be overcome in treatment, especially if orthodontic treatment is oriented toward correcting the dental occlusion more or less in spite of any jaw discrepancy. ANB, the SNA-SNB difference, is a reasonable indicator of this.

The magnitude of the ANB angle, however, is influenced by two factors other than the anteroposterior difference in

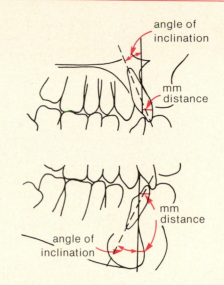

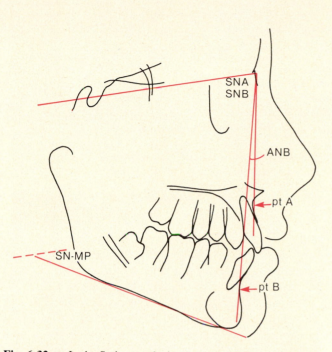

Fig. 6-32 ■ In the Steiner analysis, the angles SNA and SNB are used to establish the relationship of the maxilla and mandible to the cranial base, while the SN–MP (mandibular plane) angle is used to establish the vertical position of the mandible.

Fig. 6-33 ■ In the Steiner analysis, the relationship of the upper incisor to the NA line is used to establish the position of the maxillary dentition relative to the maxilla. Both the millimeter distance that the labial surface of the incisor is in front of the line, and inclination of the long axis of the incisor to the line, are measured. The position of the lower incisor relative to the mandible is established by similar measurements to the line NB. In addition, the prominence of the chin is established by measuring the millimeter distance from the NB line to pogonion, the most prominent point on the bony chin.

jaw position. One is the vertical height of the face. As the vertical distance between nasion and points A and B increases, the ANB angle will decrease. A second potential complication is caused by the fact that the anteroposterior position of nasion can also influence the magnitude of ANB. The validity of these criticisms has led to use of different indicators of jaw discrepancy in the later analyses presented in the following sections.

The next step in the Steiner analysis is to evaluate the relationship of the upper incisor to the NA line and both the lower incisor and the chin to the NB line, thus establishing the relative protrusion of the dentition (Fig. 6-33). Tweed had earlier suggested that the lower incisor should be positioned at 65 degrees to the Frankfort plane, thus compensating in the incisor position for the steepness of the mandibular plane.[16] In the Steiner analysis, both the angular inclination of each incisor, and the millimeter distance of the incisal edge from the vertical line, are measured. The millimeter distance establishes how prominent the incisor is relative to its supporting bone, while the inclination indicates whether the tooth has been tipped to its position or has moved there bodily. The prominence of the chin (pogonion) compared to the prominence of the lower incisor establishes the balance between them: the more prominent the chin, the more prominent the incisor can be, and vice versa. This important relationship is often referred to as the Holdaway ratio. The final measurement included in the Steiner analysis is the inclination of the mandibular plane

to SN, its only indicator of the vertical proportions of the face (Fig. 6-32). Tabulated standard values for three racial groups are given in Table 6-3.

The various measurements incorporated in the Steiner analysis from the beginning were represented graphically as "Steiner sticks," a convenient shorthand for presenting

Table 6-3 ■ Racial differences in cephalometric standard values

| Cephalometric measurement | Mean value | | |
	White	American Black	Japanese
SNA	82°	85°	81°
SNB	80	81	77
ANB	2	4	4
	4 mm	7 mm	6 mm
1̲ to NA	22°	23°	24°
	4 mm	10 mm	8 mm
1̄ to NB	25°	34°	31°
1̲ to 1̄	131	119	120
GoGn to SN	32	32	34
1̄ to mandibular plane	90°	—	—
1̄ to Frankfort plane	65°	—	—
S-Gn to Frankfort plane (Y axis)	61°	—	—

1̲, Upper incisor; 1̄, lower incisor; Go, gonion; Gn, gnathion (GoGn establishes one version of mandibular plane); S, sella; S-Gn, line from sella to gnathion.

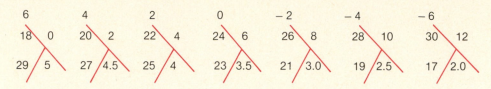

Fig. 6-34 ■ In the Steiner analysis, the ideal relationship of the incisors is expected when the ANB angle is 2 degrees, as indicated in the third diagram from the left. The inclination of the upper incisor to the NA line in degrees and its prominence in millimeters are shown on the second vertical line (22 degrees and 4 mm for an ANB of 2 degrees). The inclination of the lower incisor to the NB line and its prominence in millimeters are shown on the third line (25 degrees and 4 mm for an ANB of 2 degrees). If the ANB angle is different from 2 degrees, the different positioning of the incisors given by the inclination and protrusion figures will produce a dental compromise that leads to correct occlusion despite the jaw discrepancy. The fact that this degree of compensation in tooth position for jaw discrepancy can be produced by orthodontic treatment does not, of course, indicate that these compromises are necessarily the best possible treatment results.

the measurements. A major contribution of the Steiner analysis was that it incorporated a method for determining what compromises in incisor positions would be necessary to achieve normal occlusion when the ANB angle was not ideal. The Steiner compromises, and the method for establishing them for any given patient, are illustrated in Fig. 6-34. These figures can be helpful in establishing how much tooth movement is needed to correct any malocclusion.

However, it should not be overlooked that relying on tooth movement alone to correct skeletal malocclusion, particularly as the skeletal discrepancies become large, is not necessarily the best approach to orthodontic treatment. It is usually better to correct skeletal discrepancies at their source than to attempt only to achieve a dental compromise or camouflage (see Chapter 8 for further discussion of this important point). It is fair to say that the Steiner compromises reflect the prevailing attitude of Steiner's era, that the effects of orthodontic treatment are almost entirely limited to the alveolar process.

Sassouni analysis. The Sassouni analysis was the first cephalometric method to emphasize vertical as well as horizontal relationships, and the interaction between vertical and horizontal proportions.[17] Sassouni pointed out that the horizontal anatomic planes—the inclination of the anterior cranial base, Frankfort plane, palatal plane, occlusal plane and mandibular plane—in well-proportioned faces tend to converge toward a single point. The inclination of these planes to each other reflects the vertical proportionality of the face (Fig. 6-35).

If the planes intersect relatively close to the face and diverge quickly as they pass anteriorly, the facial proportions are long anteriorly and short posteriorly, which predisposes the individual to an open bite malocclusion. Sassouni coined the term "skeletal open bite" for this anatomic relationship. If the planes are nearly parallel, so that they converge far behind the face and diverge only slowly as they pass anteriorly, there is a skeletal predisposition toward anterior deep bite, and the condition is termed "skeletal deep bite."

In addition, an unusual inclination of one of the planes stands out because it misses the general area of intersection.

Rotation of the maxilla down in back and up in front may contribute to skeletal open bite, for instance. The tipped palatal plane reveals this clearly (Fig. 6-36).

Sassouni evaluated the anteroposterior position of the face and dentition by noting the relationship of various points to arcs drawn from the area of intersection of the planes. In a well-proportioned face, the anterior nasal spine (representing the anterior extent of the maxilla), the maxillary incisor, and the bony chin should be located along the same arc. As with vertical proportions, it could be seen visually if a single point deviated from the expected position, and in what direction.

Although the total arcial analysis described by Sassouni is no longer widely used, Sassouni's analysis of vertical facial proportions has become an integral part of the overall analysis of a patient. In addition to any other measurements that might be made, it is valuable in any patient to analyze the divergence of the horizontal planes and to examine whether one of the planes is clearly disproportionate to the others.

Harvold analysis, Wits analysis. Both the Harvold and Wits analyses are aimed solely at describing the severity or degree of jaw disharmony. Harvold, using data derived from the Burlington growth study, developed standards for the "unit length" of the maxilla and mandible.[18] The maxillary unit length is measured from the posterior border of the mandibular condyle to the anterior nasal spine, while the mandibular unit length is measured from the same point to the anterior point of the chin (Fig. 6-37). The difference between these numbers provides an indication of the size discrepancy between the jaws. In analyzing the difference between maxillary and mandibular unit lengths, it must be kept in mind that the shorter the vertical distance between the maxilla and mandible, the more anteriorly the chin will be placed for any given unit difference, and vice versa. The position of the teeth has no influence on the Harvold figures (Table 6-4).

The Wits analysis[19] was conceived primarily as a way to overcome the limitations of ANB as an indicator of jaw discrepancy. It is based on a projection of points A and B

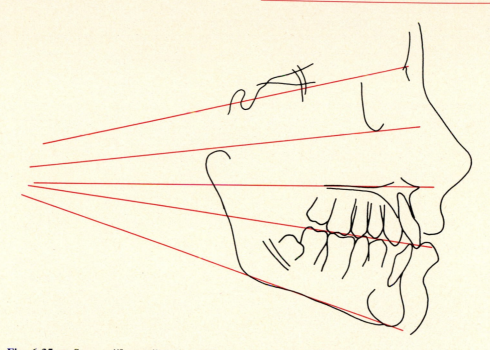

Fig. 6-35 ■ Sassouni[17] contributed the idea that if a series of horizontal planes are drawn, from the SN line at the top to the mandibular plane below, they will project toward a common meeting point in a well-proportioned face.

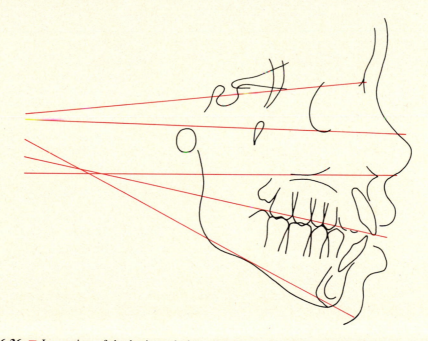

Fig. 6-36 ■ Inspection of the horizontal planes for this patient makes it clear that the maxilla is rotated downward posteriorly and the mandible rotated downward anteriorly. These rotations of the jaws contribute to an open bite tendency, so the skeletal pattern revealed here is often referred to as "skeletal open bite."

to the occlusal plane, along which the linear difference between these points is measured (Fig. 6-38). If the anteroposterior position of the jaws is normal, the projections from points A and B will intersect the occlusal plane at very nearly the same point. The magnitude of a discrepancy in the Class II direction can be estimated by how many mil-

limeters the point A projection is in front of the point B projection, and vice versa for Class III.

The Wits analysis, in contrast to the Harvold analysis, is influenced by the teeth both horizontally and vertically—horizontally because points A and B are somewhat influenced by the dentition and vertically because the occlusal

Table 6-4 ■ Harvold standard values (mm)

	Age	Male Mean Value	Male Standard Deviation	Female Mean Value	Female Standard Deviation
Maxillary length (temporomandibular point to ANS) (see Fig. 6-37)	6	82	3.2	80	3.0
	9	87	3.4	85	3.4
	12	92	3.7	90	4.1
	14	96	4.5	92	3.7
	16	100	4.2	93	3.5
Mandibular length (temporomandibular point to prognathion)	6	99	3.9	97	3.6
	9	107	4.4	105	3.9
	12	114	4.9	113	5.2
	14	121	6.1	117	3.6
	16	127	5.3	119	4.4
Lower face height (ANS-Me)	6	59	3.6	57	3.2
	9	62	4.3	60	3.6
	12	64	4.6	62	4.4
	14	68	5.2	64	4.4
	16	71	5.7	65	4.7

plane is determined by the vertical position of the teeth. It is important for Wits analysis that the functional occlusal plane, drawn along the maximum intercuspation of the posterior teeth, be used rather than an occlusal plane influenced by the vertical position of the incisors.

Neither the Harvold nor the Wits analysis is a complete measurement system. Both, properly interpreted, can add insight into the magnitude of a jaw discrepancy.

Ricketts analysis. The Ricketts analysis[20] is essentially an 11 factor summary analysis that attempts to (1) locate the chin in space, (2) locate the maxilla through the convexity of the face, (3) locate the denture in the face, and (4) evaluate the profile. In the Ricketts analysis, the major reference lines are the true Frankfort horizontal (using anatomic, not machine porion), the nasion-basion line, and the pterygoid vertical, which is established perpendicular to the Frankfort horizontal at the root of the pterygomaxillary fissure. This analysis was used in the original computerized cephalometric service and can be obtained commercially (from Rocky Mountain Data Systems).

Six of the 11 measurements in the Ricketts analysis are aimed at locating the chin in space. These measurements

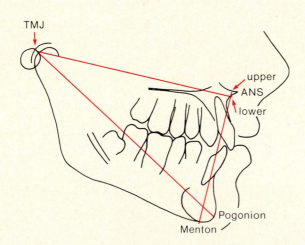

Fig. 6-37 ■ Measurements used in the Harvold analysis. Maxillary length is measured from TMJ, the posterior wall of the glenoid fossa, to lower ANS, defined as the point on the lower shadow of the anterior nasal spine where the projecting spine is 3 mm thick. Mandibular length is measured from TMJ to prognathion, the point on the bony chin contour giving the maximum length from the temporomandibular joint (close to pogonion), while lower face height is measured from upper ANS, the similar point on the upper contour of the spine where it is 3 mm thick, to menton.

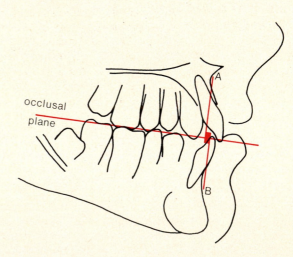

Fig. 6-38 ■ In the Wits analysis, points *A* and *B* are projected to the functional occlusal plane, which is drawn through the occlusal surfaces of the posterior teeth, and the AB difference is measured. In well-proportioned faces, the AB difference is 1 mm or less.

Table 6-5 ■ Measurements used in the Ricketts analysis*

Measurement	Mean at age 9	Age change	Measurement	Mean at age 9	Age change
1. Facial axis (angle BaN-PtmGn lines)	90° ± 3	None	8. Lower incisor to APog (mm distance APog-incisal edge)	1 ± 2 mm	None
2. Facial angle (angle FH-NPog, anatomic porion)	87 ± 3	+1°/3 yr	9. Mandibular incisor inclination (NPog–incisor axis)	22 ± 4	None
3. Mandibular plane (angle FH-GoGn)	26° ± 4	−1°/3 yr	10. Upper molar to pterygoid vertical (mm distance mesiobuccal cusp 6 to vertical line from Ptm perpendicular to Frankfort plane	14 mm	+1 mm/yr
4. Facial taper (angle NPog-GoGn)	68° ± 4	None
5. Lower face height (angle ANSXi-XiPM)	47° ± 4	None
6. Mandibular arc (angle DCXi-XiPM)	26° ± 4	+ ½°/yr
7. Convexity of point A (mm distance NPog-APog at A)	2 ± 2 mm	−1 mm/3 yr	11. Lower lip to E plane (mm distance most prominent point lower lip to line from soft tissue pogonion to tip of nose	−2 ± 2 mm	Decreases

*First six measurements locate the chin in space; last five relate the dentition to the profile. See Figs. 6-39 and 6-40.

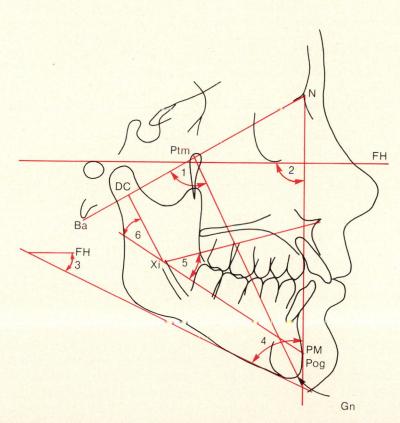

Fig. 6-39 ■ Points and measurements used in the Ricketts analysis to locate the chin in space. Points not previously described: *Xi,* geometric center of the ramus of the mandible; *PM,* point on anterior border of symphysis between point B and pogonion where the curvature changes from concave to convex; *DC,* point in the center of the condylar neck where the basion-nasion plane crosses it.

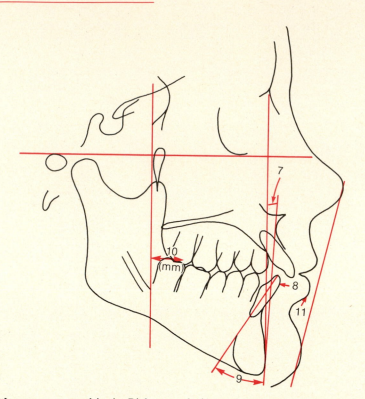

Fig. 6-40 ■ Measurements used in the Ricketts analysis to relate the dentition to the profile.

Measurements	Mean at age 9	Age change
(7) Convexity of point A (mm distance NPog-APog at A)	2 mm ± 2	−1 mm/3 yrs
(8) Lower incisor to APog (mm distance APog-incisal edge)	1 mm ± 2	None
(9) Mandibular incisor inclination (NPog-incisor axis)	22° ± 4	None
(10) Upper molar to pterygoid vertical (mm distance mesiobuccal cusp 6 to vertical line from Ptm perpendicular to Frankfort plane	14 mm	+1 mm/yr
(11) Lower lip to E plane (mm distance most prominent point lower lip to line from soft tissue pogonion to tip of nose).	−2 mm ± 2	Decreases

are illustrated and defined in Fig. 6-39. The remaining measurements, illustrated in Fig. 6-40, evaluate the other three major objectives of the analysis.

The Ricketts approach emphasizes not only an analysis of the patient's initial condition, but the prediction of future growth and treatment effects in a visualized treatment objective (VTO). Included with the tabulated normal data for the factors in the Ricketts analysis is the amount of change expected during normal growth (Table 6-5). This information is useful, of course, not only for correcting the norms for patients of different ages but also in the growth prediction phase of preparing a VTO, which is discussed in more detail in Chapter 8.

The Ricketts analysis is a contemporary synthesis based on somewhat unusual measurements and reference points. Its greatest weakness is that the normative data for many of the measurements are based on unspecified samples collected by Ricketts. It would be possible to calculate the same norms for the well-defined and intensively studied patients in the university growth studies that have been the source of normative data for most other analyses, and per-

haps such data will become available in the future. For the moment, the analysis must be interpreted cautiously, particularly when individuals whose measurements differ significantly from the norms are encountered. Nevertheless, this analysis does pull together the data in a way that facilitates establishing the positional relationships of the functional components of the face and jaws.

McNamara analysis. The McNamara analysis, originally published in 1983[21], combines elements of previous approaches (Ricketts and Harvold) with original measurements to attempt a more precise definition of jaw and tooth positions. In this method, both the anatomic Frankfort plane and the basion-nasion line are used as reference planes. The anteroposterior position of the maxilla is evaluated with regard to its position relative to the "nasion perpendicular," a vertical line extending downward from nasion perpendicular to the Frankfort plane (Fig. 6-41). The maxilla should be on or slightly ahead of this line. The second step in the procedure is a comparison of maxillary and mandibular length, using Harvold's approach. The mandible is positioned in space utilizing the lower anterior face height (ANS-

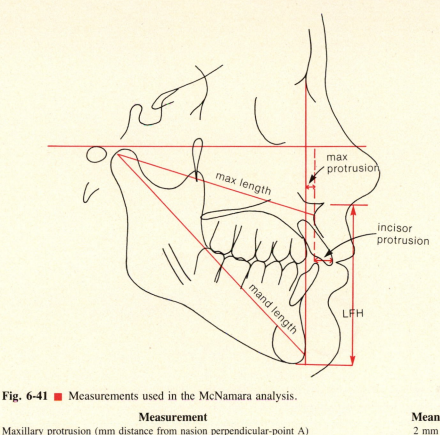

Fig. 6-41 ■ Measurements used in the McNamara analysis.

Measurement	Mean
Maxillary protrusion (mm distance from nasion perpendicular-point A)	2 mm
Maxillary incisor protrusion (mm distance from line parallel to nasion perpendicular to labial surface of incisor)	4 mm
Maxillary length	
Mandibular length	As in Harvold analysis
Lower face height (LFH)	

menton). The upper incisor is related to the maxilla using a line through point A perpendicular to the Frankfort plane, similar to but slightly different from Steiner's relationship of the incisor to the NA line. The lower incisor is related as in the Ricketts analysis, primarily using the A-pogonion line (Fig. 6-42).

The McNamara analysis has two major strengths: (1) It relates the jaws via the nasion perpendicular, in essence projecting the difference in anteroposterior position of the jaws to an approximation of the true vertical line. (Using a true vertical line, perpendicular to the true horizontal rather than anatomic Frankfort, would be better yet; the major reason for not doing so in constructing the analysis is that the cephalometric films from which the normative data were derived were not taken in natural head position.) (2) The normative data are based on the well-defined Bolton sample, which is also available in template form, meaning that the McNamara measurements are highly compatible with preliminary analysis by comparison with the Bolton templates.

Template analysis. One way to represent the data from a normative sample is to present it in terms of tabulated numbers. One of the objectives of any analytic approach based on measurements, of course, is to reduce the practically infinite set of possible measurements to a manageably small group of specific measurements that can be compared with specific norms and thereby provide useful diagnostic information. From the beginning, it was recognized that the measurements for comparison with the norms should have several characteristics. The following were specifically desired: (1) the measurements should be useful clinically in differentiating patients with skeletal and dental characteristics of malocclusion; (2) the measurements should not be affected by the size of the patient, i.e., proportions should be preserved between small and large individuals. This meant an emphasis on angular rather than linear measurements; and (3) the measurements should be unaffected, or at least minimally affected, by the age of the patient. Otherwise, a different table of standards for each age would be necessary to overcome the effects of growth.

As time passed, it became apparent that a number of measurements that fulfilled the first criterion of diagnostic usefulness did not meet either the second or third criteria.

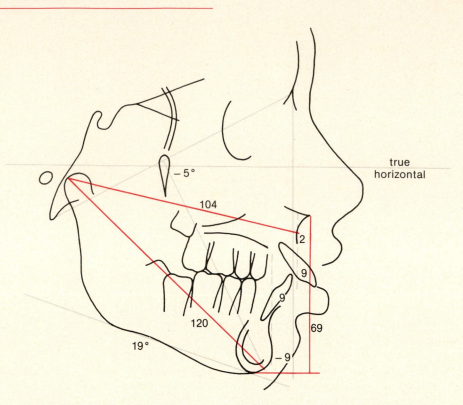

Fig. 6-42 ■ Analysis of a 12-year-old male, using the McNamara approach and including measurements from Ricketts and Harvold.

Measurement	Patient	Standard	Interpretation
Facial axis	−5°	0 (90)	Mandible growing down and back
Maxillary length	104 mm	101	Maxilla slightly prominent
Mandibular length	120 mm	114	Mandible slightly long
Lower face height	69 mm	64	Face height slightly long
Mandibular plane	19	26	Skeletal deep bite tendency
Maxillary protrusion	2 mm	2 mm	Good anteroposterior position
Maxillary dental protrusion	9 mm	4 mm	Upper incisor protrusion
Mandibular dental protrusion	9 mm	4 mm	Lower incisor protrusion
Mandibular protrusion	−9 mm	0	Mandible retrusive: skeletal Class II

Linear measurements could be used as proportions to make them size-invariant, but more and more linear measurements not used proportionally crept into diagnostic use. As excellent samples of children who had participated in growth studies became available and were used for the construction of cephalometric reference standards, it was observed that some relationships previously thought to be invariant with age changed during growth. Like it or not, it was inappropriate to compare cephalometric standards for a 9-year-old child to those of adults, or vice versa. There was obviously an advantage in using standards that changed at various ages, because this allowed a number of clinically useful linear as well as angular measurements to be included.

Any cephalometric tracing can be represented as a series of points, and each point can be located in space in terms of its coordinates on an *(x,y)* grid. If the tracings for all the individuals in a group were represented as the coordinates of a number of points (the traditional landmarks would serve nicely), it would be possible to calculate the average location for each point and then to reconstruct a composite tracing that represented the average for the group. In this way, both sex and age differences could be accommodated: an average or ideal tracing for individuals of a given sex and age could be produced. Data from the various growth studies have been treated in just this way to produce templates representing the average 9-year-old, 10-year-old, etc.

The data can be set up in schematic form to show the changing position of various landmarks with age on a single template, as has been done with the Michigan and Burlington data. Such templates are particularly useful for growth prediction, discussed in Chapter 8. Average normal templates can also be reconstructed anatomically by drawing in the lines between the averaged points, thus generating an idealized tracing of the average 9-year-old.[14] Both types of templates can be used to compare an individual patient with the norm for his or her age group, but the second type is particularly convenient for this sort of direct visual comparison. Data from the Broadbent-Bolton growth study in

Cleveland have been prepared in the idealized template form,[11] are readily available (from Kirtland Enterprises, Cleveland) and are most often used for template analysis. Anatomic templates from the Alabama growth study are also available.[13]

Even though that feature is not thought to be as important now as it was in the beginning, most measurements contained in the Ricketts, McNamara, and other analyses presented previously are minimally affected by age. Templates, on the other hand, are very much affected by age. For successful template analysis, an important preliminary step is the estimation of the patient's developmental age. Chronologic age correlates with developmental age, and it is a safe assumption that as data from a large group of children were pooled, variations in developmental age cancelled out. An individual child can be either developmentally advanced or retarded in comparison to his or her chronologic age, however, and the appropriate comparison is with children of the same developmental, not chronologic age.

Developmental age can be assessed by several methods. The state of development of secondary sexual characteristics can be helpful, particularly around adolescence; the clinical impression of relative maturity can be helpful. If warranted, more precise information can be gained from an analysis of hand-wrist radiographs.

Hand-wrist films have been used for the calculation of skeletal age for many years (see Fig. 4-23). The ossification and development of the carpal bones of the wrist, the metacarpals of the hands, and the phalanges of the fingers form a chronology of skeletal development. A satisfactory handwrist radiograph can be made utilizing a standard cephalometric cassette and a dental x-ray or the cephalometric x-ray source. In use, the overall pattern observed in the handwrist film is compared with age standards in a reference atlas[22] to obtain a skeletal age for the patient. In addition, the status of certain specific landmarks such as the ulnar sesamoid or the hamate can be used to obtain an estimate of the timing of the adolescent growth spurt.[23,24] This method is particularly valuable for children whose developmental differ markedly from their chronologic age.

The first step in template analysis, selection of the appropriate age standard, should be done from a background of knowledge of the patient's developmental age, but also taking into account his or her physical size. As a general rule, the reference template should be selected so that the length of the anterior cranial base (of which the SN distance is a good approximation) is approximately the same for the patient and the template. In almost all instances, correcting for differences between developmental and chronologic age also leads to the selection of a template that more nearly approximates the anterior cranial base length.

Analysis using a template is based on a series of superimpositions of the template over a tracing of the patient being analyzed. The sequence of superimpositions follows:

1. Cranial base superimposition, which allows the relationship of the maxilla and mandible to the cranium to be

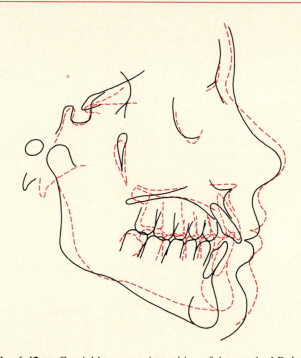

Fig. 6-43 ■ Cranial base superimposition of the standard Bolton template for age 14 (red) on the tracing of a 13-year-old boy. The age 14 template was selected because it matches cranial base length. Note that from a comparison of the template with this patient, the considerable increase in the patient's lower face height and downward rotation of his mandible can be seen clearly. It is also apparent that the patient's maxilla is rotated downward posteriorly. This comparison of a patient's tracing with a template is a direct approach toward describing the relationship of functional dentofacial units.

evaluated (Fig. 6-43). In general, the most useful approach is to superimpose on the SN line, registering the template over the patient's tracing at nasion rather than sella if there is a difference in cranial base length. For growth prediction with templates, it is important to use the posterior superimposition points described with the prediction method. For analysis, registering SN at N is usually preferable.

With the cranial base registered, the anteroposterior and vertical position of maxilla and mandible can be observed and described. It is important at this stage to look, not at the position of the teeth, but at the position of the landmarks that indicate the skeletal units, i.e., anterior nasal spine and point A for the anterior maxilla, posterior nasal spine for the posterior maxilla; point B, pogonion and gnathion for the anterior mandible, and gonion for the posterior mandible. The object is to evaluate the position of the skeletal units. The template is being used to see directly how the patient's jaw positions differ from the norm.

2. The second superimposition is on the maximum contour of the maxilla, to evaluate the relationship of the maxillary dentition to the maxilla (Fig. 6-44). Again, it is important to evaluate the position of the teeth both vertically and anteroposteriorly. The template makes it easy to see whether the teeth are displaced vertically, information often

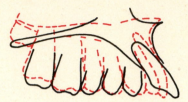

Fig. 6-44 ■ Superimposition of the Bolton template on the maxilla (primarily, the anterior palatal contour) of the patient shown in Fig. 6-43. This superimposition clearly reveals the forward protrusion of the maxillary incisors, but shows that the vertical relationship of the maxillary teeth to the maxilla for this patient is nearly ideal.

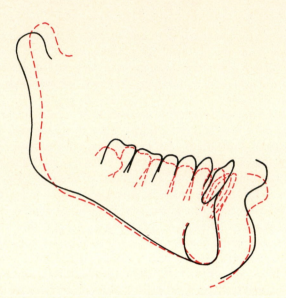

Fig. 6-45 ■ Superimposition of the Bolton template on the mandible of the patient in Fig. 6-43. This superimposition indicates that the patient's mandible is longer than the ideal, but the ramus is shorter and inclined posteriorly. All the mandibular teeth have erupted too much, especially the incisors.

not obtained in measurement analysis techniques.

3. The third superimposition is on the symphysis of the mandible along the lower border, to evaluate the relationship of the mandibular dentition to the mandible (Fig. 6-45). If the shadow of the mandibular canal is shown on the templates, a more accurate orientation can be obtained by registering along this rather than the lower border posteriorly. Both the vertical and the anteroposterior positions of the anterior and posterior teeth should be noted.

Template analysis in this fashion has two advantages: first, it allows the easy use of age-related standards and second, it quickly provides an overall impression of the way in which the patient's dentofacial structures are related. On the other hand, the template analysis is less precise and less quantitative than the measurement approaches. Sometimes, the objective of measurements, which is to gain an overall understanding of the pattern of the patient's facial relationships, is overlooked in the acquisition of the measurements themselves. Comparing the patient to a template is an excellent way to overcome this hazard and be sure that one does not miss the forest while observing the trees.

Summary of contemporary cephalometry methodology. In its early years, cephalometric analysis was correctly criticized as being just a "numbers game," leading to orthodontic treatment aimed at producing certain numbers on a cephalometric film that might or might not represent the best treatment result for that patient. Totally accepting the Steiner compromises and setting treatment goals solely in terms of producing these numbers could certainly be criticized on that basis. The problem arose, of course, not in the cephalometric measurements themselves, but in their interpretation. It must be kept in mind that all cephalometric measurements are used to estimate some anatomic relationships, so that the clinician can better understand the underlying basis for a malocclusion. To do this, he or she must look, not just at individual measurements compared to a norm, but at the pattern of relationships. The measurement is a means, not an end in itself.

At the present, each of the analytic approaches discussed previously can be said to have merit, and each can also be described as incomplete for the analysis of some patients.

A rational approach to modern cephalometrics is to focus on evaluating the relationship of the functional units and to measure whatever is necessary to establish the position, horizontally and vertically, of each of those units. Template analysis, supplemented with measurements as appropriate, is an efficient way to approach this objective and has the virtue of emphasis on the overall analysis of dentofacial relationships. There is nothing wrong with starting with one of the contemporary measurement approaches, and indeed there may be advantages in doing so, provided that the basic approach is supplemented with some other measurements when the Steiner, Ricketts, McNamara, or other method falls short of providing an adequate description for the individual patient.

■ *Orthodontic Classification*

Classification has traditionally been an important tool in the diagnosis–treatment planning procedure. An ideal classification would summarize the diagnostic data and imply the treatment plan. In our concept of diagnosis, classification can be viewed as the (orderly) reduction of the database to a list of the patient's problems (Fig. 6-46).

■ Development of Classification Systems

The first useful orthodontic classification, still an important part of orthodontic classification to the present time, was Angle's classification of malocclusion into Classes I, II, and III (see Chapter 1). The basis of the Angle classification was the relationship of the first molar teeth and the alignment (or lack of it) of the teeth relative to the line of

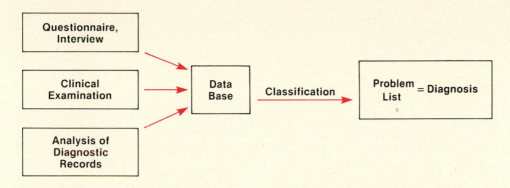

Fig. 6-46 ■ Conceptually, classification can be viewed as an orderly way to derive a list of the patient's problems from the database.

occlusion. Angle's classification thus created four groups:

Normal occlusion	Normal (Class I) molar relationship, teeth on line of occlusion
Class I malocclusion	Normal (Class I) molar relationship, teeth crowded, rotated, etc.
Class II malocclusion	Lower molar distal to upper molar, relationship of other teeth to line of occlusion not specified
Class III malocclusion	Lower molar mesial to upper molar, relationship of other teeth to line of occlusion not specified

The Angle system was a tremendous step forward, not only because it provided an orderly way to classify malocclusion, but also because for the first time it provided a simple definition of normal occlusion, and thereby a way to distinguish normal occlusion from malocclusion.

From an early stage, it was recognized that the Angle classification was not complete, because it did not include important characteristics of the patient's problem. In 1912, a committee of the British Orthodontic Society chaired by Norman Bennett suggested that although the Angle system was an adequate classification of antero-posterior relationships, it did not include information about the transverse and vertical planes and should be extended to do so.

Calvin Case, Angle's principal professional rival in the early part of the twentieth century, noted that the Angle system did not recognize protrusion of incisors as a problem, although this could be deforming for the patient. Angle classification implied a skeletal jaw relationship in the anteroposterior plane of space, because the molar relationship correlates with the skeletal jaw relationship, but it contained no information as to which jaw was at fault and was misleading if the skeletal proportions did not match the occlusal relationships.

The deficiencies in the original Angle system led to a series of informal additions at an early stage. A series of subdivisions of Class I were proposed by Martin Dewey, initially Angle's protege but later his rival. Gradually An-

gle's classification numbers were extended to refer to four distinct but related characteristics: the classification of malocclusion, as in the orginal plan; the molar relationship; the skeletal jaw relationship; and the pattern of growth (Fig. 6-47). Thus, a Class II jaw relationship actually meant a relationship in which the mandible was positioned distally relative to the maxilla, which was usually found in connection with a Class II molar relationship, but occasionally could be present despite a Class I molar relationship. Similarly, a Class II growth pattern was defined as a downward and backward growth direction of the mandible which would tend to create and maintain Class II jaw and molar relationships. Class I and Class III growth patterns show balanced and disproportionate forward mandibular growth, respectively.

In the 1930s the German orthodontist Simon proposed a new system of classification, based on a specific recording of the vertical orientation of the jaws to the cranium by what Simon called "gnathostatic" casts. In addition, Simon included an evaluation of the anteroposterior position of the incisors by specifying canine position relative to the orbits. The development of cephalometric radiology made it easier to evaluate both skeletal proportions and incisor protrusion. With the introduction of cephalometric radiology into orthodontic practice in the 1950s, Simon's concepts were incorporated into routine orthodontic diagnosis although his method of gnathostatic casts was abandoned.

In the 1960s, Ackerman and Proffit formalized the system of informal additions to the Angle method by identifying five major characteristics of malocclusion that should be considered and systematically described in classification (Fig. 6-48).[23] Although the elements of the Ackerman-Proffit scheme are often not combined exactly as originally proposed, this classification by five major characteristics is now widely used. The approach overcomes the major weaknesses of the Angle scheme. Specifically, it incorporates an evaluation of crowding and asymmetry within the dental arches and includes an evaluation of incisor protrusion and recognizes the relationship between protrusion and crowding. The Ackerman-Proffit system also includes the trans-

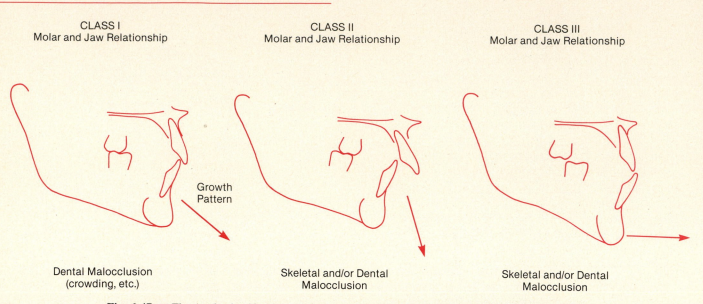

CLASS I
Molar and Jaw Relationship

CLASS II
Molar and Jaw Relationship

CLASS III
Molar and Jaw Relationship

Growth Pattern

Dental Malocclusion
(crowding, etc.)

Skeletal and/or Dental
Malocclusion

Skeletal and/or Dental
Malocclusion

Fig. 6-47 ■ The Angle classification numbers have come to describe four different characteristics: the classification of malocclusion, the molar relationship, the jaw relationship, and the pattern of growth, as shown here diagrammatically. Although the jaw relationship and growth pattern correlate with the molar relationship, the correlations are far from perfect. It is not unusual to observe a Class I molar relationship in a patient with a Class II jaw relationship, or to find that an individual with a Class I molar and jaw relationship grows in a Class III pattern, which ultimately will produce a Class III malocclusion.

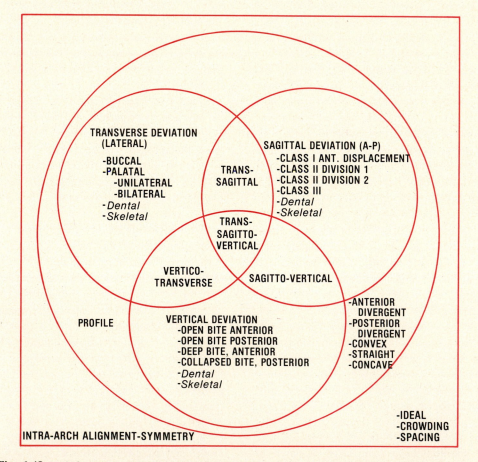

TRANSVERSE DEVIATION
(LATERAL)
-BUCCAL
-PALATAL
-UNILATERAL
-BILATERAL
-*Dental*
-*Skeletal*

SAGITTAL DEVIATION (A-P)
-CLASS I ANT. DISPLACEMENT
-CLASS II DIVISION 1
-CLASS II DIVISION 2
-CLASS III
-*Dental*
-*Skeletal*

TRANS-
SAGITTAL

TRANS-
SAGITTO-
VERTICAL

VERTICO-
TRANSVERSE

SAGITTO-VERTICAL

PROFILE

VERTICAL DEVIATION
-OPEN BITE ANTERIOR
-OPEN BITE POSTERIOR
-DEEP BITE, ANTERIOR
-COLLAPSED BITE, POSTERIOR
-*Dental*
-*Skeletal*

-ANTERIOR
DIVERGENT
-POSTERIOR
DIVERGENT
-CONVEX
-STRAIGHT
-CONCAVE

-IDEAL
-CROWDING
-SPACING

INTRA-ARCH ALIGNMENT-SYMMETRY

Fig. 6-48 ■ Ackerman and Proffit represented the five major characteristics of malocclusion via a Venn diagram. The sequential study of the major characteristics, not their graphic representation, is the key to this classification system.

verse and vertical as well as the anteroposterior planes of space, and it incorporates information about skeletal jaw proportions at the appropriate point, that is, in the description of relationships in each of the planes of space.

To utilize this classification method, the three major types of diagnostic information specified previously are required: data about the dentition itself, occlusal relationships, and skeletal jaw relationships. This is derived from clinical examination, panoramic and (if needed) intraoral radiographs, and clinical, photographic, or cephalometric evaluation of dental and facial proportions. In essence, the method of examining the five major characteristics in sequence provides a convenient way of organizing the diagnostic information to be sure that no important points are overlooked.

■ Classification by the Characteristics of Malocclusion

Step 1. Evaluation of facial proportions and esthetics. This step is carried out during the clinical examination, while facial asymmetry, anteroposterior and vertical facial proportions, and lip prominence as related to incisor protrusion are evaluated. The clinical findings can be checked against the facial photographs and lateral cephalometric film, which should confirm the clinical judgment.

Step 2. Evaluation of alignment and symmetry within the dental arches. This step is carried out by examining the dental arches from the occlusal view, evaluating first the symmetry within each dental arch and second, the amount of crowding or spacing present. Space analysis quantitates crowding or spacing, but these figures must be interpreted in the light of other findings in the total evaluation of the patient.

Step 3. Evaluation of skeletal and dental relationships in the transverse plane of space. At this stage, the casts are brought into occlusion and the occlusal relationships are examined, beginning with the transverse (posterior crossbite) plane of space. The objectives of the analysis are to accurately describe the occlusion and to distinguish between skeletal and dental contributions to malocclusion.

Posterior crossbite is described in terms of the position of the upper molars (Fig. 6-49). Thus, a bilateral maxillary lingual (or palatal) crossbite means that the upper molars are lingual to their normal position on both sides, whereas a unilateral mandibular buccal crossbite would mean that the mandibular molar was buccally positioned on one side. This terminology specifies which teeth (maxillary or mandibular) are displaced from their normal position.

It is also important to evaluate the underlying skeletal relationships, to answer the question, ''Why does this crossbite exist?'' in the sense of the location of the anatomic abnormality. If there is a bilateral maxillary palatal crossbite, for instance, is the basic problem that the maxilla itself is narrow, thus providing a skeletal basis for the crossbite, or is it that the dental arch has been narrowed although the skeletal width is correct? The width of the maxillary skeletal base can be seen by the width of the palatal vault on the

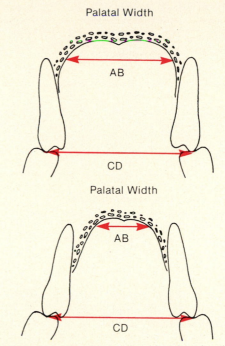

Fig. 6-49 ■ Posterior crossbite can be either *dental,* as in a patient with adequate palatal width, i.e., distance *AB* approximately equals distance *CD,* or *skeletal* because of inadequate palatal width, i.e., distance *CD* is considerably larger than distance *AB.*

casts. If the base of the palatal vault is wide, but the dentoalveolar processes lean inward, the crossbite is dental in the sense that it is caused by a distortion of the dental arch. If the palatal vault is narrow and the maxillary teeth lean outward but nevertheless are in crossbite, the problem is skeletal in the sense that it basically results from the narrow width of the maxilla. Just as there are dental compensations for skeletal deformity in the anteroposterior and vertical planes of space, the teeth can compensate for transverse skeletal problems.

Transverse displacement of the lower molars on the mandible is rare, so the question of whether the mandibular arch is too wide can be used both to answer the question of whether the mandible or maxilla is at fault in a posterior crossbite, and to implicate skeletal mandibular development if the answer is positive. Tabulated data for normal molar and canine widths are shown in Table 6-6.[24] If there is a crossbite and measurements across the arch show that the mandible is wide while the maxillary arch is normal, a skeletal mandibular discrepancy is probably present.

Step 4. Evaluation of skeletal and dental relationships in the anteroposterior plane of space. Examining the dental casts in occlusion will reveal any anteroposterior problems in the buccal occlusion or in the anterior relationships. It is important to ask whether an end-to-end, Class II, or Class III buccal segment relationship, or excessive overjet or reverse overjet of the incisors, is caused by a jaw (skeletal) discrepancy, displaced teeth on well-proportioned jaws

Table 6-6 ■ Arch width measurements*

Age	Male			Female		
	Canine	First Premolar	First Molar	Canine	First Premolar	First Molar
Maxillary arch						
6	27.5†	32.3†	41.9	26.9†	31.7†	41.3
8	29.7†	33.7†	43.1	29.1†	33.0†	42.4
10	30.5†	34.4†	44.5	29.8†	33.6†	43.5
12	32.5	35.7	45.3	31.5	35.1	44.6
14	32.5	36.0	45.9	31.3	34.9	44.3
16	32.3	36.6	46.6	31.4	35.2	45.0
18	32.3	36.7	46.7	31.2	34.6	43.9
Mandibular arch						
6	23.3†	28.7†	40.2	22.2†	28.4†	40.0
8	24.3†	29.7†	40.9	24.0†	29.5†	40.3
10	24.6†	30.2†	41.5	24.1†	29.7†	41.0
12	25.1	32.5	42.1	24.8	31.6	41.8
14	24.8	32.3	42.1	24.4	31.0	41.1
16	24.7	32.3	42.8	23.9	31.0	41.5
18	24.8	32.8	43.0	23.1	30.8	41.7

*mm distance between centers of teeth.
†Primary predecessor.
Data from Moyers, R.E., et al.: Standards of Human Occlusal Development. Monograph 5, Craniofacial Growth Series. Ann Arbor, 1976, (Center for Human Growth and Development. University of Michigan).

(dental Class II or III), or a combination of the two, as is often the case. A skeletal jaw discrepancy almost always produces an occlusal discrepancy as well, but if the jaw discrepancy is the cause, this should be described as a *skeletal* Class II or Class III (Fig. 6-50). The terminology simply means that the skeletal or jaw relationship is the cause of the Class II dental occlusion. The distinction between dental and skeletal is important, because the treatment for a skeletal Class II relationship in a child or in an adult will be different from treatment for a dental Class II problem.

If a skeletal Class II or III problem is noted on clinical examination, and if orthodontic treatment is to be undertaken, a cephalometric headfilm is required. In this circumstance, the cephalometric film has two purposes: (1) it allows a more precise definition of the nature of the problem, and (2) it provides a starting point against which the effects of treatment can be measured later. For this first purpose, a cephalometric film is desirable; for the second, it is absolutely essential. Undertaking treatment of a skeletal problem without initial and progress cephalometric films is professionally irresponsible.

Data from cephalometric analysis should be used to complete the description of a patient with significant problems in the anteroposterior plane. The object is to accurately evaluate the underlying anatomic basis of the malocclusion.

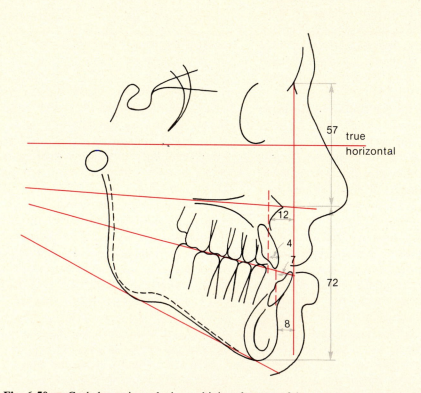

Fig. 6-50 ■ Cephalometric analysis combining elements of the measurement approaches presented earlier. A description in words of this patient's problems would be that the maxilla is quite deficient relative to the mandible and the cranial base, but the maxillary teeth are reasonably well related to the maxilla. The mandible is fairly well related in the anteroposterior plane of space to the cranial base, but the mandibular teeth protrude relative to the mandible. Vertical proportions are good.

Step 5. Evaluation of skeletal and dental relationships in vertical plane of space. With the casts in occlusion, vertical problems can be described as anterior open bite (failure of the incisor teeth to overlap), anterior deep bite (excessive overlap of the anterior teeth), or posterior open bite (failure of the posterior teeth to occlude, unilaterally or bilaterally). As with all aspects of malocclusion, it is important to ask, "Why does the open bite (or other problem) exist?" Since vertical problems, particularly anterior open bite, can result from environmental causes or habits, the "why" in this instance has two important components: at what anatomic location is the discrepancy, and can a cause be identified?

It is obvious that if the posterior teeth erupt a normal amount but the anterior teeth do not, an anterior open bite will result. This is possible but is rarely the major reason for an anterior open bite. Instead, there is usually at least some excessive eruption of posterior teeth. This can also cause anterior open bite, because if the anterior teeth erupt a normal amount but the posterior teeth erupt too much, anterior open bite is inevitable. Excessive eruption of posterior teeth requires a compensatory downward and backward rotation of the mandible. Perhaps more accurately, if the mandible rotates downward and backward, space is created into which the posterior teeth can erupt, allowing excessive posterior eruption.

This leads to an important but sometimes difficult concept: a patient with a *skeletal* open bite will usually have an anterior bite malocclusion that is characterized by normal (or even excessive) eruption of anterior teeth along with downward rotation of the mandible and excessive eruption of posterior teeth (Fig. 6-51). This facial and dental pattern is sometimes called the "long face syndrome." The reverse is true in a short face, skeletal deep bite relationship (Fig. 6-52). In that circumstance, one would expect to see a normal amount of eruption of incisor teeth but insufficient eruption of the posterior teeth. The skeletal component is revealed by the rotation of the jaws, reflected in the palatal and mandibular plane angles. If the angle between the mandibular and palatal planes is low, there is a skeletal deep bite tendency, i.e., a jaw relationship that predisposes to an anterior deep bite, regardless of whether one is present. Similarly, if the mandibular-palatal angle is high, there is a skeletal open bite tendency.

The mandibular plane angle can be measured on cephalometric films or estimated on clinical examination by placing the handle of a dental mirror or similar straight object along the lower border of the mandible, as shown in Fig.

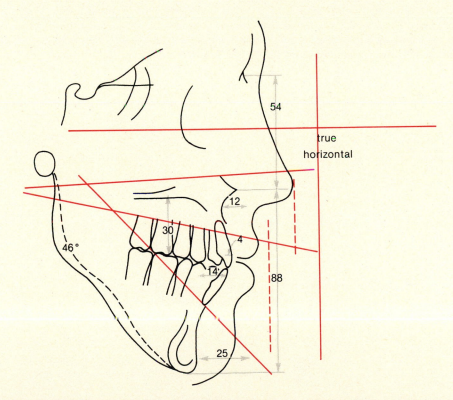

Fig. 6-51 ■ Cephalometric analysis for a patient with severe vertical problems. Note that the Sassouni lines clearly indicate the skeletal open bite pattern, and that the measurements confirm both long anterior facial dimensions and severe mandibular deficiency related to downward and backward rotation of the mandible. Measurement of the distance from the upper first molar mesial cusp to the palatal plane confirms that excessive eruption of the upper molar has occurred.

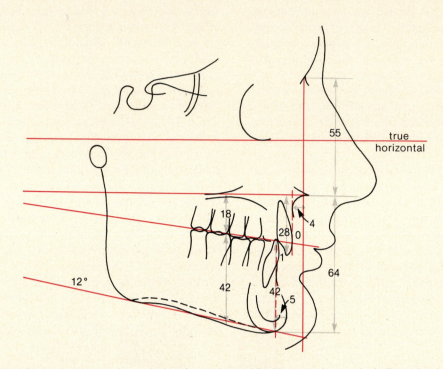

Fig. 6-52 ■ Cephalometric analysis of a patient with short anterior vertical dimensions. The measurements show excessive eruption of the lower molar compared to the upper molar and document the distal displacement of the lower incisor relative to the mandible. Note that the Sassouni planes are almost parallel, confirming the skeletal deep bite tendency.

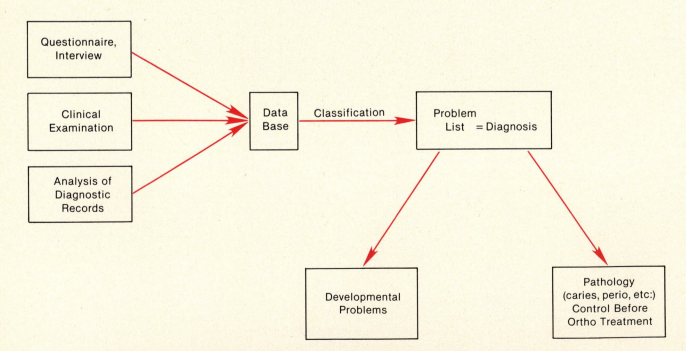

Fig. 6-53 ■ As a final step in diagnosis, the patient's problems related to pathology should be separated from the developmental problems, so that the pathology can be treated first.

6-13. It is important to remember that if the mandibular plane angle is unusually flat or steep, correcting an accompanying deep bite or open bite may require an alteration in the vertical position of posterior teeth so that the mandible can rotate to a more normal inclination. Cephalometric analysis is required for evaluation of patients with skeletal vertical problems, again with the goal of accurately describing skeletal and dental relationships.

■ *Development of a Problem List*

If positive findings from a systematic description of the patient are recorded, i.e., if the classification method described here is used, the automatic and important result is a list of the patient's problems. The step-by-step procedure is designed to ensure that the important distinctions have been made and that nothing has been overlooked.

As a final step, the problems should be divided into two groups: (1) those relating to disease or pathologic processes, and (2) those relating to the patient's malocclusion (Fig. 6-53). For any patient, disease control should receive priority. Thus, in a treatment sequence, orthodontic treatment must appear after steps to control systemic disease, periodontal treatment (at least to the extent of bringing periodontal disease under control), and restoration of dental lesions. This sequencing of different types of treatment is discussed in Chapter 7.

When the group of problems related to pathology has been set aside for priority treatment, the set of morphologic findings related to malocclusion remains as the orthodontic problem list. A morphologic problem is just that (mandibular deficiency, for instance), not the findings that indicate its presence (posterior divergence, increased facial convexity). Different aspects of the same problem should be grouped

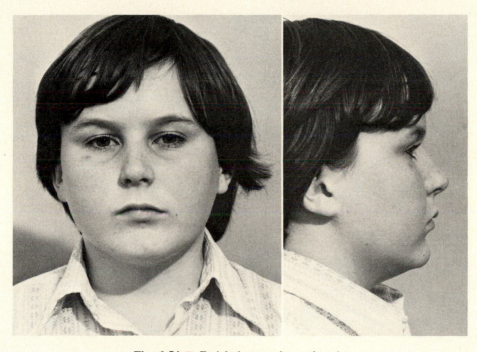

Fig. 6-54 ■ Facial photographs, patient A.

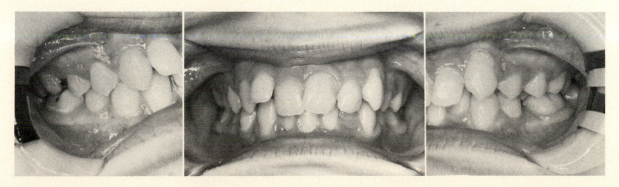

Fig. 6-55 ■ Intraoral photographs, patient A.

into a single major problem area. For instance, lingual position of the lateral incisors, labial position of the canines, and rotation of the central incisors are all the results of lack of space to properly align the incisors and should be lumped under the general problem of incisor crowding. Where possible, the problems should be indicated quantitatively, or at least classified as mild, moderate, or severe, i.e., 5 mm mandibular incisor crowding or severe mandibular deficien-

cy. This process is briefly illustrated for two patients in Figs. 6-54 through 6-65.

With the completion of a problem list, the diagnostic phase of diagnosis and treatment planning is completed, and the more subjective process of treatment planning begins. Thorough diagnostic evaluation means that all problems have been identified and characterized at this stage, omitting nothing of significance.

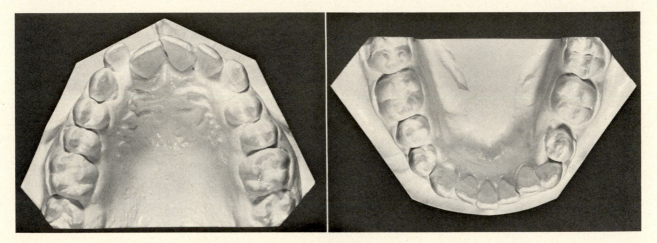

Fig. 6-56 ■ Occlusal photographs of casts, patient A.

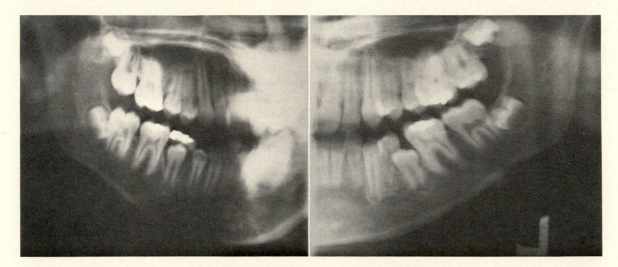

Fig. 6-57 ■ Panoramic radiograph, patient A.

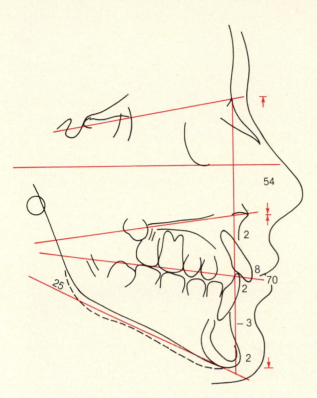

Fig. 6-58 ■ Cephalometric tracing, patient A.

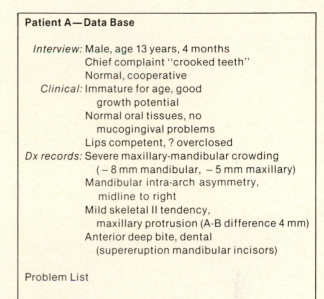

Patient A—Data Base

Interview: Male, age 13 years, 4 months
Chief complaint "crooked teeth"
Normal, cooperative
Clinical: Immature for age, good
growth potential
Normal oral tissues, no
mucogingival problems
Lips competent, ? overclosed
Dx records: Severe maxillary-mandibular crowding
(− 8 mm mandibular, − 5 mm maxillary)
Mandibular intra-arch asymmetry,
midline to right
Mild skeletal II tendency,
maxillary protrusion (A-B difference 4 mm)
Anterior deep bite, dental
(supereruption mandibular incisors)

Problem List

(1) Severe maxillary and mandibular crowding
(2) Mild skeletal Class II, II/2 dental pattern
(3) Anterior deep bite, dental

Fig. 6-59 ■ Database and problem list, patient A.

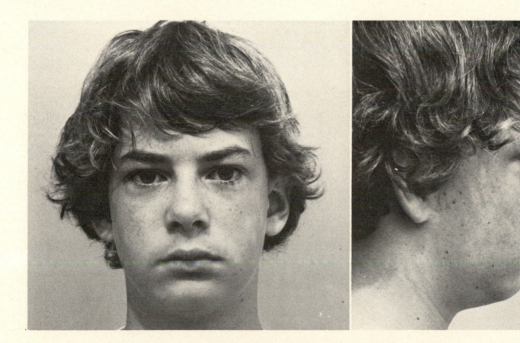

Fig. 6-60 ■ Facial photographs, patient B.

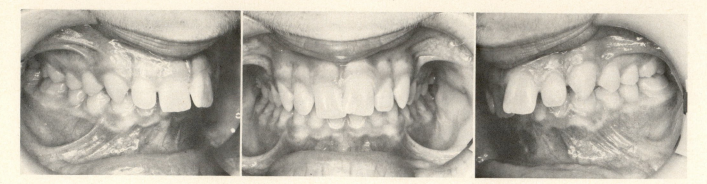

Fig. 6-61 ■ Intraoral photographs, patient B.

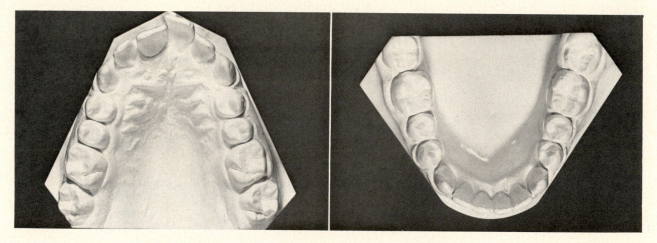

Fig. 6-62 ■ Occlusal photographs of casts, patient B.

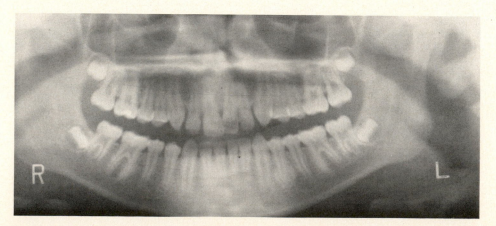

Fig. 6-63 ■ Panoramic radiograph, patient B.

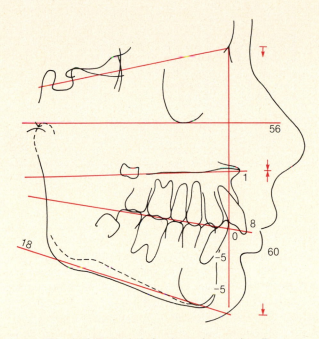

Fig. 6-64 ■ Cephalometric tracing, patient B.

Patient B—Data Base

Interview: Male, age 13 years, 4 months
         Chief complaint "teeth stick out"
         Normal, cooperative
Clinical: Early in adolescence, good
           growth potential
         Mild tetracycline staining,
           otherwise normal tissues
Dx records: Maxillary anterior irregularity, no
           maxillary or mandibular space deficiency
         Mild maxillary-mandibular incisor protrusion
         Class II: moderate skeletal mandibular
           deficiency, mild maxillary dental protrusion
         Anterior deep bite, dental
           (supereruption mandibular incisors)

Problem List

(1) Skeletal Class II, mandibular deficiency with some maxillary dental protrusion
(2) Anterior deep bite, dental
(3) Irregular maxillary incisors

Fig. 6-65 ■ Database and problem list, patient B.

■ *References*

1. Weed, L.L.: Medical Records, Medical Education and Patient Care: The Problem-oriented Record as a Basic Tool. Cleveland, 1969, Case-Western Reserve Press.
2. Moyers, R.E.: Handbook of Orthodontics, ed. 3, Chicago, 1973, Year Book Medical Publishers, Inc.
3. Hellman, M.: Variations in occlusion. Dental Cosmos **63**:608-619, 1921.
4. Tanaka, M.M., and Johnston, L.E.: The prediction of the size of unerupted canines and premolars in a contemporary orthodontic population. J. Am. Dent. Assoc. **88**:798-801, 1974.
5. Hixon, E.H., and Oldfather, R.E.: Estimation of the sizes of unerupted cuspid and bicuspid teeth. Angle Orthod. **28**:236-240, 1958.
6. Staley, R.N., and Kerber, R.E.: A revision of the Hixon and Oldfather mixed-dentition prediction method. Am. J. Orthod. **78**:296-302,1980.
7. Bolton, W.A.: The clinical application of a tooth-size analysis. Am. J. Orthod. **48**:504-529, 1962.
8. Downs, W.B.: Variations in facial relationships: their significance in treatment and prognosis. Am. J. Orthod. **34**:812, 1948.
9. Riolo, M.L., et al.: An Atlas of Craniofacial Growth. Monograph 2, Craniofacial Growth Series, Ann Arbor, 1974, University of Michigan, Center for Human Growth and Development.
10. Popovich, F., and Thompson, G.W.: Craniofacial templates for orthodontic case analysis. Am. J. Orthod. **71**:406-420, 1977.
11. Broadbent, B.H., Sr., Broadbent, B.H., Jr., and Golden, W.H.: Bolton Standards of Dentofacial Developmental Growth. St. Louis, 1975, The C.V. Mosby Co.
12. Moorrees, C.F.A., and Lebret, L.: The mesh diagram and cephalometrics. Angle Orthod. **32**:214-231, 1962.
13. Jacobson, A.: The proportionate template as a diagnostic aid. Am. J. Orthod. **75**:156-172, 1979.
14. Ackerman, R.J.: The Michigan school study norms expressed in template form. Am. J. Orthod. **75**:282, 1979.
15. Steiner, C.C.: The use of cephalometrics as an aid to planning and assessing orthodontic treatment. Am. J. Orthod. **46**:721-735, 1960.
16. Tweed, C.H.: The Frankfort-mandibular incisor angle (FMIA) in orthodontic diagnosis, treatment planning and prognosis. Angle Orthod. **24**:121-169, 1954.
17. Sassouni, V.A.: A classification of skeletal facial types. Am. J. Orthod. **55**:109-123, 1969.
18. Harvold, E.P.: The Activator in Orthodontics. St. Louis, 1974, The C.V. Mosby Co.
19. Jacobson, A.: The "Wits" appraisal of jaw disharmony. Am. J. Orthod. **67**:125-138, 1975.
20. Ricketts, R.M.: Perspectives in the clinical application of cephalometrics. Angle Orthod. **51**:115-150, 1981.
21. McNamara, J.A., Jr.: A method of cephalometric analysis. In Clinical Alteration of the Growing Face, Monograph 12, Craniofacial Growth Series, Ann Arbor, 1983, University of Michigan, Center for Human Growth and Development.
22. Greulich, W.W., and Pyle, S.L.: Radiographic Atlas of Skeletal Development of the Hand and Wrist, ed. 2, Palo Alto, 1959, Stanford University Press.
23. Ackerman, J.L., and Proffit, W.R.: The characteristics of malocclusion: a modern approach to classification and diagnosis. Am. J. Orthod. **56**:443, 1969.
24. Moyers, R.E., et al.: Standards of Human Occlusal Development. Monograph 5, Craniofacial Growth Series, Ann Arbor, 1976, University of Michigan, Center for Human Growth and Development.

Chapter 7

Orthodontic Treatment Planning: From Problem List to Final Plan

▪ *Principles of Treatment Planning*

Diagnosis is a scientific procedure. Treatment planning, in contrast, has a subjective component. Its object is not scientific truth but wisdom—the plan that a wise and prudent clinician would develop to maximize benefit to the patient. To achieve this, the potential benefit to the patient from treatment procedures must be compared to both cost and risk. Particularly when planning treatment for an adult with complex problems, the question is often asked, "Could you correct the posterior crossbite?" or "Could you develop incisal guidance for this patient?" To the question, "Could you . . ."the answer is usually yes, given an unlimited commitment to treatment. The appropriate question is not "Could you . . .?" but "Should you . . .?" Cost-benefit analysis (considering the cost in discomfort, annoyance, time, cooperation, and other such factors, as well as in money) and risk-benefit analysis are introduced appropriately when the question is rephrased.

A treatment plan in orthodontics, as in any other field, may be less than optimal if it is too ambitious or does not take full advantage of the possibilities. There is always a temptation to jump to conclusions and to proceed with a superficially obvious plan without considering all the pertinent factors. The treatment planning approach advocated here is specifically designed to avoid both missed opportunities, the false negative or undertreatment side of treatment planning, and excessive treatment, the false positive or overtreatment side. We suggest that, after a thorough diagnosis that results in a comprehensive list of the patient's problems, the treatment planning process should proceed through the following steps: (1) arranging the problem list in priority order; (2) review of treatment possibilities; (3) consideration of factors than can affect the probable result, and (4) choice of mechanotherapy (Fig. 7-1).

▪ Setting Priorities for the Problem List

Priorities for the problem list developed from analysis of the patient must be considered in two ways. First, problems that should be treated first must be separated. These are any problems related to pathologic processes, not the developmental conditions that comprise the majority of orthodontic problems. Thus periodontal disease, dental caries, and soft tissue lesions should be placed in a separate category for treatment first. Only when these disease processes have been brought under control should orthodontic treatment proceed—which is not to say that the effects of any disease-related processes must be corrected before orthodontic treatment is planned, only that the progress of acute or chronic conditions must be stopped.

The second aspect of setting priorities for the problem list is extremely important. This calls for placing the patient's remaining facial and occlusal problems in priority

168

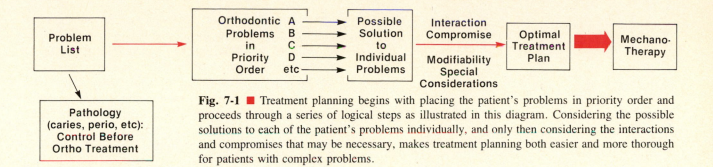

Fig. 7-1 ■ Treatment planning begins with placing the patient's problems in priority order and proceeds through a series of logical steps as illustrated in this diagram. Considering the possible solutions to each of the patient's problems individually, and only then considering the interactions and compromises that may be necessary, makes treatment planning both easier and more thorough for patients with complex problems.

order. This list does not necessarily represent the sequence of treatment, but indicates that if all problems cannot be solved, the higher-ranking problems will be addressed while lower-ranking problems will not.

The patient's perception of his or her condition is very important in setting these priorities. If the patient's major reason for seeking dental treatment is protruding and irregular incisors, this condition should receive higher priority than missing molar teeth needing prosthetic replacement. On the other hand, if the protruding and irregular incisors are no problem to the patient but occlusal function is, replacing the missing teeth should receive higher priority. It is always difficult for the clinician to avoid imposing his or her own feeling at this stage, and it is not totally inappropriate to do so; but ignoring the patient's chief complaint can lead to serious errors in planning treatment. As an example, consider the patient who complains of a protruding chin and who has a Class III malocclusion. If the clinician formulates the problem as Class III malocclusion and concentrates on bringing the teeth into correct occlusion while ignoring the protruding chin, it is not likely that the patient will be happy with the treatment result. The plan did not deal with the patient's problem.

■ **Treatment Possibilities**

Once the problem list has been placed in priority order, the next step in the planning process is to list the possibilities for treatment of each of the problems, beginning with the highest priority. At this stage, each problem is considered individually, and the total spectrum of treatment possibilities for that problem is examined as if it were the only problem the patient had. The longer the problem list, and thereby the more complex the total situation, the more valuable this step can be.

Broad possibilities, not detail, are important at this stage. As an example, consider the possibilities for correcting an anterior open bite in an adult. To bring the anterior teeth into contact, there are only three possibilities: elongating the anterior teeth, intruding the posterior teeth, or shortening the crown height of the posterior teeth. Vertical elastics to pull the anterior teeth together would probably be the method for elongating the incisors, although this could also be done by placing long crowns on them or by repositioning the

segments surgically. Intruding the posterior teeth in an adult would probably require jaw surgery. Reducing the height of the crowns, by grinding down the occlusal surfaces or making new crowns, would be a prosthetic solution.

Which of these choices would be best for the patient would depend on other items in the problem list. If the adult patient with an anterior open bite also had excessive exposure of the upper incisors and a long face, elongating the incisors would be unwise, whereas intruding the posterior teeth could also solve this problem.

If the possible solutions to the first, second, third, and other problems are listed in the same general way, it becomes apparent that some possible solutions to high priority problems also solve other problems and therefore would be of greater overall benefit to the patient. Only by considering the entire spectrum of the patient's problems can the optimal treatment plan be devised. We simply advocate doing this systematically, one problem at a time, so that treatment possibilities are not overlooked.

■ **Factors in the Choice of a Final Plan**

Four factors must now be considered in the choice of a final treatment plan:

Interaction. This refers to the interaction among possible solutions to the patient's various problems, which becomes obvious if the possible solutions to each problem are listed as described previously. Continuing with our example of the adult patient with an anterior open bite: changing the height of the posterior teeth, no matter how it is done, interacts with the anterior vertical dimension of the face (Fig. 7-2). If anterior facial height needs to be reduced to correct the long face, which is another item on the patient's problem list, intruding the posterior teeth is an appropriate way to deal with anterior open bite. On the other hand, if anterior face height is correct, intruding the posterior teeth will create another problem while correcting the anterior open bite. Looking at the possible solutions to the patient's problems taken one at the time, makes it easier to see the interaction among the possible solutions and to choose solutions that go as far as possible toward solving all the patient's problems.

Compromise. In patients with many problems, it may not be possible to solve them all. This type of compromise

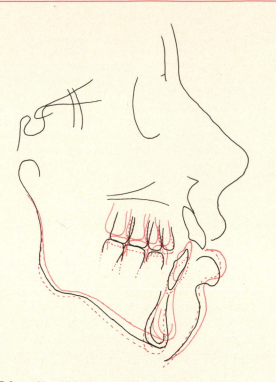

Fig. 7-2 ■ Changing the vertical position of the maxillary posterior teeth alters both the vertical and horizontal position of the mandible. *Black tracing,* original condition; *dotted red tracing,* actual growth change in this patient, showing down-back rotation of the mandible and eruption of maxillary posterior teeth; *solid pink tracing,* possible change from (surgical) intrusion of maxillary posterior teeth.

has nothing to do with the clinician's skill. It may simply be that solving one problem has no effect on another or even makes it worse, and no plan of treatment will solve all of the patient's problems. In this circumstance careful setting of priorities from the problem list is particularly important.

In a broad sense, the major goals of orthodontic treatment are ideal occlusion, functionally and statically; ideal facial esthetics; and ideal stability of result. Often it is impossible to maximize all three. In fact, attempts to achieve an absolutely ideal dental occlusion often compromise facial esthetics and may be associated with instability after treatment. In the same way, efforts to achieve the most stable result after orthodontic treatment may necessitate compromises in both occlusion and facial esthetics, whereas positioning the teeth to produce ideal facial esthetics may result in less than optimal occlusion and stability.

One way to deal with this, of course, is to emphasize one of the goals at the expense of the others. In the early twentieth century, Edward Angle, the father of modern orthodontics, solved this problem by focusing solely on the occlusion and declaring that facial esthetics and stability would take care of themselves.[1] Unfortunately, they did not. Echoes of Angle's position are encountered occasionally in contemporary dentistry, particularly among dentists strongly committed to gnathologic concepts of occlusion.

As important as dental occlusion is, it is not the most important consideration for all patients. Sometimes occlusion must be compromised, by extraction or otherwise, to gain acceptable esthetics and stability. Compromises in the other goals may also be needed. For some patients the dentist must realize that placing the teeth for optimal facial esthetics may require permanent retention because they are not stable in that position, or alternatively, that placing the teeth in a position of stability will compromise facial esthetics.

If various elements of a treatment plan are incompatible, benefit to the patient is greatest if any necessary compromises are made so that the patient's most important problems are solved, while less important problems are deferred or left untreated. If all of the three major goals of orthodontic treatment cannot be reached, those of greatest importance to that patient should be favored. Doing this successfully requires judgment and thought on the part of the clinician. The same problem list, prioritized differently for two different patients, will inevitably lead to two different final treatment plans because of these effects.

Cost-risk/benefit analysis. Practical considerations related to the difficulty of various treatment procedures as compared to the benefit to be gained from them, must be introduced in the selection of any final treatment plan. The difficulty should be considered in both risk and cost to the patient (not just in money, but also in cooperation, discomfort, aggravation, time, and other factors) and must be contrasted to the probable benefit from that procedure.

Continuing the previous example, for our patient with anterior open bite, jaw surgery must rank higher in cost and risk than elastics to elongate the incisors or occlusal reduction of the posterior teeth. On the other hand, if the less difficult procedures would provide little real benefit to the patient, while jaw surgery would provide considerable benefit, the cost-risk/benefit analysis might still favor the more difficult procedure. "Is it worth it?" is a question that must be answered not only from the point of view of what is involved, but in terms of the benefit to the patient.

Special considerations. As a final point on the mental checklist, any pertinent special considerations about this particular patient must be taken into account. Should the treatment time be minimized because of possible exacerbation of periodontal disease? Should visible orthodontic appliances be avoided because of the patient's vanity, even if this makes treatment more difficult? Should treatment options be left open as long as possible because of uncertainty of the pattern of growth? Such questions must be addressed from the perspective of the individual patient. Introducing them at this last stage of the treatment planning process, when the treatment possibilities have been clearly outlined, prevents possibilities from being overlooked.

■ Choice of Mechanotherapy

Up to this point, the treatment plan has been conceived entirely in terms of the objectives of treatment, without specific reference to the details of obtaining that result. The final step is specification of the treatment methods—in orthodontics, the mechanotherapy—that are to be used.

For a relatively simple treatment plan, the associated mechanotherapy is also reasonably simple or at least straightforward. Nevertheless, choices must be made and clearly specified in the treatment plan. For example, if the plan is to expand a narrow maxillary arch, it would be possible to do this with springs on a removable appliance, with an expansion lingual arch, or an expansion labial arch. As a final step, the treatment plan must specify which, and the relative advantages and disadvantages of the various possibilities must be considered. There is a time and a place for everything, and this last step is the place for these practical considerations of which appliance to use. The most serious errors in treatment planning are those that result from first thinking of which appliance to use, not what the appliance is supposed to accomplish.

More complex problems require more complex mechanotherapy and more careful coordination of the elements within that mechanotherapy. Here, careful speculation of the objectives of treatment helps in selecting the right treatment approach.

For instance, deep overbite is often on the problem list. Usually, it is to be corrected by leveling an excessive curve of Spee in the mandibular arch. An excessive curve of Spee, however, can be leveled in three ways (Fig. 7-3) by: (1) absolute intrusion of the mandibular incisors, literally pushing them into the alveolar process; (2) relative intrusion of the mandibular incisors, accomplished in a growing patient merely by preventing their eruption while other teeth erupt normally; or (3) elongation of the canines and premolars while holding the incisors in their original position. Since different mechanotherapy is needed to accomplish each of these types of leveling, carefully specifying the way in which leveling is to be accomplished will greatly assist in selecting the correct mechanical approach. This last step in treatment planning for patients with complex problems is discussed in more detail in Chapters 15 to 21.

The treatment planning process outlined here is applicable to all patients. In the following sections of this chapter, we present a description of how the diagnostic data can be used to separate patients with moderate problems, who have a good prognosis for treatment with simple appliances, from those with severe problems who will require complex mechanotherapy. This is followed by additional information relative to planning treatment for children at various ages and adults. Our hope is that the specific treatment planning points will be incorporated appropriately into the overall scheme, depending on the age of the patient and the complexity of the patient's problems.

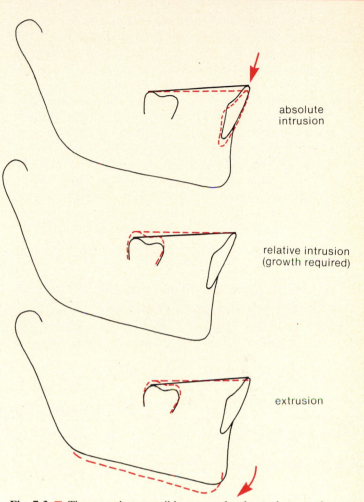

absolute intrusion

relative intrusion (growth required)

extrusion

Fig. 7-3 ■ There are three possible ways to level out a lower arch with an excessive curve of Spee: (1) absolute intrusion (2) relative intrusion, achieved by preventing eruption of the incisors while growth provides vertical space into which the posterior teeth erupt; and (3) elongation of posterior teeth, which causes the mandible to rotate downward in the absence of growth.

■ Orthodontic Triage: Distinguishing Moderate from Severe Problems

In military and emergency medicine, triage is the process used to separate casualties by the severity of their injuries.

Its purpose is twofold: to separate patients who can be treated at the scene of the injury from those who need transportation to specialized facilities, and to develop a sequence for handling patients so that those most likely to benefit from immediate treatment will be treated first.

Since orthodontic problems almost never are an emergency, the process of sorting orthodontic problems by their severity is analogous only in one sense of the word. On the other hand, it is very important for the primary care dentist to be able to distinguish moderate from severe orthodontic problems, because this process of orthodontic triage determines which patients are appropriately treated within general dental practice and which are most appropriately referred to a specialist in orthodontics. As with all components of dental practice, a generalist's decision of whether to include orthodontic treatment as a component of his services is an individual one. The principle that the less severe problems are handled within the context of general practice and the more severe problems are referred should remain the same, however, regardless of the practitioner's interest in orthodontics. Only the cutoff points for retention of a patient in the general practice or referral should change.

This section presents a logical scheme for orthodontic triage for children. It is based on the diagnostic approach developed in Chapter 5 and incorporates the principles of treatment planning discussed previously. A cephalometric radiograph is not required, but a panoramic radiograph is needed. A flow chart illustrating the steps in the triage sequence accompanies this section (Fig. 7-4). An adequate database and a thorough problem list, of course, are necessary to carry out the triage process. The first step, as Fig. 7-4, *A* illustrates, is to separate patients with syndromes or developmental abnormalities.

■ **Problems Involving Syndromes and Developmental Abnormalities** (Fig. 7-4, *A*)

From physical appearance, the medical and dental histories, and an evaluation of developmental status, some pa-

tients will be easily recognized as having a craniofacial deformity or syndrome. Examples of these disorders are cleft lip or palate, Treacher-Collins syndrome, hemifacial microsomia, and Crouzon's syndrome. The multidisciplinary treatment approach now considered as the standard of care for these patients should lead to their referral to a craniofacial team of specialists at a regional medical center for evaluation and treatment. The American Cleft Palate Association publishes a directory of these teams,[2] which now cover the whole spectrum of craniofacial problems, not just cleft palate.

A similar route of referral and medical evaluation is recommended for patients who appear to be developing either above the 97th or below the third percentiles on standard growth charts. Growth disorders may demand that any orthodontic treatment be carried out in conjunction with endocrine, nutritional, or psychologic therapy. For these patients and those with growth-related problems such as juvenile rheumatoid arthritis, the proper orthodontic therapy must be combined with identification and control of the disease process.

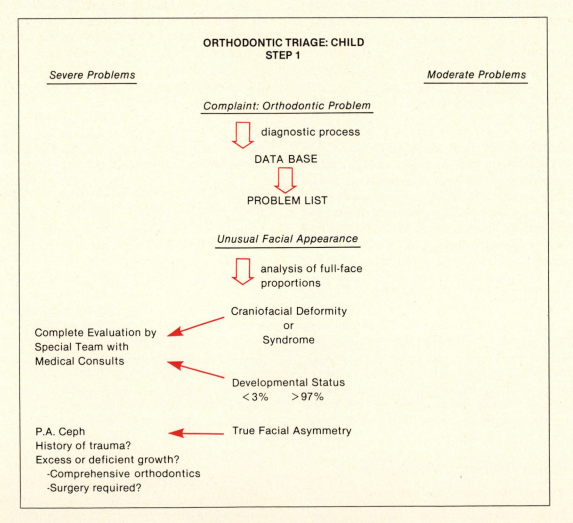

Fig. 7-4 ■ **A,** Steps in orthodontic triage.

Problems Involving Facial Disproportions and Asymmetries

Facial asymmetry (Fig. 7-4, *A*). Patients who have significant skeletal asymmetry (not necessarily those whose asymmetry results from only a functional shift of the mandible) always fall into the severe problem category. These patients require evaluation including posteroanterior and lateral cephalometric radiographs. Treatment is likely to involve surgery in addition to comprehensive orthodontics. Timing of intervention is affected by whether the cause of the asymmetry is deficient or excessive growth (Chapter 8).

Anteroposterior and vertical problems (Fig. 7-4, *B*). Skeletal Class II and Class III problems and vertical deformities of the long face and short face types, regardless of their cause, require thorough cephalometric evaluation to plan appropriate treatment and must be considered severe problems. Before puberty, these patients should have treatment aimed at modifying jaw growth, not just treatment to reposition teeth. After puberty, the amount of growth remaining is usually insufficient to allow correction of the problem, and the treatment plan must distinguish between the possibility for camouflage of the jaw discrepancy by repositioning the teeth after extraction, and surgical repositioning of the jaw.

Excessive Dental Protrusion or Retrusion (Fig. 7-4, *B*)

Severe dental protrusion or retrusion should also be recognized during the facial profile analysis. Excessive protrusion or retrusion of incisor teeth often accompanies skeletal jaw discrepancies, and if protrusion is present in a patient who also has a skeletal problem, this should be subordinated to the skeletal problem in planning treatment. It is also possible, however, for an individual with good skeletal proportions to have protrusion of incisor teeth rather than crowding. When this occurs, the space analysis will show a small or nonexistent discrepancy, because the incisor protrusion has compensated for the potential crowding.

The cardinal rule in planning treatment for patients who have incisor protrusion is that additional protrusion is extremely unlikely to be tolerated by the musculature. Conceptually, one should consider that the position of protruding incisors is similar to the titrated endpoint in a chemical reaction, that is, the incisors have aligned themselves forward at the expense of the lips as much as the musculature will allow. In many instances, the best treatment plan will be to retract the incisors, allowing better lip function and facial esthetics. If the decision in treatment planning is that the relatively protruded position of the incisors is acceptable, it is extremely important to avoid treatment procedures that will further protrude the incisors. Any further expansion in these patients is quite likely to be unsuccessful for two reasons: (1) a detrimental effect on facial esthetics and (2) probable relapse of the crowding as lip pressure pushes the incisors back toward their original position.

The problem comes, of course, in deciding how to treat a patient who has incisor protrusion and 2 or 3 mm of arch length discrepancy as judged by space analysis. Usually, extractions and bodily tooth movement are needed to reduce the problem despite the small discrepancy. If the same space management or regaining procedures employed with good success in children who do not have incisor protrusion (discussed later) are used for this patient, the arch expansion will be unstable. Once the expansion appliances are removed, a return of incisor crowding is highly likely.

To reiterate: relatively protruded incisors may be stable, although often it is better both functionally and esthetically to retract them; but treatment procedures designed to expand the arches should not be used in patients who already have incisor protrusion. Along with jaw discrepancies, this falls into the category of severe problems.

Problems Involving Dental Development (Fig. 7-4, *C*)

Abnormal sequence of dental development. An abnormal sequence of dental development constitutes a potentially severe orthodontic problem and should be planned

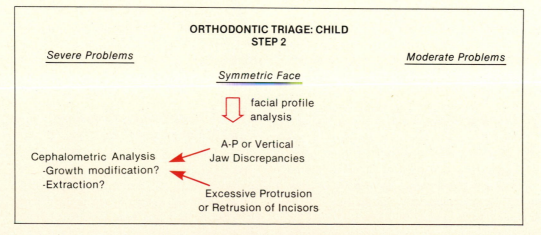

Fig. 7-4, cont'd ■ **B,** Steps in orthodontic triage.

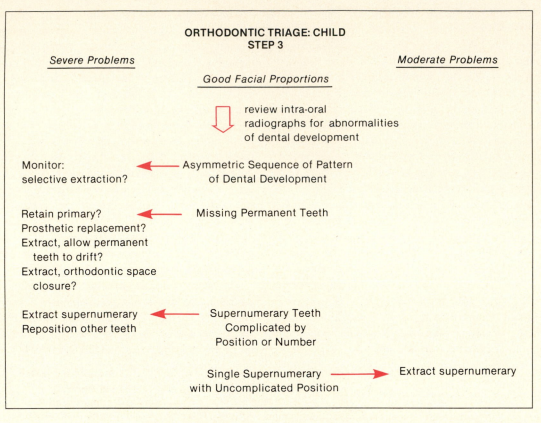

Fig. 7-4, cont'd ■ C, Steps in orthodontic triage.

for treatment only after a careful determination of the underlying cause. In a child, an asymmetry in eruption within the dental arch of greater than 6 months is a significant finding. Appropriate treatment involves careful monitoring of the situation, and in the absence of outright pathology, often requires selective extraction of primary or permanent teeth. Early intervention to promote more symmetric development of the dental arches, as for example the early extraction of the right mandibular primary canine after the left canine has been lost prematurely, can circumvent the need for treating a severe asymmetry problem at a later time, but such a step must be taken only after careful consideration of the total problem list for an individual patient.

Missing permanent teeth. A congenitally missing permanent tooth is an actual (if the primary predecessor is missing or lost) or potential (if the primary tooth is still present) problem of arch symmetry. This must be considered a severe orthodontic problem, whether or not asymmetry has developed and whether the problem is unilateral or bilateral. The permanent teeth most likely to be missing are the mandibular second premolars and the maxillary lateral incisors, but the treatment possibilities are the same whatever the missing tooth: (1) maintenance of the primary tooth or teeth; (2) replacement of the missing teeth prosthetically; (3) extraction of the overlying primary teeth, and then allowing the permanent teeth to drift; or (4) extraction of the primary teeth followed by immediate orthodontic treatment.

Making the correct decision requires a careful assessment

of facial profile, incisor position, space requirements, and the status of the primary teeth. Treatment of missing tooth problems in mixed dentition children is discussed in more detail in Chapter 13.

Supernumerary teeth. Ninety percent of all supernumerary teeth are found in the anterior part of the maxilla. Single supernumeraries that are not malformed often erupt spontaneously, causing crowding problems. If these teeth can be removed before they cause distortions of arch form, or if the supernumerary tooth erupts outside the line of the arch, extraction may be all that is needed. Multiple or inverted supernumeraries, and those that are malformed, often displace adjacent teeth or cause problems in eruption. Early removal is indicated, but this must be done carefully to minimize damage to adjacent teeth. If the permanent teeth have been displaced, surgical exposure, adjunctive periodontal surgery, and possibly mechanical traction are likely to be required to bring them into the arch.

■ Problems Involving Crowding and Malalignment (Fig. 7-4, *D*)

For children with good facial proportions who have any type of orthodontic problem, regardless of whether crowding is apparent, the results of space analysis are essential for planning treatment. Space problems may well be developing even if the teeth appear to be well aligned, and the presence or absence of adequate space for the teeth must be taken into account when other treatment is planned. It

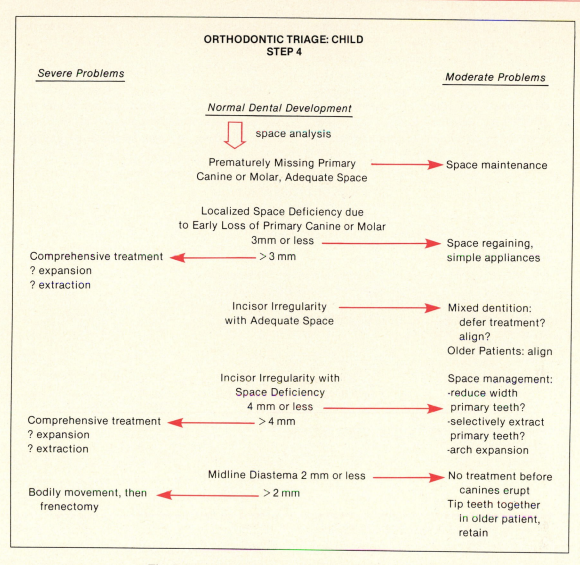

ORTHODONTIC TRIAGE: CHILD
STEP 4

Severe Problems   *Moderate Problems*

Normal Dental Development

space analysis

Prematurely Missing Primary
Canine or Molar, Adequate Space → Space maintenance

Localized Space Deficiency due
to Early Loss of Primary Canine or Molar
3mm or less → Space regaining,
Comprehensive treatment ← >3 mm   simple appliances
? expansion
? extraction

Incisor Irregularity
with Adequate Space → Mixed dentition:
                                   defer treatment?
                                   align?
                            Older Patients: align

Incisor Irregularity with
Space Deficiency   Space management:
4 mm or less →   -reduce width
Comprehensive treatment ← >4 mm   primary teeth?
? expansion   -selectively extract
? extraction   primary teeth?
                            -arch expansion

Midline Diastema 2 mm or less → No treatment before
Bodily movement, then ← >2 mm   canines erupt
   frenectomy   Tip teeth together
                             in older patient,
                             retain

Fig. 7-4, cont'd ■ **D,** Steps in orthodontic triage.

is surprisingly easy to focus so strongly on the correction of lingual displacement of a lateral incisor, for example, that the absence of adequate space to align the tooth is overlooked until during treatment it suddenly becomes painfully apparent that like all other objects, two teeth cannot occupy the same space at the same time.

In interpreting the results of space analysis for patients of any age, it is necessary to keep in mind that if space to align the teeth is inadequate, either of two conditions may develop. One possibility is that the incisor teeth may remain upright and well positioned over the basal bone of the maxilla or mandible, and then rotate or tip labially or lingually. In this instance, the potential crowding is expressed as actual crowding and is difficult to miss. The possibility, however, is that the crowded teeth may align themselves completely or partially at the expense of the lip, displacing the lip forward. Even if the space discrepancy and therefore the potential crowding are extreme, the teeth can always align themselves at the expense of interference with lip closure. This must be detected on profile examination.

If the incisors are upright and crowding is moderate, a few millimeters of arch expansion can often be carried out to solve the crowding problem. On the other hand, if there is already a degree of protrusion in addition to the crowding, it is safe to presume that the natural limits of anterior displacement of incisors have been reached.

On the basis of the space analysis results, children in the mixed dentition who do not have incisor protrusion can be divided into three groups (Fig. 7-4, *D*):

1. Those with adequate space. If a primary canine or molar has been lost prematurely, space maintenance to prevent a problem from developing is needed.

2. Those with space deficiency (localized or generalized) not more than 3 to 4 mm in either arch. These problems are the result of either (1) loss of a primary molar and drift of permanent or primary teeth or (2) a generalized tooth size–arch length problem, usually manifested as incisor crowding. These patients usually require space regaining or arch expansion respectively, as discussed below.

3. Patients with localized or generalized space deficiency

greater than 4 mm in one arch, or patients with smaller space discrepancies and incisor protrusion. These patients have space loss or a tooth size–arch length problem that often exceeds the limits of either space regaining or arch expansion and may require extraction to solve the problem.

Children in categories 1 and 2 have moderate problems and are often selected for treatment in general practice. Patients in category 3, or those with space discrepancies who also have skeletal problems, have severe problems that usually require treatment by a specialist.

■ Other Tooth Displacement (Fig. 7-4, *E*)

Whether other nonskeletal problems should be classified as moderate or severe is determined for most children by the facial form and space analysis results. A skeletal posterior crossbite, revealed by a narrow palatal vault, is a

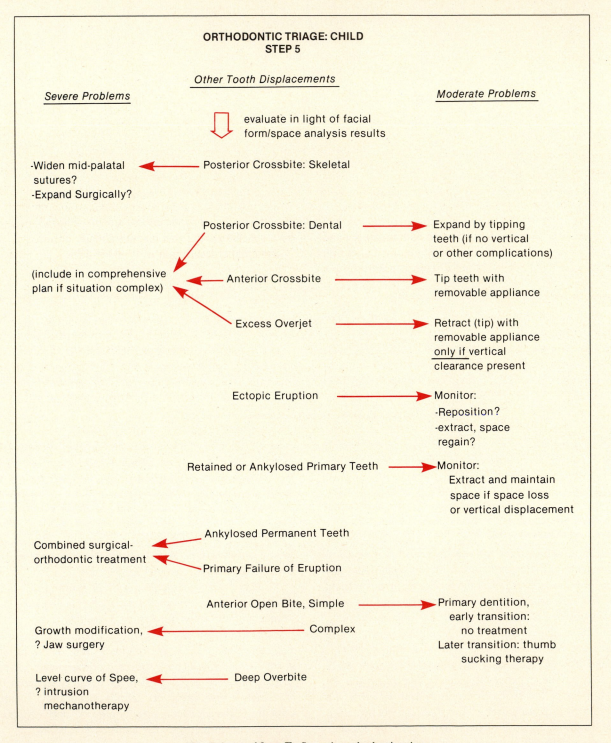

Fig. 7-4, cont'd ■ **E,** Steps in orthodontic triage.

severe problem, but a dental posterior crossbite falls into the moderate category if no other complicating factors (like severe crowding) are present. In a skeletal posterior crossbite, it is possible to widen the maxilla itself by opening the midpalatal suture, provided the patient is young enough to allow suture opening. This topic is discussed further in Chapter 8. If the crossbite is caused by maxillary posterior teeth that are tipped lingually, it is possible to tip the teeth outward into proper position with a variety of simple appliances. This approach to crossbite correction is discussed for each of the age groups in the remaining sections of this chapter.

Anterior crossbite usually reflects a jaw discrepancy, but can arise by lingual tipping of the incisors as they erupt. The use of removable appliances to correct these simple crossbites is discussed under mixed dentition treatment.

Excessive maxillary incisor overjet can also develop in patients with good jaw proportions. If adequate vertical clearance is present, the teeth can be tipped together with a simple removable appliance when the child is at almost any age. If a deep overbite is present, however, the protruding maxillary incisors can be retracted only if adequate vertical clearance is provided, and this usually involves placing a fixed orthodontic appliance on both maxillary and mandibular incisors. Treatment possibilities for correction of incisor protrusion problems are discussed briefly in this chapter below, and in more detail in Chapter 13 (children) and Chapter 16 (adults).

Ectopic eruption and ankylosed primary teeth should be monitored carefully, and space maintenance or space regaining may be required in their aftermath. Both, however, are moderate problems. Ankylosed permanent teeth or permanent teeth that fail to erupt, however, are severe problems that often require a combination of surgery and orthodontics if indeed the condition can be treated satisfactorily at all.

Anterior open bite in a young child with good facial proportions usually needs no treatment, since there is a good chance of spontaneous correction. A complex open bite (one with skeletal involvement or posterior manifestations), or any open bite in an older patient, is a severe problem, as is deep bite at all ages.

The triage scheme outlined above is primarily oriented toward children in the mixed dentition. Variations in treatment planning as they relate to different age groups are presented below.

■ *Treatment Planning for Orthodontic Problems in the Primary Dentition*

For children with a complete primary dentition (between the ages of 3 and 6), developing malocclusions can often be detected. As a general rule, little if any orthodontic treatment is indicated for preschool children. In a few circumstances, discussed in more detail following and in Chapter 13, treatment is indicated. Even if no orthodontic treatment is to be done, it is wise to discuss probable future treatment needs with parents at an early age.

The same diagnostic process used for all other patients is applicable to primary dentition children: an adequate database should be assembled and utilized to develop a problem list. The triage approach described previously can be applied without difficulty. It is important that young children who may have a facial syndrome be referred early for evaluation by a special team if this has not already occurred.

Systematic description of a malocclusion in the primary dentition also follows the same five steps as for any other malocclusion, and the comments in this and the following sections of this chapter follow the sequence in the Ackerman-Proffit approach: alignment and symmetry within the arch are examined first and the impact of the dentition on facial esthetics is considered, then problems related to the occlusal and jaw relationships in the three planes of space are noted. Systematic description of the orthodontic situation in a primary dentition child should include reference to the following special points:

Alignment problems. In the normal primary dentition, especially by age 5 and 6, spacing between the incisors is normal and in fact is necessary if the permanent incisors are to be properly aligned when they erupt. If the primary incisors contact each other proximally, one can confidently

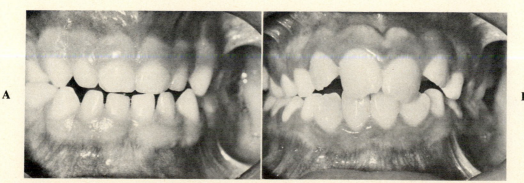

Fig. 7-5 ■ A ''Hollywood smile'' in the primary dentition, with no spaces between the primary incisors, guarantees insufficient room for the permanent incisors when they erupt and therefore, severe crowding. **A,** Age 5; **B,** age 8.

predict that the permanent incisors will be crowded and irregular (Fig. 7-5). Crowding in the primary dentition is rare. When this is observed, extremely severe crowding will be present later in the permanent dentition. The child with an adult-appearing smile at age 5 has space problems in his or her future, and the family dentist should inform the parents of this.

When teeth are lost prematurely in the complete primary dentition because of caries or trauma, there can be an impact on the position of the permanent teeth when they erupt, and crowding or malalignment may occur. At one time, it was thought that the upright primary teeth were stable in their position until a mesial component of force, such as that generated by erupting permanent first molars, was present. Evaluation of the literature[3] and clinical experience indicate that this is not the case. Treatment planning guidelines for very early loss of a primary tooth are as follows.

1. Loss of a primary incisor. In most children, spaces are present between the primary incisors, and the early loss of an incisor will cause little if any change in the dentition. Therefore, space maintenance is not necessary. On the other hand, prosthetic replacement of the teeth for esthetic reasons may need to be considered, especially since the eruption of the permanent incisors will probably be delayed if a primary incisor is lost at a very early age.

2. Loss of a primary canine. When a primary canine is lost, the incisor teeth tend to shift laterally into this space, creating a midline deviation and dental asymmetry. This tendency is accelerated at the time the permanent incisors begin to erupt, but can develop within the primary dentition. Fortunately, these teeth are infrequently lost because of caries or trauma. It is usually not necessary to institute space maintenance during the primary dentition, but it may be desirable to intervene at the time the permanent incisors begin to erupt.

3. Loss of a primary first molar. It is unlikely that the space of a first primary molar will be lost during the primary dentition because of mesial movement of posterior teeth, but particularly in the mandible, a lateral and posterior shift of the incisors may lead to development of asymmetry within the arch. Space maintenance in the primary dentition should be considered for prematurely lost primary first molars, particularly lower first primary molars, for this reason.

4. Loss of a primary second molar. The primary second molar not only reserves space for the permanent second premolars, but its distal root also guides the erupting permanent first molar into position. If the primary second molar is lost prematurely, the permanent first molar will usually migrate mesially within the bone even before it emerges into the oral cavity. A space maintaining device is needed that will both guide eruption of the permanent first molar before its emergence and then hold the first molar in proper position after occlusion is established. A distal shoe device (see Chapter 13) is indicated in this situation.

Incisor protrusion-retrusion. Sucking habits often persist throughout the primary dentition period and may cause displacement of the incisors, typically forward in the upper arch and backward in the lower. The incisor displacement produced by sucking habits is usually self-correcting if the habit stops before permanent teeth erupt. Rarely if ever is it necessary to plan any orthodontic treatment to reposition the primary incisors.

Anterior crossbite occasionally occurs in the primary dentition because of incisor interferences that cause an anterior shift of the mandible. If this occurs, it should be corrected. Usually this correction can be made merely by removing the interference, by either occlusal grinding or extracting the primary incisor if it is already near exfoliation (Fig. 7-6). It is rarely necessary to plan any orthodontic tooth movement before the permanent incisors begin to erupt.

Posterior crossbite. Transverse problems, usually manifest as posterior crossbite from a narrow upper arch, are relatively common in the primary dentition. Sucking habits tend to produce some constriction of the upper arch, particularly in the primary canine region, and occlusal interferences may then lead to a functional shift of the mandible anteriorly and laterally (Fig. 7-7). A unilateral crossbite in a preschool child almost always results, not from a true skeletal or dental asymmetry, but from a functional shift.

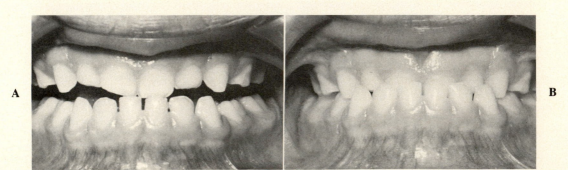

Fig. 7-6 ■ Anterior crossbite in the primary dentition can also be caused by incisor interference and a forward shift: **A,** initial contact position, **B,** habitual occlusion, after forward shift.

Since preschool children do not have well enough developed temporomandibular joints to have the equivalent of the adult's centric relation position, it can be time consuming and frustrating to try to determine where the child would occlude if the mandible were not shifted laterally, but usually a reproducible position can be identified. If this proves impossible, it is best to simply place the mandible so that the midlines are correct and plan treatment from this point. If intermolar width is satisfactory, grinding the primary canines to eliminate deflective contacts may be the only treatment required. If both molar canine widths are narrow, expansion of the upper arch (see Chapter 13) is indicated.

Anteroposterior discrepancies. Primary molar relationships are classified according to the relationship of the distal surfaces of the upper and lower second primary molars: flush terminal plane, the normal relationship; distal step, with the lower molar distally positioned relative to the upper molar; and mesial step, with the lower molar mesially positioned (see Chapter 3). Although the mesial step relationship corresponds to a Class I molar relationship in the permanent dentition, its presence at an early age indicates the possibility of excessive mandibular development and should be noted with concern. A distal step relationship correlates with a skeletal Class II jaw relationship, which in most children with a skeletal problem can be recognized by age 3.

By use of growth modification treatment methods, it is possible to correct distal step or mesial step relationships in most primary dentition children relatively easily. Unfortunately, as growth continues, the discrepancy tends to recur as quickly as it was corrected. For this reason, except in the most severe cases it is unwise to begin treatment for a skeletal Class II or Class III problem in the primary dentition. There is an adequate amount of growth remaining to obtain the necessary correction if treatment is deferred until the mixed dentition years.

Vertical problems. Both deep bite and open bite malocclusions occur in the primary dentition. Deep bite is usually associated with the skeletal proportions that predispose to this condition: a relatively short face with a square gonial angle and flat mandibular plane. Open bite, on the other hand, is often seen in children who have good skeletal proportions but sucking habits. If skeletal proportions are good, there is a strong tendency for the anterior open bite to correct spontaneously when the sucking habit ends. Vigorous efforts to prevent a preschool child from sucking, using dental appliances or other coercive approaches, are not warranted in most cases. Up to age 5 or so, sucking habits are unlikely to cause any long-term problems in children with good skeletal jaw relationships. The use of orthodontic appliances to actively close an open bite is not indicated in the primary dentition. There is no reason to place an appliance, either to alter a habit or to move teeth, if the situation is likely to correct itself without any treatment.

It is also possible that an open bite results from a skeletal jaw discrepancy of the long face type, characterized by increased lower anterior facial height. Spontaneous correction of an open bite is not likely to occur in these children. Instituting treatment for growth modification, however, is not indicated for the same reasons as for skeletal Classes II and III: if the problem is corrected in the primary dentition, it is likely to recur relatively quickly when the active treatment is discontinued. The same is true, of course, for skeletal deep bite relationships.

In summary: malposed, crowded, and irregular primary incisors are uncommon, but the absence of spaces between primary incisors often indicates that there will be crowding when permanent incisors erupt. No treatment is indicated until the mixed dentition. Posterior crossbites, particularly those with a lateral shift of the mandible upon closure, should be treated in the primary dentition, either by occlusal adjustment or by maxillary expansion. An anterior crossbite caused by a forward mandibular shift should also be treated early. Although skeletal anteroposterior and vertical problems can be detected in the primary dentition, indications for their treatment at that time are rare.

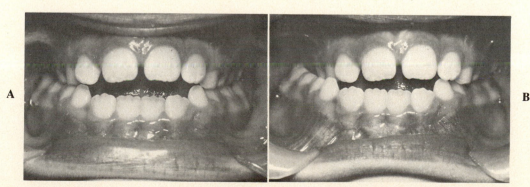

Fig. 7-7 ■ If the maxillary arch is relatively narrow, it is likely that a child will shift the jaw laterally upon closure, producing an apparent unilateral crossbite. The basic problem is usually a symmetric narrowing of the maxillary arch: **A,** initial contact position **B,** habitual occlusion.

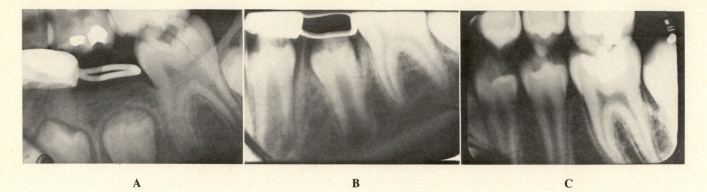

A   **B**   **C**

Fig. 7-8 ■ Space maintenance after early loss of a second primary molar. **A,** Band and loop space maintainer at age 8; **B,** same patient, age 11; **C,** same patient, age 12.

■ *Treatment Planning for Orthodontic Problems in the Early Mixed Dentition*

■ Treatment Planning for Moderate Problems

In contrast to the limited indications for primary dentition treatment, there are many indications for orthodontic treatment in the mixed dentition. For moderate problems, mixed dentition treatment may be all that is necessary, and this type of treatment can often be provided in the general practice of dentistry. Children with severe problems are often treated best with two phases of treatment, one in the mixed dentition and a second in the early permanent dentition. This treatment usually requires the expertise of a specialist.

Moderate problems in mixed dentition children, by our definition, are those selected by the triage scheme described previously. These consist entirely of dental problems resulting from misplaced permanent teeth, with skeletal problems and severe crowding problems excluded. Treatment planning for these children is discussed in the following sections and treatment procedures are described in Chapter 13.

Missing primary teeth with adequate space: space maintenance. If a primary first or second molar is missing, if there will be more than a 6 month delay before the permanent premolar erupts, and if there is adequate space (either because there has been no space loss or because space regaining has been completed) (see below); then space maintenance is needed. Although this can be done with either fixed or removable appliances, fixed appliances are preferred in most situations because they eliminate the factor of patient cooperation. If the space is unilateral, it can be managed by a unilateral fixed appliance (Fig. 7-8). If molars on both sides have been lost and the lateral incisors have erupted, it is usually better to place a lingual arch rather than two unilateral appliances. Early loss of a single primary canine in the mixed dentition requires space maintenance or extraction of the contralateral tooth to eliminate midline changes and the development of arch symmetry. If the contralateral canine is extracted, a lingual arch space maintainer may still be needed to prevent lingual movement of the incisors.

Localized space loss (3 mm or less): space regaining. Potential space problems can be created by drift of per-

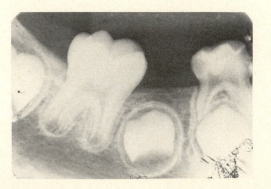

Fig. 7-9 ■ After early loss of a primary second molar, mesial drift of the permanent first molar occurs rapidly, as in this child.

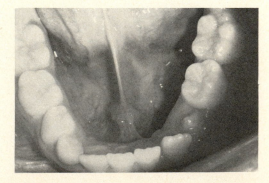

Fig. 7-10 ■ Premature loss of one primary canine leads to distal drift of the incisors toward the affected side, creating an asymmetry in the arch and a midline discrepancy.

manent incisors or molars, after premature extraction of primary canines or molars. In children who meet the criteria for moderate problems, i.e., no skeletal or dentofacial involvement, lost space can be regained by repositioning the teeth that have drifted. Then, a space maintainer is necessary to prevent further drift and space loss until the succedaneous teeth have erupted. A space maintainer alone is not adequate treatment for a space deficiency.

Space regaining is most likely to be needed when primary maxillary or mandibular second molars have been lost prematurely because of decay (Fig. 7-9) or, rarely, because of ectopic eruption of the permanent first molar. The permanent first molar usually migrates mesially quite rapidly when the primary second molar has been lost, and in the extreme case may totally close the primary second molar extraction site. If the primary second molar has been lost prematurely in a single quadrant, up to 3 mm of space may be regained by tipping the molar back distally. If space loss is bilateral, the limit of space regaining is about 4 mm for the total arch, or 2 mm per quandrant. Techniques for utilization of space regaining appliances are presented in Chapter 13.

Space within the dental arch can also be lost after premature loss of a primary canine (Fig. 7-10). In this circumstance, mesial drift of the posterior teeth is rare, but the incisor teeth do drift distally, reducing available arch length. Loss of one or both primary canines usually occurs because of root resorption caused by erupting lateral incisors without enough space, and thereby indicates a generalized crowding problem.

Generalized moderate crowding: space management. A child with a generalized arch length discrepancy up to 4 mm and no prematurely missing primary teeth can be expected to have moderately crowded incisors. If the primary canines have been exfoliated naturally or have been removed by the dentist, the incisors will be aligned with the canine spaces partially closed.

Depending on the magnitude of the space discrepancy and how crowded the incisors are, there are two treatment possibilities: (1) reduction in size of the primary canines (by disking the mesial and distal surfaces), or extraction of these teeth, and (2) gentle expansion of the arch, tipping the molars slightly distally and the incisors slightly forward while widening the arch in the premolar region. If the primary canines are extracted to allow the permanent incisors to align themselves, it is important that the incisors not be allowed to drift lingually, further increasing the space discrepancy, or that they be repositioned labially if this drift already has occurred. It must be kept in mind that severely rotated incisors will not usually correct spontaneously even if space is provided. Mild incisor crowding in the early mixed dentition can occur in children who have no arch length discrepancy, and this crowding can be relieved by disking the canines. Some expansion in addition will be necessary in children who have an arch length deficiency.

In the mandible, an adjustable lingual arch is the appliance of choice. For many patients, it is not really necessary to expand the mandibular arch much, if any. Instead, it is only necessary to prevent mesial shift of the mandibular molars at the time the second primary molars are lost (Figs. 7-11 and 7-12). On the other hand, if a lower lingual arch is used to prevent mesial shift of the mandibular molars, it will usually be necessary to move the maxillary molars or maxillary arch distally to achieve a Class I molar and canine relationship. For this purpose, a facebow with extraoral force usually is the treatment of choice (see Chapter 13).

Malpositioned incisors. In a child with spaced and flared or irregular maxillary incisors who has good molar relationships and good facial proportions, space analysis should show that the space available is excessive rather than de-

Patient: Susan C, age 11 years, 8 months	
Skeletal jaw relationship:	Normal
Lip posture:	Acceptable
Mandibular incisor position:	Acceptable
Mandibular Space Analysis	
Total space available:	68.5 mm
Space required:	69 mm
Allowance for molar shift:	3 mm
Total space required:	72 mm
Discrepancy:	−3.5 mm

Fig. 7-11 ■ Space analysis data for a patient who would be a candidate for space management. Note that the space discrepancy in the lower arch largely results from the allowance for mesial molar shift.

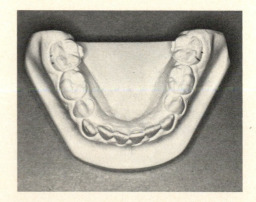

Fig. 7-12 ■ Mild incisor crowding of this extent can be corrected by utilizing leeway space at the time the second primary molars are lost, with no need to expand the arch (same patient as Fig. 7-11).

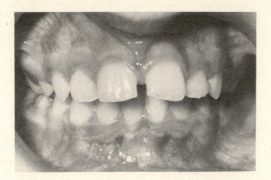

Fig. 7-13 ■ Flared and spaced maxillary incisors in a child with vertical clearance, i.e., no deep overbite, can be corrected by tipping the incisors lingually with a removable appliance. If deep overbite is present, as it is for this patient, this treatment plan is not advisable.

ficient. The presence or absence of excessive overbite, a factor not included in space analysis, however, must be evaluated to know if there is enough room.

If the upper incisors are flared forward and there is no contact with the lower incisors (Fig. 7-13), the protruding upper incisors can be retracted quite satisfactorily with a simple removable appliance. This condition is often found in the mixed dentition after prolonged thumbsucking and frequently occurs in connection with some narrowing of the maxillary arch. Physiologic adaptation to the space between the anterior teeth requires that the tongue be placed in this area to seal off the gap for successful swallowing and speech. This "tongue thrust" is not the cause of the protrusion or open bite and should not be the focus of therapy. If the teeth are retracted, the tongue thrust will disappear.

On the other hand, if there is a deep overbite anteriorly, the protruding upper incisor teeth cannot be retracted until it is corrected. The lower incisors biting against the lingual of the uppers prevents them from being moved lingually. A fixed appliance in both arches, which controls the vertical position of both the upper and lower incisors, is necessary to correct this combination of protrusion and deep overbite, even without skeletal involvement (which usually is present in these children).

A maxillary midline diastema (Fig. 7-14) can pose a special management problem. Small spaces between the maxillary incisors are normal before eruption of the maxillary canines (see Chapter 2). In the absence of deep overbite, these spaces normally close spontaneously. If the space between the maxillary central incisors is greater than 2 mm, however, spontaneous closure is unlikely.[4] Persistent spacing between the incisors is correlated with a cleft in the alveolar process between the central incisors into which fibers from the maxillary labial frenum insert (Fig. 7-14). For larger diastemas, it may be necessary to surgically remove the frenal attachment to obtain a stable closure of the midline diastema. The best approach, however, is to do nothing until the permanent canines erupt. If the space does not close spontaneously at that time, an appliance can be used to move the teeth together, and a frenectomy should be considered then if there is excessive tissue bunched up in the midline.

Anterior crossbite, particularly crossbite of all the incisors, is rarely found in children who do not have a skeletal Class III jaw relationship. A crossbite relationship of one or two anterior teeth, however, may develop in a child who has good facial proportions (Fig. 7-15). The maxillary lateral incisors tend to erupt to the lingual and may be trapped in that location, especially in the presence of severe crowding. In this situation, extracting the adjacent primary canines usually leads to spontaneous correction of the crossbite.

It is important to evaluate the space situation before attempting to correct any anterior crossbite. The prognosis for successfully pushing a 7 mm maxillary lateral incisor into a 4 mm space is not good. Frequently, even if there is enough space overall within the arch, it is necessary to remove the

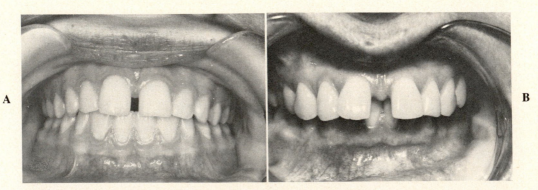

Fig. 7-14 ■ **A,** Maxillary central diastema of moderate severity, without a deep overbite. A problem of this type can be corrected with a removable appliance to bring the teeth together, because there is adequate vertical clearance of the teeth. **B,** Severe central diastema with deep overbite. Closure of this diastema will require correction of the deep overbite before the separated teeth can be brought together. A surgical frenectomy would definitely be required as part of the treatment plan for the patient in **B,** and probably would be needed for the patient in **A** also.

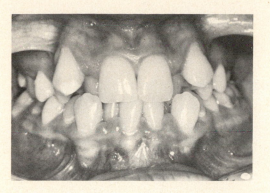

Fig. 7-15 ■ Anterior crossbite with lingual displacement of the maxillary incisors usually occurs in the presence of severe crowding, as in this 13-year-old girl.

maxillary primary canines prematurely to bring lateral incisors out of crossbite. If enough space is available to accomplish the movement, a maxillary removable appliance is usually the best mechanism to correct a simple anterior crossbite that requires tipping movement. Rotational changes and bodily movement are not effectively produced by removable appliances and require fixed appliance therapy.

Posterior crossbite. Posterior crossbites in mixed dentition children usually result from a narrowing of the maxillary arch and are often observed in children who have had prolonged sucking habits. Both removable and fixed appliances can be effective in correcting posterior crossbites (Fig. 7-16). Whether the fixed or removable appliance is used, the maxillary arch should be slightly overexpanded and then held passively in this overexpanded position for approximately 3 months before the appliance is removed.

Techniques for both removable and fixed appliances to expand the maxillary arch are illustrated in Chapter 13.

Anterior open bite. A simple anterior open bite is one that is limited to the anterior region in a child with good facial proportions. The major cause of such an open bite is

prolonged thumbsucking, and the most important step in obtaining correction is to stop sucking habits if they are present. For this purpose, behavior modification techniques are appropriate (see Chapter 3). Several approaches are possible (see Chapter 13). If an intra-oral appliance is needed, the preferred method is a maxillary lingual arch with an anterior crib device, making it extremely difficult for the child to place the thumb or other object in the mouth (Fig. 7-17). It is important that such a device be presented to the child as an aid, not as a punishment, and that psychologic support be provided to help him or her adjust to it.

In about half of the children for whom such a crib is made, thumbsucking stops immediately and the anterior open bite usually begins to close relatively rapidly thereafter. In the remaining children, thumbsucking persists for a few weeks, but the crib device is eventually effective in extinguishing thumbsucking in 85% to 90% of patients.[5] It is a good idea to leave the crib in place for 3 to 6 months after the habit has apparently been eliminated. Further details on fabrication and use of this appliance are provided in Chapter 13.

Overretained primary teeth and ectopic eruption. The eruption of a permanent tooth can be delayed if its primary predecessor is retained too long. When this happens, the obvious treatment is to remove the primary tooth. As a general guideline, a permanent tooth should erupt when approximately three-fourths of its root is completed. If root formation of the permanent successor has reached this point while a primary tooth still has considerable root remaining, the primary tooth should be extracted. This problem is most likely to arise when the permanent tooth bud is slightly displaced away from its primary predecessor (Fig. 7-18). In some children, the pace of resorption of the primary teeth is slow, for whatever reason, and occasionally almost all the primary teeth have to be removed to allow timely eruption of their permanent successors.

If a primary tooth is lost quite prematurely, a layer of relatively dense bone and soft tissue may form over the

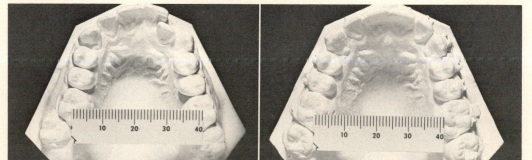

A   B

Fig. 7-16 ■ For this patient, 5 mm lateral expansion of the maxillary molars allowed correction of the posterior crossbite and also produced an increase in arch circumference that assisted in alignment of the crowded incisors (**A,** Pretreatment; **B,** post-treatment). For most patients, lateral expansion of the molars is stable, but whether this can be done for an individual patient depends on the characteristics of the malocclusion.

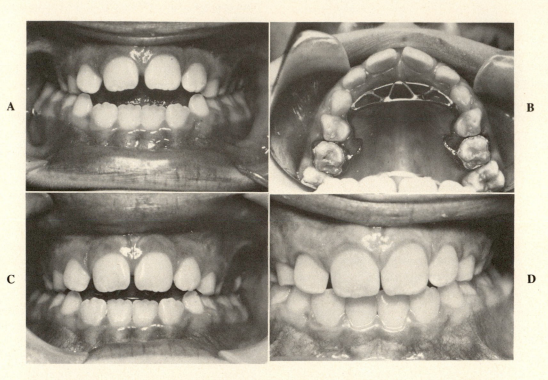

Fig. 7-17 ■ Correction of anterior open bite after cessation of thumbsucking. **A,** Open bite in an 8-year-old thumbsucking girl before treatment; **B,** crib appliance in place; **C,** improvement in open bite after 3 months; **D,** correction of open bite and crib removed after 6 months.

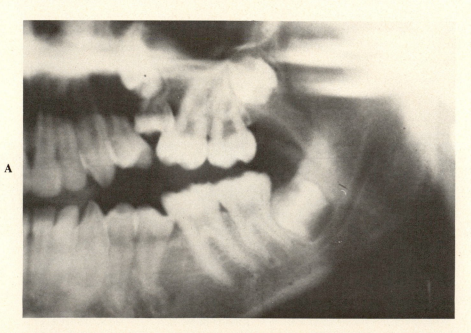

Fig. 7-18 ■ **A,** Extreme displacement of the maxillary left second premolar at age 13, after long-term ankylosis of the secondary primary molar. Note the space loss as the first molar has tipped mesially over the extraction of the ankylosed primary molar.

unerupted permanent tooth (see Fig. 7-8). This usually delays but does not prevent the eruption of the permanent tooth, and intervention is rarely indicated. If eruption of a permanent tooth has been delayed until its root formation is complete, it may still erupt on its own and should be given a chance to do so. It may be necessary, however, to place an attachment on it and gently pull it into the arch (see Chapter 13).

The eruption of maxillary first permanent molars and maxillary or mandibular lateral incisors can be delayed in the early mixed dentition by malposition of the permanent tooth and inappropriate resorption of primary molar or ca-

nine roots (ectopic eruption). The most common site is the maxillary molar region, where the second primary molar blocks the first permanent molar and suffers root resorption in the process (Fig. 7-19). If the permanent molar does not self-correct, it should be dislodged or, if all else fails, the primary molar extracted. If the primary molar is extracted, rapid space loss will result in a need for space regaining or premolar extraction. Ectopic eruption also frequently affects lateral incisors in children with severe crowding. A primary canine or canines may be lost as the lateral incisors erupt, which usually indicates that space is deficient. Maintaining symmetry after loss of one primary canine is an important consideration.

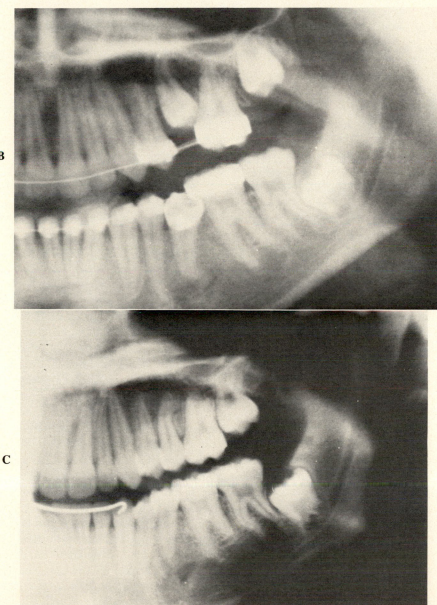

Fig. 7-18, cont'd ■ **B,** The upper left second molar has been extracted to allow the first molar to be moved distally, opening space for the premolar now erupting; **C,** second premolar in place at age 15.

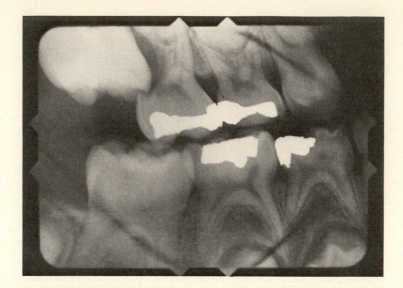

Fig. 7-19 ■ Ectopic eruption of the permanent first molar produces resorption of the distal root of the primary second molar.

■ Treatment Planning for Severe Problems

Severe problems in mixed dentition children fall into three major categories: (1) skeletal jaw discrepancies, (2) dentofacial problems related to incisor protrusion, and (3) space discrepancies of 5 mm or more. This group of patients usually requires a second stage of treatment after permanent teeth erupt, so the mixed dentition treatment is aimed at improving rather than comprehensively treating these severe problems.

Skeletal problems. Children with jaw discrepancies can often be helped considerably by application of growth modification techniques, which have become both more popular and more efficient in recent years. The key to growth modification is treatment while adequate growth remains, which means that these techniques must be applied before puberty and almost always during the mixed dentition period. Treatment planning for growth modification is discussed in Chapter 8, and the appropriate treatment techniques are described in Chapter 14.

Dentofacial problems related to incisor protrusion. Excessive protrusion of incisors (bimaxillary protrusion, not excessive overjet) is usually an indication for premolar extraction and retraction of the protruding incisors. Because of the profile changes produced by adolescent growth, it is better for most children to defer extraction to correct protrusion until late in the mixed dentition or early in the permanent dentition. It is definitely an error to begin extraction early and then allow the permanent molars to drift forward, because this will make effective incisor retraction impossible. A further discussion of this topic is presented in Chapter 8, as part of the discussion of ''the great extraction controversy.'' Techniques for controlling the amount of incisor retraction are described in Chapter 14.

Space discrepancies of 5 mm or more. Common sense indicates that the larger the space discrepancy, the greater the chance that extraction of some teeth will be necessary to align the remaining ones. It is not possible to say with certainty that any given amount of arch length discrepancy is the borderline between extraction and nonextraction treatment. As a general guideline, however, one can say that:

- Space discrepancies up to 4 mm usually can be resolved without extraction (except for third molars)
- Discrepancies in the 5 to 9 mm range sometimes are best treated without extraction, but frequently require extraction of some teeth other than third molars
- Children with space discrepancies of 10 mm or greater almost always require premolar extraction, regardless of what happens to third molars at a later date

The decision of whether more than 4 mm of arch expansion can be stable must be made on the basis of the patient's potential for lateral as well as anterior arch expansion. One possibility for arch expansion is to round out the arch form, expanding in the premolar region of the arch. Obviously, therefore, a patient with a narrow, V-shaped arch would have more potential for lateral expansion than an individual who already had oval arches. Growth potential should also be considered, since individuals who develop a rather large nose and chin can tolerate greater expansion than those who do not.

In some instances, it may be difficult to make this decision. Treatment planning for such patients should consist of an initial though relatively conservative attempt to expand the arches, while evaluating the result. If the patient tolerates arch expansion well and does not develop excessive incisor protrusion, expansion treatment may ultimately be successful in spite of a relatively large discrepancy. On the other hand, if the expansion proceeds with difficulty and the signs of excessive arch expansion, primarily incisor protrusion and labial tipping of the teeth, begin to appear, uncertainty about the correctness of a decision to extract teeth has been removed.

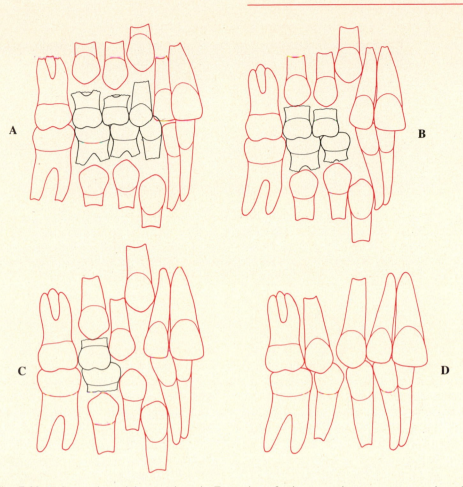

Fig. 7-20 ■ Stages in serial extraction. **A,** Extraction of primary canines as permanent laterals erupt. **B,** Extraction of primary first molars 6 to 12 months before normal exfoliation. **C,** Extraction of first premolars as they are just emerging before the canines erupt. **D,** Spontaneous space closure as the canines erupt distally and molars/premolars drift mesially. The goal is to transfer the incisor crowding posteriorly to the premolar extraction site, and the key to success is extraction of the first premolars before the canines erupt.

Serial extraction. Since the extraction of primary canines eliminates crowding of permanent incisors in the mixed dentition, it is tempting to extract these teeth when early incisor crowding develops. After the extraction of primary canines, if permanent first premolars can be extracted before the permanent canines and second premolars erupt, the permanent canines will erupt distally and the extraction spaces may all but close spontaneously. This approach, called "serial extraction," was developed in Europe in the 1930s and at times has been widely advocated as a simple way of dealing with severe space problems.

In its classic form, serial extraction applies to patients who meet the following criteria: (1) no skeletal disproportions, (2) Class I molar relationship, (3) normal overbite, and (4) large arch perimeter deficiency (10 mm or more). This procedure consists of four steps: (1) extraction of primary lateral incisors as the permanent central incisors erupt (if necessary, since this often happens spontaneously); (2) extraction of primary canines as the permanent laterals erupt; (3) extraction of primary first molars 6 to 12 months before their normal exfoliation; and (4) extraction of the permanent

first premolars before eruption of the permanent canines (Fig. 7-20).

Because an average first premolar is 7 to 8 mm wide, premolar extraction creates 14 to 16 mm space in the arch. Only when there is extremely severe crowding of 10 mm or more is there a chance that a reasonably satisfactory result can be achieved by serial extraction alone. After serial extraction, the incisors tend to drift lingually, and posterior teeth tend to drift mesially to some extent, typically leading to 2 to 3 mm of space closure in each quadrant or 4 to 6 mm total. The remainder of the space, approximately 10 mm, is available for resolution of the crowding. Residual spaces will remain at the extraction sites if the original discrepancy was small.

If it is clear that extraction is required, serial extraction in a patient with a relatively small discrepancy may simplify later treatment even though closure of residual space with fixed appliances certainly will be required (Fig. 7-21). If the space discrepancy is large enough and if everything can be timed perfectly, serial extraction can produce total space closure and reasonably good alignment of the teeth without

A   B   C

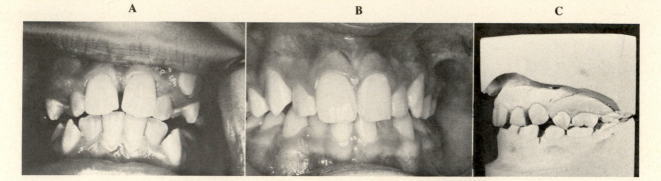

Fig. 7-21 ■ Results of early premolar extraction: **A,** severe crowding with maxillary and mandibular canines nearly blocked out of the arch; **B,** improvement in alignment after extraction of first premolars: **C,** lateral view of casts, showing failure of the extraction spaces to close completely despite the severity of the crowding. Excellent occlusion is unlikely to develop in a patient who has only extractions, despite the significant improvement in alignment that may occur.

any orthodontic appliance therapy at all (Fig. 7-22). However, such a favorable outcome is rare, and cannot be relied upon. Even with large discrepancies, the vast majority of patients undergoing serial extraction require a period of fixed appliance treatment to achieve good alignment, interdigitation, and root paralleling. Further details on management of serial extraction are given in Chapter 13.

In rare instances, a child with good skeletal proportions will have a Class II molar relationship and severe maxillary but not mandibular incisor crowding. This condition arises, of course, when upper posterior teeth have slipped mesially. In this circumstance, a modification of the serial extraction procedure to encompass only the maxillary arch can be helpful.[6] Serial extraction should be avoided in any child who has a skeletal Class II jaw discrepancy.

■ Treatment Planning for Orthodontic Problems in Adolescence (Late Mixed and Early Permanent Dentition)

Orthodontic treatment traditionally has been carried out in early adolescence, soon after the succedaneous teeth have erupted. This is the ideal time for comprehensive treatment of severe problems, but is often too late for the most effective treatment of moderate problems. Most of this treatment, therefore, is done by specialist orthodontists.

■ Alignment Problems

Crowding and protrusion. When there is crowding in the early permanent dentition, an accurate space analysis can be carried out directly, without the necessity for predicting the size of unerupted teeth. In this age group, however, it remains true that it is necessary to evaluate the amount of protrusion as well as the amount of crowding to totally evaluate the space situation. Crowding and protrusion

in the permanent dentition are interrelated, just as they are in the mixed dentition.

A significant difference between mixed dentition and early permanent dentition patients is that the simple appliances that can be used to solve space problems in the mixed dentition are no longer effective after the permanent teeth have erupted. Whether a patient in the early permanent dentition is to be treated by arch expansion or by extraction, a bonded or banded fixed appliance is needed to position the teeth correctly. Removable appliances of all types, along with lingual arches and other round wire or partially fixed appliances, are effective only for tipping teeth to new positions. If the permanent teeth have been allowed to erupt completely while still malaligned, it is rare that a satisfactory result can be obtained without using an orthodontic appliance that has the potential to change root position. Just tipping the crowns to a new location is not enough. It is also true that extraction will probably be required in the permanent dentition with relatively smaller degrees of space discrepancy than was the case with mixed dentition children, whose potential for arch development is greater.

The amount of space available for mitigation of crowding is greatest when a first premolar, canine, or incisor is extracted, because crowding usually occurs in the anterior part of the dental arch. If a more posterior tooth is selected for extraction, greater amounts of space will inevitably be lost as molars slip forward rather than canines and premolars moving distally. The amount of space available for relief of crowding after the extraction of various teeth is summarized in Table 7-1, and the general topic of extraction treatment is discussed in more detail in Chapter 8.

Tooth size discrepancies. Data from tooth size analysis become available for the first time when the succedaneous teeth erupt. A tooth size discrepancy of less than 1.5 mm is usually insignificant, but larger discrepancies create a problem that must be solved in the development of a treat-

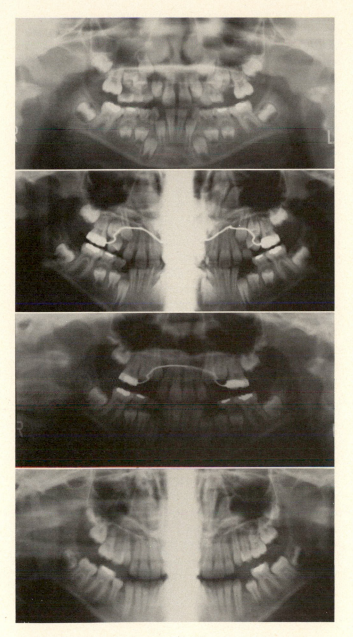

Fig. 7-22 ■ Sequential panoramic films in a child with severe crowding treated by serial extraction. Note the distal movement of the canines into the first premolar extraction spaces.

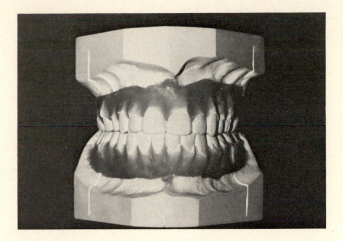

Fig. 7-23 ■ Resetting the teeth to directly evaluate how they would fit together usually is needed to verify that a plan for correcting tooth size discrepancy could succeed.

Table 7-1 ■ Space from various extractions*

Extraction	Relief of incisor crowding	Incisor retraction		Posterior forward†	
		Max.	Min.	Max.	Min.
Central incisor	5	3	2	1	0
Lateral	5	3	2	1	0
Canine	6	5	3	2	0
First premolar	5	5	2	5	2
Second pre-molar	3	3	0	6	4
First molar	3	2	0	8	6
Second molar	2	1	0	–	–

*Values given in millimeters.
†Anteroposterior plane of space in absence of crowding.

ment plan. There are five possible approaches[7]: (1) compensate in the inclination of incisors for a small size differential; (2) reduce the width of some teeth by interproximal stripping of enamel; (3) build up the width of an anomalously small tooth or teeth by adding composite resin or a crown; (4) alter the normal extraction plan to compensate for size discrepancies; or (5) accept a small space in one of the arches, usually distal to the lateral incisors.

Before one of the possible plans is accepted, it is important to determine whether the discrepancy is caused by a variation in one of the teeth or a generalized size difference between upper and lower teeth. This determination can be accomplished by Bolton analysis (see Chapter 6). The usual culprits in tooth size problems are the upper lateral incisors, but second premolars in both arches also vary in size. Reducing or building up lateral incisors if these are the source of the discrepancy is the best approach. It is less easy to alter the width of premolars, and one of the other solutions may be required. A diagnostic setup (Fig. 7-23), i.e., resetting the teeth after cutting them off the cast and modifying them, is usually needed to verify that a proposed treatment plan for tooth size discrepancy can succeed.

■ Transverse Problems

Transverse problems in the adolescent age group, as in younger patients, are most likely the result of a narrow maxillary arch. The necessary maxillary expansion may be approached either skeletally or dentally, depending on the anatomic basis of the problem. The basis of skeletal maxillary expansion is widening of the midpalatal suture by applying heavy force across the suture, producing skeletal changes either rapidly (days) or more slowly (weeks). This form of growth modification treatment is discussed in more detail in Chapter 8.

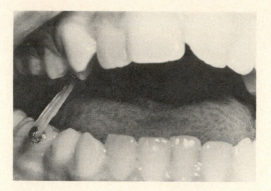

Fig. 7-24 ■ Cross-elastics from the maxillary lingual to the mandibular labial can be used to correct a single-tooth crossbite.

The maxillary arch can also be widened by dental expansion with fixed or removable appliances. Whenever a removable appliance is used for arch expansion, it is extremely important that it be tightly retained by excellent clasps. Although a screw device in a removable appliance can widen the arch, this will occur largely by tipping tooth movement and should not be considered a substitute for the fixed expansion devices used for palatal expansion. Better control of dental expansion is usually achieved with a relatively flexible lingual arch.

Single tooth crossbites or true unilateral asymmetries of the dental arch are usually best corrected by cross elastics, i.e., elastics from the lingual of one arch to the buccal of the other, in the affected area (Fig. 7-24). Reciprocal tooth movement will result if one tooth is pitted against another. Differential unilateral maxillary expansion can be achieved by placing a lower fixed appliance and using cross elastics from the stabilized lower arch to the maxillary teeth on the affected side. This concept of anchorage reinforcement for differential tooth movement is discussed in more detail in Chapter 10.

True skeletal asymmetries in the adolescent age group pose an extremely difficult problem. A possible plan for moderately severe asymmetry is a hybrid functional appliance (see Chapter 14), but surgery is often required.

■ Anteroposterior Problems

The preferred treatment for skeletal problems, whatever the plane of space, is always growth modification. For greatest success, growth modification treatment should begin before the adolescent growth spurt, and the amount of remaining growth must be evaluated carefully before treatment is planned for an adolescent. Girls mature earlier than boys, and it is especially likely that by the time a girl's permanent teeth have erupted, it is too late for effective growth modification. A second plan for correcting anteroposterior discrepancies is to camouflage them by differential movement of upper and lower incisors. If the problem is severe, a third option is surgical repositioning of the jaws. These possibilities are discussed, in Chapter 8.

Occasionally a patient who has neither a skeletal jaw discrepancy nor space problems may have excessive overjet because of maxillary incisor protrusion combined with mandibular incisor retrusion. Such cases are rare, unfortunately, since they can be described as "the orthodontist's dream." Essentially any appliance ever invented, coupled with Class II elastics or their equivalent, is capable of correcting such problems. The cases used to illustrate the wonder of many simplistic appliances will be found on close examination to fall into this category.

■ Vertical Problems

The major vertical problems of adolescents are anterior open bite and anterior deep bite, both of which are likely to be seen in combination with some anteroposterior problem. As a child becomes older, it is more and more likely that malocclusion in the vertical plane of space, as in the anteroposterior plane of space, is related to skeletal jaw proportions and not just to displacement of the teeth. Eruption problems are also likely to be more serious in this age group.

Anterior open bite. The skeletal indications of anterior open bite are increased anterior face height, a steep mandibular plane, and excessive eruption of posterior teeth. Because the mandible is rotated downward and backward in this circumstance, the patient is likely to have a Class II jaw relationship in addition to the vertical problem. Growth modification treatment, discussed in more detail in Chapter 8, is likely to include treatment aimed at intruding the maxillary molars, or at least preventing their further eruption.

In younger children, the major cause of anterior open bite is sucking habits or other environmental influences. Spontaneous correction of open bites caused by these habits often occurs during the mixed dentition and can be facilitated by relatively simple treatment. By the time adolescence is reached, however, environmental causes of anterior open bite are less important than skeletal factors (Fig. 7-25). It is rare that anterior open bite in an adolescent is solely the result of some habit, or that the open bite will correct spontaneously if the habit can be corrected.

In the past, tongue thrust swallowing was blamed for many anterior open bites in this age group, and efforts at training the patient to swallow correctly were used in an attempt to control anterior open bite problems. Contemporary research (see Chapter 3) makes it clear that tongue thrust swallow is more an adaptation to the open bite than the cause of it. Myofunctional therapy for tongue thrusting, for that reason, is ineffectual and not recommended. The appropriate growth modification therapy is discussed in Chapter 8.

Deep overbite. Anterior deep bite problems may result from an upward and forward rotation of the mandible, or from excessive eruption of mandibular incisor teeth. Supraeruption of lower incisors often accompanies a Class II malocclusion, because when there is excessive overjet, the lower incisors tend to erupt until they contact the palatal mucosa. Correction of this elongation of the lower incisors,

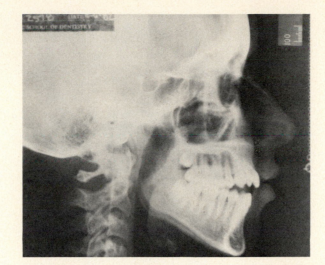

Fig. 7-25 ■ Anterior open bite in a 13-year-old girl. Every individual with this degree of anterior open bite uses the tongue to seal the anterior opening, and therefore can be labeled as having a tongue thrust swallow. It is unlikely in this age group that an open bite problem results primarily from a habit. Note the signs of skeletal vertical dysplasia, including the steep mandibular plane angle, downward rotation of the premaxilla, and increased lower face height.

by leveling out an excessive curve of Spee in the lower arch, is usually required as a part of fixed appliance orthodontic therapy. In an adolescent patient whose face height is still increasing, it is only necessary to prevent further eruption of the lower incisors as vertical growth continues, to achieve a relative intrusion. Continuous arch mechanics are appropriate. In the absence of growth, however, absolute intrusion is required (see Fig. 7-3), and segmented arch mechanics must be used to achieve this (see Chapters 10, 15, and 20).

Correction of skeletal deep bite problems requires rotating the mandible downward, increasing the mandibular plane angle and anterior face height. It must be kept in mind that in a patient with short anterior facial dimensions and a skeletal deep bite, rotating the mandible downward to correct the deep bite will reveal a skeletal mandibular deficiency. Thus the growth modification techniques necessary to deal with this problem are typically those for correction of mandibular deficiency.

Eruption problems. Failure of a permanent tooth to erupt creates a severe orthodontic problem. A localized problem is typically created either by displacement of a permanent tooth from its normal eruption path so that the tooth becomes impacted (usually a maxillary canine) (Fig. 7-26) or by trauma that leads to ankylosis (usually a maxillary incisor) (Fig. 7-27). A generalized problem implies an abnormality in the eruption mechanism.

Impacted teeth. An impacted canine or other tooth in a teenaged patient can usually be brought into the arch by orthodontic traction after being surgically exposed. In older patients, there is an increasing risk that the impacted tooth has become ankylosed. Even adolescents have a risk that surgical exposure of a tooth will lead to ankylosis. In planning treatment for an impacted permanent tooth, three treatment planning principles should be followed: (1) The prognosis should be based on the extent of displacement and the surgical trauma required for exposure. As a rule, the greater the displacement and the greater the trauma, the poorer the prognosis. Extraction of a severely impacted tooth and orthodontic space closure or prosthetic replacement may be better judgment than heroic efforts to bring the tooth into the arch. (2) During surgical exposure, flaps should be reflected so that the tooth is ultimately pulled into the arch through ketatinized tissue, not through alveolar muscosa. (3) Adequate space should be provided in the arch before attempting to pull the impacted tooth into position.

If a tooth is severely impacted, surgical transplantation is a possible treatment approach. This involves removing the tooth, creating a socket at the appropriate site in the arch, and replanting the tooth in its correct position. External root resorption often ensues after transplantation and is the major cause of failure. Approximately two-thirds of transplanted teeth are functional for 5 years, but only about one-third are retained for 10 years.[8] Orthodontic movement is preferable if it is possible.

Traumatic displacement and ankylosis. Trauma to incisor teeth can cause several types of problems, including root fractures and loss of pulp vitality. Immediate displacement of a traumatized tooth occurs because the alveolar bone compresses or fractures, allowing the tooth to move. The best treatment is to orthodontically reposition the tooth, beginning the treatment immediately but moving it slowly with light force so that the bone heals with the tooth in its proper position.[10] If even a small part of the periodontal ligament is obliterated during subsequent healing so that cementum of the root fuses to bone, neither further eruption

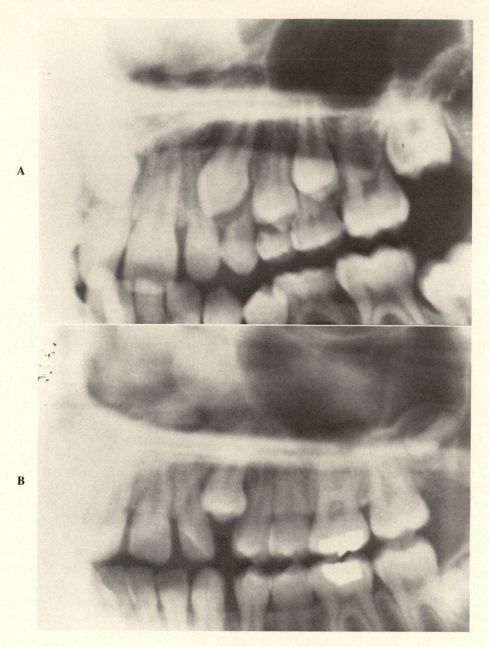

Fig. 7-26 ■ Impacted maxillary canines: **A)** mild displacement with good prognosis; **B)** impaction with minimal displacement from space shortage, with good prognosis; **C)** severe displacement with guarded prognosis for orthodontic correction.

nor orthodontic tooth movement will be possible. It is frustrating to watch helplessly as an ankylosed maxillary incisor appears to intrude while the other teeth erupt past it in a rapidly growing adolescent. Extraction followed by prosthetic replacement, however, usually is the only choice. The one possible alternative, which often is not feasible, is a small segment osteotomy to reposition both the ankylosed tooth and the adjacent alveolar bone (see Chapter 20). This procedure should not be done until growth is completed.

Generalized eruption failure. An eruption delay that affects several teeth in an adolescent patient is an ominous

sign. If the problem is a mechanical interference with eruption (see Chapter 4), the obvious treatment plan is to remove the interference and proceed with orthodontic therapy.

The condition called "primary failure of eruption"[10] (Fig. 7-28) results from a failure of the eruption mechanism itself (see Chapter 3). Unfortunately, not only do the involved teeth not erupt spontaneously, they do not respond to orthodontic force and cannot be pulled into the arch. Since prosthetic replacement is the only practical solution, it is fortunate that the condition is rare.

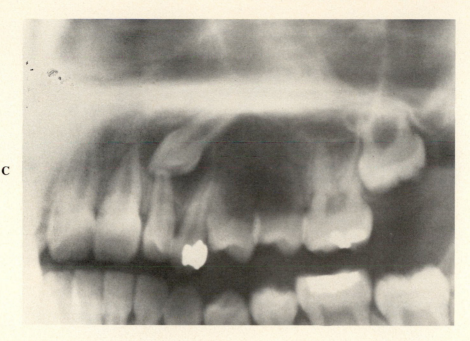

C

Fig. 7-26, cont'd ■ For legend see opposite page.

■ *Treatment Planning for Orthodontic Problems in Adults*

■ Adjunctive versus Comprehensive Treatment

Orthodontic treatment for adults can be either comprehensive in scope or limited in its objectives (adjunctive to other treatment). Adjunctive treatment is often within the scope of general dental practice and can be of considerable importance in the management of adults with periodontal disease and restorative needs.

The same triage approach used for children applies to adults for whom comprehensive orthodontic treatment is contemplated: those with skeletal discrepancies should be separated from those with dental problems, and the dental problems should be evaluated by their severity.

In adults, however, some orthodontic treatment may be needed as a part of restorative and periodontal treatment, regardless of whether major changes in the occlusion are desired. Adjunctive procedures for adults can be defined as those aimed at improving a specific occlusal characteristic, as part of an overall treatment plan usually involving major components of periodontal and restorative treatment. Relatively simple orthodontic appliances are typically involved and applied only to a specific part of the arch. Comprehensive orthodontic treatment, in contrast, nearly always involves a complete fixed appliance.

It is an error in treatment planning to overlook adjunctive treatment because the patient does not wish more comprehensive correction of malocclusion. On the other hand, the patient should receive a thorough evaluation and should be informed of treatment possibilities, including comprehensive correction if a severe malocclusion is present. As a general guideline (Fig. 7-29), most adjunctive procedures for adults are appropriately included in general practice, while comprehensive treatment of adults is usually better handled by a specialist. Treatment planning for adjunctive procedures is discussed briefly and techniques are presented in detail in Chapter 19, whereas comprehensive adult treatment is covered in Chapter 20.

The major indication for adjunctive orthodontic treatment in adults is drift of potential abutment teeth for bridges. If a permanent first molar is extracted during childhood, there is likely to be considerable mesial drift of the second molar and distal drift of premolars in the succeeding years. Periodontal defects are likely to occur on the mesial of the tipped second molar and may also be found between separated premolar teeth on the distal of the tipped molar (Fig. 7-30). In most cases, it is desirable to use a partial fixed appliance to upright the mesially tipped second molar and reposition the premolars mesially, before making a fixed bridge to replace the missing first molar. This improves the periodontal situation for most patients, and also makes it possible to fabricate a more ideal bridge (Fig. 7-31). Early loss of teeth other than the first permanent molar is less common, but drift of other permanent teeth will follow extraction of a tooth at any point in the arch. Because of this, most patients who wait to have a prosthetic replacement made until long after a tooth has been extracted will need orthodontic repositioning of abutment teeth.

If the second molar has drifted mesially, as a general rule it is preferable to upright it by tipping its crown distally and opening up space for a pontic replacing the missing first molar, rather than attempting to move the second molar

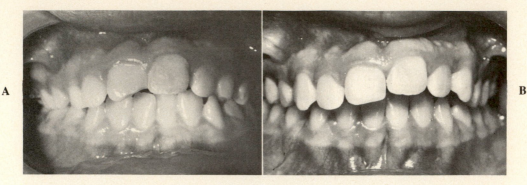

Fig. 7-27 ■ Ankylosis of maxillary incisors after trauma. **A,** At age 11; **B,** at age 13. Note the failure of the upper left central and lateral incisors to erupt. The fractured right central has been restored.

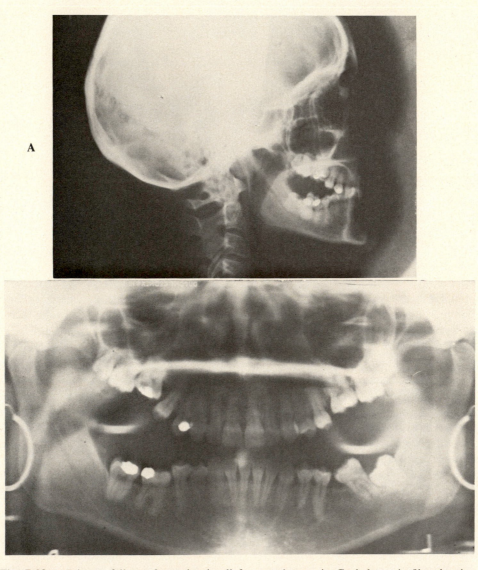

Fig. 7-28 ■ Primary failure of eruption in all four quadrants. **A,** Cephalometric film showing marked posterior open bite; **B,** panoramic film showing failure of teeth to erupt despite the lack of any obvious mechanical obstruction. Because their periodontal ligament is abnormal, the involved teeth cannot be moved orthodontically.

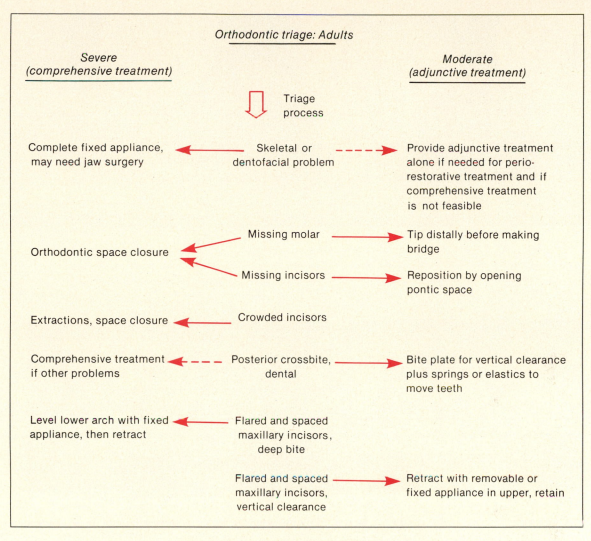

Orthodontic triage: Adults

Severe (comprehensive treatment)	Triage process	Moderate (adjunctive treatment)

Complete fixed appliance, may need jaw surgery ← Skeletal or dentofacial problem --→ Provide adjunctive treatment alone if needed for perio-restorative treatment and if comprehensive treatment is not feasible

Orthodontic space closure ← Missing molar → Tip distally before making bridge

← Missing incisors → Reposition by opening pontic space

Extractions, space closure ← Crowded incisors

Comprehensive treatment if other problems ← - - Posterior crossbite, dental → Bite plate for vertical clearance plus springs or elastics to move teeth

Level lower arch with fixed appliance, then retract ← Flared and spaced maxillary incisors, deep bite

Flared and spaced maxillary incisors, vertical clearance → Retract with removable or fixed appliance in upper, retain

Fig. 7-29 ■ Steps in orthodontic triage, adults.

mesially and close the extraction space. This is true even if the first molar space is nearly closed.

There are two reasons for this rule. The first is that it is relatively easy to tip the second molar distally, but much harder to upright the second molar by moving its roots mesially. The second reason is that if a long time has elapsed since the first molar was lost, there is almost always considerable atrophy of the alveolar ridge in the area of the original extraction site, producing a very narrow alveolar ridge. It is always difficult, and frequently impossible, to close the space and bring the second molar into good contact with the second premolar when this atrophy has occurred. Tipping the second molar distally, however, does require extraction of the third molar in most patients. When the second molar is put into its original position in the arch, there is no room for the third molar, which would have been impacted if it had not drifted mesially.

The second most common indication for repositioning abutment teeth before fabricating a fixed bridge is probably

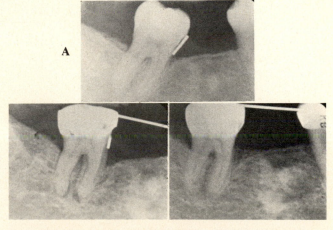

Fig. 7-30 ■ **A,** radiograph with silver point in place to the depth of the gingival sulcus before molar uprighting; **B,** silver point to the depth of the gingival sulcus immediately upon completion of molar uprighting; **C,** 3 months after uprighting, showing area of new bone fill-in on the mesial of the uprighted molar.

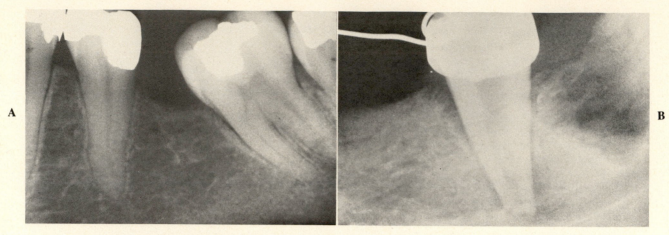

Fig. 7-31 ■ Changes in the alveolar bony architecture associated with molar uprighting. **A,** Before uprighting; **B,** after extraction of the third molar and uprighting of the second. Note the extent to which new bone has filled in on the mesial of the uprighted second molar and the upward extension of the bony attachment.

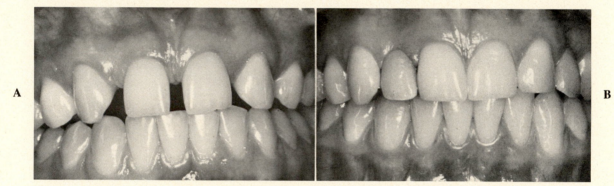

Fig. 7-32 ■ **A,** Missing maxillary lateral incisors, with drift of the central incisors making esthetic restorations impossible; **B,** same patient 1 year later, with restorations in place after adjunctive orthodontics to reposition the incisors.

in patients with missing or malformed maxillary incisors. This condition often leads to spacing between the maxillary central incisors, and the position of the maxillary canines may also be abnormal (Fig. 7-32). Adults with this problem are best treated with a fixed appliance, using an arch wire with coil springs to open space for the missing lateral incisors while simultaneously closing the central diastema. Realignment of the teeth in other areas of the dental arch, should this be indicated, would be carried out in the same way, using a fixed appliance to open space for the pontic. Closing space is considerably more difficult and falls into the category of comprehensive treatment.

Correction of crossbites in adults may also be needed as an adjunctive procedure. Since the occlusion in adults often locks teeth into a crossbite relationship, it is necessary to disengage the teeth to make tooth movement possible. This can be done either by having the patient wear a bite plate of some type to prevent occlusal contact until the orthodontic tooth movement has been completed, or by occlusal grinding to reduce interferences that would prevent the desired tooth movement.

In some adult patients, it is desirable to retract flared and spaced incisors, usually before the fabrication of fixed splints to stabilize periodontally involved teeth. If there is adequate vertical clearance, retracting flared incisors is a simple procedure with a removable appliance. If there is a deep overbite, however, it is simply not possible to retract flared and spaced upper incisors without also moving the lower incisors so that there will be proper incisor function at the end of treatment. Successful treatment almost always requires an upper and lower fixed appliance, and a relatively prolonged treatment time. These patients, whose orthodontic problems may look simple at first glance, can be extremely difficult to treat and should be placed in the category of comprehensive treatment.

■ **Periodontal considerations**

When either comprehensive or adjunctive orthodontics for an adult is planned, the periodontal management of the patient must be kept in mind. The incidence of periodontal disease rises sharply in older population groups. A number of studies have indicated that by age 30, a majority of

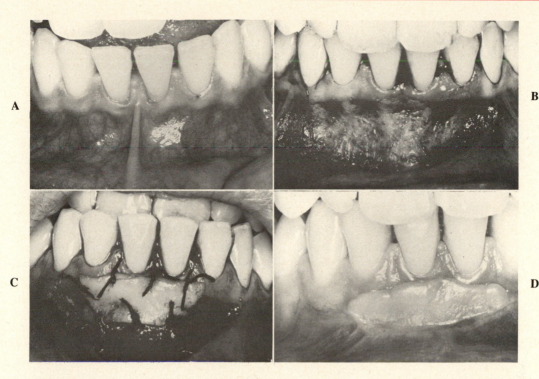

Fig. 7-33 ■ Free gingival grafts to create adequate attached gingiva may be needed before orthodontic treatment, particularly in the lower incisor area in adults. **A,** Inadequate attached gingiva and high frenum attachment create the possibility that loss of attachment will occur; **B,** preparation of a bed for free gingival graft from the palate; **C,** graft sutured into place; **D,** graft healing 6 weeks later.

patients have some periodontal problems, and by age 40 this is true for more than 75% of all patients.[11,12] Beginning or even advanced periodontal breakdown does not contraindicate orthodontic treatment, but the periodontal situation must be kept in mind whenever orthodontic treatment for adults is planned.

Periodontal findings in potential orthodontic patients are of two major types: (1) mucogingival problems, usually inadequate attached gingiva, and (2) inflammatory lesions of the gingiva or periodontium. Before any orthodontic treatment, it is important that adequate attached gingiva to withstand the stress of orthodontic tooth movement be created, if there are areas of deficiency (Fig. 7-33). Inflammatory lesions must be brought under control. Adult patients undergoing orthodontic treatment should have careful scaling on an accelerated schedule, typically at twice the frequency they would require without orthontic treatment. In other words, an adult who might be seen for scaling and polishing at 6-month intervals without orthodontic treatment probably should be seen at 3-month intervals while being treated orthodontically, while one who required care at 3-month intervals should be seen every 6 weeks while undergoing orthodontics.

Further details of periodontal management are provided in Chapters 19 and 20.

■ *References*

1. Angle, E.H.: Treatment of malocclusion of the teeth, Angle's System, ed. 7, Philadelphia, 1907, S.S. White Co.

2. American Cleft Palate Association: Membership-Team Directory. Pittsburgh, 1983, ACPA/ACPEF National Office, University of Pittsburgh School of Dentistry.

3. Owen, D.G.: The incidence and nature of space closure following extraction of deciduous teeth: a literature survey. Am. J. Orthod. **59:**37-49, 1971.

4. Edwards, J.C.: The diastema, the frenum, the frenectomy: a clinical study. Am. J. Orthod. **71:**489-508, 1977.

5. Haryett, R.D., Hansen, F.C., and Davidson, P.O.: Chronic thumb sucking. Am. J. Orthod. **57:**164-178, 1970.

6. Hotz, R.: Orthodontics in Daily Practice. Baltimore, 1974, Williams and Wilkins, pp. 185-228.

7. Fields, H.W.: Orthodontic-restorative treatment for relative mandibular anterior excess tooth-size problems. Am. J. Orthod. **79:**176-183, 1981.

8. Moss, J.P.: The unerupted canine. Dent. Pract. **22:**241-248, 1972.

9. Spalding, P.M., Fields, H.W., Torney, D., et al.: The changing role of endodontics and orthodontics in the management of traumatically intruded incisors. Ped. Dent. **7:**104-110, 1985.

10. Proffit, W.R., and Vig, K.W.L.: Primary failure of eruption: a possible cause of posterior open bite. Am. J. Orthod. **80:**173-190, 1981.

11. Betting, C.M., Massler, M., and Schour, I.: Prevalence and incidence of alveolar bone disease in men. J. Am. Dent. Assoc. **47:**190-197, 1953.

12. Marshall-Day, C.D., Stephens, R.G., and Quigley, L.F., Jr.: Periodontal disease: prevalence and incidence. J. Periodontal. **26:**185-203, 1955.

Chapter 8

Orthodontic Treatment Planning: Limitations and Special Problems

■ *Arch Expansion versus Extraction in the Treatment of Malocclusion*

Extraction of teeth for orthodontic purposes, either to correct crowding or to allow the teeth to accommodate to a jaw discrepancy, has been a controversial subject since concepts of normal occlusion were first developed in the early 1900s. The controversy has continued into the present time, exacerbated by a number of factors:

1. Concepts of occlusion held by many dentists have tended to be rigid and intolerant of anatomic deviation including both skeletal and dental discrepancy. Many of these concepts echo the feelings expressed by Edward Angle in 1907: "Every individual has the potential to have 32 teeth in normal (ideal) occlusion."[1] Modern theorists do not expect third molars in occlusion but many find it hard to accept premolar extraction in either or both arches, claiming that this can cause an impressive variety of functional problems,[2] although little if any evidence supports these claims.

2. Crowding is an exceptionally frequent problem in contemporary societies, much more so than in primitive ones. The increase in crowding with civilization is difficult to explain on a genetic basis alone and may be related in part to the change in diet (see Chapter 5). One possibility, in-

corporated into a philosophy of orthodontic treatment by Begg, is that the lack of proximal and occlusal wear of the teeth because of modern diet is largely responsible.[3] Begg advocated premolar extraction as necessary to deal with this lack of "normal development" of the dentition, implying that almost everyone would require extraction. Obviously, this concept is diametrically opposed to the first view.

3. Appropriate management of orthodontic extraction sites requires more complex orthodontic appliances than treatment by arch expansion. The greater difficulty of extraction compared to nonextraction treatment has often been a factor in the choice of modes of treatment, especially before the modern fixed appliances. In recent years in the United States, however, advocates of European-style removable appliances, which make it essentially impossible to manage extraction treatment, have attempted to bypass this disadvantage by claiming that it is of no consequence since extraction treatment is unwarranted in any event.

A realistic appraisal suggests that, as in many controversies, the extreme positions on both sides are untenable. Extraction of teeth is certainly necessary for some patients with severe crowding and is desirable in others as a way to fit the dentition into a moderate jaw discrepancy ("camouflage," discussed later). In others, even with severe crowding or a jaw discrepancy, extraction is unwarranted and harmful to the patient. Adequate diagnosis and treatment planning are the keys. A further discussion of the background and status of extraction versus nonextraction orthodontic treatment is presented in the following section to provide an appropriate perspective for current diagnosis and treatment planning.

■ The Great Extraction Controversy of the 1920s

As the occlusal concepts that culminated in his definition of normal occlusion were developed, Edward Angle struggled with both facial esthetics and stability of result as potential complications in his efforts to achieve an idealized normal occlusion. It is difficult to recreate the thought processes of a brilliant man many years ago, but it seems clear that Angle was influenced by both the philosophy of Rousseau and the biologic concepts of his time. Rousseau em-

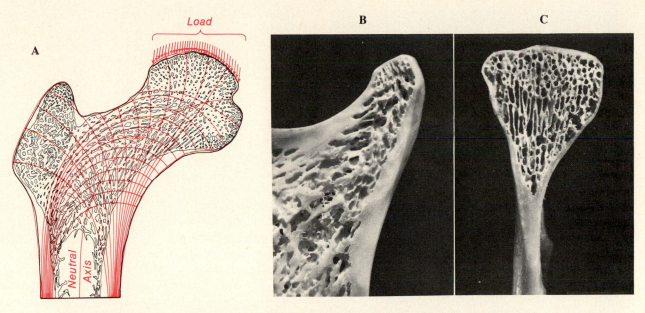

Fig. 8-1 ■ **A,** Bone trabeculae in the head of the femur follow the calculated stress lines. This observation by the German physiologist Wolff at the end of the nineteenth century led to "Wolff's law of bone," that the internal architecture of bones represents the stress pattern on them. **B,** Frontal section through the head of the mandibular condyle. **C,** Sagittal section through the head of the condyle. Note the arrangement of bony trabeculae, indicating a similar arrangement for resistance to stress as seen in the head of the femur. (**B** and **C** from DuBrul, E.L.: Sicher's Oral Anatomy, ed. 7. St. Louis, 1980, The C.V. Mosby Co.)

phasized the perfectability of man. His strong belief that many of the ills of modern man could be traced to the pernicious influences of civilization struck a responsive chord in Angle, who joined other progressive young dentists of the 1890s in their reaction to the casual attitude of that time toward extraction of teeth. In an era when teeth could be saved by dental treatment, extraction of teeth for orthodontic purposes seemed particularly inappropriate, especially if man was inherently capable of having a perfect dentition. Perfection, it appeared, required only diligent efforts to achieve. It became an article of faith for Angle and the early orthodontists that every person had the potential for an ideal relationship of all 32 natural teeth.

Secondly, Angle was impressed by the discovery that the architecture of bone responds to the stresses placed on that part of the skeleton. The demonstration by the German physiologist Wolff that bone trabeculae were arranged in response to the stress lines on the bone (the internal architecture of the head of the femur is the classic example. (Fig. 8-1) led to the concept that proper function of the dentition would be the key to maintenance of tooth position. Angle reasoned that if the teeth were placed in proper occlusion, forces transmitted to the teeth would cause bone to grow around them, thus stabilizing them in their new position even if a great deal of arch expansion had occurred. He soon saw that merely tipping the teeth to a new position might be inadequate and sought ways to move the teeth bodily. He described his first appliance capable of bodily tooth movement as the "bone growing appliance."

To Angle and his followers, relapse into crowding after expansion of the arches meant only that an adequate occlusion had not been achieved. This too became an article of faith in the nonextraction philosophy: if a correct occlusion had been produced, the result would be stable; therefore, if the orthodontic result was not stable, the fault was that of the orthodontist, not the theory.

Finally, the problem of dentofacial esthetics was solved, at least for Angle, through his interaction with a famous artist of the day, Professor Wuerpel. Early in his career, Angle devoted much effort to a search for the ideal facial form, in parallel with his search for the ideal dental occlusion (Fig. 8-2). When he consulted the art professor for advice about the perfect face, he was ridiculed—the artist's response was that the tremendous variety in human faces makes it impossible to specify any one facial form as the ideal. Reflecting on this, Angle had a moment of insight: the relationship of the dentition to the face, and with it the esthetics of the lower face, would vary, but for each individual, ideal facial esthetics would result when the teeth were placed in ideal occlusion. Whether the patient liked the outcome or not, by definition the best facial appearance for him or her would be achieved when the dental arches had been expanded so that all the teeth were in ideal occlusion.

For Angle, proper orthodontic treatment for nearly every patient involved expansion of the dental arches, and extraction for orthodontic purposes was not necessary for stability of result or for esthetics. These concepts did not go un-

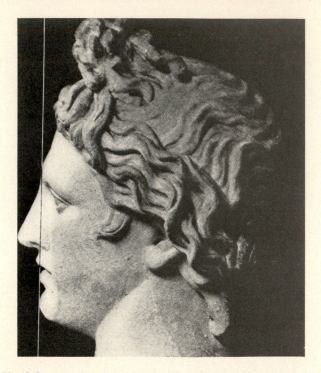

Fig. 8-2 ■ Angle originally sought an ideal profile, in parallel to his search for an ideal occlusion, and initially favored the classic Greek profile, which is often incompatible with non-extraction treatment. (From Angle, E.H.: Treatment of Malocclusion of the Teeth, ed. 7. Philadelphia, 1907, S.S. White Manufacturing Co.)

challenged. Angle's great professional rival, Calvin Case, argued that although the arches could always be expanded so that the teeth could be placed in alignment, neither esthetics nor stability would be satisfactory in the long term. The controversy culminated in a widely publicized debate between Angle and Case, carried out in the dental literature of the 1920s.[4]

Reading these papers from a current perspective leaves the impression that Case had the better argument by far. Yet Angle won the day, and extraction of teeth for orthodontic purposes essentially disappeared from the American orthodontic scene in the period between World Wars I and II. Even those who did not agree with Angle's appliance systems, particularly in the American South where removable (Crozat) or partially banded appliances (labiolingual, twin wire) were commonly used, accepted the nonextraction approach and its philosophic underpinnings.

■ Extraction in Contemporary Orthodontics

During the 1930s, relapse after nonextraction expansion treatment was frequently observed. At this time soon after Angle's death, one of his last students, Charles Tweed, decided to re-treat with extraction a number of his patients who had experienced relapse. Four first premolar teeth were removed and the teeth were aligned and retracted. After the re-treatment, Tweed observed that the occlusion was much

more stable. Tweed's dramatic public presentation of consecutively treated cases, most with premolar extraction, caused a revolution in American orthodontic thinking and led to the widespread reintroduction of extraction into orthodontic therapy by the late 1940s.

Independently of Tweed but simultaneously, another of Angle's students, Raymond Begg in Australia, also concluded that nonextraction treatment was unstable. Like Tweed, he modified the Angle-designed appliance he was using for extraction treatment, producing what is now called the Begg appliance (see Chapter 10). This was designed for extraction treatment.

The acceptance of extraction treatment and the repudiation of Angle's ideas were made easier by an intellectual climate in which the limitations of human adaptation both socially and physically, were emphasized. Breeding experiments with animals, of which Stockard's widely publicized results from cross-breeding dogs were most influential, seemed to show conclusively that malocclusion could be inherited (see Chapter 5). Rather than developing the potential within each patient, it appeared that it was necessary for the orthodontist to recognize genetically determined disparities between tooth size and jaw size, or to acknowledge that the lack of proximal wear on teeth produced tooth size–jaw size discrepancies during development. In either case, extraction was frequently necessary.

By the early 1960s, more than half the American patients undergoing orthodontic treatment had extraction of some teeth, usually but not always first premolars. Since the accepted concept was that orthodontic treatment could not affect facial growth, extraction was considered necessary to overcome discrepancies in jaw position as well as crowding from tooth-jaw discrepancies and was done for either or both purposes.

In recent years, the percentage of patients having extraction as part of orthodontic treatment has decreased from its peak in the 1960s. Experience has shown that even premolar extraction does not necessarily guarantee stability of tooth alignment. In some instances, eventual crowding after premolar extraction has been of the same magnitude as after expansion treatment.[5] With careful analysis, it now seems possible to treat some patients without extraction who would have been thought to require it earlier, and facial esthetics in these "borderline cases" are considered better without extraction by both dentists and others.

As this renewed optimism about the possibilities, not the limitations, of orthodontic treatment has appeared, the expanding and growth-guiding appliances popular in Europe for nonextraction treatment have been introduced into the United States, while American-style fixed appliances have been adopted elsewhere for extraction treatment. On the contemporary scene, every shade of opinion and practice relative to extraction can currently be found. These range from an absolute rejection of the possibility of a need for extraction, supported by arguments that seem taken word for word from Angle's era, to a rejection of the possibilities

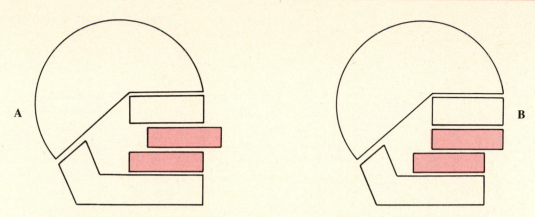

Fig. 8-3 ■ Apparently identical Class II malocclusions, viewed only in terms of the relationship of the teeth, can arise from totally different causes. The patient represented diagrammatically in block **A** has maxillary dental protrusion, best treated by extraction of upper first premolars and retraction of the protruding anterior teeth. The patient in **B,** whose problem is skeletal mandibular deficiency, would be appropriate for growth modification, camouflage or surgery, depending on the patient's age and the characteristics of the individual malocclusion.

of arch expansion and growth guidance along with a continued high percentage of extraction.

In a rational contemporary view, some orthodontic patients will require extraction. Their number varies, depending on the population being treated. The majority of patients, it seems clear, can and should be treated without removal of teeth—which is not to say that all can be. In this, as with so much else, it is necessary to understand the pertinent history to avoid repeating it.

■ *Treatment Planning for Patients with Skeletal Problems*

■ Possible Approaches

A skeletal orthodontic problem may be defined as one resulting not from malpositioned teeth on well proportioned jaws, but from a disproportion in the size or position of the jaws themselves. Skeletal problems can and do occur in all three planes of space. Skeletal problems in the anteroposterior plane of space are Angle's Class II and III, but it is important to understand that a Class II malocclusion may be either skeletal or dental depending on whether its cause is an underlying skeletal jaw discrepancy or because the teeth have been displaced relative to the jaws (Fig. 8-3). This is a critically important diagnostic distinction. There also are skeletal vertical problems, either skeletal open bite or skeletal deep bite depending on the shape and position of the jaws, and these interact with anteroposterior discrepancies, as discussed in Chapters 6 and 7. Similarly, there are skeletal crossbites, resulting from excessively wide or narrow jaws.

Only three approaches to the correction of a skeletal malocclusion are possible: (1) modification of growth so that growth corrects the problem; (2) camouflage of the skeletal jaw discrepancy by orthodontic tooth movement (which usu-

ally requires extraction), so that the dental occlusion is corrected although the skeletal discrepancy remains; or (3) surgical correction of the jaw discrepancy (Fig. 8-4).

In the appropriate circumstances, each approach has merit. The key decision in treatment planning for patients with skeletal problems is selecting the appropriate form of treatment. Growth modification, if possible, provides the ideal result. Orthodontic treatment by camouflage represents a compromise that may be quite acceptable in moderate skeletal discrepancies but is less acceptable in more severe ones. Surgical correction is reserved for the most severe problems but should not be overlooked as a possibility, especially in view of the tremendous progress in this field in recent years.

■ Growth Modification

Principles in growth modification. It seems obvious, but is sometimes overlooked, that successful growth modification treatment is possible only in patients who have a significant amount of growth remaining. Thus, for all practical purposes, growth modification must be carried out before or during the adolescent growth spurt, and therefore before attainment of the permanent dentition in most patients. Although jaw growth certainly continues after puberty, its magnitude is rarely enough to allow correction of significant skeletal jaw discrepancies.

At various times, optimism about the modifiability of jaw growth has led to efforts to correct skeletal problems by stimulating jaw growth. Growth at the temporomandibular joint in response to a forward position of the mandible can be demonstrated in experimental animals.[6,7] Since the lower jaw retains growth potential throughout life (as shown, for instance, by its growth in adults who have acromegaly), growth modification seems superficially plausible even in adults. Recent experimental studies have shown that if the mandible is positioned forward in adult monkeys, some apposition of bone at the condyle and remodeling of the

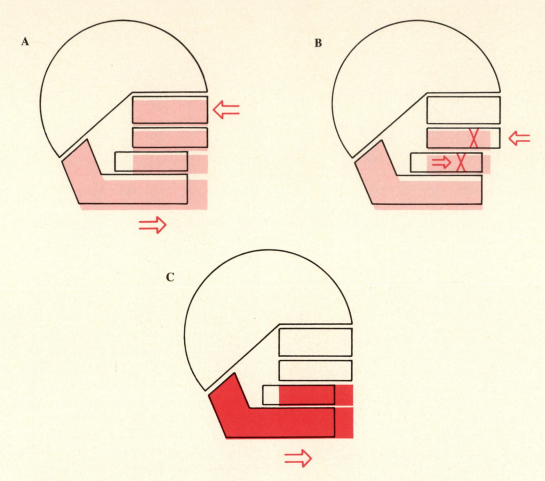

Fig. 8-4 ■ There are three major possibilities for correction of skeletal mandibular deficiency: **A,** differential growth of the lower jaw, bringing the dentition forward with it; **B,** camouflage, achieved in most cases by extracting premolars, and then closing the space by retracting the maxillary anterior teeth while bringing the mandibular posterior teeth forward. At least a small amount of vertical growth is needed because most aspects of the orthodontic mechanotherapy tend to extrude the teeth. **C,** Surgical advancement of the mandible. Growth modification is most successful in preadolescent patients; camouflage is most useful for adolescents with moderately severe problems; jaw surgery is most useful for patients with no remaining growth potential and severe problems.

temporomandibular joint occur, lending further credence to the idea that changes similar to those in normal growth can be produced in otherwise nongrowing individuals.

However, it is important to evaluate phenomena of this type quantitatively as well as qualitatively. What is significant at the microscopic level may be much less significant at the macroscopic clinical level. In fact, the magnitude of condylar change that can be produced in adult primates or humans is about 1 or 2 mm, only a small fraction of the amount necessary to correct a skeletal malocclusion. The optimistic reports that changes are possible in adults, in short, do not contradict the important principle that growth modification treatment must begin at an early age if it is to have any chance of clinical success.[9]

The pattern of normal jaw growth and its relationship to physical growth elsewhere in the body have been discussed in some detail in Chapters 2 and 3. Although the jaws are affected by the adolescent growth spurt, there is not the

same acceleration of jaw growth at puberty as in the trunk and limbs. Data from longitudinal studies of normal children suggest that in some individuals a juvenile acceleration in jaw growth, occurring at age 7 or 8, equals or exceeds the acceleration just before puberty.[10] Girls seem more likely to have a juvenile acceleration of jaw growth than boys. Since girls undergo puberty on the average 2 years before boys anyway, it is particularly important that growth modification treatment begin at an early age for girls. Beginning treatment 2 to 3 years before puberty in both sexes provides an adequate margin of safety, which means that treatment must often begin at age 8 or 9 in girls but usually can be deferred until age 10 or 11 in boys, depending in both instances on an assessment of developmental status rather than relying on chronologic age alone.

Since growth modification treatment depends on creating a differential in the rate of growth of the two jaws, and therefore should be effective at any age until growth ceases,

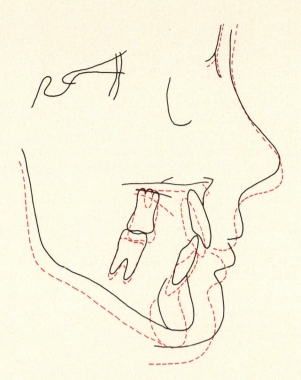

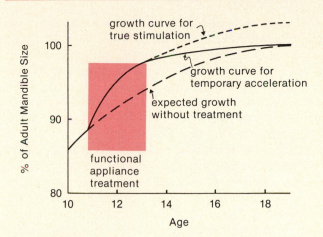

Fig. 8-6 ■ The difference between growth acceleration in response to a functional appliance and true growth stimulation can be represented using a growth chart. If growth occurs at a faster than expected rate while a functional appliance is being worn, and then continues at the expected rate thereafter so that the ultimate size of the jaw is larger, true stimulation has occurred. If faster growth occurs while the appliance is being worn, but slower growth thereafter ultimately brings the patient back to the line of expected growth, there has been an acceleration, not a true stimulation.

Fig. 8-5 ■ In this patient, excessive vertical development of the maxilla during the late teens produced a downward and backward rotation of the mandible. Orthodontic treatment with extraction of upper first premolars succeeded in maintaining normal occlusal relationships despite the unfavorable pattern of growth. Patients of this type require prolonged orthodontic retention because of the long period of vertical growth.

why not begin treatment quite early, perhaps in the preschool years? In fact, growth modification is effective in very young children. A Class II malocclusion can often be corrected with 6 to 9 months of functional appliance or headgear treatment in 4- or 5-year-old children. Unfortunately, if treatment is discontinued at that point, the condition tends to recur as the original pattern of growth reasserts itself. Growth modification treatment changes the expression of growth, but has little or no effect on the underlying growth pattern of the individual.

This leads directly to a second and important principle of growth modification treatment: treatment must continue, at least at a reduced level, until growth is essentially complete after adolescence. It is important to begin treatment early enough, but it is also important to time the treatment so that it is not begun too soon and therefore is unnecessarily prolonged. There is little advantage in beginning treatment in the primary dentition if mixed dentition treatment will be required anyway and would have been adequate to correct the problem.

Growth modification treatment is needed only for patients who have growth problems leading to skeletal jaw discrepancies. This means, of course, that growth expectations based on children with normal jaw development do not always apply perfectly. Patients with excessive growth of either jaw tend to have not only more growth, but growth

for a longer period. This prolonged growth can be seen especially clearly in two groups of patients: those with mandibular prognathism, and those with excessive vertical development of the lower face (skeletal open bite) (Fig. 8-5). In both groups, disproportionate growth may continue into the late teens, well after puberty and the normal cessation of jaw growth. Why this happens remains unclear, but it must be taken into account when planning treatment. ''Active retention'' is necessary for these patients beyond the time when treatment could normally be discontinued (see Chapter 18).

Growth modification treatment is aimed at altering the expression of growth, changing its direction, and to a lesser extent its magnitude. Can it also change the time at which growth occurs? This question bears directly on the controversy over whether mandibular growth can be stimulated when it is deficient. Stimulation can be defined in two ways (Fig. 8-6): (1) as the attainment of a final size larger than would have occurred without treatment, which may not be possible; or (2) as the occurrence of more growth during a given period of time than would have been expected without treatment, which certainly can be shown to happen.[6]

Obtaining growth more quickly, as compared with obtaining more growth than otherwise would have occurred, is a much more modest but also more realistic view of the response to growth stimulation treatment. Changing the timing of growth expression can allow more effective treatment. To the extent that functional appliances can accomplish this in the treatment of mandibular deficiency Class II problems, they offer an advantage over headgear treatment to the maxilla even though the ultimate results may be similar. This point is discussed in more detail in Chapter 14.

Although most children with a skeletal problem have some degree of discrepancy in both jaws, the problem can usually be characterized as primarily the result of deficient or excessive growth of the mandible or the maxilla. For convenience in the following discussion, it is assumed that this distinction has been made. Effects on both of the jaws and on the teeth must be expected from treatment, and this is emphasized within each section.

Mandibular deficiency. Skeletal Class II malocclusion may be caused by deficient mandibular growth, excessive maxillary growth, or (as is usually the case) a combination of the two. Several studies of the characteristics of children with Class II malocclusion reveal that the majority have a component of mandibular deficiency.[11] This was recognized from the beginning of orthodontic classification, hence Lischer's synonym "disto-occlusion" for Class II malocclusion.[12] From the beginning also, treatment methods designed to stimulate mandibular growth have been used for Class II correction. In the early years, Angle and his contemporaries thought that Class II elastics (from the lower molar to the upper incisor area) would cause the mandible to be positioned forward and therefore to grow. At a later stage in the United States, guide planes consisting of a wire framework extending down from an upper lingual arch were used to force patients to advance the mandible upon closure, also with the idea of stimulating mandibular growth[13] (Fig. 8-7).

With the advent of cephalometric analysis, it became clear that both these approaches corrected Class II malocclusion much more by mesial displacement of the mandibular teeth than by stimulating mandibular growth (Fig. 8-8). Even if the lack of desired skeletal change is overlooked, correcting a Class II problem in this way is undesirable because the resulting mandibular dental protrusion tends to be unstable. As the protruding lower incisors tend to upright after treat-

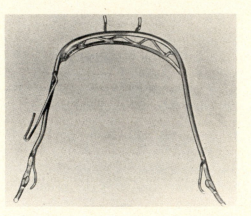

Fig. 8-7 ■ A guide plane fabricated as part of a maxillary lingual arch, to position the mandible forward. Guide planes of this type were the closest approximation to functional appliances in American fixed-appliance orthodontics until after midcentury.

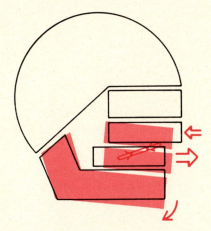

Fig. 8-8 ■ In a patient who is growing minimally, Class II elastics move the maxillary teeth back somewhat, slip the mandibular teeth forward on the mandibular base, and rotate the occlusal and mandibular planes downward. Stimulation of mandibular growth is not a consistent response.

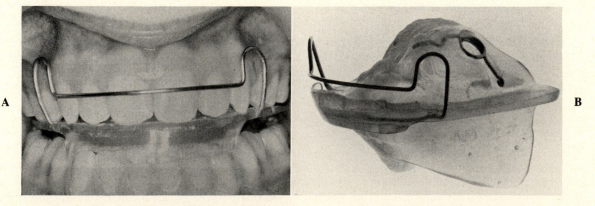

Fig. 8-9 ■ The activator appliance consists of a single block of plastic, constructed so that the lingual flanges on the lower cause the mandible to be positioned forward. Typically, the mandibular incisor teeth are capped so that forward movement is resisted, while the mandibular posterior teeth are free to erupt. **A,** Appliance in position intraorally; **B,** appliance out of the mouth.

ment, lower incisor crowding and overjet return. Because of this, these methods and with them the idea of mandibular growth stimulation fell into disrepute in the United States.

In Europe, efforts to stimulate mandibular growth led to the development of a family of "functional appliances." Their prototype was Robin's monobloc, first described in 1907, but Andresen's activator of the early 1930s and similar appliances used thereafter in Switzerland and Germany popularized this approach and provided the name[14] (Fig. 8-9). The idea was that changing the function of the mandible by forcing the patient to function with the lower jaw forward would stimulate mandibular growth, thereby correcting a Class II problem. The basic concept was thus quite similar to that of the guide plane. The activator and its successors differed from the fixed guide plane in being removable. In addition, the plastic framework provided contact with all teeth, giving better resistance to forward displacement of lower incisors and allowing control of eruption.

When the mandible is held forward, the elastic stretch of soft tissues produces a reactive effect on the structures that hold it forward. If the appliance contacts the teeth, this reactive force produces a "Class II elastics effect," moving the lower teeth forward and the upper teeth back. In addition, even if contact with the teeth is minimized, soft tissue elasticity creates a restraining force on the upper arch, so that a "headgear effect" is observed (Fig. 8-4). Thus, Class II correction by pure stimulation of mandibular growth can-

not be expected from an appliance that holds the mandible forward. There is always some restraining effect on the maxilla and usually some tooth movement. Despite this, cephalometric analysis often shows more mandibular growth in a child wearing a well-designed functional appliance than would have been expected (Fig. 8-10). This acceleration of growth is certainly growth stimulation in a relative sense, in that the growth is obtained relatively more quickly. Whether growth can be stimulated absolutely, in the sense that the lower jaw ends up larger at maturity than it would have been without treatment, is less clear. Absolute stimulation, if it does occur, is of small magnitude. There is no doubt, however, that functional appliances can be quite effective in the correction of skeletal Class II malocclusions of moderate severity.

The ideal patient for functional appliance treatment of mandibular deficiency should be prepubescent by 2 to 3 years. In addition because neither the headgear nor the Class II elastic effects can be entirely avoided with any functional appliance, this ideal patient would have:

- Normal or slightly excessive maxillary development
- Normal vertical face height (not long face)
- Slightly protrusive maxillary incisor teeth
- Normally positioned or retrusive but not protrusive lower incisors

The individual with a skeletal Class II problem who already has a protrusive lower dentition is a poor candidate

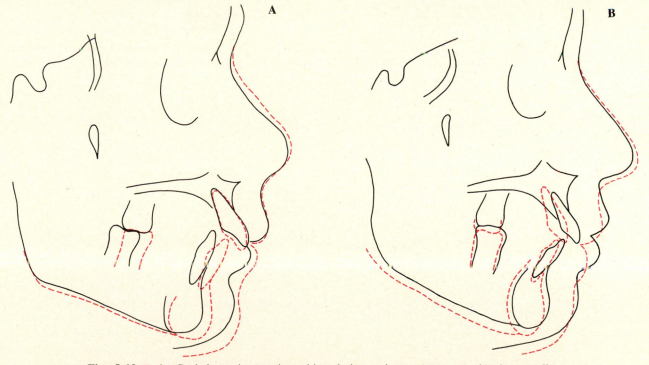

Fig. 8-10 ■ **A,** Cephalometric superimposition during activator treatment, showing excellent downward and forward mandibular growth between ages 11 and 13; **B,** cephalometric superimpositions for same patient between ages 13 and 15, during fixed appliance therapy for final positioning of teeth. For this patient, the growth response to the activator was much more an acceleration than a true stimulation, yet the activator phase of treatment was quite successful in improving the jaw relationship.

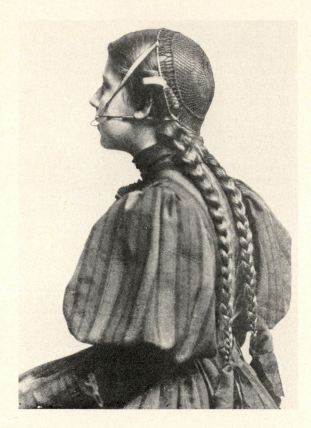

Fig. 8-11 ■ Extraoral force to the maxilla was used in the late 1800s, then abandoned, not because of ineffectiveness, but because it was thought that intraoral elastics produced the same effect. (From Angle, E.H.: Treatment of Malocclusion of the Teeth, ed. 7. Philadelphia, 1907, S.S. White Manufacturing Co.)

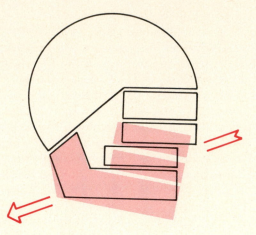

Fig. 8-12 ■ If extraoral force to the maxilla moves it downward, mandibular growth will be expressed more vertically and less horizontally, impeding the successful correction of a Class II problem. In the extreme case, with minimal mandibular growth, the downward and backward rotation of the mandible can actually cause a worsening of the problem, as in the possible response to low-pull headgear shown diagrammatically here. For this reason, an upward and backward direction of pull is usually needed.

for functional appliance treatment, since further protrusion of the lower teeth is likely to occur. Some types of appliances produce a greater headgear effect and more orthodontic tooth movement than others.

The choice of a functional appliance for any individual patient should be based on an analysis of the patient's particular problems. No one functional appliance type will prove best for all patients. This topic is discussed in detail in Chapter 14.

Maxillary excess. As the maxilla grows downward and forward, new bone is added at its upper and posterior sutural attachments, while the anterior surface is remodeled. Ample experimental evidence (see Chapter 2) indicates that the skeletal changes occur in response to soft tissue growth. The entire maxilla is translated downward and forward in accompaniment with its surrounding tissues. Growth at the sutures of the maxilla is a reactive process, not an active one. If the environment of the sutural tissues can be affected, growth will be modified. The rationale for modifying excessive maxillary growth by applying force across the sutures therefore is well established.

Extraoral force to the maxilla was utilized by the pioneer orthodontists of the late 1800s and presumably was reasonably effective (Fig. 8-11). This method of treatment was later abandoned because the orthodontists of the early 1900s came to believe that intraoral elastics could produce the same effects. Although headgear was reintroduced in the 1940s, the potential for producing skeletal change in this way was not fully appreciated until cephalometric studies clearly demonstrated effects on maxillary growth.[15]

For all practical purposes, extraoral force against the maxilla must be applied via the teeth, and tooth movement in addition to skeletal effects is the inevitable result. Applying force directly to implants in the bone has been done in experimental animals.[16] For humans, an ankylosed tooth would be the ideal implant, but since ankylosis is an irreversible procedure (at least at present), there are no practical ways to avoid force that can move the teeth when extraoral force for skeletal change is applied. With extraoral force, therefore, a combination of orthodontic tooth movement and skeletal change must always be expected.

Excessive growth of the maxilla often has both vertical and horizontal components. When extraoral force is applied, its vertical component is established by the point of application posteriorly. With a neck strap, the direction of pull will be from below the dentition, thereby extruding teeth at the point where the force is applied. Extrusion of the posterior teeth causes the mandible to rotate downward and backward, which can impede rather than help Class II correction, especially if there is minimal mandibular growth (Fig. 8-12). If the attachment is to a headcap, the direction of pull can be straight along the occlusal plane, neither elongating nor intruding, or above the occlusal plane, creating an intrusive force at the point of application. Control of the vertical component of any extraoral force system is extremely important.

Because elongation of maxillary teeth is usually unde-

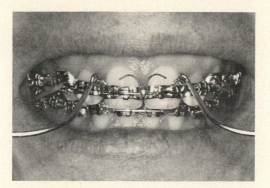

Fig. 8-13 ■ Force applied to the teeth radiates to the sutures of maxilla. For growth modification, the amount and duration of force at the sutures are important. Extraoral force is usually applied via a facebow to the first permanent molars, but can be applied to an arch wire as shown here.

sirable, in most instances cervical (neck strap) headgear alone is unsatisfactory for treatment of skeletal maxillary excess. It should be kept in mind, however, that it is the relationship of the posterior teeth to the point of attachment, not just the point of attachment itself, that determines the vertical component of force. For some patients, a neck strap attachment produces a considerable downward component of force, while for others, it produces a line of force almost along the occlusal plane. As with so many other aspects of orthodontic treatment planning, the patient's particular morphology must be considered in choosing the type of force system. It is simply impossible to always use the same extraoral force system if benefit to the patient is to be optimal.

Extraoral force applied to the maxillary teeth affects jaw growth as it is transmitted to the sutures of the maxilla in somewhat reduced form. Presumably, the sutures are influenced only by the magnitude and direction of the force when it reaches them, not by which teeth originally received the force. Skeletal effects appear to be the same whether the extraoral force is applied via a facebow to the molars or to an appliance incorporating the anterior teeth (Fig. 8-13). The facebow arrangement, however, is particularly convenient for mixed dentition patients, and most growth modification patients fall into this age group.

Although orthodontic tooth movement cannot be avoided when extraoral force is applied, it can be maximized or minimized by taking advantage of the known characteristics of optimal orthodontic force. Optimal force characteristics

for skeletal and dental effects are contrasted in Table 8-1 (see Chapter 9 for more details). From this information, it can be deduced that if the objective of treatment is to produce maximum skeletal change with minimal dental change, full-time application of extraoral force is probably undesirable. To produce maximal skeletal changes with minimal orthodontic tooth movement, the following "force prescription" is optimal:

- Heavy force (500 to 1000 grams)
- Force direction slightly above the occlusal plane (through the center of resistance of the molar teeth, if the force application is to the molars by a facebow)
- Force duration 12 to 14 hours per day, every day (10 hours minimum for significant effects)
- Typical treatment duration 12 to 18 months, depending on rapidity of growth (longer, of course, with poor cooperation)

Because excessive growth can continue into the late teens, it may be necessary to continue some use of extraoral force after the completion of active orthodontic treatment to prevent recurrence of the original problem. This is particularly true when there is a strong vertical component to the excessive maxillary growth, as in many skeletal open bite problems. Patients with these problems will have to continue wearing a headgear just at night until the cessation of growth at age 18 to 20 or will need to use a functional appliance that impedes vertical maxillary development. They cannot be left without some appliance to control maxillary growth after the typical completion of orthodontic treatment at age 14 or so. Active retention, meaning a continuation of growth modification treatment with diminished intensity, is required until growth has ceased (see Chapter 18).

Since extraoral force aimed at the maxilla inevitably produces both orthodontic and skeletal effects, the ideal patient for growth modification with extraoral force shows:

- Excessive horizontal growth of the maxilla, with or without excessive vertical changes (it is possible to produce purely horizontal forces to the maxilla, but extremely difficult to produce pure vertical forces)
- Some protrusion of maxillary teeth

Table 8-1 ■ Characteristics to produce skeletal versus dental effects of orthodontic forces

	Dental effect	*Skeletal effect*
Force magnitude	Low	High
Force duration	Long: 24 hrs/day	Shorter: 12-14 hrs/day
Force direction	Any	*Not* extrusive
Treatment time	Varies	Long
Rate of change	1 mm/month maximum	3-4 mm/year maximum

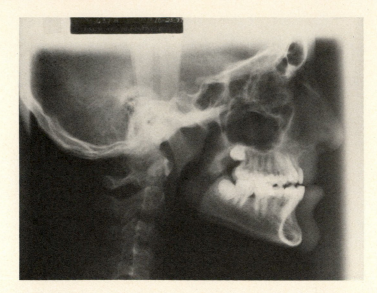

Fig. 8-14 ■ Cephalometric radiograph of a patient with a repaired cleft palate. The maxilla is deficient in both the anteroposterior and vertical planes of space (as well as in the transverse plane of space, not shown here). Failure of the maxilla to descend vertically allows the mandible to be positioned upward and forward, accentuating the Class III dental relationship.

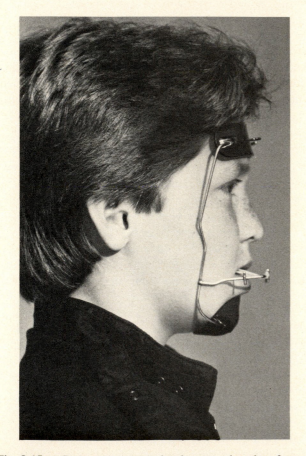

Fig. 8-15 ■ Facemask or reverse headgear, used to place forward traction against the maxilla. Such appliances can produce forward movement of maxillary teeth at any age, but are most successful in producing forward displacement of the maxilla itself at early ages.

• Reasonably good mandibular dental and skeletal morphology (since this will be minimally affected by the extraoral force)

To be effective, treatment must begin before the prepubertal growth spurt.

Maxillary deficiency. Maxillary deficiency can involve all three planes of space. In individuals with a history of cleft palate and subsequent surgical correction, maxillary deficiency in all three planes of space is often observed (Fig. 8-14). In patients without cleft palates, it is more common to observe deficiency in one of two patterns: (1) a horizontal and vertical deficiency, with reasonably normal transverse dimensions; or (2) a primarily transverse deficiency, with horizontal and particularly vertical dimensions less affected. The special problems of cleft palate patients are discussed separately later; the two patterns of deficiency in patients without cleft palates are briefly discussed here.

Horizontal-vertical deficiency. The sutures of the maxilla respond to their environment and normally develop in response to a translation of the maxilla that separates the sutures. Thus, it seems apparent that forces that pull the sutures apart should stimulate apposition of bone in those regions and thereby cause an increase in growth. Although it is relatively easy to show experimentally that exactly this result occurs when force is applied to separate the sutures,[17] it has been difficult to apply this concept to treatment of maxillary deficiency, particularly in its anteroposterior and vertical manifestations.

If headgear force compressing the maxillary sutures can inhibit forward growth of the maxilla, reverse (forward-pull) headgear separating the sutures should stimulate growth (Fig. 8-15). Until recently, however, efforts to produce maxillary growth stimulation have been impressive mainly by

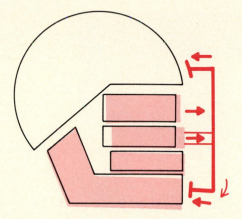

Fig. 8-16 ■ Forward traction against the maxilla and maxillary teeth typically produces more forward movement of the maxillary teeth relative to the maxilla than forward displacement of the maxilla itself, even in patients who respond favorably. In addition, the reciprocal force placed against the chin tends to rotate the mandible downward and backward.

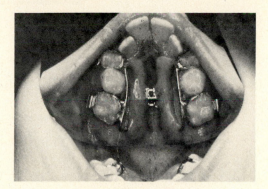

Fig. 8-17 ■ Transverse force across the maxilla in children and adolescents can open the midpalatal suture. The expansion force is usually delivered with a jackscrew mechanism fixed to maxillary teeth.

their lack of success. The usual effect of reverse headgear has been to produce forward movement of maxillary teeth, with little or no true skeletal effect on the maxilla. Reverse headgear applies a reciprocal downward and backward force to the mandible. Repositioning of the mandible in this direction is often observed and is frequently the major skeletal effect.

From the work of Delaire and coworkers in France in recent years,[18] it now appears that forward positioning of the skeletal maxilla can be achieved with reverse headgear, *if* treatment is begun at an early age. Delaire's results suggest that successful forward repositioning of the maxilla can be accomplished before age 8, but that orthodontic tooth movement overwhelms skeletal change at later ages. Skeletal maxillary deficiency can be diagnosed before age 8, but is often missed until a thorough orthodontic evaluation is done later. Fortunately, true maxillary deficiency in the anteroposterior and vertical planes of space is relatively rare in patients without cleft palates. Children who are suspected of having this problem should be referred for complete evaluation as early as possible. When growth modification is the goal, these individuals will require treatment beginning considerably earlier than orthodontic treatment has been done in the past.

Two side effects of treatment are almost inevitable when reverse headgear is used: forward movement of maxillary teeth relative to the maxilla, and downward and backward rotation of the mandible (Fig. 8-16). For this reason, in addition to the young age, the ideal patients for treatment with this method would have both:

• Normally positioned or retrusive, but not protrusive, maxillary teeth
• Normal or short, but not long, anterior facial vertical dimensions

Transverse deficiency. Maxillary deficiency in the transverse plane of space often accompanies excessive vertical

development and normal or even excessive anteroposterior development. Narrow skeletal width dimensions of the maxilla are indicated by narrow width of the palatal vault. This is one of the few skeletal jaw dimensions that can be assessed accurately from dental casts.

Separation of the midpalatal suture can be done conveniently by placing heavy force across the maxillary dental arch (Fig. 8-17). Like extraoral force to the maxilla, this method was known in the late 1800s, but was abandoned as unnecessary and potentially damaging. After demonstration of its potential in experimental animals, the method was reintroduced in the United States in the late 1950s,[19] and has been widely used since. Expansion across the suture can be done in two ways: (1) rapid expansion, the original (1950s) method, and (2) slow expansion at the rate of approximately 1 mm per week, the method advocated more recently. With both methods, the teeth are used as points of attachment, and force is applied, which separates the two halves of the maxilla, widening the midpalatal suture and leading to bone apposition at that suture. Compensatory adjustments are also required at the lateral maxillary and frontonasal sutures.

The theory of rapid palatal expansion (RPE) is that force should be applied to the maxillary teeth at a rate and magnitude beyond their capacity to respond. After some initial orthodontic movement, the teeth would be unable to move further, and a purely skeletal change would therefore be produced. Rapid expansion can be done without pain, with the application of forces that can reach 15 to 20 pounds as a jackscrew apparatus is progressively turned.[20] Occlusal radiographs make it clear than the midpalatal suture does open. This expansion is obvious clinically because a diastema appears between the maxillary central incisors (Fig. 8-18). Typically, rapid expansion is done at a rate of 0.5 to 1.0 mm per day, producing a centimeter or more of expansion in 2 to 3 weeks. With this rate of movement, the

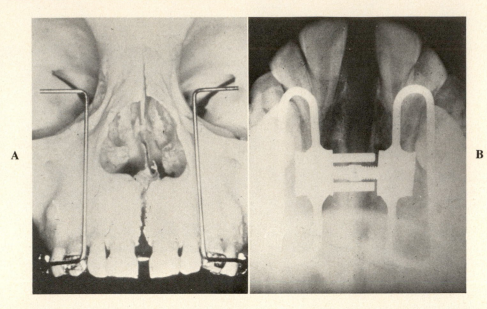

A

B

Fig. 8-18 ■ **A,** Opening of the midpalatal suture on a dried skull demonstrates the increase in width of the roof of the mouth and the floor of the nose. The maxilla opens as if on a hinge, with its apex at the bridge of the nose. **B,** The suture also opens on a hinge anteroposteriorly, separating more anteriorly than posteriorly, as shown in this radiograph of a patient.

space created at the midpalatal suture is filled initially by tissue fluids and hemorrhage. After completion of the expansion, a fixed retainer is used for 3 to 4 months. Usually, this retainer is merely the expansion device itself, stabilized so that it cannot screw itself back shut. After 3 to 4 months, new bone has filled in the space at the suture, and the expansion is complete.

The aspect of rapid expansion that was not appreciated initially was that orthodontic tooth movement continues after the expansion is completed, until bone stability is achieved. In most treatment circumstances, orthodontic forces cause the teeth to move relative to a stable bony base. It is possible, of course, for orthodontic tooth movement to allow bony segments to reposition themselves while the teeth are held stable, and this is what occurs during the approximately 3 months required for bony fill-in at the suture after rapid expansion. During this time, the dental expansion is maintained, but the two halves of the maxilla move back toward each other, a movement that can happen because at the same time the teeth move laterally on their supporting bone.

In a typical instance (Table 8-2), 10 mm of total expansion would have been produced by 9 mm of skeletal expansion and only 1 mm of tooth movement when rapid expansion ended, 2 to 3 weeks after the beginning of treatment. At 4 months, the same 10 mm of dental expansion would still be present, but at that point there would be only 5 mm of skeletal expansion, and tooth movement would account for 5 mm of the total expansion.

If force across the midpalatal suture is applied more slowly, total force buildup is less. With this method, 2 to 4 pounds of force appear optimal, depending on the age of

the patient.[21] The higher level is needed for older patients. From the beginning, the ratio of dental to skeletal expansion is about 1 to 1, so that 10 mm of expansion over a 10-week period, at the rate of 1 mm per week, would be produced by 5 mm of dental and 5 mm of skeletal expansion. It appears that approximately 1 mm per week is the maximum rate at which the tissues of the midpalatal suture can adapt, so tearing and homorrhage are minimized. With expansion at this rate, the situation at the completion of active expansion is much more stable than immediately after rapid expansion, although retention is still needed. Thus the overall result of rapid versus slow expansion is similar, but with slower expansion a more physiologic response is obtained.

Slow expansion can be accomplished either by turning the typical palate separation jackscrew less frequently, or by activating a spring to give the desired 2 to 4 pounds of force. Expansion lingual arches that deliver considerably lighter forces also produce some opening of the suture, but the lighter forces generated by these appliances probably

Table 8-2 ■ Rapid versus slow palatal expansion

	Rapid expansion*		Slow expansion*	
Weeks	Molar width increase	Palate expansion	Molar width increase	Palate expansion
1	3.5	2.5	1.0	0.5
3	10.5	9.5	3.0	1.5
5	10.5	7.5	5.0	2.5
10	10.5	5.5	10.0	5.0

*Values shown in millimeters.

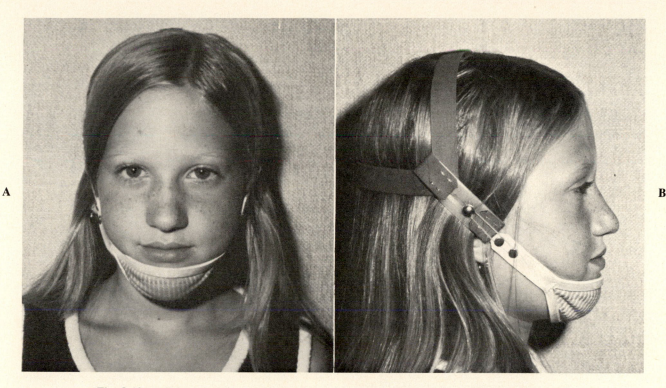

Fig. 8-19 ■ Chin cup appliance with a soft cup in clinical use. **A,** Anterior view; **B,** lateral view. The force direction is slightly below the head of the condyle.

produce a greater component of dental than skeletal expansion.

Since tooth movement in addition to skeletal expansion is inevitable when the midpalatal suture is widened, the ideal patient for this treatment should have:

- Full-cusp crossbite with a skeletal component
- Some degree of dental as well as skeletal constriction initially
- No preexisting dental expansion

Mandibular excess. Extraoral force applied via a chin cup has traditionally been used to restrain excessive growth of the mandible (Fig. 8-19). Since the mandible grows by apposition of bone at the condyle and along its free posterior border, rather dissimilarly to the sutural growth of the maxilla, a chin cup is not completely analogous to the use of extraoral force against the maxilla. If one adopts the view that the cartilage of the mandibular condyle constitutes a growth center with the capacity to grow independently, one would not expect chin cup therapy to be particularly successful. If the opposite view is adopted, that growth at the mandibular condyle is largely a response to translation of the mandible by growth of surrounding tissues, the analogy to the maxilla is much closer, and a more optimistic view of the possibilities for growth restraint would be warranted. Research in recent years (see Chapter 2) indicates that the second view of mandibular growth is the correct one. Nevertheless, results from chin cup therapy are usually discouraging.

There are two main approaches toward chin cup therapy (Fig. 8-20). The first is to apply force on a line directly through the mandibular condyle with the intent of impeding mandibular growth in exactly the same way that extraoral force against the maxilla impedes its growth.[22] Experience suggests that some changes can be produced in this way, but the changes are considerably less impressive than those that can be produced in the maxilla with headgear. The difficulty can be attributed to the nature of the temporomandibular joint, which makes it difficult to create a restraining force against the condyle, or it may reflect a more fundamental difference between maxillary and mandibular growth.

A second approach to chin cup therapy is to orient the line of force application below the mandibular condyle, so that the chin is deliberately rotated downward and backward. Less force is applied than when direct growth restriction is the objective. When the mandible is repositioned downward in this way, greater eruption of the teeth occurs. In essence, an increase in facial height is traded for a decrease in the prominence of the chin. Obviously, this approach would work best in individuals who had short facial vertical dimensions initially (Fig. 8-21). It can be quite effective within the limits established by excessive face height.

When extraoral force is applied against the chin, it is difficult to avoid tipping the lower incisors lingually. In general, an elastic type of chin cup (the sort worn by football players, adapted for orthodontic use) transfers a significant amount of force to the base of the alveolar process and

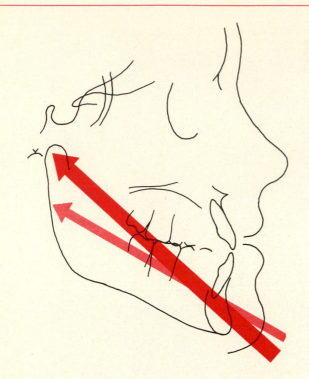

Fig. 8-20 ■ There are two main approaches to chin cup therapy, as shown diagrammatically here: heavy force aimed directly at the condylar area, or lighter force aimed below the condyle to produce downward rotation of the mandible.

causes uprighting of the lower incisors. Even when a more rigid chin cup is used, a component of dental displacement in addition to the desired skeletal change is usually observed. If the mandibular dentition was protrusive initially, of course, uprighting of the incisors is desirable. In most cases, however, the incisor uprighting is an undesirable side effect.

Functional appliances for mandibular prognathism work in exactly the same way as the second approach to chin cup therapy: they create downward and backward rotation of the mandible, achieved by increasing the vertical dimension of occlusion. The construction bite for Class III functional appliances is based on opening the mandible on a hinge, creating additional vertical space into which eruption of the teeth is guided. Although there are several types of Class III functional appliances, none of these create any direct force to restrain the mandible.

The ideal patient for chin cup or functional appliance treatment of excessive mandibular growth has:

* A mild skeletal problem, with the ability to bring the incisors end-to-end or nearly so
* Short vertical face height
* Normally positioned or protrusive but not retrusive lower incisors

A patient with severe mandibular prognathism, even at an early age, can be labeled as eventually requiring surgical correction. Modification of growth in this circumstance can be successful only within narrow limits, whatever the appliance system.

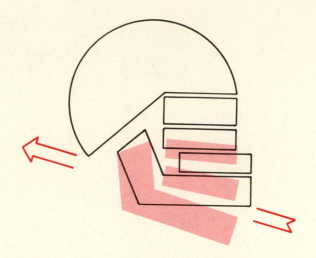

Fig. 8-21 ■ Diagrammatic representation of a typical response to chin cup therapy, showing the downward and backward rotation of the mandible accompanied by an increase in facial height.

■ Orthodontic Camouflage for Skeletal Discrepancies

Goals and limitations of camouflage. With extraction of teeth, it is possible to obtain correct molar and incisor relationships despite an underlying skeletal Class II or III jaw relationship (Fig. 8-4). This is the basic idea of camouflage as treatment for a skeletal jaw discrepancy. The method was developed as extraction treatment was reintroduced into orthodontics in the 1930s and 1940s and was the major approach to treatment of skeletal problems in that era. Inherent in this approach is the concept that major changes in skeletal jaw relationships are not possible, and that the role of the orthodontist therefore is to achieve the best possible occlusion, given the limitations established by the jaw relationships. At the time that extraction treatment became popular, growth modification as a treatment approach had been largely rejected as ineffective, and surgical techniques to correct skeletal problems had barely begun to be developed. It seemed appropriate, therefore, for the orthodontist to accept the limitations in skeletal relationships and concentrate on the dental occlusion.

Camouflage also implies that repositioning of the dentition will have a favorable effect on facial esthetics. For patients with mild to moderate skeletal Class II problems, displacement of the teeth relative to their bony bases to achieve good occlusion is compatible with reasonable facial esthetics, and the camouflage can be quite successful. Considerable retraction of the upper incisors can be accomplished for most patients before an increasing prominence of the nose and an unestheticly obtuse nasolabial angle signal the effective limits of camouflage.

In more severe Class II problems, it may be possible to obtain good occlusion only at considerable expense to facial esthetics. The upper incisors must be displaced far distally to compensate for mandibular deficiency. The esthetic result is increased prominence of the nose and an overall appearance of lower facial deficiency (Fig. 8-22). Ironically, im-

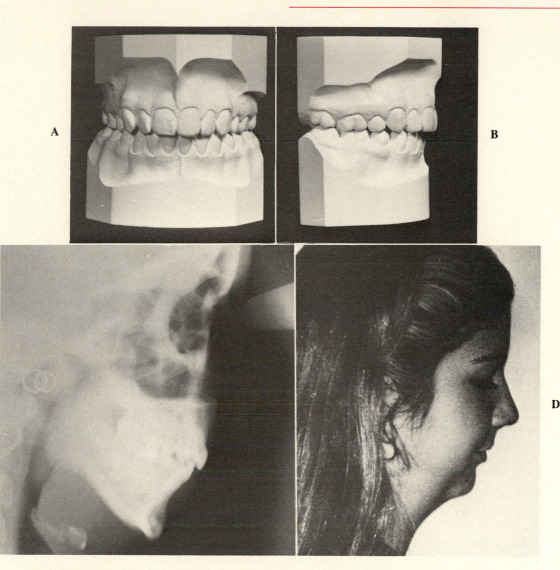

Fig. 8-22 ■ Orthodontic camouflage for Class II malocclusion caused by a severe mandibular deficiency may result in reasonably satisfactory occlusal relationships but poor facial esthetics. **A** and **B,** occlusal relationships after premolar extractions 4 years of orthodontic treatment; **C** and **D,** profile relationships after treatment. The orthodontic treatment has resulted in backward positioning of the maxilla and maxillary teeth to an undesirable extent.

provements in orthodontic mechanotherapy that allow greater displacement of the teeth have made it possible to obtain occlusal correction of Class II problems that goes beyond the limits of successful camouflage from an esthetic sense.

In Class III problems, camouflage is much less successful. Retraction of lower incisors makes the chin more prominent, and even minimal retraction often magnifies the facial esthetic problems associated with Class III malocclusion (Fig. 8-23). Although premolar extraction combined with Class III elastics and extraoral force can produce good dental occlusion for many Class III patients, the treatment rarely produces successful camouflage and frequently makes esthetics worse. For this reason, camouflage treatment is largely limited to Class II problems.

Extraction of teeth provides space for deliberate displacement of the remaining teeth only in the anteroposterior plane

of space. If a patient has vertical or transverse skeletal problems, extractions for camouflage are not helpful. A patient whose primary problem is excessive vertical development is also likely to have excessive overjet and a tendency toward Class II relationships of posterior teeth, simply because the mandible has been rotated downward and backward. Applying interarch elastics after extracting teeth, the classic approach to Class II camouflage, usually produces disastrous esthetic results in these patients. Not only do the extractions not help in dealing with the basic vertical problem, the force systems used to reposition dental segments tend to extrude posterior teeth and may actually make the vertical component of the problem worse.

Camouflage as a treatment plan implies that growth modification to overcome the basic problem is not feasible. Because of the extrusive nature of most orthodontic mechanics, however, it helps to have some vertical growth

A

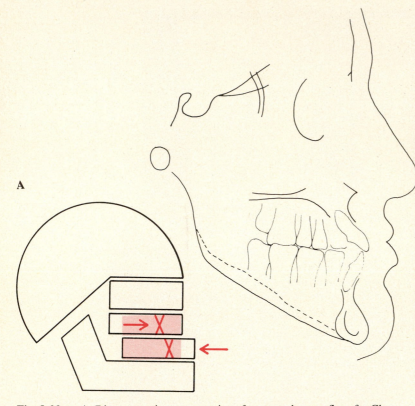

B

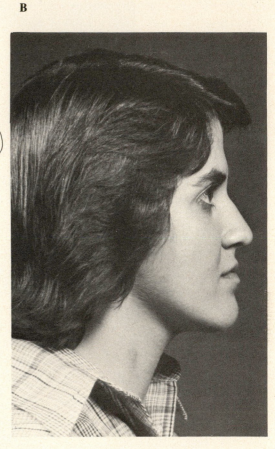

C

Fig. 8-23 ■ **A,** Diagrammatic representation of attempted camouflage for Class III relationships, showing the obvious chin prominence created by retracting mandibular incisor teeth; **B** and **C,** profile relationships for a patient after treatment in which lower incisors were retracted and upper incisors were tipped forward. The patient was unhappy with the appearance of her chin and requested further treatment.

during treatment to avoid downward and backward rotation of the mandible. At present, camouflage treatment is most useful in patients in the early permanent dentition years, who are past the pubertal growth spurt but still have some growth remaining.

Although this type of treatment is possible for nongrowing adults, it is more difficult because the potentially extrusive components of any mechanical system must be much more carefully controlled than is necessary in adolescent patients who still have some vertical growth to be completed.

The characteristics of a patient who would be a good candidate for camouflage treatment could be listed as follows:

- Too old for successful growth modification
- Mild to moderate skeletal Class II jaw relationship
- Reasonably good alignment of teeth (so that the extraction spaces would be available for controlled anteroposterior displacement and not used to relieve crowding)
- Good vertical facial proportions, neither extreme short face (skeletal deep bite) or long face (skeletal open bite)

Conversely, camouflage treatment designed to correct the occlusion despite jaw relationship problems should be avoided in:

- Severe Class II, Class III, and vertical skeletal discrepancies
- Patients with severe crowding or protrusion of incisors, in whom the extraction spaces will be required to achieve proper alignment of the incisors
- Patients with excellent remaining growth potential (in whom growth modification treatment should be used) or nongrowing adults with more than mild discrepancies (in whom surgical jaw repositioning usually offers better long-term results)

Growth prediction and visualized treatment objective as treatment planning tools. To compensate for an anteroposterior jaw discrepancy, it is necessary to retract the maxillary incisors and protract the mandibular incisors. Specification of the desired change in incisor position in each arch in advance defines the extent to which the extraction spaces are to be closed by retracting the incisors versus slipping the posterior teeth forward. In turn, this specification makes it possible to plan the degree of posterior anchorage conservation necessary in each arch, the mechanism to be used for space closure, the extent of interarch elastic wear, and other pertinent factors in appliance design (see Chapter 10).

The incisor position desired at the end of treatment can be expressed cephalometrically, and indeed this was incorporated in the Steiner analysis at an early stage in cephalometrics. Steiner developed a table of appropriate positions for the incisors as a function of the magnitude of the ANB angle (see Fig. 6-32), thereby indicating the position for the incisors needed to produce any given degree of camouflage for jaw discrepancy. However, to use the Steiner tables, it is obviously necessary to predict the ANB angle at the end of treatment. Steiner's original assumption was that the ANB angle for any given patient would not change much if at all during orthodontic treatment, but clinical experience quickly showed that improvements in the ANB angle often did occur during treatment, especially when growth modification was attempted. To use the Steiner compromises as a cephalometric treatment objective, therefore, it was necessary to predict the amount of change that would be produced by growth and the additional impact of any growth modification treatment.

The clinical usefulness of this type of growth prediction and the need to develop estimates of treatment response as well as changes produced by growth alone were recognized by Ricketts in the 1950s.[23] Ricketts and coworkers have focused strongly on cephalometric prediction methods since that time. The cephalometric analysis advocated by Ricketts incorporates a visualized treatment objective (VTO) as a treatment planning tool in addition to its diagnostic component. The contemporary VTO, discussed in more detail later, goes beyond Steiner's compromise position of incisors by including growth prediction to indicate the expected final position of both skeletal and dental structures.

Methods for clinical growth prediction. Prediction of growth changes requires specification of the *amount* of growth change at a given point during a given period of time, and the *direction* of growth. It is also necessary to specify a baseline or reference point against which the magnitude and direction of growth are projected. As might be expected, whatever the chosen reference point, both the magnitude and direction of growth at various landmarks are rather variable. An additional problem is that growth, particularly in the position of the chin, does not follow a straight line, but appears to project along a segment of an arc.

From experimentation with cephalometric data from his own patients, Ricketts developed a method for projecting the arc of mandibular growth and used this as the basis for his first growth prediction methods.[23] The Ricketts approach has been refined in recent years,[24] but is still based on changes observed during the treatment of orthodontic patients and so may incorporate some treatment effects.

Data from several major studies of growth in children who did not receive orthodontic treatment have also been treated statistically to allow their use in growth prediction. The most complete and best known of such data sets are those based on the Burlington (Ontario) growth study, conducted under the auspices of the University of Toronto,[25] the Michigan growth study, at the Center for Human Growth

and Development at the University of Michigan,[26] and the Bolton growth study, conducted at Case Western Reserve University in Cleveland.[27]

In each of these studies, cephalometric radiographs were taken at regular intervals during the growth of normal children, and the resultant data were grouped to provide a picture of the average, normal growth changes. A convenient way to show the average growth changes is with templates that show the expected direction and increment of growth at specified points and ages[25,26] or as a series of complete templates from which change at given points can be deduced.[27]

The major difficulty with growth prediction is that an individual patient may have neither the average amount nor the average direction of growth, and thus there is the possibility of significant error. The more the individual whose growth one is attempting to predict is representative of the sample from which the average changes were derived, the more accurate one would expect the prediction to be, and vice versa. Ideally, separate growth standards would be established for the two sexes, the major racial groups, and important subgroups within each of the major categories. The existing data sets simply are too small to allow this sort of subdivision and because it is no longer considered ethically acceptable to make repeated x-rays on children who will not be treated, it is unlikely that the necessary quantity of data ever will be available.

Data from the Bolton study are not subdivided in any way. The Michigan data are subdivided by sex, providing different male and female predictive values; the Burlington data have been subdivided on the basis of facial pattern, with different growth predictions for individuals with short, normal, and long vertical facial dimensions.

Estimation of treatment response. There have been almost no well-controlled and well-defined studies of the response to specific orthodontic treatment procedures. Distilled clinical experience offers some guidelines, and Ricketts and coworkers have used this information to provide some reasonable estimates of treatment effects.[28] Because of the variability in response, it is particularly difficult to predict what the effect of growth modification treatment will be, but estimates must be incorporated into a visualized treatment objective (see later). When the variable for growth is eliminated, as is the case for adults who are treated by a combination of orthodontics and orthognathic surgery, prediction of the effect of treatment becomes easier and more reliable. Tabulated data for surgical prediction are provided in the standard text on this subject,[29] and these prediction methods are discussed in Chapter 21.

Combination of growth prediction and estimated treatment response into a visualized treatment objective. A visualized treatment objective combines the changes that would be produced by normal growth in the absence of treatment, with the changes in jaw relationship and tooth position that are expected to result from treatment. Despite the limitations and inaccuracies in both the estimate of

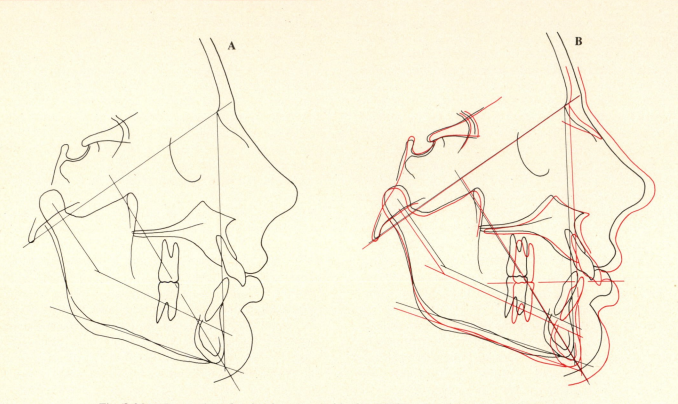

Fig. 8-24 ■ Preparation of a visual treatment objective (VTO), using the method of Ricketts. **A,** Cephalometric tracing of a 13-year-old boy with maxillary dental crowding and Class II malocclusion with mandibular deficiency. **B,** Growth prediction (red) for the next 2 years superimposed on the original tracing. The growth prediction is based on lengthening the basion-nasion line 2 mm/year (1 mm increment at basion and nasion), and on lengthening the mandibular condylar axis and corpus axis 2 mm/year. The maxilla is predicted to move down and forward two thirds as much as the mandible (see Ricketts[28] for details).

growth and the estimate of treatment response, a VTO can be quite helpful in understanding the treatment procedures needed to produce a desired response. Steps in the development of a VTO, using the method advocated by Ricketts, are shown in brief outline in Fig. 8-24 and presented in detail by Ricketts et al.[28]

Treatment response as an aid in treatment planning. Even when growth prediction and treatment response are combined into a visualized treatment objective, there is an initial element of uncertainty in the treatment plan for many preadolescent or adolescent orthodontic patients with a jaw discrepancy. As a general principle, if the patient exhibits good skeletal growth and cooperates well, it should be possible to achieve a good result without extractions for camouflage. On the other hand, if growth, cooperation, or both are poor, extractions and camouflage would be the best approach.

A practical problem in treatment planning, then, is what to do in the presence of this uncertainty. Proceed with growth modification, regardless? Go ahead with extractions for camouflage, on the theory that this would assure success whatever the patient's growth? Use the estimates underlying the VTO as an aid in making the decision? Each of these approaches has been advocated seriously by respected orthodontic clinicians, but each has limitations. Attempted growth modification in a poorly growing patient produces an unstable and generally unsatisfactory result. Camouflage can provide an acceptable result in a poorly growing patient, but extractions for this purpose in a patient with good growth are undesirable esthetically and functionally. Growth prediction works satisfactorily for average patients, but not so well for the ones whose growth has already produced an orthodontic problem.

One way to reduce the amount of uncertainty in planning treatment for this type of patient is to use the initial treatment response as an aid in treatment planning, deferring the adoption of a definitive treatment plan until some experience has been achieved with the patient. This approach, sometimes called "therapeutic diagnosis," allows a better evaluation of both growth response and cooperation with treatment than can be obtained by prediction alone.[30]

In practice, the therapeutic diagnosis approach involves implementing a conservative, i.e., nonextraction, treatment plan initially, and scheduling a reevaluation of the patient

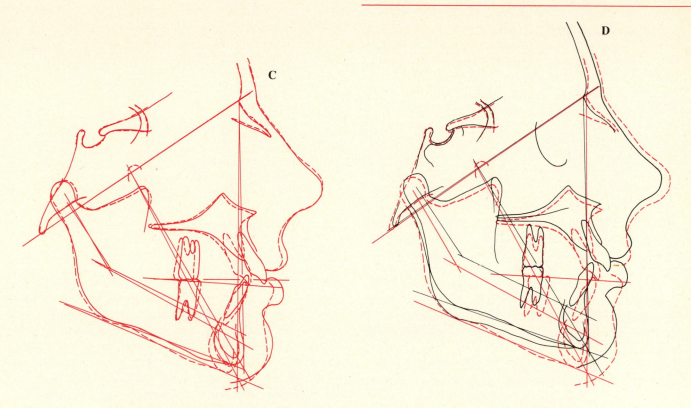

Fig. 8-24, cont'd ■ **C,** VTO (dashed red) superimposed on growth prediction. Guidelines for rotation of the mandible (changes in the facial axis) are that a 1 degree opening of the facial axis *(arrow)* can be expected for each 3 mm of molar correction, 4 mm of overbite reduction, and/or 5 mm convexity reduction. A reduction in point *A* can be achieved with headgear (maximum 8 mm) or Class II elastics (maximum 3 mm). Tooth movement relative to supporting bone is predicted in terms of spaces created by extraction or transition of the dentition. For this patient, a combination of headgear and elastics for Class II correction was projected, without extractions, producing the changes shown here. **D,** VTO superimposed on the original tracing, showing the estimated combined effect of growth and treatment.

after 6 to 9 months to observe the response to this treatment. Typically, a child with a skeletal Class II malocclusion might be placed on a functional appliance or extraoral force to the maxilla, with minimal use of fixed appliances for tooth movement. If a good response is observed after 6 to 9 months, this treatment approach is continued, with the odds of long-term success greatly improved.

On the other hand, if a poor response is observed, whether because of poor cooperation or poor growth, the growth modification therapy might be dropped in favor of extractions and a fixed appliance, camouflage-oriented approach. The disadvantage of the evaluation period in the latter instance is that treatment may take longer than it would have if the extraction decision had been made initially. The advantage, however, is that with this approach, it will prove possible to treat a number of children without the necessity for extracting teeth, who might well have had extraction if the decision were based on prediction.

No method of pretreatment prediction is as accurate for establishing the appropriate treatment plan as an observation of the actual response to treatment. Whatever the treatment plan, of course, it is important at all stages of all types of

treatment to carefully monitor the patient's response and to make appropriate adjustments in the original plan to deal with unexpected variations in response.

■ Surgical Correction

Although surgical procedures to correct mandibular prognathism date back to the beginning of the twentieth century, rapid progress in orthognathic surgery began only in the 1950s. Since that time, surgical techniques have been developed which allow severe problems of any type to be corrected. Excellent results require careful coordination of the orthodontic and surgical phases of treatment. The principles of combined surgical and orthodontic treatment are discussed in some detail in Chapter 21.

The characteristics of a patient who would best be treated surgically are:

- Severe skeletal discrepancy or extremely severe dentoalveolar problem
- Adult patient (little if any remaining growth), or younger patient with extremely severe or progressive deformity
- Good general health status (mild, controlled systemic disease acceptable)

An important principle of treatment planning is that orthodontic treatment for camouflage and orthodontic preparation for surgery often require exactly opposite tooth movements. The reason is found in the concept of "dental compensation for skeletal discrepancy." This can occur naturally as well as being created by orthodontic camouflage treatment. In a patient with mandibular prognathism, for instance, the upper incisors tend to protrude while the lower incisors incline lingually, so that the dental discrepancy is smaller than the jaw discrepancy. Tooth position has compensated at least partially for the jaw discrepancy. Some degree of dental compensation accompanies most skeletal jaw discrepancies, even without treatment. Orthodontic treatment for camouflage, of course, consists of accentuating the dental compensation (Fig. 8-4). If the jaws are to be repositioned surgically, however, this dental compensation must be removed. Otherwise, when the jaws fit, the teeth will not. Orthodontic preparation for surgery usually involves removing, not creating, dental compensation, and therefore is just the opposite of conventional orthodontic treatment.

The result is that vigorous orthodontic treatment to correct a difficult skeletal problem may eventually make surgical correction all but impossible without another session of orthodontic treatment to undo the results of the original orthodontics. The patient, of course, is not likely to be pleased by this news. It is appropriate to attempt growth modification in younger patients with severe problems. As a general rule, however, an attempt at camouflage in a patient who may well need surgery should be avoided unless a successful outcome can be clearly predicted.

■ *Treatment Planning in Special Circumstances*

■ Sequence of Treatment for Patients with Multiple Dental Problems

For patients with multiple dental problems including malocclusion, the appropriate sequencing of treatment is important (Table 8-3). Whether the patient is a child or adult, the principles are the same:

- Dental disease should be brought under control initially
- Orthodontic treatment, including skeletal as well as dental changes, should be carried out next
- Definitive restorative and periodontal treatment should be completed after the orthodontic phase of treatment

Control of dental disease includes a number of treatment procedures: tooth extractions if necessary, endodontic treatment if required, periodontal treatment procedures necessary to bring the patient to a point of satisfactory maintenance, and restorative treatment to eliminate the progression of dental caries.

At one time, there was concern that endodontically treated teeth could not be moved orthodontically. It is now clear that as long as the periodontal ligament is normal, endo-

Table 8-3 ■ Sequence of treatment in patients with multiple problems

1. Disease Control
   Caries control
   Endodontics
   Initial periodontics (no osseous surgery)
   Initial restorative (no cast restoration)
2. Establishment of occlusion
   Orthodontics
   Orthognathic surgery
   Periodontal maintenance
3. Definitive periodontics (including osseous surgery)
4. Definitive restorative
   Cast restoration
   Splints, partial dentures

dontically treated teeth respond to orthodontic force in the same way as do teeth with vital pulps, except that the nonvital teeth appear somewhat more subject to root resorption.[31] For some adults, hemisection of a posterior tooth, with removal of one root and endodontic treatment of the remaining root, may be needed before orthodontic treatment is instituted. It is perfectly feasible to orthodontically reposition the remaining root of a posterior tooth, should this be necessary. Prior endodontic treatment does not contraindicate orthodontic tooth movement.

Essentially all periodontal treatment procedures may be used in bringing a preorthodontic patient to the point of satisfactory maintenance, with the exception of osseous surgery. Scaling, curettage, flap procedures, and gingival grafts should be employed as appropriate before orthodontic treatment, so that progression of periodontal problems during orthodontic treatment can be avoided. Children or adults with mucogingival problems, most commonly a lack of adequate attached gingiva, should have free gingival grafts to create attached gingiva before the beginning of orthodontics. Since research findings indicate that 5% to 10% of children and 20% to 25% of adults who need orthodontic treatment have mucogingival problems,[32] periodontal treatment to deal with this before orthodontic therapy is needed relatively frequently (see Fig. 7-33).

Further details in the sequencing of treatment for adults with multiple problems are provided in Chapters 19 and 20.

■ Patients with Systemic Disease Problems

Patients who are suffering from systemic disease are at greater risk for complications during orthodontic treatment, but can have successful orthodontic treatment as long as the systemic problems are under control.

In adults or children, the most common systemic problem that may complicate orthodontic treatment is diabetes or a prediabetic state. The rapid progression of periodontal disease in patients with diabetes is well recognized, and the indication for orthodontic treatment in these individuals is often a series of occlusal problems related to previous periodontal breakdown and loss of teeth.

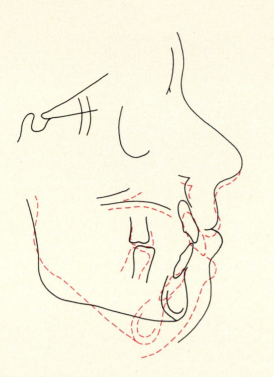

Fig. 8-25 ■ Cephalometric superimpositions for a patient with severe degeneration of the condylar process of the mandible because of rheumatoid arthritis. Age 18, after uneventful orthodontic treatment (black); age 29 (dotted red). (Courtesy Dr. J.R. Greer.)

If the diabetes is under good control, periodontal responses to orthodontic force are essentially normal and successful orthodontic treatment, particularly the adjunctive procedures most often desired for adult diabetics, can be carried out successfully. If the diabetic condition is not under good control, however, there is a real risk of accelerated periodontal breakdown. For this reason, careful monitoring of a diabetic patient's compliance with medical therapy is essential during any phase of orthodontic treatment. Prolonged comprehensive orthodontic treatment should be avoided in these patients if at all possible.

Arthritic degeneration may also be a factor in orthodontic planning. Juvenile rheumatoid arthritis frequently produces severe skeletal mandibular deficiency, and adult onset rheumatoid arthritis can destroy the condylar process and create a deformity (Fig. 8-25). In milder arthritic or similar problems, long-term administration of steroids as part of the medical treatment may increase the possibility of periodontal problems during orthodontics. In adults, degenerative changes in the temporomandibular joint (TMJ) accompanying osteoarthritis may be related to occlusal problems in some instances, although this is not always or even usually the case. If repositioning of teeth in adults with evidence of TMJ changes is needed as part of treatment, orthodontic treatment will not accelerate the joint degeneration. In this instance, orthodontic repositioning of teeth may be helpful and is not likely to accentuate the patient's problems (see Chapter 20).

Comprehensive orthodontic treatment for children with other systemic diseases is also possible if the disease is controlled, but requires careful judgment about whether the benefit to the patient warrants the orthodontic treatment.[33] It is not uncommon for the parents of a child with a severe systemic problem, for example, cystic fibrosis, to seek orthodontic consultation in their bid to do everything possible for the unfortunate child. With the increasing long-term survival after childhood leukemia, children with this medical background are now also being seen as potential orthodontic patients. Although the treatment is technically feasible, it is usually good judgment to limit the scope of treatment plans, accepting some compromise in occlusion to limit treatment time and intensity. Orthodontic tooth movement should be avoided in patients who have received significant radiation to the jaws.

■ Anomalies and Injuries of the Mandibular Condyles

Asymmetric mandibular deficiency. If the mandibular condyles are affected by either a congenital condition or an injury at birth or later, facial asymmetry is likely to result. Since the appropriate treatment is quite different if the restriction of mandibular growth is from an injury rather than a congenital anomaly, this is an important diagnostic decision.

In the congenital syndrome of hemifacial microsomia, there is an absence of tissue in the region of the mandibular condyle. In more severe cases, the entire distal portion of the mandible may be missing, along with associated soft tissues (see Chapter 3). In less severe cases, the size of the affected area may simply be diminished, with slower growth on that side and a resulting asymmetry. An apparently similar situation of reduced growth on one side can also result from an injury to the mandibular condyle, with subsequent scarring and fibrosis of the area that restricts movement. In hemifacial microsomia, the problem is a lack of tissue, so that normal growth potential is not present. In postinjury problems, there is potential for normal growth, but restriction from fibrotic tissue prevents expression of this growth.

In planning treatment, it is important to evaluate whether the affected condyle can translate normally. If it can, as one would expect in a mild form of hemifacial microsomia, a functional appliance could be helpful and should be tried first. If translation of the condyle is restricted by posttraumatic scarring, a functional appliance will be ineffective and should not be attempted until the restriction on growth has been removed.

Asymmetry problems are a particular indication for custom-designed "hybrid" functional appliances (Fig. 8-26) because requirements for the deficient side will be different from those for the normal or more normal side. Often it is desirable to incorporate a bite block between the teeth on the normal side while providing space for eruption on the deficient side, so that the vertical component of the asymmetry can be addressed. In the construction bite, the mandible would be advanced more on the deficient side than on

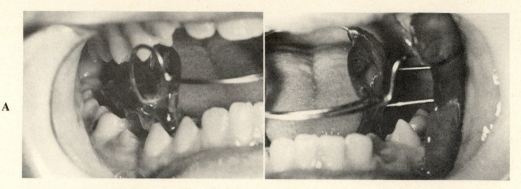

Fig. 8-26 ■ A "hybrid" functional appliance can be used to correct vertical and transverse jaw asymmetries. For this patient, **(A)** the appliance consists of a bite block on the right side, and **(B)** shields on the left that allow free eruption of teeth. The construction bite, swinging the jaw to one side, is designed to correct the transverse asymmetry by producing more growth on the deficient side, while differential eruption corrects the vertical asymmetry.

the normal side. Further details on fabrication of hybrid functional appliances are presented in Chapter 14.

The restriction of growth that accompanies reduced translation of the condyle often leads to a progressively more severe deformity as growth of other parts of the face continues. Progressive deformity of this type is an indication for early surgical intervention. There is nothing to be gained by waiting for such a deformity to become worse.

Condylar hyperplasia. Mandibular and facial asymmetry can also be caused by excessive growth of the mandibular condyle on one side. Growth problems of this type are almost never symmetric. They appear to be caused by an escape of the growing tissues on one side from normal regulatory control, the exact mechanism of which is not understood. The condition typically appears in the late teens, but may begin at an earlier age.

There are two possible modes of treatment, both surgical: (1) a ramus osteotomy to correct the asymmetry resulting from unilateral overgrowth, after the excessive growth has ceased; and (2) condylectomy to remove the excessively growing condyle and reconstruct the joint. The reconstruction is usually done with a section of rib incorporating the costochondral junction area, but occasionally can be accomplished just by recontouring the condylar head ("condylar shave"). Since surgical involvement of the temporomandibular joint should be avoided if possible, the first treatment plan is preferable. This treatment plan implies, however, that the abnormal growth has stopped or in a younger patient, will stop within reasonable limits. As a practical matter, removal of the condyle is likely to be necessary in the more severe and more rapidly growing cases, while a ramus osteotomy is preferred for the less severe problems.

The bone seeking isotope ^{99m}Tc can be used to distinguish an active rapidly growing condyle from an enlarged condyle that has ceased growing.[34] This short-lived gamma-emitting isotope is concentrated in areas of active bone deposition.

^{99m}Tc imaging of the oral structures typically shows high activity in areas around the alveolar ridge, particularly in areas where teeth are erupting. The condyles are not normally areas of intense imaging. A "hot" condyle is evidence of active growth at that site (Fig. 8-27).

Unfortunately, though false positive images are rare, false negatives may occur, so a negative bone scan of the condyles

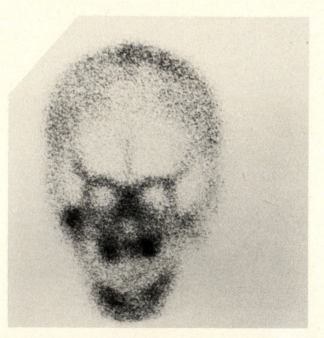

Fig. 8-27 ■ Image (anterior Towne's view with the mouth open) from bone scan with ^{99m}Tc in a 10-year-old boy with suspected hyperplasia of the right mandibular condyle. Note the "hot spot" in the area of the right condyle and the difference in uptake of the isotope between the right and left sides. Eruption of teeth and apposition of bone at the alveolar processes normally create heavy imaging along the dental arches.

cannot be taken as evidence that hyperplastic growth of one condyle is not occurring. In a younger patient, a prolonged positive unilateral condylar response on a growth scan indicates that condylectomy will probably be required, whereas a negative response means that further observation for continuing growth is indicated.

■ Treatment Planning for Cleft Lip and Palate Patients

Patients with cleft lip and palate routinely require extensive and prolonged orthodontic treatment. Orthodontic treatment may be required at any or all of four separate stages: (1) in infancy before the initial surgical repair of the lip, (2) during the late primary and early mixed dentition, (3) during the late mixed and early permanent dentition, and (4) in the late teens after the completion of facial growth, in conjunction with orthognathic surgery.

Infant orthopedics. An infant with a cleft lip and palate will have a distorted maxillary arch at birth in nearly every instance. In patients with a bilateral cleft, the premaxillary segment is often displaced anteriorly while the posterior maxillary segments are lingually collapsed behind it (Fig. 8-28). Less severe distortions occur in infants with unilateral palatal clefts. If the distortion of arch form is extremely severe, surgical closure of the lip, which is normally carried out in the early weeks of life, can be extremely difficult. Orthodontic intervention to reposition the segments and to bring the protruding premaxillary segment back into the arch may be needed to obtain a good surgical repair of the lip. This "infant orthopedics" is one of the few instances in which orthodontic treatment for a newborn infant, before eruption of any teeth, may be indicated.

Infant orthopedics of this type was pioneered by Burston in Liverpool in the late 1950s[35] and was carried out on a large scale at many cleft palate centers in the 1960s. In a child with a bilateral cleft, two types of movement of the maxillary segments are needed (Fig. 8-29). First, the lin-

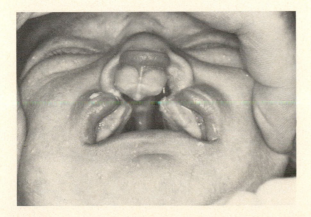

Fig. 8-28 ■ A forward displacement of the premaxillary segment and medial collapse of the lateral maxillary segments can be seen clearly in this photograph of a newborn infant with a bilateral cleft of the lip and palate.

gually collapsed maxillary posterior segment must be brought back into the arch. If the posterior segments are expanded laterally, pressure against the premaxilla will reposition it lingually into its approximately correct position in the arch. This movement can be accomplished by a light elastic strap across the anterior segment, by an orthodontic appliance pinned to the segments that applies a contraction force, or even by pressure from the repaired lip if lip repair is done after the lateral expansion. In patients with extremely severe protrusion, an appliance held to the maxillary segments by pins might be required, while an elastic strap or the pressure of the lip itself would be adequate with less severe problems.

In infants, the segments can be repositioned surprisingly quickly and easily, so that the period of active treatment is a few weeks at most. If presurgical movement of maxillary segments is indicated, this typically would be done beginning at 3 to 6 weeks of age, so that the lip closure could be carried out at approximately 10 weeks. A passive plate, similar to an orthodontic retainer, is then used for a few months after lip closure.

Even in children with unilateral clefts and relatively slight distortion of the arch, an improvement in the position of the premaxillary segment can be noted if a passive plate is placed, because there is a molding effect on the arch after lip closure. For these patients, the passive appliance would be placed before lip closure, then maintained for perhaps 3 months after the lip closure. Acceptance of such an appliance by the infant is surprisingly good. It serves as a "feeding plate," apparently making it easier for the infant to swallow normally. A passive plate can be left in position for most of the first year of life if desired.

After 20 years of experience with presurgical infant orthopedics, the present consensus is that these procedures offer less long-term benefit than was originally expected.[36] For this reason, the method is used less frequently than when enthusiasm was at a peak. Soon after this treatment, the infants who have had presurgical orthopedics look much better than those who have not had it. With each passing year, however, it becomes more difficult to tell which patients had segments repositioned in infancy and which did not. The short-term benefit is more impressive than the long-term benefit.

At some centers, bone grafts were placed across the cleft alveolus soon after the infant orthopedics to stabilize the position of the segments. Although some controversy still surrounds this procedure,[37] the consensus is that early grafting of the alveolar process is contraindicated because it tends to interfere with later growth.[38] Alveolar bone grafts are better deferred until the early mixed dentition.

For some infants with extremely malpositioned segments, which occur almost exclusively in bilateral cleft lip and palate, presurgical infant orthodpedics remains useful. For the majority of patients with cleft lip or palate however, the orthodontist is no longer called to reposition segments in infants. Instead, if the segments protrude, the lip repair may

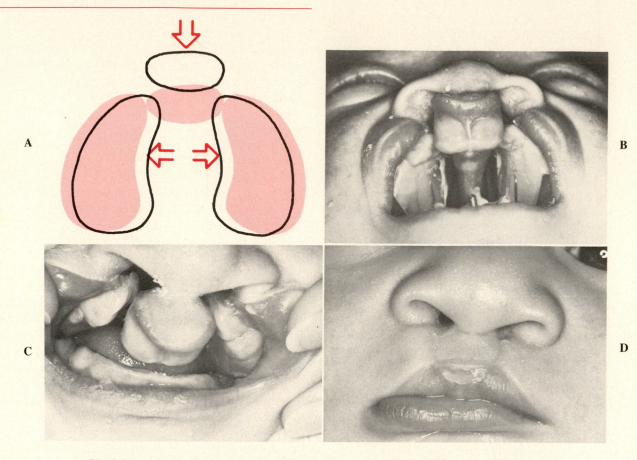

Fig. 8-29 ■ **A,** Diagrammatic representation of the movements needed to place maxillary segments in their proper position. The posterior segments must be moved laterally so that the premaxillary segment can move lingually. **B,** Infant with bilateral cleft and appliance in place to widen the posterior segments. **C,** Same infant after an elastic strap has been used to reposition the premaxillary segment lingually. **D,** Same infant, after surgical repair of the cleft lip.

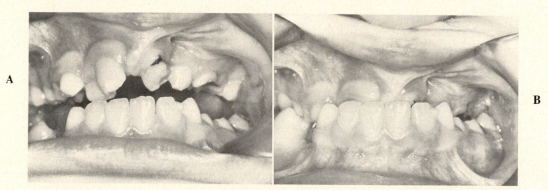

Fig. 8-30 ■ In a patient with a repaired cleft palate, the permanent incisors usually erupt severely rotated and tipped toward the cleft site (**A**), and are often in anterior crossbite (**B**).

be carried out in two stages, first with a lip adhesion to provide an elastic force from the lip itself, followed at a somewhat later stage by definitive lip repair. Rather than presurgical orthopedics being recommended for nearly all infants with cleft lop or palate, at present a minority are treated with presurgical orthopedics.

Late primary and early mixed dentition treatment.
Many of the orthodontic problems of cleft palate children in the late and early mixed dentition result not from the cleft itself, but from the effects of surgical repair. Although the techniques for repair of cleft lip and palate have improved tremendously in recent years, closure of the lip inevitably

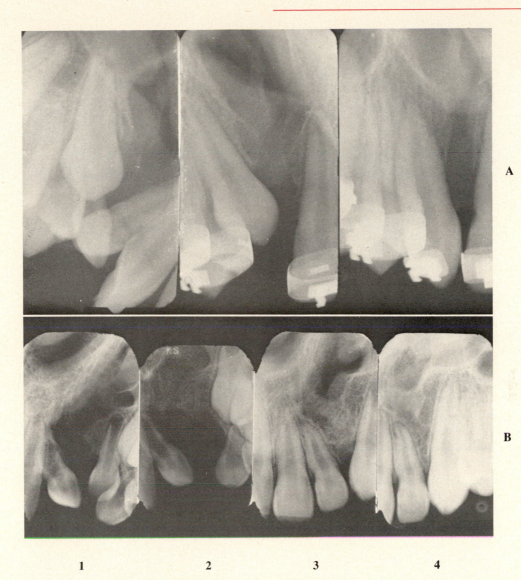

1   2   3   4

Fig. 8-31 ■ **A,** Eruption of the maxillary canine in a patient who did not accept the recommendation for a bone graft to the alveolus. After orthodontic alignment of the teeth (right), a severe defect persists in the alveolus. Uncorrected defects of this type jeopardize the long-term retention of teeth on either side. **B,** Eruption of the canine after placement of a bone graft at age 8 (*1,* pretreatment, age 8; *2,* immediately after grafting; *3,* after eruption of the canine; *4,* after orthodontic treatment). Note the excellent fill-in of bone in the graft site. Best results are obtained if the graft is placed before eruption of the canine tooth, so that it erupts through the grafted area (from Turvey and Vig[40]).

creates some constriction across the anterior part of the maxillary arch, and closure of a cleft palate causes at least some degree of lateral constriction. As a result, surgically treated cleft palate patients have a tendency toward both anterior and lateral crossbite, which is not seen in patients with untreated clefts.[39] This result is not an argument against surgical repair of the lip and palate, which is necessary for esthetic and functional (speech) reasons. It simply means that orthodontic treatment must be considered a necessary part of the habilitation of such patients.

Orthodontic intervention is often unnecessary until the permanent incisor teeth begin to erupt, but is usually imperative at that point. As the permanent teeth come in, there is a strong tendency for the first molars to erupt into crossbite, and for the maxillary incisors to erupt severely rotated and in crossbite (Fig. 8-30). Orthodontic correction of these problems is usually done best with a removable appliance. The orthodontist must expect that even if anterior and lateral crossbites are corrected at this stage, they will recur as the mandible and mandibular arch develop normally while the maxillary arch lags behind because of the congenital defect and surgical treatment.

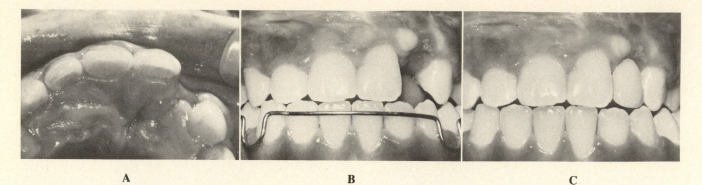

A   B   C

Fig. 8-32 ■ In fixed appliance orthodontics for patients with repaired clefts, it is often necessary to open space for a prosthetic replacement tooth (**A** and **B**). It is better to place a semipermanent acid-etch bridge, as in **C**, than to have a patient wear an orthodontic retainer that incorporates a replacement tooth for longer periods.

Alveolar bone grafts in infancy appear to be contraindicated. However, placing a bone graft in the alveolar cleft area after eruption of the lateral incisors (if present), but before eruption of the permanent canines, is advantageous in stabilizing the cleft area and creating a healthy environment for the permanent teeth, particularly the canines.[40] Ideally, the canines should erupt through the graft (Fig. 8-31), which means that the best time to place such a graft is between 8 and 10 years. Any necessary alignment of incisors or expansion of posterior segments should be completed before the alveolar grafting.

Early permenent dentition treatment. As the canine and premolar teeth erupt, there is a tendency for crossbite problems, particularly on the cleft side in a unilateral situation. In essentially every instance, fixed appliance orthodontic treatment is necessary at this time. A major objective of this phase of treatment may be the positioning of teeth as abutments for eventual fixed prosthodontics to replace missing incisors and stabilize the maxillary anterior segment (Fig. 8-32).

At the conclusion of active orthodontic treatment, a resin-bonded bridge to provide a semipermanent replacement for missing teeth can be extremely helpful. Orthodontic treatment is often completed at age 14, but a permanent bridge in many instances cannot be placed until age 17 or 18. The semipermanent fixed bridge is preferable to prolonged use of a removable retainer with a replacement tooth.

Orthognathic surgery for patients with cleft lip and palate. In approximately 10% of patients with cleft lip and palate, but more often in males than females, continued mandibular growth after the completion of active orthodontic treatment leads to the return of anterior and lateral crossbites. This result is not so much from excessive mandibular growth as from deficient maxillary growth, both anteroposteriorly and vertically. Failure of the maxilla to grow vertically allows the mandible to rotate upward and forward, creating a relative deficiency in face height and with it, increased protrusion of the mandible. Orthognathic surgery

to bring the deficient maxilla downward and forward may be a necessary last stage in treatment of a patient with cleft lip or palate typically at about age 18. Occasionally, surgical mandibular setback may also be needed. After this, the definitive restorative work to replace any missing teeth can be carried out.

■ *References*

1. Angle, E.H.: Treatment of Malocclusion of the Teeth, ed. 7, Philadelphia, 1907, S.S. White Manufacturing Co.
2. Witzig, J.W., and Yerkes, I.M.: Functional jaw orthopedics: mastering more than technique. In Gelb, H., editor: Clinical Management of Head, Neck, and TMJ Pain and Dysfunction, ed. 2, Philadelphia, 1985, W.B. Saunders.
3. Begg, P.R.: Stone age man's dentition. Am. J. Orthod. **40**:298-312, 1954.
4. Case, C.S.: The question of extraction in orthodontics. Reprinted in Am J. Orthod. **50**:658-691, 1964.
5. Little, R.M., Walker, T.R., and Riedel, R.A.: Stability and relapse of mandibular anterior alignment: first premolar extraction cases treated by traditional edgewise orthodontics. Am. J. Orthod. **80**:349-364, 1981.
6. Stockli, P.W., and Willert, H.G.: Tissue reactions in the temporomandibular joint resulting from anterior displacement of the mandible in the monkey. Am. J. Orthod. **60**:142, 1971.
7. Petrovic, A.G., Stutzmann, J.J., and Gasson, N.: The final length of the mandible: is it genetically predetermined? In Carlson, D.S., editor: Craniofacial Biology. Ann Arbor, 1981, University of Michigan Center for Human Growth and Development.
8. McNamara, J.A.: Neuromuscular and skeletal adaptations to altered function in the orofacial regions. Am. J. Orthod. **64**:578-606, 1973.
9. McNamara, J.A.: Dentofacial adaptations in adult patients following functional regulator therapy. Am. J. Orthod. **85**:57-71, 1984.
10. Woodside, D.G.: The activator. In Salzmann, J.A., editor: Orthodontics in Daily Practice. Philadelphia, 1974, J.B. Lippincott Co.
11. McNamara, J.A.: Components of Class II malocclusion in children 8-10 years of age. Am. J. Orthod. **51**:177-202, 1981.

12. Lischer, B.E.: Time to Tell: A Comment on Orthodontic Orthodoxy, and Other Essay, New York, 1955, Vantage Press.

13. Oliver, O.A., and Oliver, W.H.: The occlusal guide plane: an auxiliary with any type of orthodontic appliance. In Kraus, B.F., and Riedel, R.A., editor: Vistas in Orthodontics, Philadelphia, 1962, Lea and Febiger.

14. Graber, T.M., and Neumann, B.: Removable Orthodontic Appliances, ed. 2, Philadelphia, 1984, W.B. Saunders.

15. Weislander, L.: The effect of orthodontic treatment on the concurrent development of the craniofacial complex. Am. J. Orthod. **49:**15-27, 1963.

16. Turley, P.: The loading of bioglass implants to produce premaxillary expansion in *M. mulatta*. Seattle, 1978, Univeristy of Washington, MSD Thesis.

17. Stutzmann, J.J., and Petrovic, A.G.: Experimental analysis of general and local extrusive mechanisms controlling upper jaw growth. In McNamara, J.A., editor: Factors Affecting the Growth of the Midface. Ann Arbor, 1977, University of Michigan Center for Human Growth and Development.

18. Verdon, P.: Professor Delaire's facial orthopedic mask. Denver, 1982, Rocky Mountain Orthodontic Products.

19. Haas, A.J.: Rapid expansion of the maxillary dental arch and nasal cavity by opening the midpalatal suture. Angle Orthod. **31:**73-90, 1961.

20. Isaacson, R.J., Wood., J.L., and Ingram, A.H.: Forces produced by rapid maxillary expansion. Angle Orthod. **34:**256-270, 1964.

21. Hicks, E.P.: Slow maxillary expansion: a clinical study of the skeletal versus dental response to low-magnitude force. Am. J. Orthod. **73:**121-141, 1978.

22. Graber, T.M.: Dentofacial orthopedics. In Graber, T.M., and Swain, B.F., editors: Current Orthodontic Concepts and Techniques, ed. 2, Philadelphia, 1975, W.B. Saunders.

23. Ricketts, R.M.: Planning treatment on the basis of the facial pattern and an estimate of its growth. Angle Orthod. **27:**14-37, 1957.

24. Bench, R.W., Gugino, C.F., and Hilgers, J.J.: Bioprogressive therapy. Part 3. Visual treatment objective (VTO). J. Clin. Orthod. **11:**744-763, 1977.

25. Popovich, F.P., et al.: Burlington growth study templates. Toronto, 1981, University of Toronto Department of Orthodontics.

26. Johnston, L.E.: A simplified approach to prediction. Am J. Orthod. **67:**253-257, 1975.

27. Broadbent, B.H., Sr., Broadbent, B.J., Jr., and Golden, W.H.: Bolton Standards of Dentofacial Developmental Growth. St. Louis, 1975, The C.V. Mosby Co.

28. Ricketts, R.M., et al.: Bioprogressive Therapy. Denver, 1979, Rocky Mountain Orthodontics.

29. Bell, W.H., Proffit, W.R., and White, R.P.: Surgical Correction of Dentofacial Deformities, Philadelphia, 1980, W.B. Saunders.

30. Ackerman, J.L., and Proffit, W.R.: Treatment response as an aid in diagnosis and treatment planning. Am J. Orthod. **57:**490-496, 1970.

31. Wickwire, N.A., et al.: The effects of tooth movement upon endodontically treated teeth. Angle Orthod. **44:**235-242, 1974.

32. Coatoam, G.W.: The width of keratinized gingiva during orthodontic treatment: its significance and impact on periodontal status. J. Periodontol. **52:**307-313, 1981.

33. vanVenrooy, J.R., and Proffit, W.R.: Orthondontic care for medically compromised patients. J. Am. Dent. Assoc. **111:**262-266, 1985.

34. Matteson, S.R., Proffit, W.R., and Terry, B.T.: Bone scans as a diagnostic procedures for hyperplasia of the mandibular condyles. Oral Surg. Oral Med. Oral Pathol. **60:**356-367, 1985.

35. Burston, W.R.: The pre-surgical orthopaedic correction of the maxillary deformity in clefts of both primary and secondary palate. In Wallace, A.B., editor: Transactions of the 2nd International Congress on Plastic Surgery, Baltimore, 1960, Williams & Wilkins.

36. Vargervik, K.: Growth characteristics of the premaxilla and orthodontic treatment principles in bilateral cleft lip and palate. Cleft Palate J. **20:**289-302, 1983.

37. Jacobson, B.N., and Rosenstein, S.W.: Early maxillary orthopedics for the newborn cleft lip and palate patient. Angle Orthod. **54:**247-263, 1984.

38. Friede, H., and Johanson, B.: A follow-up study of cleft children treated with primary bone grafting. Scan. J. Plast. Reconstr. Surg. **8:**88-103, 1974.

39. Ross, R.B., and Johnston, M.C.: Cleft Lip and Palate. Baltimore, 1972, Williams & Wilkins.

40. Turvey, T., Vig, K., Moriarty, J., et al.: Delayed bone grafting in the cleft maxilla and palate: A retrospective multidisciplinary analysis. Am. J. Orthod. **86:**244-256, 1984.

41. DuBrul, E.L.: Sicher's Oral Anatomy, ed. 7, St. Louis, 1980, The C.V. Mosby Co.

BIOMECHANICS AND MECHANICS

Orthodontic therapy depends on the reaction of the teeth, and more generally the facial structures, to gentle but persistent force. In an orthodontic context, the term biomechanics is commonly used in discussions of the reaction of the dental and facial structures to orthodontic force, whereas the term mechanics is reserved for the properties of the strictly mechanical components of the appliance system. In this section, the biologic responses to orthodontic force that underlie biomechanics are discussed in Chapter 9. Chapter 10, which is concerned with the design and application of orthodontic appliances, is largely devoted to mechanics, but includes some biomechanical considerations as well.

The Biologic Basis of Orthodontic Therapy

Orthodontic treatment is based upon the principle that if prolonged pressure is applied to a tooth, tooth movement will occur as the bone around the tooth remodels. Bone is selectively removed in some areas and added in others. In essence, the tooth moves through the bone carrying its attachment apparatus with it, as the socket of the tooth migrates. Because the bony response is mediated by the periodontal ligament, tooth movement is primarily a periodontal ligament phenomenon.

Forces applied to the teeth can also affect the pattern of bone apposition and resorption at sites distant from the teeth, particularly the sutures of the maxilla and bony surfaces on both sides of the temporomandibular joint. Thus, the biologic response to orthodontic therapy includes not only the response of the periodontal ligament but also the response of bone surfaces distant from the dentition. In this chapter, the response of periodontal structures to orthodontic force is discussed initially, and then the response of skeletal areas distant from the dentition is considered briefly, drawing on the background of normal growth provided in Chapters 2 and 3.

■ *Periodontal and Bone Response to Normal Function*

■ Periodontal Ligament Structure and Function

Each tooth is attached to and separated from the adjacent alveolar bone by a heavy collagenous supporting structure, the periodontal ligament (PDL). Under normal circumstances, the periodontal ligament occupies a space approximately 0.5 mm in width around all parts of the root. By far the major component of the ligament is a network of parallel collagenous fibers, inserting into cementum of the root surface on one side and into a relatively dense bony plate, the lamina dura, on the other. These supporting fibers run at an angle, attaching farther apically on the tooth than on the adjacent alveolar bone. This arrangement, of course, resists the displacement of the tooth expected during normal function (Fig. 9-1).

Although the vast majority of the periodontal ligament space is taken up with the collagenous fiber bundles that constitute the ligamentous attachment, two other major components of the ligament must be considered. These are (1) the cellular elements, including mesenchymal cells of various types along with vascular and neural elements, and (2) the tissue fluids. Both play an important role in normal function and in making orthodontic tooth movement possible.

The principal cellular elements in the periodontal ligament are undifferentiated mesenchymal cells and their progeny in the form of fibroblasts and osteoblasts. The collagen of the ligament is constantly being remodeled and renewed during normal function. It appears that the same cells can serve as both fibroblasts, producing new collagenous matrix materials, and fibroclasts, destroying previously produced collagen.[1] Remodeling and recontouring of the bony socket and the cementum of the root is also constantly being carried out, though on a smaller scale, as a response to normal function. Bone and cementum are removed by specialized osteoclasts and cementoclasts, respectively. These multinucleated giant cells are quite different from the osteoblasts and cementoblasts that produce bone and cementum and are derived from monocytes in the blood-lymphatic system, not from the local osteoprogenitor cells.[2]

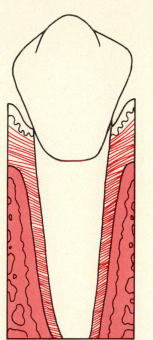

Fig. 9-1 ■ Diagrammatic representation of periodontal structures (bone in pale red). Note the angulation of the periodontal ligament fibers.

Although the periodontal ligament is not highly vascular, it does contain blood vessels and cells from the vascular system. Nerve endings are also found within the ligament, both the unmyelinated free endings associated with perception of pain and the more complex receptors associated with pressure and positional information (proprioception).

Finally, it is important to recognize that the periodontal ligament space is filled with fluid; this fluid is the same as that found in all other tissues, ultimately derived from the vascular system. A fluid filled chamber with retentive but porous walls could be a description of a shock absorber, and in normal function, the fluid allows the periodontal ligament space to play just this role.

■ Response to Normal Function

During masticatory function, the teeth and periodontal structures are subjected to intermittent heavy forces. Tooth contacts last for 1 second or less; forces are quite heavy, ranging from 1 or 2 kg while soft substances are chewed up to as much as 50 kg against a more resistant object. When a tooth is subjected to heavy loads of this type, quick displacement of the tooth within the periodontal ligament space is prevented by the incompressible tissue fluid. Instead, the force is transmitted to the alveolar bone, which bends in response.

The extent of bone bending during normal function of the jaws (and other skeletal elements of the body) is often not appreciated. The body of the mandible bends as the mouth is opened and closed, even without heavy masticatory loads. Upon wide opening, the distance between the mandibular molars decreases by 2 to 3 mm.[3] In heavy function,

Table 9-1 ■ Physiologic response to heavy pressure against a tooth

Time (seconds)	Event
<1	PDL* fluid incompressible, alveolar bone bends, piezoelectric signal generated
1-2	PDL fluid expressed, tooth moves within PDL space
3-5	PDL fluid squeezed out, tissues compressed; immediate pain if pressure is heavy

*PDL, periodontal ligament.

individual teeth are slightly displaced as the bone of the alveolar process bends to allow this to occur, and bending stresses are transmitted over considerable distances. As discussed more completely later, bone bending in response to normal function generates piezoelectric currents that appear to be an important stimulus to skeletal regeneration and repair. This is the mechanism by which bony architecture is adapted to functional demands.

Very little of the fluid within the periodontal ligament space is squeezed out during the first second of pressure application. If pressure against a tooth is maintained, however, the fluid is rapidly expressed, and the tooth displaces within the PDL space, compressing the ligament itself against adjacent bone. Not surprisingly, this hurts. Pain is normally felt after 3 to 5 seconds of heavy force application, indicating that the fluids are expressed and crushing pressure is applied against the PDL in this amount of time (Table 9-1). The resistance provided by tissue fluids allows normal mastication, with its force applications of 1 second or less, to occur without pain.

Although the periodontal ligament is beautifully adapted to resist forces of short duration, it rapidly loses its adaptive capability as the tissue fluids are squeezed out of its confined area. Prolonged forces, even of low magnitude, produce a different physiologic response. Orthodontic tooth movement is made possible by the application of prolonged forces. In addition, light prolonged forces in the natural environment—forces from the lips, cheeks, or tongue resting against the teeth—have the same potential as orthodontic forces to cause the teeth to move to a different location.[4]

■ Role of the Periodontal Ligament in Eruption and Stabilization of the Teeth

The phenomenon of tooth eruption makes it plain that forces generated within the periodontal ligament itself can produce tooth movement (see Chapter 3). The eruption mechanism appears to depend on metabolic events within the PDL, probably related to formation, cross-linkage, and maturational shortening of collagen fibers.[5] This process continues, although at a reduced rate, into adult life. A tooth whose antagonist has been extracted will often be observed to begin to erupt again after many years of apparent qui-

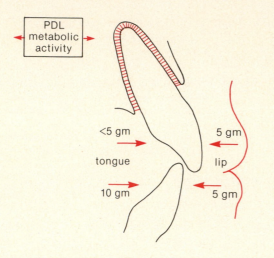

Fig. 9-2 ■ Resting pressures from the lips or cheeks and tongue are usually not balanced. In some areas, as in the mandibular anterior, tongue pressure is greater than lip pressure. In other areas, as in the maxillary incisor region, lip pressure is greater. Active stabilization produced by metabolic effects in the periodontal ligament probably explains why teeth are stable in the presence of imbalanced pressures that would otherwise cause tooth movement.

escence. The continuing presence of this mechanism indicates that it may serve to produce not only eruption of the teeth under appropriate circumstances but also active stabilization of the teeth against prolonged forces of light magnitude. It is commonly observed that light prolonged pressures against the teeth are not in perfect balance, as would seem to be required if tooth movement were not to occur (Fig. 9-2). The ability of the periodontal ligament to produce active, not just passive, stabilization of the teeth probably explains this.

Active stabilization also implies a threshold for orthodontic force, since forces below the stabilization level would be expected to be ineffective. The threshold for outside force, of course, would vary depending on the extent to which existing soft tissue pressures were already being resisted by the stabilization mechanism. In some experiments, the threshold for orthodontic force, if one existed at all, appeared extremely low. In other circumstances, a somewhat higher threshold, but still one of only a few grams, seemed to exist.[6] Current data suggest that active stabilization can overcome prolonged forces of a few grams at most, perhaps up to the 5 to 10 gm/cm^2 often observed as the magnitude of unbalanced soft tissue resting pressures.

■ *Periodontal Ligament and Bone Response to Sustained Orthodontic Force*

The response to sustained force against the teeth is a function of force magnitude: heavy forces lead to rapidly developing pain, necrosis of cellular elements within the periodontal ligament, and the phenomenon (discussed in more detail later) of "undermining resorption" of alveolar

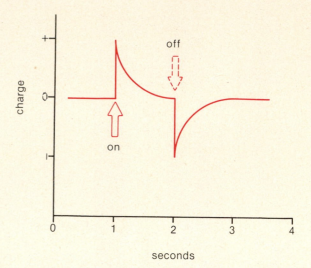

Fig. 9-3 ■ When a force is applied to a crystalline structure (like bone or collagen), a flow of current is produced that quickly dies away. When the force is released, an opposite current flow is observed. This effect results from migration of electrons within the crystal lattice of the structure.

bone near the affected tooth. Lighter forces are compatible with survival of cells within the PDL and a remodeling of the tooth socket by a relatively painless "frontal resorption" of the tooth socket. In orthodontic practice, the objective is to produce tooth movement as much as possible by frontal resorption, recognizing that some areas of PDL necrosis and undermining resorption will probably occur despite efforts to prevent this.

■ Biologic Control of Tooth Movement

Before discussing in detail the response to orthodontic force, it is necessary to consider the biologic control mechanisms that lead from the stimulus of sustained force application to the response of orthodontic tooth movement. Two possible control elements, biologic electricity and blood flow, are contrasted in the two major theories of orthodontic tooth movement. The newer piezoelectric theory relates tooth movement at least in part to changes in bone metabolism controlled by the electric signals produced from flexing and bending of the alveolar bone.[7] The blood flow theory relates tooth movement to cellular changes produced by alterations in blood flow through the periodontal ligament. Pressure and tension within the PDL, by reducing (pressure) or increasing (tension) the diameter of blood vessels in the ligament space, could certainly alter blood flow.[8]

The two theories are neither incompatible nor mutually exclusive. From a contemporary perspective, it appears that both mechanisms may play a part in the biologic control of tooth movement.

Piezoelectricity is a phenomenon observed in many crystalline materials in which a deformation of the crystal structure produces a flow of electric current as electrons are displaced from one part of the crystal lattice to another. The

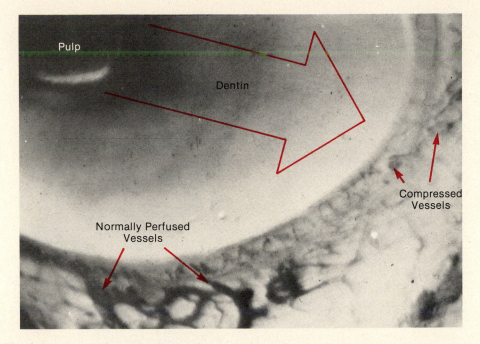

Fig. 9-4 ■ In experimental animals, changes in blood flow in the periodontal ligament can be observed by perfusing India ink into the vascular system while the animal is being sacrificed. The vessels are filled with India ink, so that their size can be seen easily. This specimen is seen in horizontal section, with the tooth root on the left and the pulp chamber just visible in the upper left. The periodontal ligament is below and to the right. Note that vessels have been compressed in the area of the periodontal ligament toward which the tooth is being moved. Cells disappear in the compressed areas, and the area is sometimes said to be "hyalinized" because of its resemblance to hyaline connective area. (Courtesy Dr. F.E. Khouw.)

piezoelectricity of many inorganic crystals has been recognized for many years and has been used in everyday technology, for instance, the crystal pickup found in inexpensive phonographic systems. Only in the last few years has it been recognized that organic crystals can also have piezoelectric properties. Not only is bone mineral a crystal structure with piezoelectric properties, collagen itself is piezoelectric. Thus, force against skeletal elements that produce bone bending would also of necessity produce piezoelectric signals.

Piezoelectric signals have two unusual characteristics: (1) a quick decay rate, i.e., when a force is applied, a piezoelectric signal is created in response that quickly dies away to zero even though the force is maintained, and (2) the production of an equivalent signal, opposite in direction, when the force is released (Fig. 9-3).

Both these characteristics are explained by the migration of electrons within the crystal lattice as it is distorted by pressure. When the crystal structure is deformed, electrons migrate from one location to another and an electric charge is observed. As long as the force is maintained, the crystal structure is stable and no further electric events are observed. When the force is released, however, the crystal returns to its original shape, and a reverse flow of electrons is seen. With this arrangement, rhythmic activity would produce a constant interplay of electric signals, whereas occasional

application and release of force would produce only occasional electric signals.

There is also a reverse piezoelectric effect. Not only will the application of force cause distortion of crystalline structure and with it an electric signal, application of an electric field can cause deformation of crystal structure and produce force in doing so. Reverse peizoelectricity has no place in natural control systems, at least as far as is presently known, but if biologically important signals are produced by normal piezoelectricity, the potential for using reverse piezoelectricity therapeutically is immediately intriguing.

There is no longer any doubt that piezoelectric signals are important in the general maintenance of the skeleton. Without such signals, bone mineral is lost and general skeletal atrophy ensues—a situation that has proved troublesome for astronauts whose bones no longer flex in a weightless environment as they would under normal gravity. Piezoelectric signals are certainly generated by the bending of alveolar bone during normal chewing, and they are very probably important for maintenance of the bone around the teeth. On the other hand, sustained pressures of the type used to induce orthodontic tooth movement do not produce prominent piezoelectric signals. When a force is applied, a brief signal is created; when it is removed, the reverse signal appears. As long as the force is sustained, however, nothing happens.

Electric fields affect membrane permeability, and thereby can easily serve to trigger cellular changes. It is possible that this effect can be utilized in the future to enhance orthodontic tooth movement, even if the electrical signals are quite different from those produced by biologic piezoelectricity. If piezoelectric signals were important in producing the bone remodeling associated with orthodontic tooth movement, a vibrating application of pressure would be advantageous. Experiments indicate little or no advantage in vibrating over sustained force for the movement of teeth;[9] in fact, there may be disadvantages.

It appears that piezoelectricity, important as it is for normal skeletal function, probably has little if anything to do with the response to orthodontic tooth movement. One should not conclude from this that other electrical signals could not be used advantageously to alter the events associated with tooth movement. Animal experiments suggest that applying low voltage direct current, a type of signal very different from piezoelectricity, can increase the rate of tooth movement.[10] Perhaps a fair conclusion is that even though piezoelectric signals do not explain tooth movement, electric influences can modify the situation and may yet prove useful therapeutically.

The blood flow theory, the classic theory of tooth movement, relies on chemical rather than electric signals as the stimulus for cellular differentiation and ultimately tooth movement. In this theory, an alteration in blood flow within the periodontal ligament is produced by the sustained pressure that causes the tooth to shift position within the periodontal ligament space, compressing the ligament in some areas while stretching it in others. Blood flow is decreased where the PDL is compressed (Fig. 9-4), while it is maintained or increased where the PDL is under tension (Fig. 9-5). Alterations in blood flow quickly create changes in the chemical environment. For instance, oxygen levels certainly would fall in the compressed area, but might increase on the tension side. The relative proportions of other metabolites would also change in a matter of minutes or hours, and these chemical changes certainly could cause cellular changes.

This theory does explain reasonably well the events associated with tooth movement. It remains the basis for the following discussion.

■ Effects of Force Magnitude

The heavier the pressure, the greater should be the reduction in blood flow through compressed areas of the periodontal ligament, up to the point that the vessels are totally collapsed and no further blood flows (Fig. 9-6). That this theoretic sequence actually occurs has been demonstrated in animal experiments, in which increasing pressure against a tooth causes decreasing perfusion of the PDL on the compression side (see Figs. 9-4 and 9-5). Let us consider the time course of events after application of orthodontic force, contrasting what happens with heavy versus light force (Table 9-2).

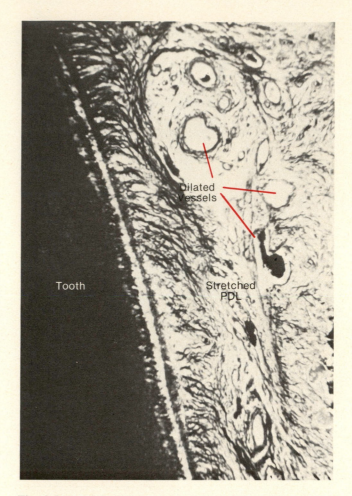

Fig. 9-5 ■ On the side away from the direction of tooth movement, the periodontal ligament space is enlarged and blood vessels dilate. Expanded vessels on the tension side of the periodontal ligament, in an animal perfused at the time of death, are shown here. (Courtesy Dr. F.E. Khouw.)

When light force is applied, blood flow through the partially compressed periodontal ligament decreases in a matter of minutes. Within a few hours at most, the resulting change in the chemical environment produces a different pattern of cellular activity. Animal experiments indicate that increased levels of cyclic AMP, the "second messenger" for many important cellular functions including differentiation, appear after about 4 hours of sustained pressure.[11] This amount of time to produce a response correlates rather well with the human response to removable appliances. If a removable appliance is worn less than 4 to 6 hours per day, it will produce no orthodontic effects. Above this duration threshold, tooth movement does occur.

For the tooth to move, osteoclastic cells must be formed, which will remove bone from the area adjacent to compression of the periodontal ligament. Osteoblasts also must form new bone on the tension side, but the timing of osteoclastic, not osteoblastic, activity is critical. With decreased blood flow, monocytes in the periodontal ligament area are stimulated to form osteoclasts. The first osteoclasts appear within

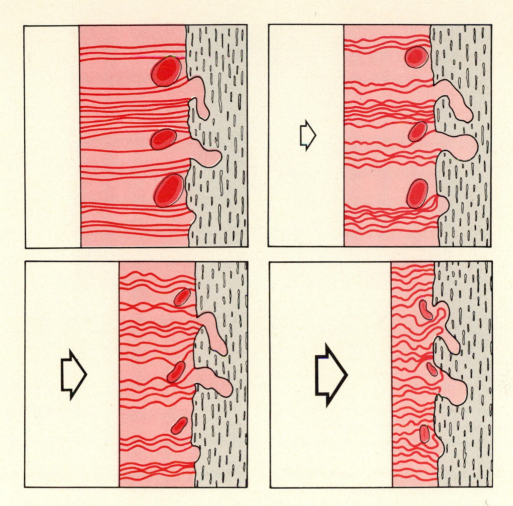

Fig. 9-6 ■ Diagrammatic representation of the increasing compression of blood vessels as pressure within the periodontal ligament increases. At a certain magnitude of continuous pressure, blood vessels are totally occluded and a sterile necrosis of periodontal ligament tissue ensues.

Table 9-2 ■ Physiologic response to sustained pressure against a tooth

Light pressure	Time		Event
		Heavy pressure	
	<1 sec		PDL* fluid imcompressible, alveolar bone bends, piezoelectric signal generated
	1-2 sec		PDL fluid expressed, tooth moves within PDL space
3-5 sec			Blood vessels within PDL partially compressed on pressure side, dilated on tension side
Minutes			Blood flow altered, oxygen tension begins to change
Hours			Metabolic changes occurring
~4 hours			Increased cAMP levels detectable, cellular differentiation begins within PDL
~2 days			Tooth movement beginning as osteoclasts/osteoblasts remodel bony socket
		3-5 sec	Blood vessels within PDL occluded cn pressure side
		Minutes	Blood flow cut off to compressed PDL area
		Hours	Cell death in compressed area
		3-5 days	Cell differentiation in adjacent narrow spaces, undermining resorption begins
		7-14 days	Undermining resorption removes lamina dura adjacent to compressed PDL, tooth movement occurs

*PDL, periodontal ligament.

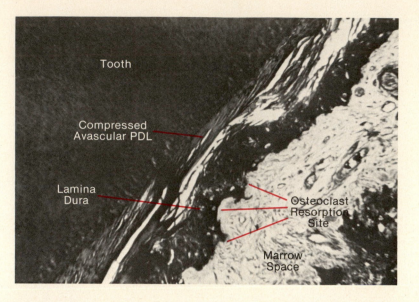

Fig. 9-7 ■ Histologic specimen of compressed periodontal ligament area after several days. When the periodontal ligament is compressed to the point that blood flow is totally cut off, differentiation of osteoclasts within the periodontal ligament space is not possible. After a delay of several days, osteoclasts within adjacent marrow spaces attack the underside of the lamina dura in the process called "undermining resorption." (Courtesy Dr. F.E. Khouw.)

the compressed ligament 36 to 72 hours after force was applied. These cells attack the adjacent lamina dura, removing bone in the process of "frontal resorption," and tooth movement begins.

The course of events is different if forces are great enough to totally occlude blood vessels and cut off the blood supply to an area within the periodontal ligament. When this happens, rather than cells within the PDL being stimulated to develop into osteoclasts, a sterile necrosis ensues within the compressed area. Because of the histologic appearance as the cells disappear, such an avascular area has traditionally been referred to as "hyalinized" (see Fig. 9-4). Despite the name, the process has nothing to do with the formation of hyaline connective tissue, but represents the inevitable loss of all cells when the blood supply is interrupted. When this happens, remodeling of bone adjacent to the necrotic area must be accomplished by cells derived from adjacent undamaged areas.

After a delay of several days, cellular elements from other areas of periodontal ligament begin to invade the necrotic (hyalinized) area. More importantly, osteoclasts differentiate within the adjacent bone marrow spaces and begin an attack on the underside of the bone immediately adjacent to the necrotic PDL area (Fig. 9-7). This process is appropriately described as "undermining resorption," since the attack is from the underside of the lamina dura. When hyalinization and undermining resorption occur, an inevitable delay in tooth movement results. This is caused first by a delay in stimulating differentiation of cells within the marrow spaces, presumably because the chemical stimulus to differentiation must diffuse across the lamina dura; and second, because a considerable thickness of bone must be re-

moved from the underside before tooth movement occurs. The different time course of tooth movement when frontal resorption is compared to undermining resorption is shown graphically in Fig. 9-8.

Not only is tooth movement more efficient when areas of periodontal ligament necrosis are avoided, but pain is also lessened. Clearly, it is better to avoid excessive orthodontic force. However, despite the desirability of producing tooth movement by frontal resorption, it can be extremely difficult to do in clinical practice. Even with light forces, small avascular areas are likely to develop in the PDL and tooth movement will be delayed until these can be removed by undermining resorption. The smooth progression of tooth movement with light force shown in Fig. 9-8 is probably an unattainable ideal. In clinical practice, tooth movement usually proceeds in a more stepwise fashion because of the inevitable areas of undermining resorption. Nevertheless, too much force is not helpful.

■ Effects of Force Distribution and Types of Tooth Movement

From the previous discussion, it is apparent that the optimal force levels for orthodontic tooth movement should be just high enough to partially but not completely occlude blood vessels in the periodontal ligament. Both the amount of force delivered to a tooth and also the area of the periodontal ligament over which that force is distributed are important. The PDL response is determined not by force alone, but by force per unit area, or pressure. Since the distribution of force within the PDL, and therefore the pressure, differs with different types of tooth movement, it is necessary to specify the type of tooth movement as well as

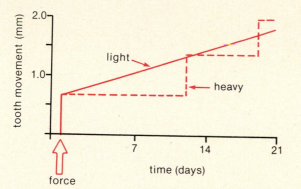

Fig. 9-8 ■ Diagrammatic representation of the time course of tooth movement with frontal resorption versus undermining resorption. With frontal resorption, a steady attack on the outer surface of the lamina dura results in smooth continuous tooth movement. With undermining resorption, there is a delay until the bone adjacent to the tooth can be removed. At that point, the tooth "jumps" to a new position, and if heavy force is maintained, there will again be a delay until a second round of undermining resorption can occur.

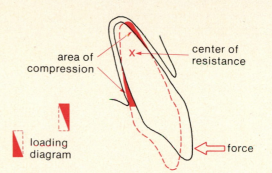

Fig. 9-9 ■ Application of a single force to the crown of a tooth creates rotation around a point approximately halfway down the root. Heavy pressure is felt at the root apex and at the crest of the alveolar bone, but pressure decreases to zero at the center of resistance. The loading diagram, therefore, consists of two triangles as shown.

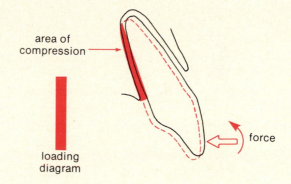

Fig. 9-10 ■ Translation or bodily movement of a tooth requires that the periodontal ligament space be loaded uniformly from alveolar crest to apex, creating a rectangular loading diagram. Twice as much force applied to the crown of the tooth would be required to produce the same pressure within the PDL for bodily movement as compared to tipping.

the amount of force in discussing optimal force levels for orthodontic purposes.

The simplest form of orthodontic movement is tipping. Tipping movements are produced when a single force (for instance, a spring extending from a removable appliance) is applied against the crown of a tooth. When this is done, the tooth rotates around its "center of resistance," a point located about halfway down the root. (A further discussion of the center of resistance and its control follows in Chapter 10.) When the tooth rotates in this fashion, the periodontal ligament is compressed near the root apex on the same side as the spring, and at the crest of the alveolar bone on the opposite side from the spring (Fig. 9-9). Maximum pressure in the PDL is created at the alveolar crest and at the root apex. Progressively less pressure is created as the center of resistance is approached, and there is minimum pressure at that point.

In tipping, only one-half the PDL area that could be loaded actually is. As shown in Fig. 9-9, the "loading diagram" consists of two triangles, covering half the total PDL area. On the other hand, pressure in the two areas where it is concentrated is high in relation to the force applied to the crown. For this reason, forces used to tip teeth must be kept quite low. Both experiments with animals and clinical experience with humans suggest that tipping forces should not exceed approximately 50 gm.

If two forces are applied simultaneously to the crown of a tooth, the tooth can be moved bodily (translated), i.e., the root apex and crown move in the same direction the same amount. In this case, the total periodontal ligament area is loaded uniformly (Fig. 9-10). It is apparent that to produce the same pressure in the PDL and therefore the same biologic response, twice as much force would be required for bodily movement as for tipping. To move a tooth

so that it was partially tipped and partially translated would require forces intermediate between those needed for pure tipping and bodily movement (Table 9-3).

In theory, forces to produce rotation of a tooth around its long axis could be much larger than those to produce other tooth movements, since it might be possible to distribute the force over the entire periodontal ligament rather than a narrow vertical strip. In fact, however, it is essentially impossible to apply a rotational force so that the tooth does not also tip in its socket, and when this happens, an area of severe compression is created, just as in any other tipping movement. For this reason, appropriate forces for rotation are relatively low, intermediate between those for pure tipping and bodily movement.

Extrusion and intrusion are also special cases. Extrusive movements ideally would produce no areas of compression within the periodontal ligament, only tension. Like rotation, this is probably more a theoretic than a practical possibility,

Table 9-3 ■ Optimal forces for orthodontic tooth movement

Type of movement	Force* (gm)
Tipping	50-75
Bodily movement (translation)	100-150
Root uprighting	75-125
Rotation	50-100
Extrusion	50-100
Intrusion	15-25

*Values depend in part on the size of the tooth; smaller values appropriate for incisors, higher values for posterior teeth.

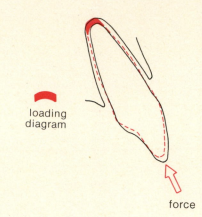

loading
diagram

force

Fig. 9-11 ■ When a tooth is intruded, the force is concentrated over a small area at the apex. For this reason, extremely light forces are needed to produce appropriate pressure within the periodontal ligament during intrusion.

since if the tooth tipped at all while being extruded, areas of compression would be created. Even if compressed areas could be avoided, heavy forces in pure tension would be undesirable unless the goal was to extract the tooth rather than to bring alveolar bone along with the tooth. Extrusive forces should be of about the same magnitude as those for tipping.

For many years, it was considered essentially impossible to produce orthodontic intrusion of teeth. Clinically successful intrusion has been demonstrated in recent years, and it has become clear that doing this requires careful control of force magnitude so that very light forces are applied to the teeth. The reason is that intrusive force will be concentrated in a small area at the tooth apex (Fig. 9-11). As with extrusion, the tooth probably will tip somewhat as it is intruded, but the loading diagram nevertheless will show high force concentration at the apex. Only if the force is kept very light, can intrusion be expected.

■ Effects of Force Duration and Force Decay

The key to producing orthodontic tooth movement is the application of sustained force, which does not mean that the force must be absolutely continuous. It does mean that the force must be present for a considerable percentage of the time, certainly hours rather than minutes per day. As indicated previously, animal experiments suggest that only after force is maintained for approximately 4 hours do cyclic nucleotide levels in the periodontal ligament increase, indicating that this duration of pressure is required to produce the "second messengers" needed to stimulate cellular differentiation.

Clinical experience suggests that there is a threshold for force duration in humans, probably at about 6 hours, and that increasingly effective tooth movement is produced if force is maintained for longer durations. Although no firm experimental data are available, a plot of efficiency of tooth movement as a function of force duration would probably look like Fig. 9-12. Continuous forces, produced by fixed appliances that are not affected by what the patient does, produce the most efficient tooth movement. Removable appliances present almost all the time are almost as effective, but removable appliances worn for decreasing fractions of time produce decreasing amounts of tooth movement.

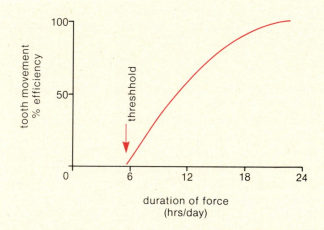

Fig. 9-12 ■ Theoretic plot of tooth movement efficiency versus duration of force in hours per day. Continuous force, 24 hours per day, produces the most efficient tooth movement, but successful tooth movement can be produced by shorter durations, with a threshold at about 6 hours.

Duration of force has another aspect, related to how force magnitude changes as the tooth responds by moving. Only in theory is it possible to produce a perfect spring, one that would deliver the same continuous force day after day, no matter how much or how little the tooth moved in response to that force. In reality, every spring has a rate of decay. Some decline in force magnitude is noted with even the springiest device. After the tooth has moved even a short distance, the force delivered by some mechanisms may drop all the way to zero. From this perspective, orthodontic force duration is classified (Fig. 9-13) by the rate of decay as:

Continuous—force maintained at some appreciable fraction of the original from one patient visit to the next

Interrupted—force levels decline steadily to zero between activations

Intermittent—force levels decline abruptly to zero intermittently, when the orthodontic appliance is removed by the patient.

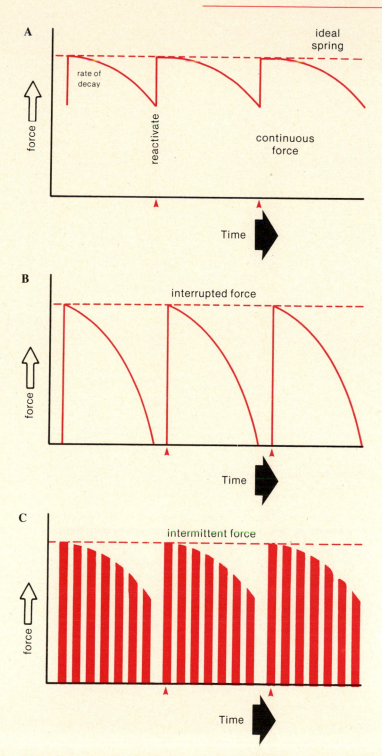

Fig. 9-13 ■ Diagrammatic representation of force decay. **A,** An ideal spring would maintain the same amount of force regardless of the distance a tooth had moved. Forces that are maintained between activations of an orthodontic appliance, even though the force declines, are defined as continuous. In contrast, **B,** interrupted forces drop to zero between activations. **C,** Intermittent forces fall to zero when a removable appliance is taken out, only to resume when the appliance is reinserted into the mouth.

Both continuous and interrupted forces can be produced by fixed appliances that are constantly present.

Intermittent forces are produced by all patient-activated appliances, such as removable plates, headgear, and elastics. Forces generated during normal function can be viewed as a special case of intermittently applied forces, most of which are not maintained for enough hours per day to have significant effects on the position of the teeth.

There is an important interaction between force magnitude and how rapidly the force declines as the tooth responds. Consider first the effect of a nearly continuous force. If this force is quite light, there will be a relatively smooth progression of tooth movement resulting from frontal resorption. If the continuous force is heavy, however, tooth movement will be delayed until undermining resorption can remove the bone necessary to allow the tooth movement. At that time, the tooth will change its position rapidly, and the constant force will again compress the tissues, preventing repair of the periodontal ligament and creating the need for further undermining resorption, and so on. Such a heavy continuous force can be quite destructive, to both the periodontal structures and the tooth itself (see the following discussion).

Consider now the effect of forces that decay fairly rapidly, so that the force declines to zero after the tooth moves only a short distance. If the initial force level is relatively light, the tooth will move a small amount by frontal resorption and then will remain in that position until the appliance is activated again. If the force level is heavy enough to produce undermining resorption, the tooth will move when the undermining resorption is complete. Then, since the force has dropped to zero at that point, it will remain in that position until the next activation. Although the original force is heavy, after the tooth movement there is a period for regeneration and repair of the PDL before force is applied again.

Theoretically, there is no doubt that light continuous forces produce the most efficient tooth movement. Despite the clinician's best efforts to keep forces light enough to produce only frontal resorption, some areas of undermining resorption are probably produced in every clinical patient. The heavier forces that produce this response are physiologically acceptable, only if force levels decline so that there is a period of repair and regeneration before the next activation, or at least if the force decreases to the point that no second and third rounds of undermining resorption occur.

Heavy continuous forces are to be avoided; heavy intermittent forces, though less efficient, can be clinically acceptable. To say it another way: the more perfect the spring in the sense of its ability to provide continuous force, the more careful the clinician must be that only light force is applied. Some of the cruder springs used in orthodontic treatment have the paradoxic virtue of producing forces that rapidly decline to zero and are thus incapable of inflicting the biologic damage that can occur from heavy continuous forces.

Undermining resorption requires 7 to 14 days (longer on the initial application of force, shorter thereafter). When this is the mode of tooth movement and when force levels decline rapidly, tooth movement is essentially complete in this length of time. Experience has shown that orthodontic appliances should not be reactivated more frequently than at 3-week intervals. A 4-week appointment cycle is more typical in clinical practice. The wisdom of this interval between adjustments now becomes clear. If the appliance is springy and light forces produce continuous frontal resorption, there is no need for further activation. If the appliance is stiffer and undermining resorption occurs, but then the force drops to zero, the tooth movement occurs in the first 10 days or so, and there is an equal or longer period for periodontal ligament regeneration and repair before force is applied again. This repair phase is highly desirable, and needed with many appliances. Activating an appliance too frequently, short circuiting the rapair process, can produce damage to the teeth or bone that a longer appointment cycle would have prevented or at least minimized.

■ *Deleterious Effects of Orthodontic Force*

■ Effects on the Pulp

In theory, the application of light sustained force to the crown of a tooth should produce a periodontal ligament reaction but should have little if any effect on the pulp. In fact, although pulpal reactions to orthodontic treatment are minimal, there is probably a modest and transient inflammatory response within the pulp, at least at the beginning of treatment.[12] This may contribute to the discomfort that patients often experience for a few days after appliances are activated, but the mild pulpitis has no long-term significance.

There are occasional reports of loss of tooth vitality during orthodontic treatment. Rarely, this reaction occurs for no apparent reason. Usually, however, poor control of orthodontic force is the culprit. If a tooth is subjected to extremely heavy continuous force, a sequence of abrupt movements occurs, as undermining resorption allows increasingly large increments of change. Such highly traumatic movements could sever the blood vessels as they enter the root apex. Loss of vitality has also been observed when incisor teeth were tipped distally to such an extent that the root apex, moving in the opposite direction, was actually moved outside the alveolar process. Again, such movements would sever the blood vessels entering the pulp canal (Fig. 9-14).

Since the response of the periodontal ligament, not the pulp, is the key element in orthodontic tooth movement, moving endodontically treated teeth is perfectly feasible. Especially in adults receiving adjunctive orthodontic treatment (see Chapter 18), it may be necessary to treat some teeth endodontically, and then reposition them orthodontically. There is no contraindication to this practice. Some

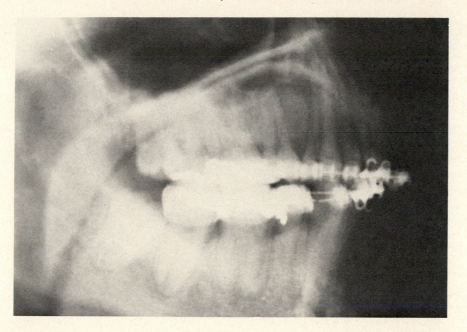

Fig. 9-14 ■ Extreme tipping of maxillary incisor teeth from excessive and poorly controlled orthodontic forces. In this patient, the apex of all four maxillary incisors was carried through the labial cortical plate, and pulp vitality was lost.

evidence indicates that endodontically treated teeth are slightly more prone to root resorption during orthodontics than are teeth with normal vitality.[13] In evaluating this finding, it should be kept in mind that in general, endodontically treated teeth are more prone to root resorption. Severe root resorption should not be expected as a consequence of moving a nonvital tooth that has had proper endodontic therapy.

■ Effects on Root Structure

Orthodontic treatment requires resorption and apposition of bone adjacent to the root structure of teeth. For many years, it was thought that the root structure of the teeth was not remodeled in the same way as bone. More recent research has made it plain that when orthodontic forces are applied, there is usually an attack on the cementum of the root, just as there is an attack on adjacent bone.[14] Root remodeling, in other words, is a constant feature of orthodontic tooth movement, a finding that does not mean that permanent loss of root structure must necessarily occur during orthodontic treatment. A careful examination of the root surface of teeth that have been moved orthodontically reveals areas of resorption of both cementum and dentin of the root (Fig. 9-15). These areas tend to fill in with new cementum, so that the original form of the root is retained. It appears that cementum (and dentin, if resorption penetrates through the cementum) is removed from the root surface while active force is present, then cementum is restored during periods of relative quiescence.

Only if the attack on the root surface produces large defects at the apex that eventually become separated from the root surface is repair of the damaged root impossible.

Once an island of cementum or dentin has been cut totally free from the root surface, it will be resorbed and will not be replaced. On the other hand, even deep defects in the form of craters into the root surface will be filled in again with cementum once orthodontic movement stops. Therefore, permanent loss of root structure related to orthodontic treatment occurs only at the apex.

Despite the potential for repair, careful radiographic examination of individuals who have undergone orthodontic treatment shows some loss of root length in nearly every patient. Some teeth are more prone to root resorption than others: maxillary central and lateral incisors, mandibular incisors, and mandibular first molars are more likely to lose root length than other teeth (Table 9-4). In almost all patients, however, the loss of root structure is minimal and clinically insignificant.

For a few patients, the risk of permanent root shortening during orthodontic treatment is much greater. Above-

Table 9-4 ■ Average root length change during premolar extraction treatment

	Maxillary	*Mandibular*
Central incisor	−2.0 mm	−1.0 mm
Lateral incisor	−2.5 mm	−1.5 mm
Canine	−1.5 mm	−1.0 mm
Second premolar	−1.5 mm	−1.5 mm
First molar	−1.0 mm	−1.5 mm
Second molar	0	−1.5 mm

From Kennedy, D.B. et al. Am. J. Orthod. **84**:183, 1983.

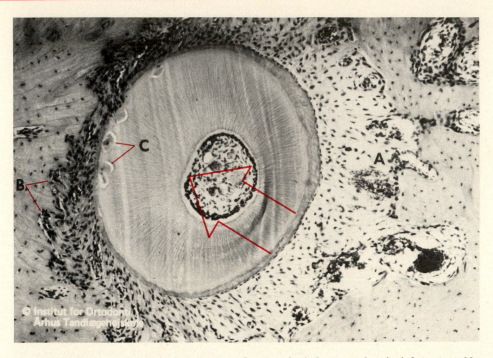

Fig. 9-15 ■ Coronal section through the root of a premolar being moved to the left *(arrow)*. Note the zone of periodontal ligament compression to the left and tension to the right. Dilation of blood vessels and osteoblastic activity **(A)** can be seen on the right. Osteoclasts removing bone are present on the left **(B).** Areas of beginning root resorption that will be repaired by later deposition of cementum also can be seen on the left **(C).** (Courtesy Prof. B. Melsen.)

average resorption can be anticipated if the teeth have conical roots with pointed apices, distorted tooth form (dilaceration),[15] or a history of severe trauma (whether or not endodontic treatment was required).[16]

Excessive force during orthodontic treatment increases the risk of root resorption, particularly if heavy continuous forces are used. Prolonged duration of orthodontic treatment also increases the amount of resorption. Occasionally, loss of one-third or one-half the root structure is observed in patients who received only routine orthodontic therapy (Fig. 9-16). Some individuals are prone to root resorption, even without orthodontic treatment. If there is evidence of root resorption before orthodontic treatment, the patient is at considerable risk of further resorption during orthodontic treatment, much more so than a patient with no pretreatment resorption. Although various hormonal imbalances and other metabolic derangements have been suspected in these susceptible patients, little evidence supports these theories. Why a few patients are extremely susceptible to root resorption simply remains unknown.

■ Effects of Treatment on the Height of Alveolar Bone

At the root apex, if the balance between apposition and resorption of the root surface tips too far toward resorption, irreversible shortening of the root may occur. It seems logical to suspect that this might also happen at the alveolar bone crest, and that another effect of orthodontic treatment might

be loss of alveolar bone height. Since the presence of orthodontic appliances increases the amount of gingival inflammation, even with good hygiene, this potential side effect of treatment would seem even more likely. Careful examination of patients who have undergone orthodontic treatment shows that a very small but measurable reduction in alveolar crest height does occur. Loss of alveolar crest height in one large series of patients averaged less than 0.5 mm and almost never exceeded 1 mm.[17] Fortunately, excessive loss of crestal bone height is almost never seen as a complication of orthodontic treatment. Adults who have had bone loss from periodontal disease can have orthodontic treatment, if the periodontal disease is well controlled. (See Chapter 19.)

The relationship between the position of a tooth and alveolar bone height can be seen clearly when teeth erupt too much or too little. A supraerupted tooth carries alveolar bone with it, often for considerable distances. In the absence of pathology, a tooth that erupts too much simply does not gradually move itself out of the bone. On the other hand, unless a tooth erupts into an area of the dental arch, alveolar bone will not form there. If a tooth is congenitally absent or extracted at an early age, a permanent defect in the alveolar bone will occur unless another tooth is moved into the area relatively rapidly. This finding becomes an argument against very early extraction, as for instance, the enucleation of an unerupted premolar. Early removal of teeth poses a risk of creating an alveolar bone defect that cannot

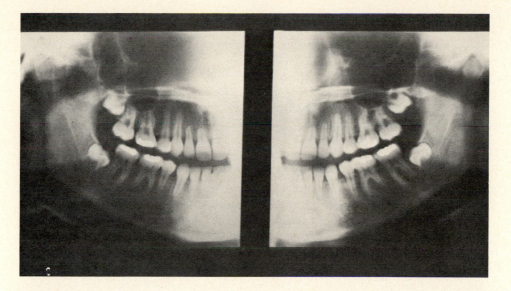

Fig. 9-16 ■ Resorption of incisor or other roots occasionally accompanies routine orthodontic therapy, for no apparent reason, as in this patient. Some individuals appear unusually susceptible to root resorption.

be overcome by later orthodontic treatment.

The same effects on alveolar bone height are seen with orthodontic extrusion as with eruption: as long as the orthodontic treatment is carried out with reasonable force levels and reasonable speed of tooth movement, a tooth brought into the dental arch by extrusive orthodontic forces will bring alveolar bone with it. The height of the bone attachment along the root will be about the same at the conclusion of movement as at the beginning. If a tooth is intruded, bone height tends to be lost at the alveolar crest, so that about the same percentage of the root remains embedded in bone as before, even if the intrusion was over a considerable distance.

In most circumstances, this tendency for alveolar bone height to stay at the same level along the root is a therapeutic plus. Occasionally, it would be desirable to change the amount of tooth embedded in bone. For instance, it would be nice to be able to improve the bone support around periodontally involved teeth by intruding the teeth and forcing the roots deeper into the bone. There are a few reports of therapeutic benefit from intruding periodontally involved teeth, but lack of soft tissue reattachment and simultaneous reduction of alveolar crest height prevent dramatic improvement. On occasion, it is desirable to elongate the root of a fractured tooth, to make it possible to use it as a prosthetic abutment without crown-lengthening surgery. If heavy forces are used to extrude a tooth quickly, a relative loss of attachment may occur, and this deliberately nonphysiologic type of extrusion may be helpful for a few adult patients (see Chapter 19). As a general rule, however, physiologic extrusion or intrusion that keeps the alveolar bone height at the same level is desirable.

■ Pain and Mobility Related to Orthodontic Treatment

If heavy pressure is applied to a tooth, pain develops almost immediately as the periodontal ligament is literally crushed. There is no excuse for using force levels for orthodontic tooth movement that produce immediate pain of this type. If appropriate orthodontic force is applied, the patient feels little or nothing immediately. Several hours later, however, pain usually appears. The patient feels a mild aching sensation, and the teeth are quite sensitive to pressure, so that biting a hard object hurts. The pain typically lasts for 2 to 4 days, then disappears until the orthodontic appliance is reactivated. At that point, a similar cycle may recur.

The source of the pain appears to be the creation of ischemic areas within the periodontal ligament, probably areas that will undergo sterile necrosis (hyalinization). The increased tenderness to pressure suggests inflammation at the apex, and the mild pulpitis that usually appears soon after orthodontic force is applied probably contributes to this. There does seem to be a relationship between the amount of force used and the amount of pain: the greater the force, the greater the pain, all other factors being equal. It is commonly noted that pain of any type involves a great deal of individual variation, and this observation is certainly true for the response to orthodontic treatment. Some patients report little or no pain even with relatively heavy forces, whereas others experience considerable discomfort with quite light forces.

If the source of pain is the development of ischemic areas, strategies to temporarily relieve pressure and allow blood flow through compressed areas should help. In fact, if light forces are used, the amount of pain experienced by patients can be decreased by having them engage in repetitive chewing (of gum, a plastic wafer placed between the teeth, or whatever) during the first 8 hours after the orthodontic appliance is activated. There is no doubt that this technique works clinically. Presumably the effect results from temporarily displacing the teeth enough to allow some blood flow through compressed areas, thereby preventing buildup of metabolic products that stimulate pain receptors. Light forces, however, are the key to avoiding pain as a concomitant of orthodontic treatment.

Orthodontic tooth movement requires not only a remodeling of bone adjacent to the teeth, but also a reorganization of the periodontal ligament itself. Fibers become detached from the bone and cemental surfaces, then reattach at a later time. Radiographically, it can be observed that the PDL space widens during orthodontic tooth movement. The combination of a wider ligament space and a somewhat disorganized ligament means that an increase in mobility will be observed in every patient.

A moderate increase in mobility is an expected response to orthodontic treatment. The heavier the orthodontic forces, however, the greater the amount of undermining resorption expected, and the greater the mobility that will develop. Excessive mobility is an indication that excessive forces were used. If a tooth becomes extremely mobile during orthodontic treatment, all force should be discontinued until the mobility decreases to moderate levels. Unlike root resorption, excessive mobility will usually correct itself without permanent damage.

Skeletal Effects of Orthodontic Force

In the early years of the twentieth century, orthodontists were confident that orthodontic treatment could modify jaw proportions as well as dental relationships. Early cephalometric studies demonstrated that skeletal effects from intraoral forces were much less than those the orthodontic pioneers had expected and taken for granted. Just as the effectiveness of orthodontic appliances in producing skeletal change had become an article of faith earlier, it became the accepted dogma by midcentury that orthodontic treatment effects were limited to the dentoalveolar process. If the 1920s represented a peak of optimism about the possible skeletal effects of orthodontic treatment and the 1950s the depths of pessimism about skeletal change, one might expect a 30-year cycle to produce a new height of optimism in the 1980s.

In recent years, new concepts of facial developments, notably the functional matrix theory discussed in more detail in Chapter 2, have provided a stronger theoretic rationale for growth modification treatment than ever existed before, and it has been demonstrated clinically that changes in the pattern of facial growth can be produced by orthodontic treatment. Orthodontic forces are indeed felt at sites distant from the teeth and can have important therapeutic benefits at these remote locations. The possibilities for inducing skeletal change are discussed in Chapter 7; the biologic principles underlying these clinical guidelines are discussed more fully here.

■ Effects on the Maxilla and Midface

During normal development, the maxilla grows in size as new bone is added at the sutures that attach it to the zygoma, the pterygoid plates, and the frontonasal area. Bone is added when growth in other areas literally pulls the sutures apart. An additional force pulling the sutures apart should create a stimulus to additional growth, whereas forces tending to prevent the bones from separating should serve to restrain or redirect growth. This, in fact, is exactly what happens when heavy forces applied to the teeth radiate outward to be felt at locations where bone growth is occurring (Fig. 9-17).

The sutures of the maxilla are similar in some respects to the periodontal ligament, but are neither as complex in their structure nor nearly as densely collaginous. It is difficult to measure pressure at the sutures, although it is easy to demonstrate that when the PDL is compressed, force will be transmitted to them. Clinical experience suggests that forces against the upper teeth as light as 300-400 gm total (6-8 oz per side) can retard and redirect maxillary growth. The amount of pressure at the sutures is only a fraction of the pressure within the PDL because the suture area is so much larger.

Both animal experiments and experience with patients suggest that force levels to separate the sutures in a way that leads to apposition of new bone must be much greater than those to retard growth. Although maxillary growth can be restrained by relatively small force levels, it is difficult to produce forward displacement of the maxilla with a "re-

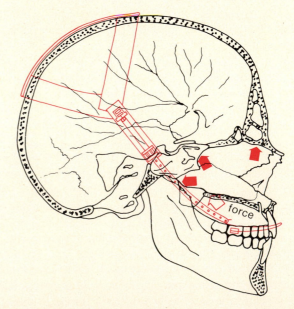

Fig. 9-17 ■ Extraoral force applied to the maxillary teeth radiates to the sutures of the maxilla, where it can affect the pattern of skeletal maxillary growth.

verse headgear'' that pulls the maxilla forward. To separate the midpalatal suture in prepubertal children requires about 1000 gm, and 2000 gm is needed in adolescence.[18] Obviously, greater force would be needed to move the entire maxilla.

The difficulty in stimulating the entire maxilla to grow forward probably reflects our inability to produce the necessary force levels at the sutures to separate them, but probably is also conditioned by the extent of interdigitation of bony spicules across the sutural lines. As sutures become more and more highly interdigitated with increasing age, it becomes more and more difficult to separate them without producing crushing force against some areas of the suture. An analogy can be drawn to the difficulty of extruding a tooth without tipping it in its socket so that some area of the PDL is strongly compressed. With a long and complexly structured suture, of course, this would be even more difficult.

The response of sutures to orthodontic force is analogous to the periodontal ligament response in another sense, in that the duration (hours per day) of force necessary to produce a response seems to be similar. Clinical experience suggests that if anything, the threshold to produce a skeletal response may be higher and the response curve flatter, i.e., once the threshold is reached, more time produces less dramatic improvements than with tooth movement, but this is difficult to quantitate. Skeletal changes can be produced with 8 to 10 hours per day of force application. Below that, little response can be expected.

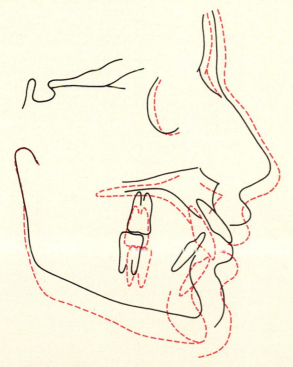

Fig. 9-18 ■ Cephalometric superimposition showing growth modification produced by extraoral force to the maxilla. Note that the maxilla has moved downward and backward, not in the expected downward and forward direction shown by the mandible.

Often it is desirable to produce as much skeletal effect as possible, while minimizing tooth movement. When force is applied to the teeth, regardless of whether dental effects desired, it is impossible to avoid some tooth movement. Forces applied against the teeth when skeletal change is desired should be relatively heavy (500-1000 gm) if they are to have appreciable effects at distant locations. As indicated previously, heavy continuous forces can create damage to both root and periodontal structures. Heavy intermittent forces are a less effective way to induce tooth movement, probably because the stimulus for undermining resorption is diluted during the times that the heavy force is removed.

For this reason, if maximal skeletal but minimal dental change is desired, full-time wear of a headgear or other device to restrain maxillary growth is unwise. If the patient wears a headgear 12 to 16 hours per day, a considerable skeletal effect can be produced (Fig. 9-18). Some tooth movement will certainly occur also, but the amount of tooth movement is much less than would be seen with 24-hour wear, while the skeletal effect produced by 24-hour wear is not that much greater than the effect produced by 12 to 16 hours. Sometimes extraoral force is used with the aim of promoting tooth movement, and then, of course, the force levels should be lighter and the duration of wear longer.

Theoretically, it should be possible to produce skeletal effects by applying force directly against the jaw, bypassing the teeth entirely. Experiments with implants placed directly in the bones of experimental animals[19] have demonstrated that this can be done. Whether similar implants in human patients would ever be feasible is doubtful, even in exceptional instances. It is possible, however, that an ankylosed primary molar could be used like an implant to deliver force that would produce a purely skeletal response. Deliberately inducing ankylosis of primary molars during the mixed dentition and then applying headgear to these teeth might be possible. Eventually, the primary molar would resorb or would have to be extracted, but its permanent successor would be unharmed. Inducing ankylosis of a permanent tooth, on the other hand, would never be feasible because vertical growth, and with it the continuing eruption of the permanent teeth, continues into the late teens. If ankylosis of a permanent tooth occurred before vertical growth was completed, this tooth would end up out of occlusion in adult life.

Further research is needed to explore this presently entirely theoretic approach. Whether it will become a practical clinical procedure in the future remains to be seen.

■ Effects on the Mandible

The attachment of the mandible to the rest of the facial skeleton via the temporomandibular joint is very different from the sutural attachment of the maxilla. The response of the mandible to force transmitted to the joint is also quite different.

Efforts to restrain mandibular growth by applying a compressive force to the mandibular condyle have been largely unsuccessful. The problem may be related to a different mechanism of growth control of the mandible or may result from the difficulty of creating appropriate force levels within the joint.

A restraining force applied at the chin can be directed upward and backward to the temporomandibular joint. However, there are two problems in loading the growing surfaces within the joint. The first is that the presence of the articular disk complicates the situation, making it difficult to determine exactly what areas are being loaded. The second, perhaps more important, is that the geometry of the rounded joint surfaces makes it difficult to load the entire area (Fig. 9-19). A force aimed at the top of the condyle might well restrain growth there, but growth only a few millimeters away would be unaffected, since that area would experience little or no force. If the force were aimed at the back of the condyle, the top would be minimally affected. Animal experiments suggest that restraining forces may cause remodeling within the temporal fossa. Despite the theoretic possibility of mandibular growth restraint, it is difficult to demonstrate significant clinical effects in humans.

On the other hand, the condyle translates forward away from the temporal bone during normal function, and the mandible can be pulled into a protruded position and held there with minimal force. Arguments have raged for many years over whether holding the mandible in a protruded position causes stimulation or acceleration of growth. Contemporary research indicates that accelerated growth does occur when the mandible is constantly protruded. There are two mechanisms for protrusion. One is passive, that is, the mandible is held forward by some apparatus. The other is active, that is, the mandible is held forward by the protrusive muscles, including the lateral pterygoid. Some research suggests that activation of the lateral pterygoid is a key to stimulation of growth,[20] implying that active rather than passive protrusion would be desired for maximal growth effects. Why active protrusion should produce a greater effect, if indeed it does, is unknown.

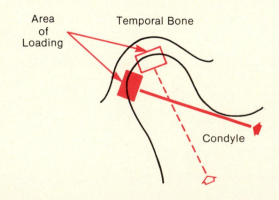

Fig. 9-19 ■ Extraoral force aimed at the condyle of the mandible tends to load only a small portion of the rounded surface, which is one explanation for the relative ineffectiveness of this type of attempted growth modification.

Holding the mandible forward passively requires a force of a few hundred gm. If this force is distributed to the maxillary and mandibular teeth, a force system is created which would move the upper teeth backward, move the lower teeth forward, and restrain maxillary growth. All these responses, in addition to changes in the pattern of mandibular growth, can be seen when appliances that hold the mandible forward are used. To maximize skeletal effects and minimize dental effects, it is clear that the reactive forces should be kept away from the teeth, in so far as possible. It is probably for this reason that the tissue-borne Frankel appliance (discussed in more detail in Chapter 14) seems capable of producing the greatest amount of skeletal change in proportion to dental change.

■ *References*

1. Ten Cate, A.R.: The role of fibroblasts in the remodeling of periodontal ligament during physiologic tooth movement. Am. J. Orthod. **69**:155-168, 1976.
2. Bonucci, E.: New knowledge on the origin, function and fate of osteoclasts. Clin. Orthoped. **158**:252-269, 1981.
3. Burch, J.G., and Paterson, R.: Intra-arch dimensional changes of the mandible during jaw movement. San Francisco, 1968, 46th General meeting, International Association for Dental Research Abstract 561.
4. Proffit, W.R.: Equilibrium theory revisited: factors influencing position of the teeth. Angle Orthod. **48**:175-186, 1978.
5. Thomas, N.R.: The process and mechanism of tooth eruption. Bristol, 1965, Ph.D. Thesis, Bristol University.
6. Weinstein, S., et al.: On an equilibrium theory of tooth position. Angle Orthod. **33**:1-26, 1963.
7. Baumrind, S.: A reconsideration of the propriety of the "pressure-tension" hypothesis. Am. J. Orthod. **55**:12-22, 1969.
8. Giannelly, A.A.: Force-induced changes in the vascularity of the periodontal ligament. Am. J. Orthod. **55**:5-11, 1969.
9. Shapiro, E.: Orthodontic movement using pulsating force-induced piezoelectricity. Am. J. Orthod. **73**:59-66, 1979.
10. Davidovitch, Z., et al.: Electric currents, bone remodeling, and orthodontic tooth movement. II. Increase in rate of tooth movement and periodontal cyclic nucleotide levels by combined force and electric current. Am. J. Orthod. **77**:33-47, 1980.
11. Davidovitch, Z., and Shamfield, J.L.: Cyclic nucleotide levels in alveolar bone of orthodontically treated cats. Arch. Oral Biol. **20**:567-574, 1975.
12. Anstendig, H., and Kronman, J.: A histologic study of pulpal reaction to orthodontic tooth movement in dogs. Angle Orthod. **42**:50-55, 1972.
13. Wickwire, N.A., et al.: The effects of tooth movement upon endodontically treated teeth. Angle Orthod. **44**:235-242, 1974.
14. Reitan, K.: Biomechanical principles and reactions: In Graber, T.M., and Swain, B.F.: Orthodontics: Current Principles and Technique. St. Louis, 1985, The C.V. Mosby Co.
15. Phillips, J.R.: Apical root resorption under orthodontic therapy. Angle Orthod. **25**:1-22, 1955.
16. Hines, F.B.: A radiographic evaluation of the response of previously avulsed teeth and partially avulsed teeth to orthodontic movement. Am. J. Orthod. **75**:1-18, 1979.

17. Kennedy, D.B., et al.: The effect of extraction and orthodontic treatment on dentoalveolar support. Am. J. Orthod. **84:**183-190, 1983.

18. Hicks, E.: Slow maxillary expansion: a clinical study of the skeletal versus dental response to low-magnitude force. Am. J. Orthod. **73:**121, 1978.

19. Turley, P.: The loading of bioglass implants to produce pre-maxillary expansion in *M. mulatta*. 1978, MSD Thesis, University of Washington.

20. Petrovic, A.: Control processes in the postnatal growth of the condylar cartilage of the mandible. In McNamara, J.A., editor: Determinants of Mandibular Form and Growth, Ann Arbor, 1975, University of Michigan Center for Human Growth and Development.

Chapter 10

Mechanical Principles in Orthodontic Force Control

Optimal orthodontic tooth movement is produced by light, continuous force. The challenge in designing and using an orthodontic appliance is to produce a force system with these characteristics, creating forces that are neither too great nor too variable over time. It is particularly important that the light forces do not decrease rapidly, decaying away either because the material itself loses its elasticity or because a small amount of tooth movement causes a larger change in the amount of force delivered. Both the behavior of elastic materials and mechanical factors in the response of the teeth must be considered in the design of an orthodontic appliance system through which mechanotherapy is delivered.

■ *Elastic Materials and the Production of Orthodontic Force*

■ The Basic Properties of Elastic Materials

The elastic behavior of any material is defined in terms of its stress-strain response to an external load. Both stress and strain refer to the internal state of the material being studied: stress is the internal distribution of the load, defined as force per unit area, whereas strain is the internal distortion produced by the load, defined as deflection per unit length.

For analysis purposes, orthodontic archwires and springs can be considered as beams, supported either only on one end (for example, a spring projecting from a removable appliance) or on both ends (the segment of an archwire spanning between attachments on adjacent teeth) (Fig. 10-1). If a force is applied to such a beam, its response can be measured as the deflection (bending or twisting) produced by the force (Fig. 10-2). Force and deflection are external measurements. Internal stress and strain can be calculated from force and deflection by including the considerations of area and length of the beam.

For orthodontic purposes, three major properties of beam materials are critical in defining their clinical usefulness: strength, stiffness/springiness, and range. Each can be defined by appropriate reference to a force-deflection or stress-strain diagram (Figs. 10-2 and 10-3).

Three different points on a stress-strain diagram can be taken as representative of the strength of a material (Fig. 10-3). Each represents, in a somewhat different way, the

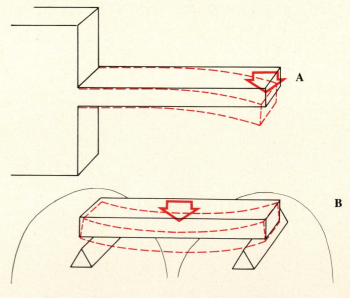

Fig. 10-1 ■ Cantilever (**A**) and supported (**B**) beams.

maximum load that the material can resist. The most conservative measure is the proportional limit (also called the elastic limit), the point at which any permanent deformation is first observed. A more practical indicator is the point at which a deformation of 0.1% is measured; this is defined as the yield strength. The maximum load the wire can sustain, the ultimate tensile strength, is reached after some permanent deformation and is greater than yield strength. Since this ultimate strength determines the maximum force the wire can deliver if used as a spring, it is important clinically, especially since yield strength and ultimate strength differ much more for the newer titanium alloys than for steel wires. Strength is measured in stress units (gm/cm²).

Stiffness and springiness are reciprocal properties:

$$\text{Springiness} = 1/\text{Stiffness}.$$

Each is proportional to the slope of the elastic portion of the force-deflection curve (Fig. 10-2). The more horizontal the slope, the springier the wire; the more vertical the slope, the stiffer the wire.

Range is usually determined from the 0.1% offset point on the force-deflection diagram. It is defined as the distance that the wire will bend elastically before permanent deformation occurs. This distance, of course, is measured in millimeters (or other length units) (Fig. 10-2). If the wire is deflected beyond its yield strength, it will not return to its original shape, but clinically useful springback will occur unless the failure point is reached. This springback is measured along a segment of the horizontal axis to the right of the range, as shown in Fig. 10-2. In many clinical situations,

orthodontic wires are deformed beyond their elastic limit. Their springback properties in the portion of the load-deflection curve between the elastic limit and the ultimate strength, therefore, are important in determining clinical performance.

These three major properties have an important relationship:

$$\text{Strength} = \text{Stiffness} \times \text{Range}$$

Two other characteristics of some clinical importance can also be illustrated with a stress-strain diagram: resilience and formability (Fig. 10-4). Resilience is the area under the stress-strain curve out to the proportional limit. It represents the energy storage capacity of the wire, which is a combination of strength and springiness. Formability is the amount of permanent deformation that a wire can withstand before failing. It represents the amount of permanent bending the wire will tolerate (while being formed into a clinically useful spring, for instance) before it breaks.

The properties of an ideal wire material for orthodontic purposes can be described largely in terms of these criteria: it should possess (1) high strength, (2) low stiffness (in most applications), (3) high range, and (4) high formability. In addition, the material should be weldable or solderable, so that hooks or stops can be attached to the wire. It should also be reasonable in cost. In contemporary practice, no one archwire material meets all these requirements, and the best results are obtained by using specific archwire materials for specific purposes.

■ Orthodontic Archwire Materials

Precious metal alloys. Before the 1950s, precious metal alloys were used routinely for orthodontic purposes, primarily because nothing else available would tolerate tolerate

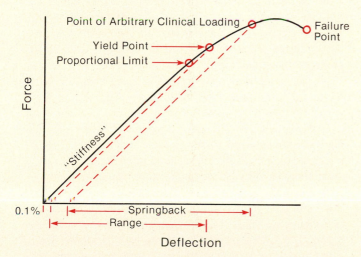

Fig. 10-2 ■ A typical force-deflection curve for an elastic material like an orthodontic arch wire. The stiffness of the material is given by the slope of the linear portion of the curve. The range is the distance along the X-axis to the yield point, at which 0.1% permanent deformation has occurred. Clinically useful springback occurs if the wire is deflected beyond the yield point, but of course it no longer returns to the original shape. At the failure point, the wire breaks.

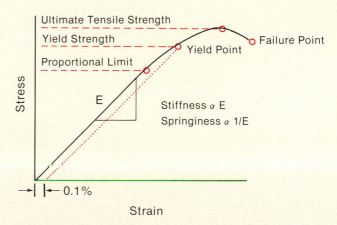

Fig. 10-3 ■ Stress and strain are internal characteristics that can be calculated from measurements of force and deflection, so the general shapes of force-deflection and stress-strain curves are similar. Three different points on a stress-strain diagram can be taken as representing the strength. The slope of the stress-strain curve, *E*, is the modulus of elasticity to which stiffness and springiness are proportional.

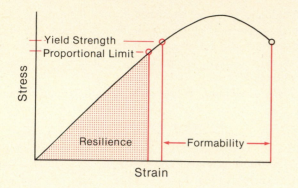

Fig. 10-4 ■ Resilience and formability are defined as an area under the stress-strain curve and a distance along the X-axis respectively, as shown here.

Table 10-1 ■ Properties of Nitinol and TMA compared to stainless steel

	Stainless steel or Elgiloy	TMA	Nitinol
Modulus of elasticity (10^6 psi)	28.5	10.0	4.8
Yield strength (10^3 psi)	260	170	>180
Ultimate tensile strength (10^3 psi)	330	180	240
Load at given deflection	1.0	0.35	0.17
Deflection at given load	1.0	2.85	5.94
Deflection at yield	1.0	1.90	3.95
Springback after 90° bend	15°	20°	48°*
Weldable	Yes	Yes	No

*Many fractured.

intraoral conditions. Gold itself is too soft for nearly all dental purposes, but alloys (which often included platinum and palladium along with gold and copper) could be useful orthodontically. Their marginal properties had made precious metal alloys obsolete for orthodontic purposes before the price increases of the 1970s made them also prohibitively expensive. Only the Crozat appliance is still occasionally made from gold, following the original design of the early 1900s (see Chapter 11).

Stainless steel and chrome-cobalt alloys. Since midcentury, almost all orthodontic practice has relied on stainless steel or on a chrome-cobalt alloy (Elgiloy; Rocky Mountain Co.) with very similar properties. Stainless steel's rust resistance results from a relatively high chromium content. A typical formulation for orthodontic use has 18% chromium and 8% nickel (thus the material is often referred to as an 18-8 stainless steel).

The properties of these steel wires can be controlled over a reasonably wide range by varying the amount of cold working and annealing during manufacture. Steel is softened by annealing and hardened by cold working. Fully annealed stainless steel wires are quite soft and highly formable. The ligatures used to tie orthodontic archwires into brackets on the teeth are made from such "dead soft" wire. Steel archwire materials are offered in a range of partially annealed states, in which yield strength is progressively enhanced at the cost of formability. The steel wires with the most impressive yield strength are almost brittle and will break if bent sharply. The "regular" grade of orthodontic steel wire can be bent to almost any desired shape without breaking. If sharp bends are not needed, the "super" wires can be useful.

Elgiloy, the chrome-cobalt alloy, has the advantage that it can be supplied in a softer and therefore more formable state, and then can be hardened by heat treatment after being shaped. The heat treatment increases strength significantly. After heat treatment, the softest Elgiloy becomes equivalent to regular stainless steel, while harder initial grades are equivalent to the "super" steels.

Titanium alloys. Two new archwire materials, both with a major component of titanium, became available in the late

1970s. The first of these, a nickel-titanium alloy marketed as Nitinol (Unitek Corp.), was developed for the space program (Ni, nickel; Ti, titanium; NOL, Naval Ordnance Laboratory) but has proved very useful in clinical orthodontics. The second, a beta-titanium material sold as TMA (titanium-molybdenum alloy) (Ormco/Sybron), was developed primarily for orthodontic use. It offers a highly desirable combination of strength and springiness. (i.e., excellent resilience) and reasonably good formability. Comparative properties of stainless steel, chrome-cobalt (Elgiloy), nickel-titanium (Nitinol), and beta titanium wires are illustrated in Table 10-1.

In the space program, it was possible to take advantage of the temperature transition from an austenite to a martensite grain (crystal) structure within the Nitinol alloy to produce a shape memory effect. A Nitinol wire with an appropriate transition temperature can be formed to a desired shape (ideal dental arch form, for instance) when it is in its martensite form; cooled (or heated, depending on the precise alloy) to produce a transition to an austenite form; deformed to a different shape (by tying it to malaligned teeth, for instance); and caused to spring back to its original shape by again going through the transition temperature. The alloy remembers its shape in the martensite form.

To this point, it has not been possible to take advantage of temperature transition and shape memory in Nitinol for orthodontic purposes, but this remains a possibility for the future. The Nitinol originally offered for orthodontic use is in the martensite form at room temperature and, as prepared, is exceptionally springy and quite strong but has poor formability. A martensitic alloy marketed more recently (Titanal, Lancer Pacific) has very similar strength and spring characteristics to Nitinol but also has very high formability (Table 10-2).

Recently, new nickel-titanium wires with a primarily austenite grain structure have appeared. Burstone et al.[1] report

Table 10-2 ■ Comparative fatigue resistance
of wire materials

Material	Number of bend cycles to fracture
Stainless steel	3
TMA	3
Nitinol	1
Titanal	10

From Kusy, R.P., Elastic property ratio of orthodontic arch wires.[3]

that such a NiTi alloy developed in China has the type of force-deflection curve shown in Fig. 10-5. Note that over a considerable range of deflection, force hardly varies. This means that an initial arch wire would exert about the same force whether it were deflected a relatively small or a large distance, which is a unique and extremely desirable characteristic.

The unique force-deflection curve for the Chinese NiTi wire occurs because of a partial transition in grain structure from austenite to martensite, in response not to a temperature change but to applied force. The result is "superelasticity," which means that the elasticity possible from the martensite structure is added to that from the austenite structure as the wire deforms. In other words, the new alloy takes advantage of the transition in internal structure without requiring a significant temperature change to accomplish this.

The Chinese NiTi is also unusual in that its unloading curve differs from its loading curve (Fig. 10-6), i.e., the force that it delivers is not the same as the force applied to activate it. This produces the even more remarkable effect that the force delivered by a NiTi wire can be changed during clinical use merely by releasing and retying it (Fig. 10-7). The Chinese wire is not yet available commercially, but a similar Japanese material with superelastic properties (Ni-Ti, Ormco/Sybron; Sentinol, GAC) was marketed in 1985.

At this writing, the superelastic alloys are so new that ways to fully exploit them clinically are still being developed. Additional progress in orthodontic arch materials, including composite plastic "wires" as well as new metal alloys, can be anticipated.

■ Comparison of Contemporary Archwires

The chrome-cobalt (Eligiloy) and stainless steel wires used in recent years have had remarkably similar strength, stiffness, and range properties. Nickel-titanium and beta-titanium are quite different, both from stainless steel and from each other. A useful method for comparison of two archwires of various materials, sizes, and dimensions is the use of ratios of the major properties (strength, stiffness, and range):

Strength A/Strength B = Strength ratio
Springiness A/Stiffness B = Stiffness ratio
Range A/Range B = Range ratio

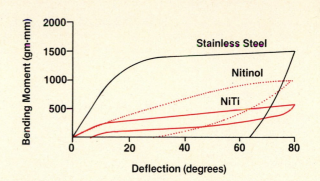

Fig. 10-5 ■ Bending moment versus deflection plotted for .016 orthodontic wires (*black*, stainless steel; *dashed red*, martensitic NiTi (Nitinol); *red*, austenitic NiTi (Chinese NiTi). Note that Chinese NiTi produces lower moments and forces than Nitinol. Both the nickel-titanium wires are much more flexible than steel. (From Burstone, C.J., et al.: Am. J. Orthod. **87**:445-452, 1985.)

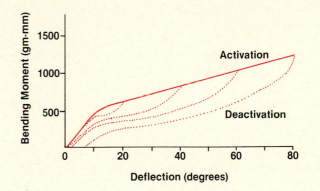

Fig. 10-6 ■ Activation *(solid)* and deactivation *(dashed)* curves for austenitic NiTi wire. Note that the unloading curves change at different activations, i.e., the unloading stiffness is affected by the degree of activation. The unloading stiffness for steel, TMA, and Nitinol wires is the same for all activations. (From Burstone, C.J., et al.: Am. J. Orthod. **87**:445-452, 1985.)

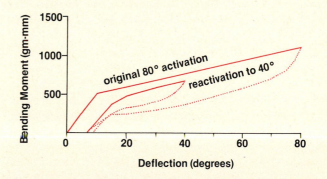

Fig. 10-7 ■ Activation (to 80 degrees) and reactivation (to 40 degrees) curves for austenitic NiTi wire. In each case, the loading curve is solid and the unloading curve dashed. The unloading curve indicates the force that would be delivered to a tooth. Note that the amount of force exerted by a piece of austenitic NiTi wire that had previously been activated to 80 degrees could be considerably increased by untying it from a bracket and then retying it—again, a unique property of this alloy. (From Burstone, C.J., et al.: Am. J. Orthod. **87**:445-452, 1985.)

Table 10-3 ■ Elastic property ratios: .016 and .018 wire in bending

	Strength		Stiffness		Range	
	.016	*.018*	*.016*	*.018*	*.016*	*.018*
Stainless steel	1.0		1.0		1.0	
TMA	0.6	0.6	0.3	0.3	1.8	1.8
Nitinol	0.6	0.6	0.2	0.2	3.9	3.9

These ratios have been calculated for many different wires by Kusy[2] and the data presented here are taken from his work.

Three points must be kept in mind when ratios are compared:

1. These ratios are functions of both physical properties and geometric factors, hence the importance of specifying both in the comparison. Geometric factors relate to both the size of the wire and its shape, whether it is round, rectangular, or square. These are discussed in more detail following.

2. Bending describes round wires reasonably completely in orthodontic applications, but both bending and torsional stresses are encountered when rectangular wires are placed into rectangular attachments on teeth. The fundamental relationships for torsion are analogous to those in bending but are not the same. Appropriate use of the equations for torsion, however, allows torsion ratios to be computed in the same way that bending ratios can be.

3. The ratios apply to the linear portion of the load-deflection curve and thus do not accurately describe the behavior of wires that are stressed beyond their elastic limit but still have useful springback. This limitation is especially significant with TMA and superelastic NiTi wires, which have a considerable distance between their elastic limit and ultimate strength. The nonlinear response of these materials makes calculation of the ratios difficult. Nevertheless, the ratios offer an initial understanding of the properties of traditional steel wires as compared to the new titanium alloys.

In the beginning, tabulated comparative data are easiest to understand. Note in Tables 10-3 and 10-4 the comparative properties of .016, 018 and .019 × .025 wires in stainless steel (or Elgiloy), Nitinol, and TMA. In each case, the steel wire has been given an arbitrary value of 1. Note that the new wires in each case provide a gain in springiness and range that is greater than the loss in strength.

From Table 10-3, it can be seen that:

1. The strength of .016 and .018 Nitinol and TMA wires are the same: both are 60% as strong as steel.

2. Stiffness of the small round titanium wires is also similar, less than one-third that of steel.

3. TMA has nearly twice the range of steel, and Nitinol has twice the range of TMA and nearly four times the range of steel.

For alignment of teeth, all other factors being equal, a small round Nitinol wire could move a tooth considerably

Table 10-4 ■ Elastic property ratios: .019 × .025 wire in bending (B) and torsion (T)

	Strength		Stiffness		Range	
	B	T	B	T	B	T
Stainless steel	1.0		1.0		1.0	
TMA	0.6	0.6	0.3	0.3	1.8	2.0
Nitinol	0.6	0.8	0.2	0.1	4.0	5.4

Table 10-5 ■ Wires of equivalent stiffness

Bending			
Nickel-titanium NiTi	Beta-titanium	Stainless steel	
Nitinol Titanal Sentinol NiTi	TMA	Steel or Elgiloy	Relative springiness
.016*†	–	.0175″ (3 × .008)	6.6
.019‡	.016	.012	3.3
–	.018	.014	1.9
.017 × .025	–	.016	1.0
.021 × .025	–	.018	0.70
–	.019 × .025	–	0.37
–	–	.019 × .026	0.12

*Greatest range for NiTi.
†.015 Nitinol = .016 NiTi (approx.)
‡Greatest range.

Table 10-6 ■ A sequence of increasingly stiff wires in torsion

Wire	Stiffness index
.018 × .018 Nitinol	1.0
.017 × .025 Nitinol	1.7
.021 × .025 Nitinol	2.8
.017 × .025 TMA	3.5
.019 × .025 TMA	4.6
.017 × .025 Steel	12
.019 × .025 Steel	16

further than either of its competitors before requiring reactivation. The same is true of the other NiTi alloys. (The term NiTi is used subsequently in this book to refer to the family of nickel-titanium wire materials. Reference to a specific material is by its trademark name.)

Table 10-4 shows that properties of rectangular wire in bending and torsion are quite different. Note that at this common wire size, both TMA and Nitinol have greater springiness and range than steel. Nitinol in torsion must bend more than twice as far as TMA to deliver the same load (because of its great springiness), and thus is at a disadvantage when small precise adjustments are needed. TMA would be a better choice for making final adjustments

in tooth inclination (torque), but if alignment were needed with this larger wire size, Nitinol's properties are much better (the same is true for the other NiTi alloys).

Table 10-5 shows wires of equivalent stiffness, with .016 stainless steel as the index value. Table 10-6 illustrates a sequence of rectangular wires that are increasingly stiff in torsion. The application of this information to the selection of archwires at various stages of fixed appliance treatment is covered in detail in Chapters 15 to 17.

A more graphic and efficient method for comparing different wire materials and sizes is the use of nomograms: fixed charts that display mathematic relationships via appropriately adjusted scales. In the preparation of a nomo-

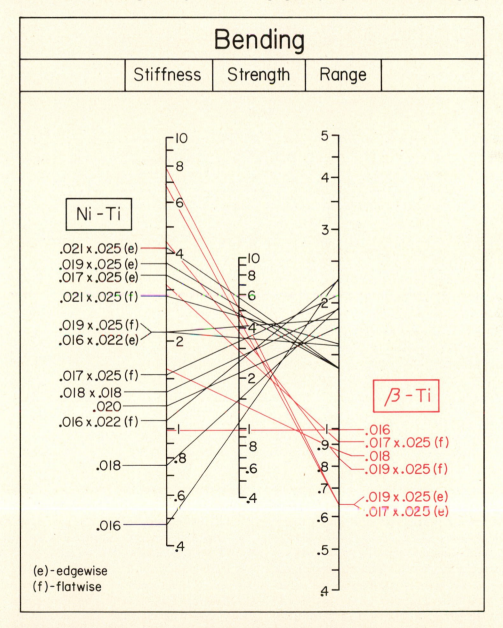

Fig. 10-8 ■ Nomogram comparing nickel-titanium (Nitinol) and beta-titanium (TMA) wires in bending. Note that the index wire, with an assigned value of 1, is .016 TMA. (From Kusy, R.P.: Elastic property ratios of orthodontic arch wires. Chapel Hill, NC, 1982, University of North Carolina Department of Orthodontics/Dental Research Center.)

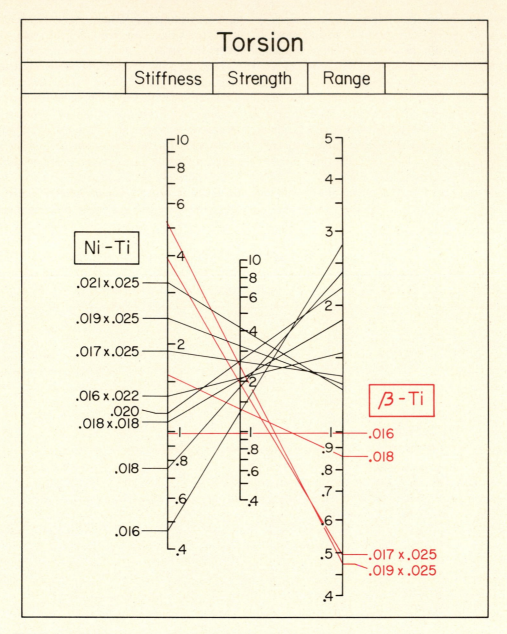

Fig. 10-9 ■ Nomogram comparing titanium (Nitinol) and beta-titanium (TMA) in torsion. (From Kusy, R.P.: Elastic property ratios of orthodontic arch wires. Chapel Hill, NC, 1982, University of North Carolina Department of Orthodontics/Dental Research Center.)

gram, a reference wire is given a value of 1, and many other wires can then be located appropriately in reference to it. Nomograms developed by Kusy[3] to provide a generalized comparison of Nitinol and TMA in bending and torsion are shown in Figs. 10-8 and 10-9.

The nomograms are particularly helpful in allowing one to assess at a glance a whole set of relationships that would require pages of tables. For example, using Fig. 10-9 to compare .017 × .025 Nitinol to .017 × .025 TMA in torsion (the appropriate comparison if the wires would be used to produce a torquing movement of the root of a tooth): .017 × .025 TMA has a stiffness value of 4, while .017 × .025 Nitinol has a value of 1.9, so the TMA would

deliver more than twice the force at a given deflection; the strength value for .017 × .025 TMA wire is 2, while the value for this size Nitinol wire is 2.6, so the Nitinol wire is slightly stronger in torsion; the range value for .017 × .025 TMA is 0.5, while the same size Nitinol has a value of 1.4, so the Nitinol has nearly three times the range. The nomogram contains the information to allow a similar comparison of any one of the wire sizes listed to any other wire shown on the chart.

■ Effects of Size and Shape on Elastic Properties

Each of the major elastic properties—strength, springiness, and range—is substantially affected by a change in

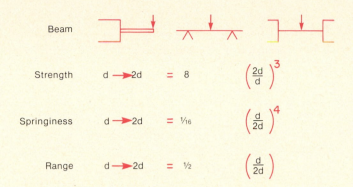

Fig. 10-10 ■ Changing the diameter of a beam, no matter how it is supported, greatly affects its properties. Doubling the diameter of a cantilever beam makes it 8 times as strong, but it is then only 1/16 as springy and has half the range. More generally, when two sizes of round wire are compared, strength changes as a cubic function of the ratio of the two diameters; springiness changes as the fourth power of the ratios; range changes as a direct proportion.

the geometry of a beam. Both the diameter (or cross-section if the beam is rectangular) and length of a beam are of great significance in determining its properties. Changes related to size and shape, of course, are independent of material, but the performance of a beam, whether beneath a highway bridge or between two teeth in an orthodontic appliance, is determined by the combination of material properties and geometric factors.

Effects of diameter or cross-section. Let us begin by considering a cantilever beam, supported on only one end. In orthodontic applications, this is the type of spring often used in removable appliances, in which a wire extends from the plastic body of the removable appliance as a fingerspring. When a round wire is used as a fingerspring, doubling the diameter of the wire increases its strength eight times, i.e., the larger wire can resist eight times as much force before permanently deforming, or can deliver eight times as much force. Doubling the diameter, however, decreases springiness by a factor of 16 and decreases range by a factor of two.

More generally, for a round cantilever beam, the strength of the beam changes as the third power of the ratio of the larger to the smaller beam; springiness changes as the fourth

power of the ratio of the smaller to the larger; and range changes directly as the ratio of the smaller to the larger (Fig. 10-10).

The situation is somewhat more complex for a beam supported on both ends, as is the case for a segment of archwire between two teeth. Supporting both ends makes the beam stronger and less flexible, particularly if the ends are tightly anchored as compared to being free to slide. If a rectangular beam is evaluated, its dimension in the direction of bending is the primary determinant of its properties. The principle with any supported beam, however, is the same as with a cantilever beam: as the beam size increases, strength increases as a cubic function, while springiness decreases as a fourth power function and range decreases proportionately, not exponentially.

Although round beams are placed in torsion in engineering applications, torsion is of practical importance in orthodontics only for rectangular wires that can be twisted into rectangular slots. In torsion, the analytic approach is basically similar to that in bending, but shear stress rather than bending stress is encountered, and the appropriate equations are all different. The overall effect is the same, however: decreasing the size of a wire decreases its strength in torsion while increasing its springiness and range, just as in bending.

As the diameter of a wire decreases, its strength decreases so rapidly that a point is reached at which the strength is no longer adequate for orthodontic purposes. As the diameter increases, its stiffness increases so rapidly that a point is reached at which the wire is simply too stiff to be useful. These upper and lower limits establish a range of orthodontically useful wire sizes. The phenomenon is the same for any material, but the range of useful sizes varies considerably from one material to another (Table 10-7). As Table 10-7 indicates, useful gold wires are considerably larger than the steel wires that replaced them. The titanium wires are much springier than steel wires of equal sizes, but not quite as strong. Their useful sizes, therefore, are slightly larger than steel.

Effects of length and attachment. Changing the length of a beam, whatever its size or the material from which it is made, also dramatically affects its properties. If the length of a cantilever beam is doubled, its bending strength is cut

Table 10-7 ■ Useful wire sizes in various materials

	Gold	*Steel*	*Elgiloy*	*TMA*	*Nitinol*
Stranded archwire	–	.007-.010	–	–	–
Archwire					
Round	.020-.022	.012-.020	.012-.020	.016-.022	.016-.022
Rectangular	.022 × .028	.016 × .016- .019 × .025	.016 × .016- .019 × .025	.017 × .025- .021 × .025	.017 × .025- .021 × .025
Removable appliance	.030-.040	.022-.030	.022-.030	–	–
Lingual arch	.040	.030-.036	.030-.036		
Headgear, auxiliary expansion arches	–	.045-.051	–		

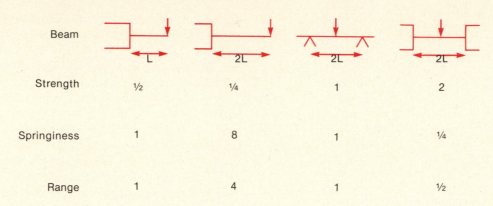

Beam	L	2L	2L	2L
Strength	½	¼	1	2
Springiness	1	8	1	¼
Range	1	4	1	½

Fig. 10-11 ■ Changing both the length of a beam and the way in which it is attached dramatically affects its properties. Doubling the length of a cantilever beam cuts its strength in half, but makes it 8 times as springy and gives it 4 times the range. More generally, strength varies inversely with length, whereas springiness varies as a cubic function of the length ratios, and range as a second power function. Supporting a beam on both ends makes it much stronger but also much less springy than supporting it on only one end. If a beam is rigidly attached on both ends, it is twice as strong but only one fourth as springy as a beam of the same material and length that can slide over the abutments.

in half, but its springiness is increased eight times and its range four times. More generally, when the length of a cantilever beam increases, its strength decreases proportionately, while its springiness increases as the cubic function of the ratio of the length and its range increases as the square of the ratio of the length (Fig. 10-11). Length changes affect torsion quite differently from bending: springiness and range in torsion increase proportionally with length, while torsional strength is not affected by length.

Changing from a cantilever to a supported beam, though it complicates the mathematic expressions, does not affect the big picture: as beam length increases, there are proportional decreases in strength but exponential increases in springiness and range.

The way in which a beam is attached also affects its properties. An archwire can be tied tightly or loosely, and the point of loading can be any point along the span. As Fig. 10-11 shows, a supported beam like an archwire is four times as springy if it can slide over the abutments (in clinical use, through a bracket into which it is loosely tied) than if the beam is firmly attached (tied tightly). With multiple attachments, as with an archwire tied to several teeth, the gain in springiness from loose ties of an initial archwire is less dramatic but still significant.

Controlling orthodontic force by varying materials and size-shape. Obtaining enough orthodontic force is never a problem. The difficulty is in obtaining light but sustained force. A spring strong enough to resist permenent deformation may be too stiff, so that the force is heavy initially but decays rapidly when the tooth begins to move. A flexible spring may nevertheless fail to provide a sustained force if it distorts the first time the patient has lunch. The best balance of strength, springiness, and range must be sought among the almost innumerable possible combinations of beam materials, diameters, and length.

The first consideration in spring design is adequate strength: the wire size selected must not deform permanently in use. As a general rule, fingersprings for removable appliances are best constructed using steel wire. Great advantage can be taken of the fact that springiness increases as a cubic function of the increase in length of the beam, while strength decreases only in direct proportion. Thus, a relatively large wire, selected for its strength, can be given the desired spring qualities by increasing its length.

In practice, this lengthening often means doubling the wire back on itself or winding a helix into it, to gain length while keeping the spring within a confined intraoral area (Fig. 10-12). The same technique can be used with archwires, of course; the effective length of a beam is measured along the wire from one support to the other, and this does not have to be in a straight line (Fig. 10-13). Bending a loop into an archwire segment between two teeth greatly increases the springiness and range of that segment, much more so than it decreases strength. Bending loops in archwires can be a time-consuming chairside procedure, which is the major disadvantage.

Another way to increase strength while retaining springiness is to combine two or more strands of a small, and therefore springy wire. Two .010 steel wires in tandem, for instance, could withstand twice the load as a single strand before permanently deforming, but if each strand could bend without being restrained by the other, springiness would not be affected. The genesis of the "twin wire" appliance system (see following) was just this observation, that a pair of .010 wires offered excellent springiness and range for aligning teeth, and that two wires gave adequate strength although one did not. More recently, three or more strands of smaller wires, twisted into a cable, have come into common use (Fig. 10-13). The properties of the multistrand wire depend both on the characteristics of the individual wire strands and

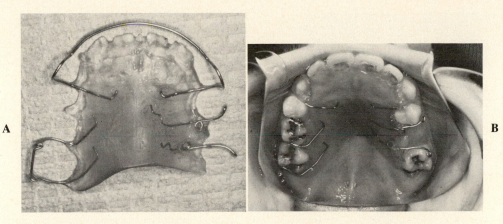

Fig. 10-12 ■ **A** and **B,** A removable appliance incorporating cantilever springs to reposition an upper molar and upper first premolar. Note that a helix has been bent into the base of the cantilever springs, effectively increasing their length to obtain more desirable mechanical properties.

on how tightly they have been woven together. Current multistrand wires offer an impressive combination of strength and spring qualities (Table 10-8).

The exceptional springiness of NiTi makes it a particularly attractive alternative to steel wires in the initial phases of treatment when the teeth are severely malaligned. A continuous NiTi archwire will have better properties than multistrand steel wires and properties similar to a steel archwire with loops. Nitinol's lack of formability, of course, means that it is essentially impossible to make it even springier by bending loops into it, and this procedure is rarely done with any of the NiTi wires. For the same reason, NiTi does not lend itself to the formation of springs for closing spaces. TMA, as an intermediate between NiTi and steel, is less useful than either in the first stage of full-appliance treatment. Its excellent overall properties, however, make it quite useful in space closure and finishing. It is possible, and frequently desirable, to carry out orthodontic treatment with a series of wires of approximately the same size, using a sequence from NiTi to TMA to steel.[4] Archwire selection

in varying circumstances is discussed in more detail later in this chapter and in Chapters 15 to 17.

■ Rubber and Plastic Sources of Elastic Force

From the beginning, rubber bands were used in orthodontics to transmit force from the upper arch to the lower. More recently, rubber and plastic elastomers have also been used to close spaces within the arches. Rubber has the particularly valuable quality of a great elastic range, so that the extreme stretching produced when a patient opens the mouth while wearing rubber bands can be tolerated without destroying the appliance. Rubber bands are also easier for a patient to remove and replace than, for instance, a heavy coil spring would be.

From a materials point of view, the greatest problem with all types of rubber is that they absorb water and deteriorate under intraoral conditions. Gum rubber, which is used to make the rubber bands commonly used in households and

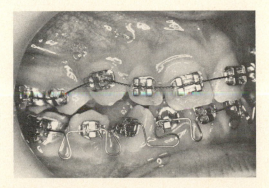

Fig. 10-13 ■ In fixed appliance orthodontics, improved flexibility of initial archwires can be obtained by either of two strategies: bending loops into the archwire, as shown in the lower arch here, to increase the length of the beam segments between adjacent teeth; or using multiple strands of small diameter wires, as shown in the upper arch.

Table 10-8 ■ Comparison of multistrand (3 × .008) with single-strand orthodontic wires

Properties compared to 3 × .008 steel*	Strength	Stiffness	Range
Steel:			
.010	0.78	1.0	0.76
.012	1.4	2.2	0.63
.014	2.2	4.0	0.54
.016	3.2	6.8	0.47
.016 × .016	5.5	12.0	0.47
Nitinol†:			
.016	1.8	1.2	1.6
.018	2.6	1.9	1.4
.017 × .025	8.1	8.1	1.0
TMA‡:			
.016	1.7	2.4	0.71
.018	2.5	3.9	0.63

From Kusy, R.P., Dilley, G.J. Am. J. Orthod. **86:**177, 1984.
*Wildcat .0175 (GAC Corp.)
†Unitek Corp.
‡Ormco/Sybron.

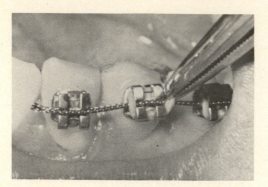

Fig. 10-14 ■ Elastomeric module used to hold an archwire in a bracket.

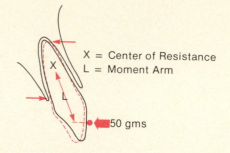

X = Center of Resistance
L = Moment Arm

50 gms

Fig. 10-15 ■ The center of resistance for any tooth is at the approximate midpoint of the embedded portion of the root. If a force is applied to the crown of a tooth, the tooth will tend to rotate around the center of resistance, and a moment, which is a force acting at a distance, is created. The distance from the point of force application to the center of resistance is the moment arm.

offices, begins to deteriorate in the mouth within a couple of hours, and much of its elasticity is lost in 12 to 24 hours. Although orthodontic elastics made from this material are still offered, they have been largely superceded by latex elastics, which have a useful performance life 4 to 6 times as long. In contemporary orthodontics, only latex rubber elastics should be used.

Elastomeric plastics developed in the 1960s became available for orthodontic purposes during the following decade and are marketed under a variety of trade names. Small elastomeric modules replace wire ligature ties to hold archwires in the brackets in many applications (Fig. 10-14), and can also be used to apply a force to close spaces within the arches. Like rubber materials, however, these elastomers tend to deteriorate in elastic performance after a relatively short period in the mouth. This feature does not prevent them from performing quite well in holding arch wires in place, nor does it contraindicate their use to close small spaces. It simply must be kept in mind that when elastomers are used, the forces decay rapidly, and so can be characterized better as interrupted than continuous. Progress in the development of elastomeric materials is reducing this deficiency, and it may well be that elastomers capable of providing light sustained forces will become available in the future.

■ *Design Factors in Orthodontic Appliances*

■ Two Point Contact and Control of Root Position

Definition of terms. Before beginning to discuss control of root position, it is necessary to understand some basic physical terms that must be used in the discussion:

Force—a load applied to an object that will tend to move it to a different position in space. Force, though rigidly defined in units of Newtons (mass times the acceleration of

gravity), is usually measured in mass units of grams or ounces.

Center of resistance—a point at which resistance to movement can be concentrated for mathematic analysis. For an object in free space, the center of resistance is the same as the center of mass. If the object is partially restrained, as is the case for a fencepost extending into the earth or a tooth root embedded in bone, the center of resistance will be determined by the nature of the external constraints. The center of resistance for a tooth is at the approximate midpoint of the embedded portion of the root, i.e., about halfway between the root apex and the crest of the alveolar bone (Fig. 10-15).

Moment—a force acting at a distance. A moment is defined as the product of the force times the distance to the center of resistance and thus is measured in units of gm-mm (or equivalent). If the point at which a force is applied to an object is not directly opposite the center of resistance, a moment is necessarily created (Fig. 10-15). Not only will the force tend to translate the object, moving it to a different position, it will also tend to rotate the object around the center of resistance. This effect, of course, is precisely the situation when a force is applied to the crown of a tooth. Not only is the tooth displaced in the direction of the force, it also rotates around the center of resistance—thus there is a tipping tooth movement.

Couple—two forces equal in magnitude and opposite in direction. The result of applying two forces in this way is a pure moment, since the translatory effect of the forces cancels out. A couple will produce pure rotation, spinning the object around its center of resistance, while the combination of a force and a couple can change the way an object rotates while it is being moved (Fig. 10-16).

Center of rotation—the point around which rotation actually occurs when an object is being moved. If a force and a couple are applied to an object, the center of rotation can be controlled and made to have any desired location. The application of a force and a couple to

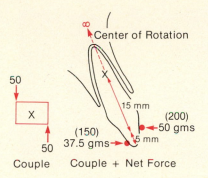

Fig. 10-16 ■ A couple is defined as two forces equal in magnitude and opposite in direction. This produces pure rotation. If a 50 gm force were applied to a point on the labial surface of an incisor tooth 15 mm from the center of resistance, a 750 gm-mm moment would be produced, tipping the tooth. To obtain bodily movement, it is necessary to create a moment equal in magnitude and opposite in direction to the original movement. One way to do this would be to apply a force of 37.5 gm pushing the incisal edge labially at a point 20 mm from the center of resistance. This creates a force system equivalent to a couple creating a 750 gm-mm movement in the opposite direction and a 12.5 gm lingual force. With this force system, the tooth would not tip, but there would be only a net 12.5 gm to move the incisor lingually. To achieve a net 50 gm for effective movement, it would be necessary to use 200 gm against the labial surface, and 150 gm in the opposite direction against the incisal edge. Controlling forces of this magnitude without a fixed appliance is difficult.

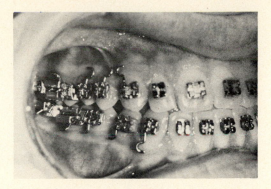

Fig. 10-17 ■ Attachments extending toward the center of resistance, seen here on canines and premolars, can be used to decrease the amount of tipping when teeth are moved mesiodistally. This idea from the 1920s has recently been reintroduced into contemporary fixed appliances.

the crown of a tooth, in fact, is the mechanism by which bodily movement of a tooth, or even greater movement of the root than the crown, can be produced (Fig. 10-16).

Forces, moments, and couples in tooth movement. Consider the clinical problem posed by a protruding maxillary central incisor. If a single force of 50 gm is applied against the crown of this tooth, as might happen with a spring on a maxillary removable appliance, a force system will be created that includes a 750 gm-mm moment (Fig. 10-16). The result will be that the crown will be retracted, but the root apex will not and might actually move slightly in the opposite direction. (Remember that a force will tend to displace the entire object, despite the fact that its orientation will change via simultaneous rotation around the center of resistance.) If it is desired to maintain the inclination of the tooth while retracting it, it will be necessary to overcome the moment inadvertently created when the force was applied to the crown.

One way to decrease the magnitude of the moment is to apply the force closer to the center of resistance. In orthodontics, it is impractical to apply the force directly to the root, but a similar effect could be achieved by constructing a rigid attachment that projected upward from the crown, so that the force could be applied to that attachment. If the attachment were perfectly rigid, the effect would be to re-

duce the length of the moment arm and thereby the amount of tipping. As Fig. 10-17 illustrates, this approach is used in some contemporary orthodontic appliances to reduce tipping. Since it is difficult to make the arms long enough to totally eliminate tipping, this procedure is only a partial solution.

Another way to control or eliminate tipping is to create a second moment opposite in direction to the first one. If a second counterbalancing moment could be created equal in magnitude to the moment produced by the first force application, the tooth would remain upright and move bodily. A moment can be created only by application of a force at a distance, however, so this would require that a second force be applied to the crown of the tooth.

In our example of the protruding central incisor, one way to correct the problem would be to apply a second force on the lingual surface of this tooth, perhaps with a spring pushing outward from the lingual edge near the incisal edge (Fig. 10-16). As a practical matter, it can be difficult to maintain removable appliances in place against the displacing effects of a pair of springs with heavy activation. The usual orthodontic solution is a fixed attachment on the tooth, constructed so that forces can be applied at two points. With round wires, an auxiliary spring is needed (Fig. 10-18). A rectangular archwire fitting into a rectangular bracket slot on the tooth is most widely used because the entire force system can be produced with a single wire (Fig. 10-19).

It should be noted that with this approach, the two points of contact are the opposite edges of the rectangular wire. The moment arms of the couple, therefore, are quite small, which means that the forces at the bracket necessary to create a countervailing moment are quite large. If a rectangular archwire is to be used to retract a central incisor bodily, the net retraction force should be small, but the twisting forces on the bracket must be large in order to generate the moment.

Moment-to-force ratios and control of root position. The previous analysis demonstrates that control of root position during movement requires both a force to move the

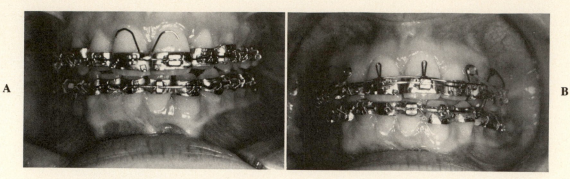

Fig. 10-18 ■ **A,** Auxiliary springs soldered to a round archwire to create a torquing moment on the maxillary central incisors. The springs that extend gingivally provide a second point of contact on the labial surface. **B,** Auxiliary springs used to be supplement the effect of rectangular archwires in moving the roots of maxillary incisor teeth lingually. In contemporary orthodontics, auxiliary springs of this type rarely are used. Instead, a tightly fitting rectangular arch wire in a rectangular bracket is used.

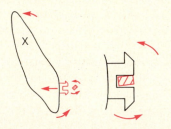

Fig. 10-19 ■ A rectangular archwire fitting into a rectangular slot can generate the moment necessary to control root position. The wire is twisted (placed into torsion) as it is put into the bracket slot. The two points of contact are at the edge of the wire, where it contacts the bracket. The moment arm, therefore, is quite small, and forces must be large to generate the necessary moment.

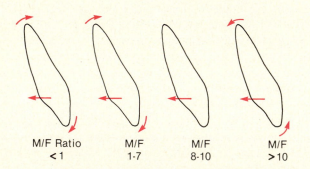

Fig. 10-20 ■ The ratio between the force applied to move a tooth, and the counterbalancing moment used to control root position, determines the type of tooth movement. If the ratio between the counterbalancing moment and the retraction force is less than one, the tooth will tip just apically to its center of resistance. As the moment-to-force ratio increases, the center of rotation is displaced further away from the center of resistance, producing controlled tipping. With a moment-to-force ratio of 8 to 10, bodily movement occurs. If the moment-to-force ratio is greater than 10, the root apex will be retracted more than the crown, producing lingual root torque.

tooth in the desired direction, and a couple to produce the necessary counterbalancing moment for control of root position. The ratio of the moment produced by this couple to the net force in the direction of desired tooth movement can be used to predict the type of tooth movement that will occur. The heavier the force, the larger the counterbalancing movement must be to prevent tipping, and vice-versa.

Clinical experience has shown that bodily movement of a tooth requires a moment-to-force ratio of 8:1 to 10:1, depending on the length of the root. In other words, if a 100 gm net force is used to move the tooth, a moment of 800 to 1000 gm-mm will be needed to obtain the same amount of root movement as crown movement. Moment-to-force ratios smaller than this allow some tipping but less than would occur without the application of a countervailing moment. Higher moment-to-force ratios produce more root movement than crown movement (Fig. 10-20). In the example presented previously, if a 50 gm net force was used to retract of a central incisor, a 500 gm-mm moment would be needed to keep the tooth from tipping. To produce a moment of this magnitude within the confines of a 0.4 mm bracket would require a twisting force of 1250 gm from the archwire (Fig. 10-19). This force at the bracket produces only a pure moment, but the necessary magnitude can come as a considerable surprise. The wire must literally snap into the bracket.

■ Narrow Versus Wide Brackets in Fixed Appliance Systems

Control of root position with an orthodontic appliance is especially needed in two circumstances: when the root of a tooth needs to be torqued faciolingually (as in the previous example), or when mesiodistal root movement is needed for proper paralleling of teeth at extraction sites. In the former instance, the necessary moment is generated within the bracket; in the latter circumstance, the moment is generated across the bracket.

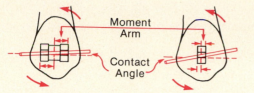

Fig. 10-21 ■ The width of the bracket on a tooth determines the length of the moment arm for control of mesiodistal root position. Bracket width also influences the contact angle at which the corner of the bracket meets the archwire. The wider the bracket, the smaller the contact angle.

The wider the bracket, all other things being equal, the easier it will be to generate the moments needed to bring roots together at extraction sites or to control mesiodistal position of roots in general. Consider a canine tooth in which the root must be retracted into a first premolar extraction site (Fig. 10-21). With a retraction force of 100 gm, a 1000 gm-mm moment will be needed. If the bracket on this tooth is 1 mm wide, 1000 gm of force will be needed at each corner of the bracket, but if the bracket is 4 mm wide, only 250 gm of force at each corner will be necessary.

This assumes even greater practical significance when the extraction site is to be closed by sliding teeth along an archwire, and friction between the wire and bracket is encountered. Frictional resistance to sliding (discussed more fully following) is affected by the force with which the bracket contacts the archwire and the contact angle between the wire and the bracket (Fig. 10-21). The wider bracket reduces both the amount of force and the contact angle, and is thus advantageous for space closure by sliding.

Despite their advantage when spaces are to be closed by sliding teeth on an archwire, wide brackets also have a partially offsetting disadvantage. The wider the bracket on a tooth, the smaller the interbracket span between adjacent teeth, and therefore the shorter the effective length of the archwire segments between supports. Reducing the span of the wire segments in this way, of course, greatly decreases both the springiness of the archwire and its range of action, and this reduction makes it more difficult to control forces exerted by the archwire. For this reason, the use of extremely wide brackets is contraindicated. The maximum practical width of a wide bracket is about half the width of a tooth, and even narrower brackets have an advantage when teeth are malaligned because the greater interbracket span gives more flexibility.

■ Effect of Bracket Slot Size in the Edgewise System

The use of rectangular archwires in rectangular bracket slots was introduced by Edward Angle in 1930 with his edgewise arch mechanism, hailed as the ''latest and best in orthodontics.''[5] The original appliance was designed for use with gold archwires, and the .022 × .028 inch bracket slot size was designed to accommodate rectangular archwires of approximately the same dimension. In Angle's concept of treatment, sliding teeth along archwires to close extractions sites was rarely necessary, because extractions for orthodontic purposes were simply not done. Torquing movements, on the other hand, were important, and a major goal of the appliance design was efficient torque. Gold archwires of .022 × .028 dimension, used with narrow brackets, had a reasonable range of action in torsion.

When steel archwires replaced gold, some of the advantage of the rectangular wire in the rectangular slot was lost because steel wire of the same size was so much stiffer. With steel archwires of .021 as the smaller dimension, close enough to the original .022 bracket slot size to give a good fit, springiness and range in torsion are so limited that effective torque with the archwire is essentially impossible. Exaggerated inclinations of smaller rectangular wires, for example, .019 × .025, are one alternative, but torquing auxiliaries (Fig. 10-18) are often necessary with undersize steel wires in .022 slot edgewise brackets. Another alternative was to redesign the edgewise appliance, optimizing the bracket slot size for steel. A reduction in slot size from .022 to .018 was advocated for this purpose. Even with this smaller slot size, full dimension steel wires still produce slightly greater forces than the original edgewise system did, but the properties of the appliance system are much closer to the original. Good torque is possible with steel wires and .018 edgewise brackets.

On the other hand, using undersized archwires in edgewise brackets is a way to reduce friction if teeth are to slide along the archwire, an important consideration by the time steel wire replaced gold. As a practical matter, sliding teeth along an archwire requires at least .002 inch clearance, and even more clearance may be desirable. The greater strength of an .018 archwire as compared with an .016 wire can be an advantage in sliding teeth. The .018 wire would, of course, offer excellent clearance in an .022 slot bracket, but fits too tightly for sliding space closure in an .018 slot bracket. The original .022 slot size, therefore, might have some advantage during space closure but would be a definite disadvantage when torque was needed later. Using wide brackets to help with space closure would make the latter problem worse.

In this situation, a role for the new titanium archwires becomes clearer. If only steel wires are to be used, the .018 slot system has considerable advantage over the larger bracket slot size. With their excellent flexibility, NiTi alloys overcome some of the limitations of steel wires in wide .022 slot brackets for alignment, while rectangular TMA wires would be much better than steel for the finishing phases of treatment and torque control. In short, the new titanium archwires greatly help to overcome the major problems associated with continued use of the original edgewise slot size.

■*Anchorage and Its Control*

■ Anchorage: Resistance to Unwanted Tooth Movement

The term anchorage, in its orthodontic application, is defined in an unusual way: the definition as "resistance to unwanted tooth movement" includes a statement of what the dentist desires. The usage, though unusual, is clearest when presented that way. The dentist or orthodontist is always in the position of constructing an appliance that is to produce certain desired tooth movements. For every (desired) action there is an equal and opposite reaction. Inevitably, reaction forces can move other teeth as well if the appliance contacts them. Anchorage, then, is the resistance to reaction forces that is provided by other teeth or by structures outside the mouth.

In planning orthodontic therapy, it is simply not possible to consider only the teeth whose movement is desired. Reciprocal effects throughout the dental arches must be carefully analyzed, evaluated, and controlled. The goal of mechanotherapy can be expressed most clearly as maximizing the tooth movement that is desired, while minimizing undesirable side effects.

Relationship of tooth movement to force. An obvious strategy for anchorage control would be to concentrate the force needed to produce tooth movement where it was desired, and then to dissipate the reaction force over as many other teeth as possible. Force against a tooth is biologically effective as pressure (force per unit area) in the periodontal ligament. Different types of tooth movement concentrate or distribute the force, producing varying pressures. Tipping, for example, loads only one-half the periodontal ligament area that bodily movement does (see Chapter 9). Not only

the amount of force, but also the way it will be distributed, must be considered in determining the pressure that will be produced.

A threshold, below which pressure would produce no reaction, could provide perfect anchorage control, since it would only be necessary to be certain that the threshold for tooth movement was not reached for teeth in the anchorage unit. A differential response to pressure, so that heavier pressure produced more tooth movement than lighter pressure, would make it possible to move some teeth more than others even though some undesired tooth movement occurred.

In fact, the threshold for tooth movement appears to be quite low, but there is a differential response to pressure, and so this strategy of "divide and conquer" is reasonably effective. As Fig. 10-22 indicates, teeth behave as if the response is proportional to the magnitude of the pressure, up to a point. When that point is reached, the amount of tooth movement becomes more or less independent of the magnitude of the pressure, so that a broad plateau of orthodontically effective pressure is created. Eventually, the response may begin to decline, as the pressure becomes intolerably large. The optimal force level for orthodontic movement would be the lightest force and resulting pressure that would produce a maximal response. Forces greater than that, though equally effective in producing tooth movement, would be unnecessarily traumatic and, as we will see, unnecessarily stressful to anchorage.

From the background of this chart, we can now define several anchorage situations:

Reciprocal tooth movement. In a reciprocal situation, the forces applied to teeth and to arch segments would be equal, and so would the force distribution in the periodontal ligament. A simple example is what would occur if two maxillary central incisors separated by a diastema were connected by an active spring (Fig. 10-23). The essentially identical teeth would feel the same force distributed in the same way through the periodontal ligament and would move toward each other by the same amount.

A somewhat similar situation would arise if a spring were placed across a first premolar extraction site, pitting the central incisor, lateral incisor, and canine in the anterior arch segment against the second premolar and first molar

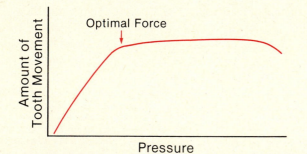

Fig. 10-22 ■ Theoretic representation of the relationship of pressure within the periodontal ligament to the amount of tooth movement. Pressure in the PDL is determined by the force applied to a tooth divided by the area of the PDL over which that force is distributed. The threshold for tooth movement is very small. Tooth movement increases in relation to pressure up to a point, remains at about the same level over a fairly broad range, and then may actually decline with extremely heavy pressure. The best definition of the optimal force for orthodontic purposes is the lightest force that produces a maximal or near-maximal response. The magnitude of this optimal force will vary depending on the way it is distributed in the PDL.

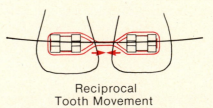

Fig. 10-23 ■ Reciprocal tooth movement is produced when two teeth or resistance units of equal size pull against each other, as in this example of the reciprocal closure of a maxillary midline diastema.

posteriorly (Fig. 10-24). Whether this technique would really produce reciprocal tooth movement requires some thought. Certainly the same force would be felt by the three anterior teeth and the two posterior teeth, since the action of the spring on one segment has an equal and opposite reaction on the other. Reciprocal movement would require that the total periodontal ligament (PDL) area over which the force was distributed be the same.

Conceptually, the "anchorage value" of a tooth, that is, its resistance to movement, can be thought of as a function of its root surface area, which is the same as its periodontal ligament area. The larger the root, the greater the area over which a force can be distributed, and vice versa. As Fig. 10-24 shows, the PDL area for the two posterior teeth in this example is slightly larger than the total anterior PDL area. Therefore, with a simple spring connecting the segments, the anterior teeth would move slightly more than the posteriors. The movement would not be truly reciprocal, but would be close to it.

Reinforced anchorage. Continuing with the extraction site example: if it was desired to retract the anterior teeth, the anchorage of the posterior teeth could be reinforced by adding the second molar to the posterior unit (Fig. 10-24). This would change the ratio of the root surface areas and would thereby produce relatively more retraction of the anterior segment than forward movement of the posterior segment.

Reinforcement of anchorage by adding more resistance units is effective because with more teeth (or extraoral structures) in the anchorage, the reaction to the force against the movement unit is distributed over a larger periodontal ligament area in the anchorage unit. This reduces the pressure on the anchor units, moving them down the slope of the pressure-response curve (Fig. 10-25). As the graph shows, however, using unnecessarily high force on the movement unit would be ineffective in causing more of the desired tooth movement but would cause more movement of the anchor teeth. Keeping the force light, in other words, would be more efficient from an anchorage conservation point of view, as well as making the tooth movement as atraumatic as possible.

Stationary anchorage. This term, traditionally used though inherently less descriptive than reinforced anchorage, refers to the advantage that can be obtained by pitting bodily movement of one group of teeth against tipping of another (Fig. 10-26). Using our same example of a premolar extraction site, if the appliance were arranged so that the anterior teeth could tip lingually while the posterior teeth could only move bodily, the optimal pressure for the anterior segment would be produced by about half as much force as if the anterior teeth were to be retracted bodily. This would mean that the reaction force distributed over the posterior teeth would be reduced by half, and as a consequence, these teeth would move much less.

If periodontal ligament areas were equal, tipping the an-

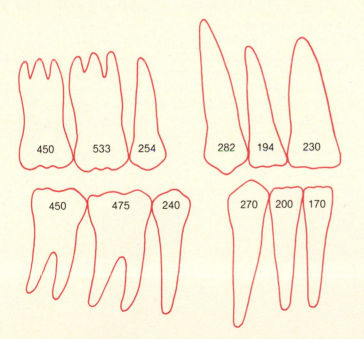

Fig. 10-24 ■ The "anchorage value" of any tooth is roughly equivalent to its root surface area. As this diagram shows, the first molar and second premolar in each arch are approximately equivalent in surface area to the canine and three incisors. (Modified from Freeman, D.C.: Root surface area related to anchorage in the Begg technique. Memphis, 1965, University of Tennessee, Department of Orthodontics, M.S. Thesis.)

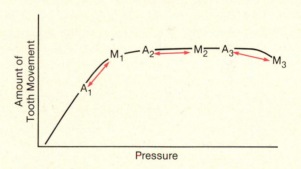

Fig. 10-25 ■ Consider the response of anchor teeth (*A* on the chart) and teeth to be moved *(M)* in three circumstances. In each case, the pressure in the periodontal ligament of the anchor teeth is less than pressure in the periodontal ligaments of teeth to be moved because there are more teeth in the anchor unit. In the first case *(A1↔M1)*, the pressure on the roots to be moved is at the optimal level, whereas pressure in the anchor unit is suboptimal. In the second example *(A2↔M2)*, although the force on the anchor teeth is less than the force on the teeth to be moved, both are on the plateau of the force-response curve, and the anchor teeth can be expected to move as much as the teeth that are desired to move. With extremely high force *(A3↔M3)*, there might be more movement of the anchor teeth than of the teeth it was desired to move. Although the third possibility is theoretic and may not be encountered clinically, it is clear that both the first and second situations are seen in clinical orthodontics. This principle explains the efficacy of light forces in controlling anchorage.

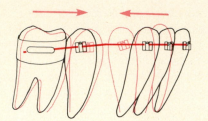

Fig. 10-26 ■ Displacement of anchor teeth can be minimized by arranging the force system so that anchor teeth must move bodily if at all, while movement teeth are allowed to tip, as in this example of retracting incisors by tipping them posteriorly. The approach is called "stationary anchorage." In this example, treatment is not complete because the roots of the lingually tipped incisors will have to be uprighted at a later stage, but two-stage treatment with tipping followed by uprighting can be used as a means of controlling anchorage.

terior segment while holding the posterior segment for bodily movement would have the effect of doubling the amount of anterior retraction as compared to posterior forward movement. It is important to note again, however, that successful implementation of this strategy would require that forces be kept light. If the force were large enough to bring the posterior teeth into their optimal movement range, it would no longer matter whether the anterior segment tipped or was moved bodily. Using too much force would disastrously undermine this method of anchorage control.

Differential force. If tooth movement were actually impeded by very high levels of pressure, it might be possible to structure an anchorage situation so that there was more movement of the arch segment with the larger periodontal ligament area. This result could happen, of course, if such high force were used that the smaller segment was placed beyond the tooth movement range, while the larger segment was still on it (Fig. 10-25). Because the effect would be

highly traumatic, it would be an undesirable way to deliberately manage anchorage.

In fact, it is not certain that the amount of tooth movement in response to applied force really decreases with very high force levels in any circumstance, and so this type of differential movement may not really exist. By using too much force, however, it is certainly possible to produce more movement of the anchor segment than was expected even if the mechanism is merely a differential movement of the anchor segment up the slope of the force-response curve rather than a decline in the response of the movement segment. Differential force is understood best in terms of the plateau portion of the curve in Fig. 10-25, not the questionable decline at the far right.

Cortical anchorage. A final consideration in anchorage control is the different response of cortical compared to medullary bone. Cortical bone is more resistant to resorption, and tooth movement is slowed when a root contacts it. Some authors have advocated torquing the roots of posterior teeth outward against the cortical plate as a way to inhibit their mesial movement when extraction spaces are to be closed.[6] Since the mesial movement would be along rather than against the cortical plate, it is doubtful that this technique greatly augments anchorage. However, a layer of dense cortical bone that has formed within the alveolar process can certainly affect tooth movement. This situation may be encountered at an old extraction site, for example, in an adult in whom a molar or premolar was lost many years previously (Fig. 10-27). It can be almost impossible to close such an extraction site, because tooth movement is slowed to a minimum as the roots encounter cortical bone along the resorbed alveolar ridge.

As a general rule, torquing movements are limited by the facial and lingual cortical plates. If a root is persistently forced against the cortical plate, tooth movement is greatly slowed, root resorption is likely, and eventual penetration of the cortical bone may sometimes occur (Fig. 10-28). It is possible to torque the root of a tooth labially or lingually

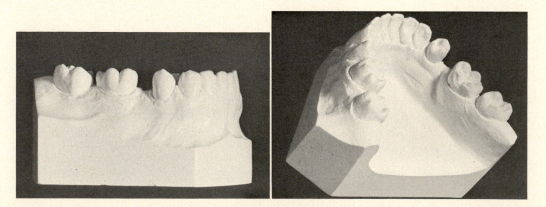

Fig. 10-27 ■ Loss of alveolar bone at an old extraction site can create an area of cortical bone between adjacent teeth, as the alveolar process narrows. This is one situation in which "cortical anchorage" can definitely be a factor. Closing such an extraction site is extremely difficult because of the resistance of the cortical bone to remodeling.

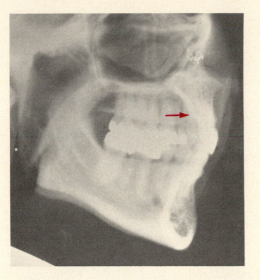

Fig. 10-28 ■ When the root of a maxillary incisor is torqued lingually until it contacts the lingual cortical plate, further tooth movement is often all but impossible because of the resistance of this cortical bone. For this patient, although the upper incisor might be judged to be too upright and in need of root torque, further lingual movement of the root will be impeded by the lingual cortical plate.

out of the bone, but fortunately, exceedingly difficult to do so.

■ Frictional Effects on Anchorage

When one moving object contacts another, friction at their interface produces resistance to the movement. The frictional resistance is dependent upon (1) the area of contact, (2) the force with which the contacting surfaces are pressed together, and (3) the type of surface at the interface (rough or smooth, modified by lubricants, etc.). Frictional resistance can be reduced by modifying any or all of these major factors, but it cannot be totally eliminated. To a surprisingly large extent, friction is a factor in orthodontic anchorage control, particularly for space closure with fixed appliances.

Consider the magnitude of frictional resistance when a bracket attached to a tooth slides along an archwire, or when an archwire slides through a bracket as other teeth are moved. All the factors described previously would come into play: the total frictional resistance would be determined by the area of contact between the wire and the bracket, the force with which the wire was pressed against the bracket, and the quality of the surfaces in contact. It is possible in the laboratory to measure the actual friction between various wires and brackets, and then to compare the magnitude of frictional resistance to the force levels needed to produce tooth movement. Results show that the force needed to overcome friction is of the same magnitude as force needed to move teeth.[7,8]

As noted earlier, when teeth slide along an archwire, it is easier to generate the moments needed to control root

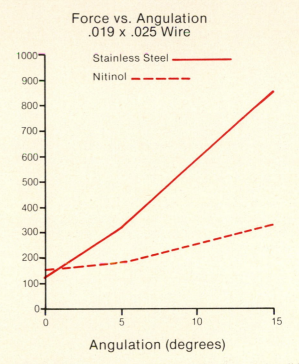

Fig. 10-29 ■ The amount of friction produced as a wire slides through a bracket increases as a function of the angulation of the wire across the bracket. Nitinol has an inherently slicker surface than stainless steel and is less affected by the angulation change (from Peterson L., et al.: Quintessence Int., pp. 563-571, 1982).

position with a wide bracket because the wider the bracket, the smaller the force needed at its edges to generate any necessary moment. With respect to friction, the wider bracket would also have the advantage of reducing the force on the wire as it slides through the bracket, thus decreasing friction from that source. However, a wider bracket provides a larger area at the base of the bracket that the wire can touch, thus increasing the contact area. Apparently, these factors tend to balance each other out, since laboratory data indicate that bracket width has surprisingly little effect on friction.[8]

The amount of force between the wire and the bracket strongly influences the amount of friction. If a tooth is pulled along an archwire, it will tip until the corners of the bracket contact the wire and the wire bends enough to generate a moment preventing further tipping (see Fig. 10-21). If the initial tipping is to be prevented and true bodily movement produced, the wire initially must cross the bracket at an angle. The greater the angle, the greater the initial moment and the greater the force between the wire and the bracket. As can be seen from Fig. 10-29, friction goes up rapidly as a function of the angle, and thereby the force, between the bracket and the wire.

Orthodontic wires and brackets have smooth, polished surfaces, and in the mouth, saliva serves as a reasonably good lubricant. Interestingly, NiTi has an inherently slick surface compared to stainless steel, so that all other factors

Friction, No Angulation

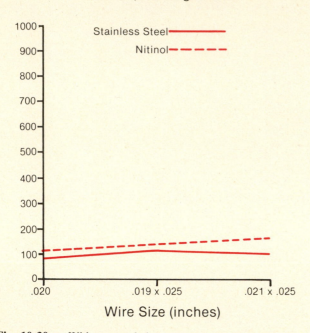

Fig. 10-30 ■ Without angulation, there is about 100 gm of friction when three commonly used wire sizes slide in 0.022 in edgewise brackets (from Peterson, L., et al.: Quintessence Int., pp. 563-571, 1982).

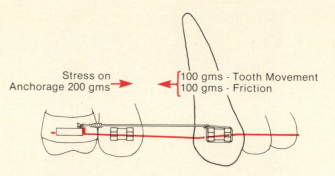

Fig. 10-31 ■ To retract a canine tooth by sliding it along an archwire, a frictional resistance equal to the force necessary to move the tooth must be overcome.

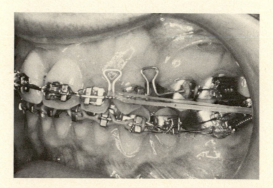

Fig. 10-32 ■ A closing loop is being used to retract the maxillary incisors, while a spring to slide the archwire through the molar tube is used for space closure in the lower arch. The Class II elastic from lower posterior to upper anterior also provides force to close both the upper and lower spaces.

being equal, there is less frictional resistance to sliding a tooth along a NiTi wire than a stainless steel one. This theoretic advantage may not be a practical one, but it does illustrate that changes in surface qualities can be significant. Certainly it would be unwise to attempt to slide teeth along unpolished or irregular wire surfaces. It is interesting to note that the irregular surface of a twisted or braided archwire can increase resistance to sliding.

Perhaps the most important information to be gained from a consideration of friction is an appreciation of its magnitude, even under the best of circumstances. Note that if an .019 × .025 steel wire is placed in an .022 slot bracket, the minimum frictional resistance to sliding a single bracket is about 100 gm (Fig. 10-30). In other words, if a canine tooth is to slide along an archwire as part of the closure of an extraction space, and a 100 gm net force is needed for tooth movement, at least another 100 gm will be needed to overcome friction (Fig. 10-31). The total force needed to slide the tooth, therefore, is twice as great as might have been expected, and the 200 gm reaction force will be felt by the anchor teeth.

Friction in the appliance system can be avoided if a spring loop is bent into the archwire, so that archwire segments move, taking the teeth with them instead of the teeth moving relative to the wire. Springs of this type are called retraction springs if they attach to only one tooth, or closing loops if they connect two archwire segments (Fig. 10-32). Incorporating springs into the archwire makes the appliance more complex to fabricate and to use clinically, but eliminates

the difficulty in anchorage control caused by frictional resistance.

■ Methods to Control Anchorage

From the previous discussion, it is apparent that several potential strategies can be used to control anchorage. Nearly all the possible approaches are actually used in clinical orthodontics, and each method is affected by whether friction will be encountered. Considering them in more detail:

Reinforcement. Reinforcement of anchorage typically involves including as many teeth as possible in the anchorage unit. For reasonable control, the ratio of periodontal ligament area in the anchorage unit to PDL area in the tooth movement unit should be at least 2 to 1 without friction, 4 to 1 with it. Anything less produces something close to reciprocal movement. Obviously, larger ratios are desirable if they can be obtained.

Satisfactory reinforcement of anchorage may require the addition of teeth from the opposite dental arch to the anchor unit. Reinforcement may also include forces derived from structures outside the mouth. Using our same example of a mandibular premolar extraction site: it would be possible to

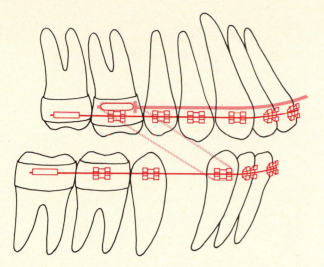

Fig. 10-33 ■ Reinforcement of anchorage can be produced by adding additional teeth within the same arch to the anchor unit, or by using elastics from the opposite arch to help produce desired tooth movement, as with the interarch elastic here. Additional reinforcement can be obtained with extraoral force, as with the facebow to the upper molar here, which resists the forward pull of the elastic.

stabilize all the teeth in the maxillary arch, so that they could only move bodily as a group, and then to run an elastic from the upper posterior to the lower anterior, thus pitting forward movement of the entire upper arch against distal movement of the lower anterior segment (Fig. 10-33). This addition of the entire upper arch would greatly alter the balance between retraction of the lower anteriors and forward slippage of the lower posteriors.

This anchorage could be reinforced even further by having the patient wear an extraoral headgear appliance that placed backward force against the upper arch. The reaction force from the headgear is dissipated against the bones of the cranial vault, thus adding the resistance of these structures to the anchorage unit. The only problem with reinforcement outside the dental arch is that springs within an arch provide constant forces, while elastics from one arch to the other tend to be intermittent, and extraoral force is likely to be even more intermittent. Although this time factor can significantly decrease the value of cross-arch and extraoral reinforcement, both can be quite useful clinically.

Subdivision of desired movement. A common way to improve anchorage control is to pit the resistance of a group of teeth against the movement of a single tooth, rather than dividing the arch into more or less equal segments. In our same extraction site example, it would be perfectly possible to reduce the strain on posterior anchorage by retracting the canine individually, pitting its distal movement against mesial movement of all other teeth within the arch (Fig. 10-34). After the canine tooth had been retracted, one could then add it to the posterior anchorage unit, and retract the four incisors individually. This approach would have the

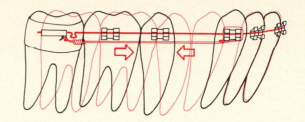

Fig. 10-34 ■ Retraction of the canine by itself, as the first step in a two-stage space closure, is often used to conserve anchorage, particularly when sliding teeth along an archwire.

advantage that the reaction force would always be dissipated over a large periodontal ligament area in the anchor unit. Its disadvantage is that closing the space in two steps rather than one would take nearly twice as long.

Subdivision of tooth movement improves the anchorage situation whether or not friction is involved, and no matter where a space in the arch is located. If it is desired to slip all the posterior teeth forward (in which case the anterior teeth are the anchor unit), bringing them forward one at a time is the most conservative way to proceed. Moving them one at a time without friction, of course, will put less strain on anchorage than sliding them one at a time.

Tipping/uprighting. Another possible strategy for anchorage control is to tip the teeth and then upright them, rather than moving them bodily. In our familiar extraction site example, this would again require two steps in treatment. First, the anterior teeth would be tipped distally by being pitted against mesial bodily movement of the posterior segment (Fig. 10-26). As a second step, the tipped teeth would be uprighted, moving the canine roots distally and torquing the incisor roots lingually, again with stationary anchorage in the posterior segments. It would be extremely important to keep forces as light as possible during both steps, so that the teeth in the posterior segment were always below the optimal force range while the anterior teeth received optimal force.

The desired amount of incisor retraction for any patient should be carefully planned, and the mechanotherapy should be selected to produce the desired outcome. This subject is discussed in considerably more detail in Chapter 16.

At this point, however, it is interesting to consider a relatively typical extraction situation, in which it is desired to close the extraction space 60% by retraction of the anterior teeth and 40% by forward movement of the posterior segments (Fig. 10-35). This outcome would be expected from any of three possible approaches: (1) one-step space closure with a frictionless appliance; (2) a two-step closure sliding the canine along the archwire, then retracting the incisors (as in the original Tweed technique); or (3) two-step space closure, tipping the anterior segment with some friction, then uprighting the tipped teeth (as in the Begg technique). The example makes the cost of friction in a clinical setting more apparent: the greater strain on anchorage when brackets slide along an archwire must be compensated by a more

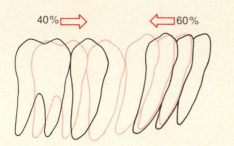

Fig. 10-35 ■ Closure of a premolar extraction site is often desired in a ratio of 60% retraction of incisors, 40% forward movement of molar and second premolar. This result can be obtained straight-forwardly in three ways: (1) a one-step space closure with a frictionless (closing loop) mechanism; (2) a two-step space closure with sliding mechanics, retracting the canine individually, and then retracting the four incisors in a second step; or (3) a two-step sliding space closure involving distal tipping of the canine and incisors initially, followed by uprighting of these teeth. The cost of friction in space closure, with well-managed orthodontic appliances, is more in treatment time rather than quality of result.

conservative approach to anchorage control. The price is usually paid, therefore, in increased treatment time. The frictionless appliance, though more difficult to fabricate and manipulate, will result in the same space closure significantly faster.

■ *The Development of Contemporary Orthodontic Appliances*

■ Angle's Progression to the Edgewise Appliance

Edward Angle's position as the "father of modern orthodontics" is based not only on his contributions to classification and diagnosis but also on his creativity in developing new orthodontic appliances. With few exceptions, the fixed appliances used in contemporary orthodontics are based on Angle's designs from the early twentieth century. Angle developed four major appliance systems:

The E-arch. In the late 1800s, a typical orthodontic appliance depended on some sort of rigid framework to which the teeth were tied so that they could be expanded to the arch form dictated by the appliance. Angle's first appliance, the E-arch, was of this type (Fig. 10-36). Bands were placed only on molar teeth, and a heavy labial archwire extended around the arch. The end of the wire was threaded, and a small nut placed on the threaded portion of the arch allowed the archwire to be advanced, building in a mechanism for arch expansion. Individual teeth were simply ligated to this expansion arch.

Pin and tube. The E-arch was capable only of tipping teeth to a new position. It was not possible to precisely position any individual tooth. To overcome this difficulty, Angle began placing bands on other teeth and used a vertical tube on each tooth into which a soldered pin from a smaller archwire was placed. With this appliance, tooth movement

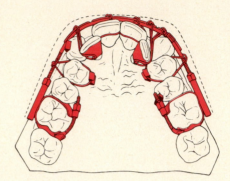

Fig. 10-36 ■ Edward Angle's E-arch, from the early 1900s. Ligatures from a heavy labial arch were used to bring malposed teeth to the line of occlusion.

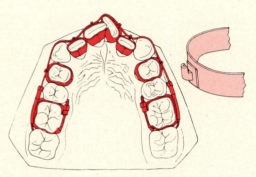

Fig. 10-37 ■ Angle's ribbon arch appliance, introduced about 1910, was well adapted to bring teeth into alignment but was too flexible to allow precise positioning of roots.

was accomplished by repositioning the individual pins at each appointment.

Obviously, an incredible degree of craftsmanship was involved in constructing and adjusting this pin and tube appliance, and although it was theoretically capable of great precision in tooth movement, it proved impractical in clinical use. It is said that only Angle himself and one of his students ever mastered the appliance. The relatively heavy base arch meant that spring qualities were poor, and the problem therefore was compounded because many small adjustments were needed.

Ribbon arch. Angle's next appliance modified the tube on each tooth to provide a vertically positioned rectangular slot behind the tube. A ribbon arch of .010 × .020 gold wire was placed into the slot and held with pins (Fig. 10-37). The ribbon arch was an immediate success, primarily because the archwire, unlike any of its predecessors, was small enough to have good spring qualities and was quite efficient in aligning malposed teeth. Although the ribbon arch could be twisted as it was inserted into its slot, the major weakness of the appliance was that it provided relatively poor control of root position. The resiliency of the ribbon archwire simply did not allow generation of the moments necessary to torque roots to a new position.

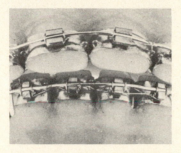

Fig. 10-38 ■ Angle's edgewise appliance received its name because the archwire was inserted at a 90 degree angle to the plane of insertion of the ribbon arch. With the rectangular wire in a rectangular slot, excellent control of root position was possible.

Edgewise. To overcome the deficiencies of the ribbon arch, Angle reoriented the slot from vertical to horizontal and inserted a rectangular wire rotated 90 degrees to the orientation it had with the ribbon arch, thus the name "edgewise" (Fig. 10-38). The dimensions of the slot were altered to .022 × .028, and an .022 × .028 precious metal wire was used. These dimensions, arrived at after extensive experimentation, did allow excellent control of crown and root position in all three planes of space.

After its introduction in 1928, this appliance became the mainstay of multibanded fixed appliance therapy, although the ribbon arch continued in common use for another decade.

■ Other Early Appliance Systems

Before Angle, placing attachments on individual teeth simply had not been done, and Angle's concern about precisely positioning each tooth was not widely shared during his lifetime. In addition to a variety of removable appliances utilizing fingersprings for repositioning teeth, the major competing appliance systems were the labiolingual appliance, which used bands on first molars and a combination of heavy lingual and labial archwires to which fingersprings were soldered to move individual teeth (Fig. 10-39), and the twin-wire appliance (Fig. 10-40). This appliance used bands on incisors as well as molars, and featured twin .010 archwires for alignment of the incisor teeth. These delicate wires were protected by long tubes extending forward from the molars to the vicinity of the canines. None of these appliances, however, was capable of more than tipping movements except with special and unusual modifications.

■ The Begg Appliance

Given Angle's insistence on expansion of the arches rather than extraction to deal with crowding problems, it is ironic that the edgewise appliance finally provided the control of root position necessary for successful extraction treatment, and that the appliance was being used for this purpose within a few years of its introduction. Charles Tweed, one

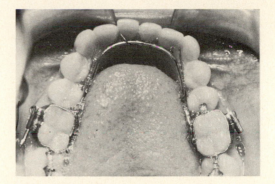

Fig. 10-39 ■ The labiolingual appliance, widely used until recent years but now obsolete, combined a heavy maxillary labial arch like Angle's E-arch with a heavy mandibular and occasionally maxillary lingual arch to which fingersprings and ligature ties were attached, as shown here. Only the first molar teeth were banded.

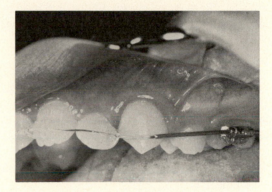

Fig. 10-40 ■ The twin-wire appliance used two strands of .010 wire for initial alignment of the incisor teeth. Incisors and first molars had fixed attachments, but canines and premolars were not usually banded. A heavy tube extending forward from the first molar was used to protect the delicate twin wires.

of Angle's last students, was the leader in the United States in adapting the edgewise appliance for extraction treatment. In fact, little adaptation of the appliance was needed. Tweed moved the teeth bodily and used the subdivision approach for anchorage control, first sliding the canines distally along the archwire, then retracting the incisors.

Raymond Begg had been taught the ribbon arch appliance at the Angle school before his return to Australia in the 1920s. Working independently in Adelaide, Begg also concluded that extraction of teeth was often necessary, and set out to adapt the ribbon arch appliance so that it could be used for better control of root position.

Begg's adaptation took three forms: (1) he replaced the precious metal ribbon arch with high strength .016 stainless steel wire as this became available in the late 1930s; (2) he retained the original ribbon arch bracket, but turned it upside down, so that the bracket slot pointed occlusally rather than gingivally; and (3) he added auxiliary springs to the appliance for control of root position. In the resulting Begg

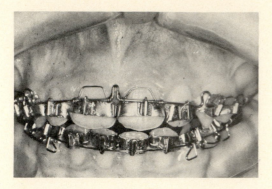

Fig. 10-41 ■ The Begg appliance is a modification of the ribbon arch attachment, into which round archwires are pinned. A variety of auxiliary archwires is used in this system to obtain control of root position.

appliance (Fig. 10-41), friction was minimized because the area of contact between the narrow ribbon arch bracket and the archwire was very small and the force of the wire against the bracket was also small. Begg's strategy for anchorage control was tipping/uprighting (Fig. 10-26).

Although the progress records with his approach looked vastly different, it is not surprising that the overall result in anchorage control was similar to Tweed's, since both used two steps to overcome some frictional problems. The Begg appliance is still seen in contemporary use though it has declined in popularity. It is a complete appliance in the sense that it allows good control of crown and root position in all three planes of space.

■ Contemporary Edgewise: the Straight-Arch Appliance

The contemporary edgewise appliance has evolved far beyond the original design while retaining the basic principle of a rectangular wire in a rectangular slot. Despite many variations, the contemporary appliances have many features in common. Major steps in the evolution of edgewise appliances include:

Automatic rotational control. This is accomplished either by using twin brackets on the labial surface (Fig. 10-42), or single brackets with extension wings that contact the archwire to control and correct rotations (Lewis brackets).

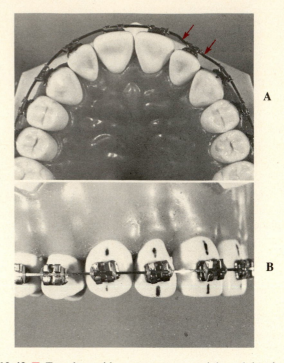

Fig. 10-42 ■ Typodont with contemporary straight arch brackets on the right side and conventional twin brackets on the left. **A,** Bends in the archwire to compensate for the lateral incisor position are required on the conventional side *(arrows),* whereas on the straight arch side, a thicker base for the lateral bracket provides the same positioning without a bend in the wire. **B,** On the straight arch side, each bracket slot is also angulated individually and cut at an angle, eliminating angulating and torquing bends.

Alteration in bracket slot dimensions. Edgewise bracket slots are now routinely deeper than Angle originally proposed, either .022 × .030 or .018 × .030. The significance of reducing slot width from .022 to .018 has been discussed earlier. The deeper bracket slot allows better engagement of large archwires and the possibility of placing two smaller archwires simultaneously if desired.

Variation in bracket thickness to compensate for the varying thickness of individual teeth. In the original edgewise appliance, faciolingual bends in the archwires (first-order bends) were necessary to compensate for variations

Table 10-9 ■ A generalized torque/angular prescription for ''straight arch'' edgewise

	Maxillary		Mandibular	
	Angulation	Torque	Angulation	Torque
Central	+5°	+14°	0°	−1°
Lateral	+8°	+7°	0°	−1°
Canine	+10°	−3°	+6°	−7°
First premolar	0°	−7°	0°	−14°
Second premolar	0°	−7°	0°	−17°
First molar	+10°	−10°	0°	−25°
Second molar	+10°	−10°	0°	−30°

in the contour of labial surfaces of individual teeth. In the contemporary appliance, this compensation is built into the base of the bracket itself (Fig. 10-42, *A*).

Angulation of bracket slots. Angulation of brackets relative to the long axis of the tooth is necessary to achieve proper positioning of the roots of most teeth. Originally, this mesiodistal root positioning required angled bends in the archwire, called second-order bends. Angulating the bracket or bracket slot removes the necessity for these bends in archwires (Table 10-9, Fig. 10-42, *B*).

Torque in bracket slots. Because the facial surface of individual teeth varies markedly in inclination to the true vertical, in the original edgewise appliance it was necessary to place a varying twist (referred to as third-order bends) in segments of each rectangular archwire, to avoid inadvertent torquing movements of properly positioned teeth. The bracket slots in the contemporary edgewise appliance are inclined to compensate for the inclination of the facial surface, so that third order bends are unnecessary.

With the elimination of the need to routinely place first, second, and third-order bends in nearly every archwire, without the necessity to tie for rotation control, and with the availability of new archwire materials, the edgewise system has become considerably easier to manage clinically. The combination of the alterations listed previously, particularly the last three described, has produced the group of modern edgewise appliances referred to as the straight-arch systems. Contemporary fixed appliances are discussed more fully in Chapter 12, and the clinical use of the contemporary edgewise appliance is described in detail in Chapters 15 to 17.

■ Lingual Appliances

A major objection to fixed orthodontic appliances has been their visible placement on the facial surface of the teeth. Improving esthetics by using an invisible appliance has been one goal of orthodontic appliance design for many years. This has always been one reason for the use of removable appliances.

The development of techniques for bonding brackets directly to the enamel surface, rather than attaching them to metal bands, was a potent step toward improving the esthetic qualities of fixed appliances. A bonded metal bracket is much less obtrusive than a metal band around an anterior tooth. Bonded plastic brackets further improve esthetics, but unfortunately these brackets tend to discolor and break after prolonged use, and so offer less esthetic advantage than was hoped originally.

With bonding techniques, it is also possible to place fixed attachments on the lingual rather than the labial surface of teeth, producing an invisible fixed appliance (Fig. 10-43). In theory, it should be possible to obtain the same three-

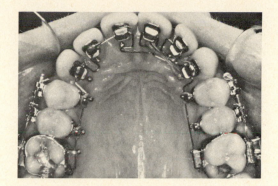

Fig. 10-43 ■ Adaptation of the edgewise appliance so that it can be placed on the lingual surface requires drastic alterations in the shape of the brackets, but the principle of a rectangular wire in a rectangular slot remains.

dimensional control of crown and root position from the lingual surface as the labial, and considerable progress has been made toward this goal. The small interbracket span between lingual attachments is a considerable problem with fixed lingual appliances. The situation is somewhat reminiscent of Edward Angle's problems with the pin and tube appliance: the reduced resilience of the lingual appliance means that it requires more frequent adjustments, but the appliance is relatively inaccessible and quite difficult to adjust. It is probable that significant changes in lingual appliance designs will occur. An adaptation of the Begg rather than the edgewise appliance, or a totally new design, may be the answer to present problems. At this writing, it is fair to say that the initial promise of lingual appliances has not yet been fulfilled.

■ *References*

1. Burstone, C.J., Qin, B., and Morton, J.Y.: Chinese NiTi wire: a new orthodontic alloy. Am. J. Orthod. **87**:445-452, 1985.
2. Kusy, R.P.: On the use of nomograms to determine the elastic property ratios of orthodontic arch wires. Am. J. Orthod. **83**:374-381, 1983.
3. Kusy, R.P.: Elastic property ratios of orthodontic arch wires. Chapel Hill, NC, 1982, University of North Carolina Department of Orthodontics/Dental Research Center.
4. Burstone, C.J.: Variable-modulus orthodontics. Am. J. Orthod. **80**:1-16, 1981.
5. Angle, E.H.: The latest and best in orthodontic mechanism. Dental Cosmos **70**:1143-1158, 1928.
6. Ricketts, R.M., et al.: Bioprogressive Therapy. Denver, 1979, Rocky Mountain Orthodontics, p. 100.
7. Andreasen, G.F., and Quevedo, F.R.: Evaluation of friction forces in the 0.022 × 0.028 edgewise bracket in vitro. J. Biomechanics **3**:151-160, 1970.
8. Peterson, L., Spencer, R., and Andreasen, G.: A comparison of friction resistance for Nitinol and stainless steel wire in edgewise brackets. Quintessence Int., pp. 563-571, 1982.

FIXED AND REMOVABLE APPLIANCES

Contemporary orthodontic treatment involves the use of both fixed and removable appliances. It is important to understand both the potential contribution and the limitations of removable appliances, and Chapter 11 is written from this perspective. Although removable appliances tend to play only a supporting role in comprehensive treatment, they are an important part of preliminary treatment for preadolescents, adjunctive treatment for adults, and retention for all types of patients. Contemporary fixed appliance treatment is built around the modern edgewise appliances that use offset, angulated, and torqued bracket slots to eliminate routine first, second, and third order bends in arch wires. In Chapter 12, banding and bonding as methods for attaching fixed appliances are described and illustrated, and the characteristics of the contemporary edgewise appliances are discussed in detail.

Chapter 11

Removable Appliances

Removable orthodontic appliances have two immediately apparent advantages: they can be removed on socially sensitive occasions, which makes them (at least initially) more acceptable to patients, and they are fabricated in the laboratory rather than directly in the patient's mouth, reducing the dentist's chair time during the initial part of treatment. In addition, as described in Chapter 14, they allow some types of growth guidance treatment to be carried out more readily than is possible with fixed appliances. These advantages for both the patient and the dentist have ensured a continuing interest in removable appliances.

There are also obvious disadvantages: the response to treatment is heavily dependent on patient compliance, since the appliance can be effective only when the patient chooses to wear it, and it is difficult to obtain the two-point contacts on teeth necessary to produce complex tooth movements, which means that the appliance itself may limit the possibilities for treatment. Because of these limitations, contemporary comprehensive treatment is dominated by fixed, not removable appliances.

The goals of this chapter are to describe the development of removable appliances, to discuss the fabrication, adjustment, and use of contemporary removable appliances, and to describe both their indications and contraindications in the movement of teeth.

■ The Development of Removable Appliances

Any removable appliance has three major components (Fig. 11-1): (1) a retentive component, consisting of various clasps to hold it in place, (2) a framework or baseplate, and (3) tooth-moving elements, typically either springs or screws. The story of the development of removable appliances is one of continuing improvements in each of these components. The limitations of removable appliances are usually their retentive components, and advances have centered around improvements in clasps. The best spring is useless unless it can be held in proper position against the tooth. As discussed in Chapter 10, the forces that must be applied to the crown of a tooth to produce root movement are surprisingly large, and retaining a removable appliance while it delivers these forces can be a real challenge.

In the United States, Victor Hugo Jackson was the chief proponent of removable appliances among the pioneer orthodontists of the early twentieth century. At that time, neither the modern plastics for baseplate materials nor stainless steel wires for clasps and springs were available, and the appliances were rather clumsy combinations of vulcanite bases and precious metal or nickel-silver wires.

In the early 1900s, George Crozat developed a removable appliance fabricated entirely of precious metal that is still used occasionally. The appliance consisted of an effective clasp for first molar teeth modified from Jackson's designs, heavy gold wires as a framework, and lighter gold fingersprings to produce the desired tooth movement (Fig. 11-2). At the time the Crozat appliance was developed, a typical

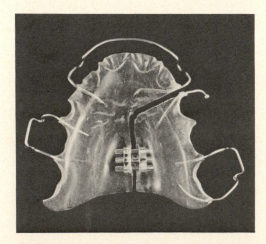

Fig. 11-1 ■ A typical maxillary active removable appliance, showing the three major components: clasps, framework, and tooth moving elements.

fixed appliance consisted of bands only on first molars, with wire ligatures tied to a heavy labial or lingual arch wire to align malposed teeth. The Crozat appliance was a removable but more flexible version of the same device.

The Crozat appliance attracted a small but devoted and loyal following, primarily in the area around New Orleans. It is still used by some practitioners, but had little impact on the mainstream of American orthodontic thought and practice. From the beginning, the emphasis in American orthodontics was on fixed appliances, and the steady progression of fixed appliance techniques has been illustrated in Chapter 10.

For a variety of reasons, development of removable appliances continued in Europe despite their neglect in the United States. It appears that there were three major reasons for this trend: (1) Angle's dogmatic approach to occlusion,

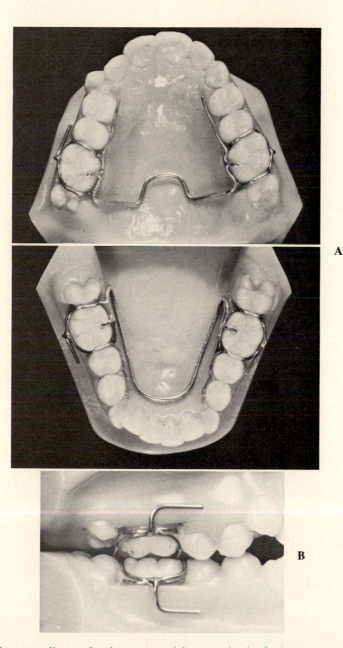

A

B

Fig. 11-2 ■ Crozat appliances for the upper and lower arch. **A,** Occlusal view, showing the transverse connectors that allow lateral expansion; **B,** closeup of the Crozat clasps, which utilize fingers extending into the mesiobuccal and distobuccal undercuts.

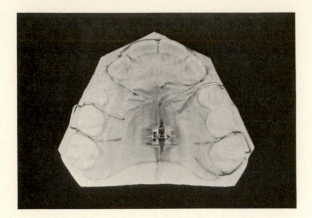

Fig. 11-3 ■ A "split-plate" appliance of the type popularized by Martin Schwartz in Vienna and widely used in the European orthodontics of the midtwentieth century.

odontics of this period was functional appliances for guidance of growth. The development of these appliances is discussed in Chapter 14. In addition to the functional appliance pioneers, two European orthodontists deserve special mention for their contributions to removable appliance techniques for moving teeth. Martin Schwartz in Vienna developed and publicized a variety of "split plate" appliances (Fig. 11-3), which could produce most types of tooth movements.[1] Philip Adams in Belfast modified the arrowhead clasp favored by Schwartz into the Adams crib, which became the basis for English removable appliances and is still the most effective clasp for orthodontic purposes[2] (Fig. 11-4).

Despite the ingenious designs of the European removable appliances, however, the essential limitations remained. Although treatment with these appliances was less expensive and more available, orthodontic tooth movement was neither as efficient nor as precise as with fixed appliances. Within the past 20 years, the dichotomy between European and American orthodontics has largely disappeared. European-style removable appliances, particularly for first-stage mixed dentition treatment, have become widely used in the United States, while fixed appliances have largely replaced removables for comprehensive treatment in Europe and elsewhere throughout the world. This trend has been accelerated by the replacement of orthodontic bands with bonded attachments, which makes the placement of fixed appliances easier for both the dentist and the patient.

In contemporary practice, the decision of whether a fixed or a removable appliance is to be used should be made, not on the basis of the national system for orthodontic treatment, but on the needs of the individual patient. Although most patients will require fixed appliances for satisfactory comprehensive treatment, removable appliances still have a place, particularly for growth modification during the mixed dentition, simple tooth movement in children or adults (including some adjunctive treatment to facilitate periodontal or restorative treatment), and retention after fixed appliance treatment.

with its emphasis on precise positioning of each tooth, had less impact in Europe than in the United States. (2) Social welfare systems developed much more rapidly in Europe, which meant that the emphasis tended to be on widespread if limited orthodontic treatment, often delivered by general practitioners rather than orthodontic specialists. (3) Precious metal for fixed appliances was less available in Europe, both as a consequence of the social systems and because the use of precious metal in dentistry was banned in Nazi Germany, forcing German orthodontists to emphasize removable appliances that could be made with available materials. (Precision steel attachments were not available until long after World War II; fixed appliances required precious metal.)

The interesting result was that in the 1925 to 1965 era, American orthodontics was based almost exclusively on the use of fixed appliances, while fixed appliances were essentially unknown in Europe and all treatment was done with removables, not only for growth guidance but also for tooth movement of all types.

A major part of European removable appliance orth-

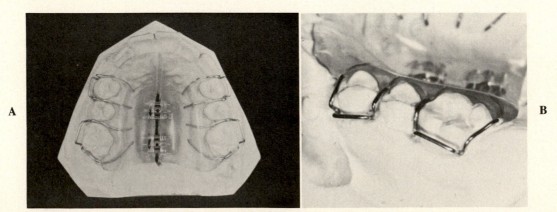

A   **B**

Fig. 11-4 ■ Adams cribs used as clasps for a maxillary expansion plate. This clasp is the most effective retention device for removable appliances. **A,** Occlusal view; **B,** lateral view.

■ *Indications for Removable Appliances*

Removable appliances are indicated for three major uses:

- Limited (tipping) tooth movements, especially for arch expansion or correction of individual tooth malposition; this treatment is the focus of the remainder of this chapter
- Growth modification during the mixed dentition, discussed in Chapter 14
- Retention after comprehensive treatment, discussed in Chapter 18

■ Arch Expansion with Active Plates

In the European approach of the midtwentieth century, removable appliances were typically divided into "activators" or functional appliances aimed at modifying growth, and "active plates" aimed at moving teeth. The framework of an active plate is a baseplate, usually made of acrylic. It serves as a base to which both clasps and springs are attached. Typically, the baseplate is also used to control anchorage by preventing the unwanted movement of some teeth. If screws or springs are embedded within the baseplate, the edges of the plate can become an active part of the appliance.

The indications for arch expansion as a method of treatment for crowding and malalignment are presented in Chapters 7 and 8. Obviously, a careful diagnostic evaluation is required to summarize all the characteristics of an individual malocclusion, and the treatment plan must be calculated to achieve maximum benefit for the patient. Because of the necessity to individualize treatment, it is neither wise nor practical to reduce the diagnosis and treatment planning to simple generalities. However, the greater the extent of crowding, the greater the chance of relapse after expansion treatment. Gaining more than a few millimeters of space by arch expansion is rarely desirable.

Anterior expansion of maxillary incisors. One of the simplest uses of an active plate for expansion is to correct a maxillary anterior crossbite when there is room to accommodate the teeth in their appropriate position within the arch (Fig. 11-5). In this circumstance, the baseplate material is usually brought up over the occlusal surface of the teeth, creating a bite plane that separates the teeth vertically and allows clearance for the upper incisors to move out of crossbite. In children, the bite plane to separate the teeth may not be necessary, but in older patients it is almost always needed. The bite plane must be supported by the teeth, not just the underlying soft tissue, which would be the case if the bite plane were lingual to the upper incisors that are being advanced.

Retention for a plate of this type can sometimes be obtained simply by allowing the acrylic material to flow slightly into buccal and lingual undercuts. Alternatively and more typically, clasps are incorporated, which extend into buccal undercuts of posterior teeth. A flexible spring behind the incisors completes the appliance.

Transverse expansion of the arches. Another common circumstance in which arch expansion is appropriate is a constricted maxillary arch, with a tendency toward crossbite. A split-plate removable appliance (Fig. 11-6) will expand the arch almost totally by tipping the posterior teeth buccally, not by opening the midpalatal suture and widening the maxilla itself, and for this reason, removable plates are not indicated for skeletal crossbites or for dental expansion of more than 4 to 5 mm. To achieve bilateral maxillary expansion, excellent clasping is required, and the mesiobuccal and mesiolingual undercuts of the maxillary posterior teeth are used for this purpose.

The active element of a split expansion plate is almost always a screw placed in the midline so that it holds the two parts of the plate together. Opening the screw with a

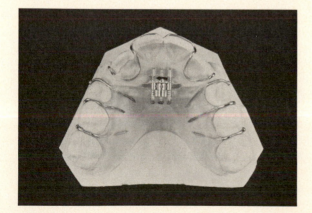

Fig. 11-5 ■ An active plate for forward positioning of the maxillary incisors, to correct an anterior crossbite. An active plate of this type, though reasonably effective in tipping the incisors forward, must be activated very slowly to prevent excessive force against the teeth and displacement of the plate.

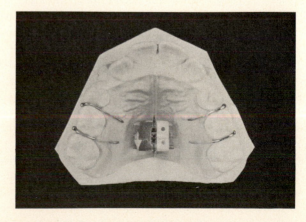

Fig. 11-6 ■ A split-plate removable appliance for correction of posterior crossbite. A plate of this type can tip the posterior teeth buccally, provided the screw is opened slowly and excellent retention is available. Usually, clasps that provide more retention than the ball clasps shown here are needed (see Fig. 11-4).

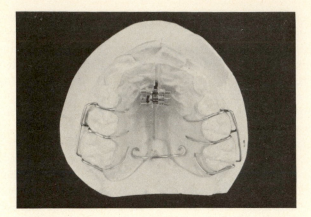

Fig. 11-7 ■ An expansion plate designed to produce more expansion anteriorly than posteriorly. Asymmetric opening of the plate is possible because of a certain amount of twisting within the screw itself. Note the double Adams cribs posteriorly, which provides much firmer retention than the ball clasps shown in Fig 11-6.

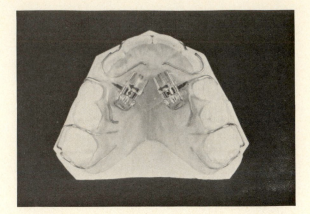

Fig. 11-8 ■ The "Y-plate" designed by Schwartz to simultaneously expand the maxillary posterior teeth laterally and the incisors anteriorly. As with all screw-activated appliances, very slow and careful activation of the screws is required. As a general rule, appliances of this type are no longer recommended in contemporary use.

key then separates the two halves of the plate, widening the arch and tipping the posterior teeth buccally. The use of a screw offers the advantage that the amount of movement can be controlled, and the baseplate remains rigid despite being cut into two parts. The disadvantage is that the force system is very different from the ideal one for moving teeth. Rather than providing a light but continuous force, activation of the screw produces a heavy force that decays rapidly.

As discussed in Chapter 9, heavy intermittent forces are acceptable for production of orthodontic tooth movement, provided adequate time is allowed for remodeling and repair between activations. Heavy force and damage could result from activating the screw too rapidly. In bilateral expansion of the maxillary arch, however, the force from the screw is distributed over a number of teeth, thereby reducing the amount of force felt by any individual tooth. In addition, even with the best clasps, if the force levels become too high, the appliance will be displaced before damage could occur, so that damage is unlikely. This displacement is the most common problem with expansion plates: activating the screw too rapidly results in the appliance being progressively displaced away from the teeth rather than the arch being expanded as desired.

Most screws open 1 mm per complete revolution, so that a single quarter turn produces 0.25 mm of tooth movement. The rate of active tooth movement should not exceed 1 mm per month. A screw used for expansion of the maxillary arch should under no circumstance be activated more than twice a week, a rate that would produce movement of 1 mm per month bilaterally. With the plates of this type, it is usually preferable to place the appliance in the mouth, turn the screw with the appliance held firmly in position, and not remove it for several hours after activation. This maximizes the chance that the removable appliance will continue to fit.

If it is desired to expand the maxillary arch more anteriorly than posteriorly, a wire can be placed holding the posterior parts of the split plate together (Fig. 11-7). The screw itself will allow a certain amount of twisting, and up to 4 mm of opening anteriorly can be achieved with an ordinary screw in a plate that is wired posteriorly. Special screws that allow greater fanwise expansion are available, if indicated—which is rarely the case.

Lateral expansion of the mandibular arch with a removable appliance is much more difficult than maxillary expansion, simply because the screw must be placed more anteriorly. Expanding the mandibular intercanine distance with an anteriorly positioned screw in a removable appliance is not recommended, because excessive forces can easily be produced and because mandibular intercanine expansion is notoriously unstable.

Simultaneous anterior and posterior expansion. It is also possible to expand, particularly in the maxillary arch, by dividing the baseplate into three rather than two segments. This design was the basis of Schwartz's original "Y plate," used to simultaneously expand the maxillary posterior teeth laterally and the incisors anteriorly (Fig. 11-8). If plates of this type are activated slowly and carefully, they can be quite effective in arch expansion, and differential activation of the screws would provide a way to deal with asymmetries within the arch. The major problem with such a plate, as with any screw-activated device, is the heavy intermittent force system, which requires that the tooth movement proceed extremely slowly.

A variant of the Y plate divides the baseplate into only two sections, one large and one small (Fig. 11-9). With an asymmetrically divided plate, activation of the screw will produce more force per unit area in the smaller baseplate segment than in the larger, and therefore there should be more movement of the teeth in the small segment. Carrying

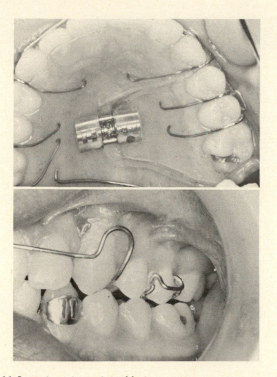

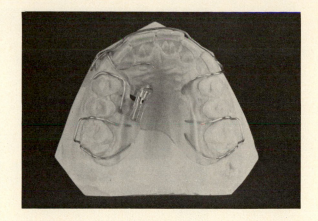

Fig. 11-10 ■ A split-plate appliance designed to expand the dental arch anteroposteriorly, creating additional space for crowded teeth. An appliance of this type is sometimes called a ''sagittal appliance,'' because of its direction of force along the sagittal plane. This appliance produces much more forward tipping of incisors than posterior movement of molars and also creates extremely unphysiologic force levels. Although appliances of this type were frequently used in Europe a generation ago, they have little or no place in contemporary orthodontics and are not recommended.

Fig. 11-9 ■ A variant of the Y-plate, used to produce more expansion on the left than the right side in this patient with a unilateral crossbite tendency. Differential expansion occurs because the teeth on the patient's left side, adjacent to the small section of the plate, receive more force from opening the screw than teeth adjacent to the large segment.

this idea to an extreme would lead to putting a single tooth in the small segment, with all other teeth contained in the large segment. This approach is not recommended, because too much force is produced by an activation if it is concentrated against a single tooth. The practical limit for the number of teeth in a small segment is two or three. As a general rule, springs rather than screws should be used if the movement of only one or two teeth is required.

It is also possible to use a split-plate design and a screw to expand an arch in an anteroposterior direction, as for example with an appliance to open space for a blocked out canine or a premolar; this device is sometimes called a sagittal appliance (Fig. 11-10). The same objection to screws applies to this circumstance: the force system is just the opposite of what is desired for physiologic tooth movement. For this reason, screw-activated appliances cannot be recommended for intra-arch expansion. Using a screw for this purpose is at best obsolete and at worst positively dangerous.

All split-plate appliances produce only tipping tooth movement, because the edge of the plate contacts each tooth at only one point. There is no way to produce the couple necessary for labial or buccal root torque without modifying the design to include a second spring (see Chapter 10), and even then, movements other than tipping are extremely difficult. Even when tipping is an acceptable result in expan-

sion, a fixed appliance with only a few teeth banded, for example, a lingual arch, produces similar effects and is often a better choice. Removable appliances for arch expansion, in short, have limited indications in children and adults.

■ Active Springs for Positioning Individual Teeth

The springs used in removable appliances must combine strength, springiness, and range of action to be effective. Strength is an important criterion for any component of an orthodontic appliance, but is especially critical for the springs in a removable appliance, which are activated and deactivated frequently. If the spring distorts permanently the first time the appliance is removed and replaced, it will be totally unsuccessful clinically. This necessity to obtain adequate strength usually means that the wires for springs in a removable appliance must be larger than would be ideal for good spring properties. This increased wire size, in turn, means that it is necessary to increase the length of the spring wires in most applications, recurving the wire on itself, bending a helical loop into the wire, and/or supporting the spring wire on only one end as opposed to both ends (Fig 11-11). The relationships between wire size and configuration on one hand, and the properties of strength, stiffness, and range on the other, are discussed in some detail in Chapter 10.

In contrast to the heavy, rapidly decaying forces produced by a screw, nearly optimal light continuous forces can be produced by the springs incorporated in removable appliances. Like the edges of an active plate, however, these springs contact the tooth surface at only one point, and it is difficult to use them for anything but tipping tooth movements. Root movements are not impossible, but generating

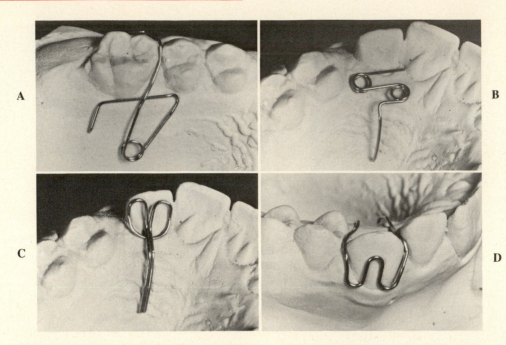

Fig. 11-11 ■ A variety of springs for possible use with a removable appliance: **A,** helical spring for distal tipping of a molar; **B,** double helical spring for labial tipping of a lateral incisor; **C,** paddle spring for labial movement of an incisor. Note that this design provides better control over the position of the part of the spring that contacts the tooth, at the cost of greater potential occlusal interference; **D,** buccal loop spring, to tip a canine lingually. The attachment portion of a spring of this type must be contoured carefully as it extends into the baseplate so that it does not interfere with the desired tooth movement.

the necessary moments requires either the application of two springs applying forces in opposite directions to the same tooth (see Chapter 10), or the attachment of a tube to the tooth surface into which the spring of the removable appliance can insert. Neither solution is very practical. The guideline for tooth movement with a simple spring from a removable appliance, therefore, is that this device is acceptable for a few millimeters of tipping movement. Root control is needed for more than 3 to 4 mm of crown movement.

One possible use of a removable appliance is to retract flared incisors, and for this purpose, a long labial bow with loops for greater flexibility and adjustment is normally used. The classic labial bow was designed by Charles Hawley in the 1920s (Fig. 11-12) and a removable appliance incorporating it is still often called a Hawley appliance or (since it is frequently used as a retainer after comprehensive treatment) a Hawley retainer. A wire labial bow is usually included in split plate appliances, even if there is no desire to reposition the anterior teeth, because it provides some anterior stabilization for the appliance and allows the position of the incisor teeth to be adjusted if necessary.

■ Combined Functional-Active Plate Appliances

A functional appliance by definition is an appliance that produces all or part of its effect by altering the position of the mandible. Nearly all functional appliances are remov-

able. Their purpose is to modify the pattern of jaw growth, change the direction and amount of tooth eruption, or both, to correct jaw discrepancies. In theory, there is no reason that growth guidance with a functional removable appliance cannot be combined with active tooth movement produced by springs or screws. A number of European removable appliance systems do incorporate active elements into a functional appliance. The original activators did not use any springs or screws, but essentially all of the modified activators developed in Europe after World War II were modified largely in the sense that the elements of active plates were added to an activator framework so that teeth could be moved while jaw growth was controlled.

Incorporating active elements into a functional removable appliance is a decidedly mixed blessing. There are two problems. The first is that correcting the occlusal relationships by actively moving teeth is not the goal of functional appliance therapy, and in fact active tooth movement may prevent the modification in jaw position that is desired as a result of functional treatment. To take Class II malocclusion as an example, the more the occlusion is corrected by springs that move the lower incisors forward relative to the mandible, the less the skeletal change that will be produced (Fig. 11-13). Adding springs or screws to push the teeth toward the desired occlusion does make the treatment proceed faster, but the result may be worse than that achieved by a functional appliance without active springs.

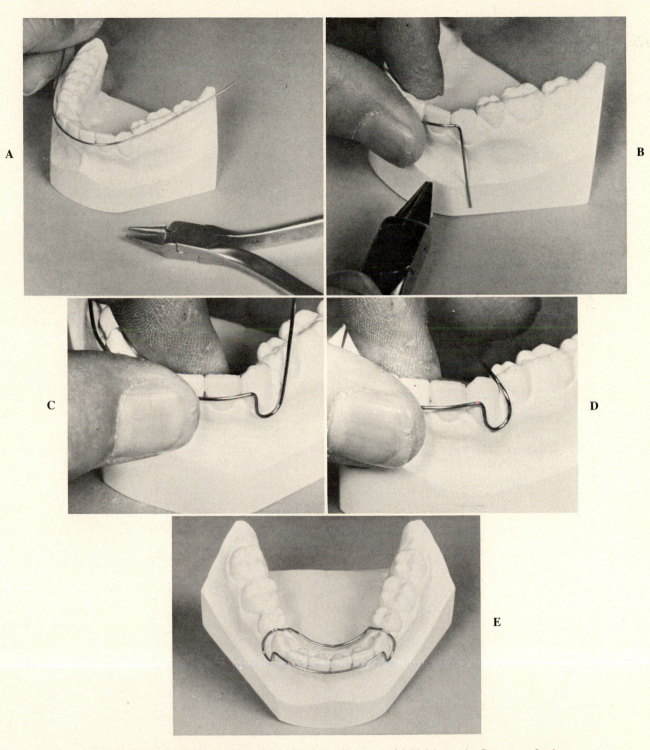

Fig. 11-12 ■ Steps in the fabrication of the Hawley type of labial bow. **A,** Segment of wire contoured to the labial surface of the incisors; **B,** bending the adjustment loop, which should cover the distal two-thirds of the canine; **C,** the loop completed, extending gingivally 6 to 8 mm; **D,** wire contoured across the canine-premolar contact; **E,** the completed labial bow, showing the wire contoured to the alveolar process behind the incisors, where it will be incorporated into the acrylic framework of the appliance.

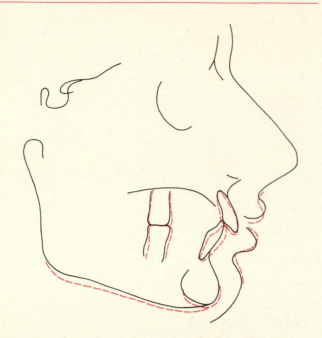

Fig. 11-13 ■ Cephalometric superimposition showing an unsatisfactory response to a removable functional appliance for a skeletal Class II malocclusion. Note the forward movement of the lower incisors, slight retraction and elongation of the upper incisors, and downward and backward rotation of the mandible. Adding springs to a functional appliance, if it accentuates this pattern of tooth movement, makes the treatment response worse rather than better.

The second problem with active functional appliances relates to the long-term stability, or lack of it, from arch expansion. Functional appliances are less successful in correcting crowding and irregularity within the arches than in improving a Class II open bite or deep bite occlusal relationship. A major motivation for including active elements in a functional appliance is that this provides a way to correct crowding within the arches at the same time that jaw discrepancies are being treated. It does not follow logically, however, that more arch expansion can be tolerated by patients whose jaw growth is being manipulated.

A combination of active springs with a functional appliance can achieve a spectacular expansion of the dental arch at the same time that a Class II jaw relationship is being improved. What is not so obvious initially is that the relapse into crowding can be equally spectacular if the arch was overexpanded. The indications for active functional appliances, particularly as a means of providing comprehensive treatment, are extremely limited (see Chapter 14). In contemporary orthodontics, there are few indications for removable appliances designed to provide all aspects of treatment like those commonly used in Europe a generation ago.

■ *Components of Removable Appliances*

■ Clasps

Adams clasp. By far the most useful and versatile clasp for contemporary removable appliances is the Adams crib. This clasp, a modification of Schwartz's arrowhead clasp, is designed to engage the mesiobuccal and distobuccal undercuts of individual posterior teeth. It has the significant advantage over the arrowhead clasp that it does not tend to separate the teeth, and it has excellent retentive properties.

The Adams clasp is made of .028 inch (0.7 mm) wire, except that .024 inch (0.6 mm) wire is preferred for clasps on canines. The first step in fabricating an Adams clasp, establishing the distance between the retentive points, is critically important, since there is no way to compensate for a significant error. Partially performed clasps with varying bridge lengths and preformed retentive points are available commercially (Fig. 11-14), but the clasp must be fabricated individually from that point. The retentive points of the clasp must fit well into the undercuts for good retention.

When this clasp is used for children, it may be necessary for the points to slip slightly into the gingival crevice. This step is accomplished by trimming away stone interproximally on the laboratory cast, so that the clasp can fit far enough down the tooth. Steps in the fabrication of an Adams clasp are illustrated in Fig. 11-15.

When a new removable appliance is received from the lab-

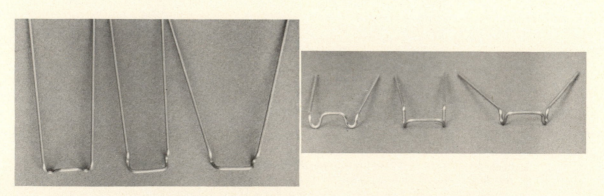

Fig. 11-14 ■ Commercially available preformed Adams cribs. Although the retentive points have been formed, the clasps must be fabricated individually for each tooth beyond that point.

oratory, or when a patient returns for adjustments, it is often necessary for the dentist to tighten the clasps. Most of the time, this adjustment is done as illustrated in Fig. 11-16, *A*, by simply bending the clasp slightly gingivally from its point of attachment. It is also possible to bend the retentive points inward to obtain better contact in the undercut areas (Fig. 11-16, *B*), which really should be necessary only if the laboratory fabrication of the clasps was imperfect.

As a general principle, the more active a removable appliance is to be and the greater the force applied during its use, the more clasping is required to hold it in place. It is possible to modify the Adams clasp by soldering an exten-

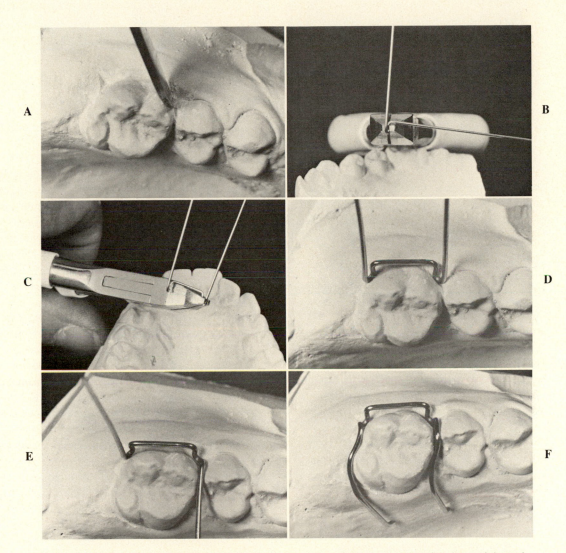

Fig. 11-15 ■ Steps in the fabrication of Adams crib. **A,** Carving the cast, exposing the mesiobuccal and distobuccal undercuts into which the retentive points will insert. This is a critically important step in fabricating a clasp for a young child. **B,** Forming a retentive point from .028 inch (0.7 mm) wire. If preformed components are used, this step can be omitted. **C,** Angulation of the retentive points, which must sit at about 45 degrees to the bridge portion of the clasp that connects the retentive points. This adjustment is required if preformed components are used. **D,** The partially formed clasp, showing the retentive points in position, with the bridge portion of the clasp at least 1 mm away from the buccal surface. **E,** Contouring the attachment portion of the clasp over the top of the contacts. It is important that the wire be contoured as close to the occlusal surface of the teeth as possible to minimize occlusal interferences. **F,** Completed clasp, showing the clearance between the bridge portion and the buccal surface of the tooth, and the contouring of the attachment portion of the clasp on the lingual side of the contact point. If the clasp wire is not bent down sharply into the lingual embrasure, interference with the buccal cusps of the lower teeth is almost inevitable. Note also that the wire ends are bent toward the palate, ensuring a small space beneath the wires so that acrylic will surround the portion of the wire contained in the baseplate.

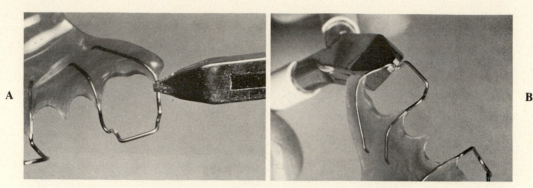

A   B

Fig. 11-16 ■ Clinical adjustments of an Adams clasp. **A,** Tightening the clasp by bending it gingivally at the point where the wire emerges from the baseplate. This is the usual adjustment for a clasp that has become loose after repeated insertions and removals of an appliance. **B,** Adjustment of the clasp by bending the retentive points inward. This alternative method of tightening a clasp is particularly useful during the initial fitting of an appliance.

sion to the buccal bridge portion of the clasp, which allows an additional retentive point to be placed in the next embrasure. As shown in Fig. 11-17, this is particularly useful as a means of gaining retention from a second molar as well as a first molar, in an older patient. The same approach can be used to clasp both premolars if needed. The Adams clasp is so effective, however, that three or four retentive points on each side will support almost any practical type of movement with a removable appliance.

Of the dozens of other clasp designs that can be used, three deserve brief mention here:

Circumferential clasp (Fig. 11-18, A, and B). The circumferential clasp is particularly useful for second molars, and occasionally for canines. This clasp's greatest virtue is that it is easier to keep out of occlusal contact than the Adams clasp, but it does not compare to the Adams clasp in retentive ability and should be considered only a supporting rather than a truly retentive element. For practical purposes, the circumferential clasp might be adequate for a retainer but not for an active removable appliance.

Ball clasp (Fig. 11-18, C). The ball clasp, like the Adams clasp, extends across the embrasure between adjacent teeth and uses undercuts on the buccal surface. These clasps are easy to fabricate, which is their major advantage, but because of their short span they are relatively stiff and unable to extend as deeply into the undercuts as an Adams clasp. Ball clasps should be considered only when the demands on them will be limited.

Lingual extension clasp (Fig. 11-18, D). Any wire that crosses the occlusal table can interfere with occlusion, so it would be ideal to have a clasp that operated only from the lingual. In theory, extending a spring element into the lingual embrasures should provide retention, but in fact, it is difficult to develop and use clasping of this type. A short loop of .016 inch (0.4 mm) wire can be placed into the first molar–second premolar embrasure from the lingual on most patients and can provide enough retention for a maxillary removable retainer.

Offsetting the advantage of no wire crossing the occlusal surface, these clasps have several disadvantages: they are difficult or impossible to adjust, prone to breakage, may cause tissue irritation, and if too active can separate the teeth. They are recommended, therefore, only for retainers and then only in unusual circumstances.

■ Framework (Baseplate)

The framework or baseplate of removable appliances can be fabricated from a variety of contemporary plastic materials. Self-curing acrylic resins, if used, should be cured in a pressure pot to improve their density. Newer light-cured or thermoplastic materials have significant advantages and are replacing the older acrylic resins. There is no advantage to a metal framework such as that employed in the Crozat appliance, even if it is made of precious metal as in the original design. The increased cost and complexity have made metal frameworks obsolete for contemporary orthodontic use.

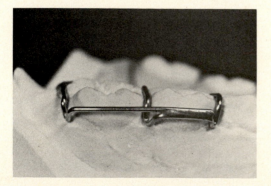

Fig. 11-17 ■ A double Adams crib, used to clasp two adjacent teeth. The bridge portion of the second clasp section is soldered to the bridge of the first clasp.

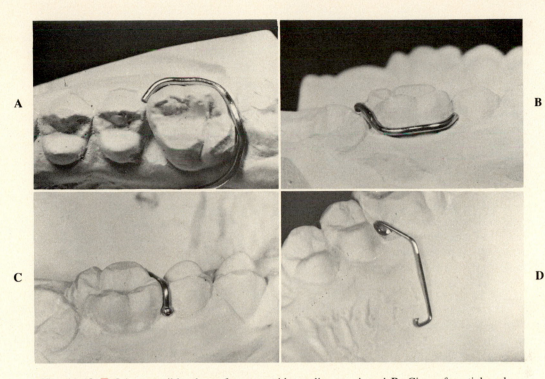

Fig. 11-18 ■ Other possible clasps for removable appliances. **A** and **B,** Circumferential molar clasp, extending into the mesiobuccal undercut; **C,** ball clasp, extending into the buccal embrasure; **D,** lingual extension clasp, made from fine wire extending into the lingual embrasure.

The fit of any removable appliance depends on the stability of its framework or baseplate. For this reason, maxillary removable appliances tend to be both better tolerated by patients and more successful than mandibular removables. The maxillary appliance is stabilized by the direct connection across the arch between the molar teeth, while the horseshoe-shaped mandibular removable appliance is inevitably somewhat flexible, making it less stable and prone to breakage.

A second complication with mandibular appliances is the frequent presence of lingual undercuts in the molar region. The lower molars tend to be inclined lingually, particularly in older patients, and the mylohyoid ridge is relatively high in many patients, preventing the baseplate from extending far gingivally. The combination of an inherently less stable framework and a tendency for a loose fit posteriorly makes mandibular removables less comfortable for patients and generally less effective in producing tooth movement than maxillary removables.

■ **Active Elements (Springs)**

For the reasons previously described, screws are not recommended for active tooth movement with removable appliances, except occasionally for lateral expansion of the maxillary arch. The extremely heavy force application provided by a screw, which then decays to zero very rapidly, is almost the exact opposite of what is desired for optimal tooth movement. Although teeth can certainly be moved with screws, what was an acceptable practice 50 years ago is difficult to justify now. Screws do not provide appropriate orthodontic forces.

Two important principles must be kept in mind when designing springs for a removable appliance: (1) the design must ensure adequate springiness and range while retaining acceptable strength, which usually means recurved or looped wires for additional length, and (2) the spring must be guided so that its action is exerted only in the appropriate direction.

Spring design for acceptable properties. Because of the first of these principles, it is unwise to fabricate springs for removable appliances from steel wire smaller than .020 inch (0.5 mm), and larger diameter wires are usually used. In general, it is better to use a larger wire for its (considerably) greater strength, and then gain springiness and range by increasing the length of the spring, than to use a smaller wire initially. Examples of springs for specific purposes are shown in Fig. 11-11.

Guidance for springs. The major problem with long flexible springs is that the spring can deflect three-dimensionally even though tooth movement in only one direction is usually desired. If a spring is placed against a lingually positioned incisor, it will be ineffective if it distorts vertically, sliding down the lingual surface toward the incisal edge. This is a problem with any spring against any tooth surface: unless the spring remains in its planned position, its action will be unpredictable.

This difficulty can be overcome in three ways:

1. Place the spring in an undercut area of the tooth, so

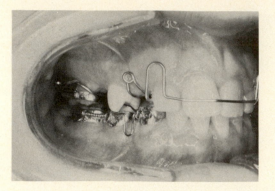

Fig. 11-19 ■ The end of this helical spring to tip the first premolar posteriorly is held in position because it engages the mesial undercut of the premolar. Placing the end of the spring in an undercut also aids in retention of the appliance, whereas a spring not held in position tends to displace itself and the appliance.

that it cannot slip toward the occlusal surface (Fig. 11-19). The spring may then have an extrusive as well as a horizontal component of force, but this usually does not cause a practical problem. For posterior teeth, this approach is the preferred solution.

2. Use a guide to hold the spring in its proper position (Fig. 11-20). This approach is often necessary with active springs to move canines and incisors labially, because no undercuts are available on the lingual surface. The guide can be either a rigid wire over the spring, or a shelf of baseplate material extending over the top of the spring to prevent its displacement.

3. Bond an attachment to the tooth surface, to provide a point of positive attachment for the spring. This approach is more practical now than it was before the development of direct bonding. On the other hand, there is a risk of isolated bonded attachments being swallowed, which does not exist when a series of bonded attachments are tied to an arch wire, and it is no more difficult to bond a bracket for fixed appliance technique than to bond a stop against which a removable spring would rest. Tooth movements

that can be accomplished with removable appliances only by bonding attachments for springs, in other words, may be an indication for using a fixed appliance technique.

Limitations of springs. The problem of controlling exactly where a spring contacts a tooth, more than any other factor, makes it difficult to control root position in removable appliance treatment. As an example, consider the problem of torquing a maxillary central incisor with a removable appliance. To move the root back while maintaining the crown in approximately the same position, it is necessary to generate a moment by applying two forces against the crown of the tooth. If a spring is applied from the lingual against the incisal edge, while a wire labial bow is applied above the point at which the lingual spring contacts the tooth, the necessary force system can be achieved (see Chapter 10, Fig. 10-13). It is almost impossible to keep the lingual spring from slipping out of position without bonding material to the lingual surface, creating a ledge toward the incisal edge into which the spring can fit securely.

For all practical purposes, then, torquing the roots of incisors with a removable appliance can be done only if the tooth surface is modified so that a spring with a heavy activation will stay in place. Even this technique does not end the difficulty, because if forces of the magnitude necessary to produce the root-moving moments are applied, the best of clasps may be unable to resist displacement of the baseplate.

Exactly the same problems arise if spaces within the arch are closed using a removable appliance. It is possible, with a removable appliance, to tip teeth together at an extraction site or large diastema, but virtually impossible to generate the moments necessary for proper root paralleling. In theory, one could place a spring on each side of the teeth being moved together, one high and the other low, to create a root paralleling moment (Fig. 11-21). In practice, it is difficult to keep the springs in position without either notching the teeth or bonding an attachment. Furthermore, the forces necessary to generate the moments are high enough that it is very difficult to keep them from displacing a removable

A   **B**

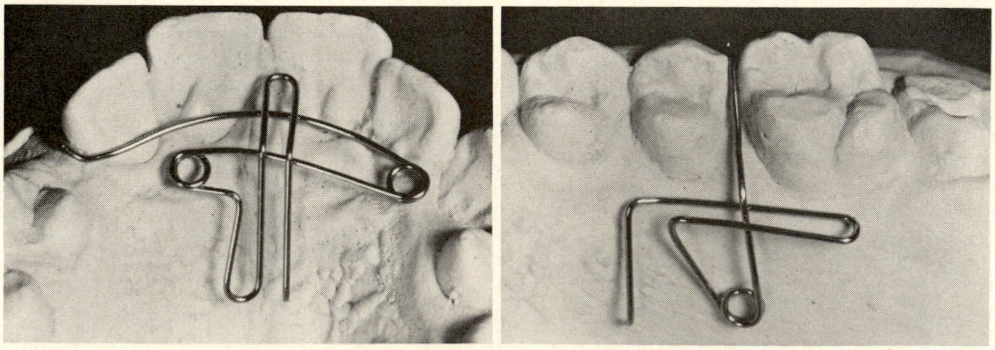

Fig. 11-20 ■ A long spring requires a guide to hold the spring in proper position. **A,** Wire guide for spring to tip the upper incisors forward. If a removable appliance is used to tip incisors for correction of an anterior crossbite, a spring of this type, rather than the screw arrangement shown in Fig 11-5, is preferred. **B,** Wire guide for spring to tip upper molar distally.

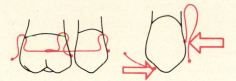

Fig. 11-21 ■ Diagrammatic representation of the spring assembly necessary for bodily retraction of a canine with a removable appliance. The mesial spring exerts a heavier force than the distal spring, leaving a net force to move the canine distally, while the couple necessary for control of root position is created by the opposing action of the two springs. Although bodily movement with a removable appliance is theoretically possible with spring arrangements of this type, the spring adjustments become too complex for practical clinical use. A fixed appliance is necessary if bodily tooth movement is needed.

appliance. Using screws instead of springs, so that a section of the baseplate contacts the teeth, slightly improves the ability to control the point of force application. This approach does not overcome the initial disadvantages, however, and introduces the additional complication of totally inappropriate force magnitude–duration characteristics.

This inability to control root position is, therefore, a major limitation of removable appliances. If tooth movement requirements go beyond simple tipping of teeth, a fixed rather than removable appliance is almost always indicated.

■ Clinical Adjustments

Three adjustments are necessary when an active removable appliance is being used appropriately: tightening of clasps when they become loose, activation of the spring or springs, and removal of material from the baseplate. Clasps usually require a minor adjustment at each appointment, bending them as described previously (see Fig. 11-16). Baseplate material must not be removed near a clasp, since this would allow that tooth to move and retention of the appliance would be lost. On the other hand, it is immediately obvious that unless baseplate material is removed, it will not be possible for any spring to move a tooth lingually. Nevertheless, failure to relieve the baseplate near a spring is a common error. Only a small amount of baseplate material should be removed at one time, because excessive removal lessens the fit of the appliance and decreases control.

A patient who is wearing an active removable appliance should be seen at 4 to 6 week intervals. Springs should be adjusted to produce approximately 1 mm of tooth movement (which may require slightly more activation of the spring than that) and the baseplate should be relieved to allow a similar amount of clearance (Fig. 11-22). At the next appointment, the spring is reactivated and the baseplate is again relieved by a similar amount. This has the advantage that the appliance "fails safe" if the patient does not return

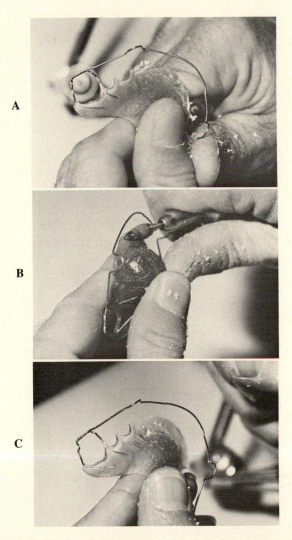

Fig. 11-22 ■ Removal of baseplate material is necessary to allow lingual movement of teeth, as with this maxillary removable appliance to tip the incisors lingually. **A,** Removal of acrylic at the incisal edge; **B,** removal of baseplate material above the incisal edge, to accommodate the expected tipping tooth movement; **C,** the appliance after trimming, in which 1 mm of baseplate material has been removed.

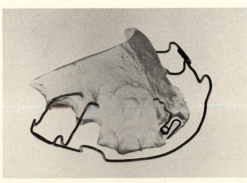

Fig. 11-23 ■ Maxillary removable appliance with a lingual spring to move one lateral incisor labially and a labial bow to control the amount of labial movement. As a design principle, an active component of a removable appliance should be restrained by the baseplate or by a restraining wire after the desired tooth movement has occurred, producing a fail-safe effect.

for the next appointment at the expected time. An overactivated spring, with nothing to check its action, could produce an excessive response.

Preventing an excessive response by limiting the relief of the baseplate is possible only when a tooth is being moved lingually, not labially. The same fail safe effect, however, can be achieved by placing a labial or buccal restraining wire. For example, it may be a good idea to incorporate both a lingual spring and a labial restraining wire in an appliance to move a single tooth labially. The spring is activated to produce the tooth movement, and the restraining wire is adjusted to prevent excessive movement if the spring becomes distorted (Fig. 11-23). Split-plate appliances cannot be made to fail safe in this way, but since it is necessary for the patient to activate a screw and because the rate of activation is quite slow, these appliances have less danger of an excessive response.

Their inherent limitations mean that removable appliances are rarely indicated for comprehensive treatment. Removables are most indicated for phase one mixed dentition treatment, as adjuncts in the early stages of comprehensive treatment, for limited tooth movement in adolescents and adults, and as retainers after comprehensive treatment. For these purposes, however, removable appliances do form an essential component of contemporary treatment.

■ *References*

1. Graber, T.M., and Neumann, B.: Removable Orthodontic Appliances, ed. 2, Philadelphia, 1983, W.B. Saunders.
2. Adams, C.P.: The Design and Construction of Removable Appliances, ed. 4, Bristol, England, 1970, John Wright & Sons, Ltd.

Chapter 12

Contemporary Fixed Appliances

Contemporary fixed appliances are predominantly variations of the edgewise appliance system. The only current fixed appliance system that does not incorporate the ability to use rectangular arch wires in a rectangular slot is the Begg appliance, and even in the Begg system, there is renewed interest in the use of rectangular arch wires at the finishing stage of treatment. The focus in this and the succeeding chapters, therefore, is almost entirely on use of the contemporary edgewise appliance, with occasional reference to Begg technique.

The mechanical principles underlying the use of any fixed appliance are discussed in detail in Chapter 10. The historical development of fixed appliances, including the progression from original edgewise to the contemporary edgewise appliance, is presented at the end of that chapter. This chapter is devoted to methods by which fixed attachments are placed, i.e., banding and bonding techniques, and to the characteristics of the appliance itself. Chapters 15 to 17 cover fixed appliance treatment techniques during the three major stages of comprehensive treatment.

■ *Bands for Attachments*

■ Indications for Banding

Until recently, the only practical way to place a fixed attachment was to put it on a band that could be cemented to a tooth. The pioneer orthodontists of the early 1900s used clamp bands, which were tightened around molar teeth by screw attachments. Only with the advent of custom-fitted pinched bands was it practical to place fixed attachments on more than a few teeth. For the fabrication of pinched bands, a special plier was used to stretch thin gold band material around the tooth, and the seam on the lingual surface was soldered and then ground smooth (Fig. 12-1).

When steel replaced gold as the common orthodontic material, pinched bands were welded rather than soldered, with the welded seam bent over on the lingual surface and welded flat. The first preformed steel bands were a byproduct of the manufacture of anatomically shaped steel crowns for restorative purposes. Preformed steel bands came into widespread use during the 1960s and are now available in anatomically correct shapes for all teeth.

There are definite advantages to bonding attachments directly to the tooth surface. Bonded attachments have no interproximal component, and therefore require no separation of teeth and are less painful. They are easier both to put on and to remove than bands, and they are also more esthetic because the highly visible metallic band material is eliminated. They make it easier to handle tooth-size problems during treatment, by leaving the interproximal surfaces accessible for modification if needed. Bonded attachments are less irritating to the gingiva and less prone to produce decalcification and white spots on the teeth, although they do not totally eliminate this problem. For these reasons, it is no longer appropriate to routinely place bands on all teeth that are to receive fixed attachments. However, a number of indications still exist for use of a band rather than a bonded attachment, including

1. Teeth that will receive heavy intermittent forces against the attachments. An excellent example is an upper first molar against which extraoral force will be placed via a headgear. The twisting and shearing forces often encountered when the facebow is placed or removed are better resisted by a steel band than by a bonded attachment.

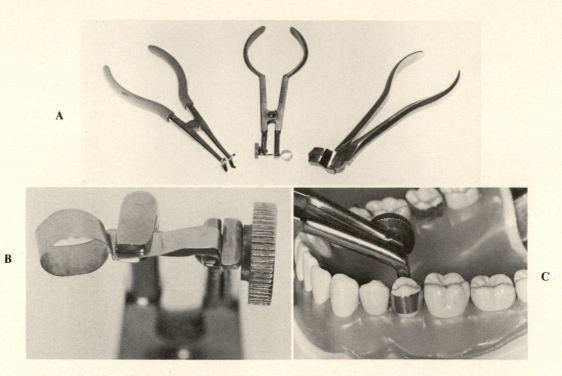

Fig. 12-1 ■ Band-forming pliers. **A,** Three types of pliers to stretch band material for a tight fit around the teeth; **B,** closeup view of band in the plier; **C,** band being formed on a lower premolar.

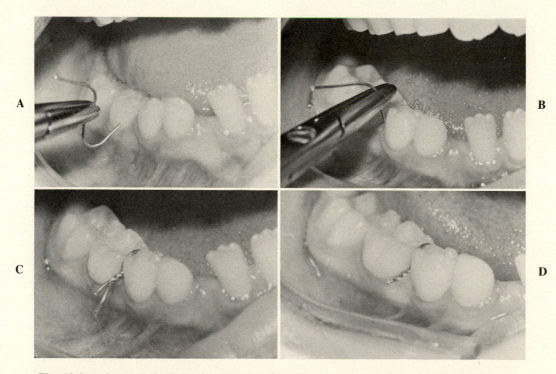

Fig. 12-2 ■ Separation with brass wire. **A,** .020 soft brass wire bent in an open hook shape; **B,** wire passed beneath the contact; **C,** wire brought back over the contact and twisted slightly; **D,** wire pigtail cut to 3 mm length and tucked in the gingival crevice. A brass wire separator of this type is normally left in place 5 to 7 days.

2. Teeth that will need both labial and lingual attachments, especially if the lingual will not be tied to some other part of the appliance. Although it is possible to bond on both sides of a tooth, it is usually easier for both the dentist and the patient to place a band with welded labial and lingual attachments, than to go through two separate bonding procedures. More importantly, banded lingual attachments are less likely to be swallowed or aspirated if something comes loose.

3. Teeth with short clinical crowns. Bands can be placed subgingivally, and as a general rule, the gingival margin of a band should either go slightly subgingival or should clear the gingival margin by at least 2 mm, so that the area of exposed enamel can be cleaned. If attached to a band, a tube or bracket can slightly displace the gingiva as it is carried into proper position. It is much more difficult to do this with bonded attachments. The decision to band rather than bond second premolars is often based on the length of the clinical crown.

4. Tooth surfaces that are incompatible with successful bonding. Tooth surfaces that have been restored in amalgam or precious metal are impossible to bond, and such teeth require banding. Porcelain restorations are difficult to bond, although this can be done by breaking the glaze on the porcelain surface and using a coupling agent to improve the adhesion of the bonding agent.[1] In the best of circumstances, bond strengths for attachment to porcelain are poor. Some nonrestored surfaces are also extremely difficult to prepare for bonding; teeth affected by fluorosis are the primary example. A good band initially is better than a series of unsuccessful bonds in these circumstances.

Although there are exceptions, the rule in contemporary orthodontics is that bonded attachments are almost always preferred for anterior teeth; bonds or bands may be used on premolars, depending on the height of the clinical crown and whether lingual attachments are needed; bands are preferred for molars, especially if both buccal and lingual attachments are needed.

This rule suggests that preformed molar and premolar bands should be available in a contemporary orthodontic practice. Incisor and canine bands are needed so rarely and in such unusual circumstances that pinching a band from band material, rather than relying on preformed anterior bands, may be the most appropriate approach.

■ Separation

Tight interproximal contacts make it impossible to properly seat a band, which means that some device to separate the teeth must usually be used before banding. Although separators are available in many varieties, the principle is

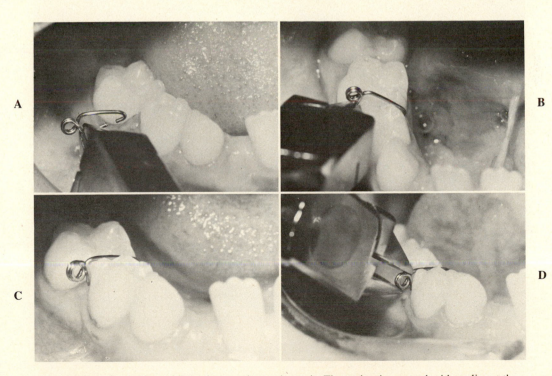

Fig. 12-3 ■ Separation with steel separating springs. **A,** The spring is grasped with a plier at the base of its shorter leg; **B,** the bent-over end of the longer leg is placed in the lingual embrasure, and the spring is pulled open as the shorter leg can slip beneath the contact; **C,** the spring in place, with the helix to the buccal; **D,** the spring can be removed most easily by squeezing the helix, forcing the legs apart.

the same in each case: a device to force or wedge the teeth apart is left in place long enough for initial tooth movement to occur, so that the teeth are slightly separated by the appointment at which bands are to be fitted. Separation can be painful, particularly for anterior teeth, and the necessity for separation must be considered a disadvantage of banding and its absence an advantage of bonding.

Three main methods of separation are used for posterior teeth: (1) brass wire, which is twisted tightly around the contact as shown in Fig. 12-2 and left in place for 5 to 7 days; (2) separating springs (Fig. 12-3), which exert a scissors action above and below the contact, typically opening enough space for banding in approximately 1 week; and (3) elastomeric separators ("doughnuts"), applied as shown in Fig. 12-4, which surround the contact point and squeeze the teeth apart over a period of several days.

Both brass wire and steel spring separators tend to come loose and may fall out as they accomplish their purpose, which is the main reason for leaving them in place only a few days. Brass wire and elastomeric separators are more difficult to insert, but are usually retained well when they are around the contact, and so may be left in position for somewhat longer times. Because elastomeric separators are radiolucent, however, a serious problem can arise if one is lost into the interproximal space. It is wise to use a brightly colored elastomeric material to make a displaced separator more visible, and these separators should not be left in place for more than 2 weeks.

■ Fabricating and Fitting Bands

It is possible to purchase preformed bands and to weld attachments to them in the dental office. However, it is cost-

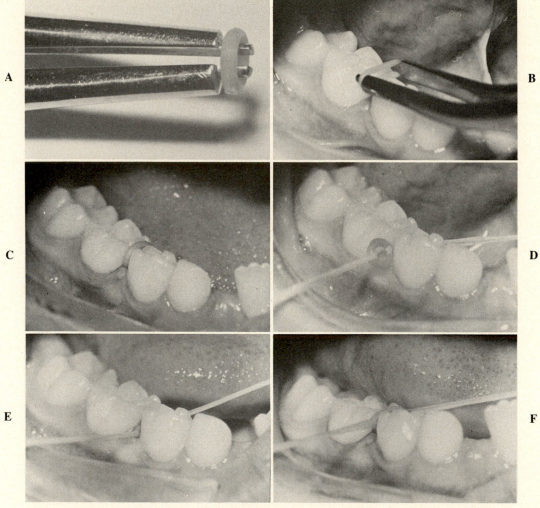

Fig. 12-4 ■ Separation with an elastomeric ring or "doughnut." **A,** The elastomeric ring is placed over the beaks of a special plier; **B,** the ring is stretched, then one side is snapped through the contact; **C,** the separator in place; **D,** an alternative to the special plier is two loops of dental floss, placed so they can be used to stretch the ring. The dental floss is snapped through the contact; **E,** the doughnut is pulled underneath the contact point, then; **F,** the doughnut is snapped into position. At that point, the dental floss is removed.

effective to obtain preformed bands with prewelded attachments, especially if a contemporary edgewise appliance with precisely angulated attachments is selected, since production jigs to assure accurate placement are needed to weld the attachments.

Fitting a preformed band involves stretching the stainless steel material over the tooth surface. This simultaneously contours and work-hardens the initially rather soft band material. It follows that heavy force is needed to seat a preformed band, stretching it to place. The necessary force

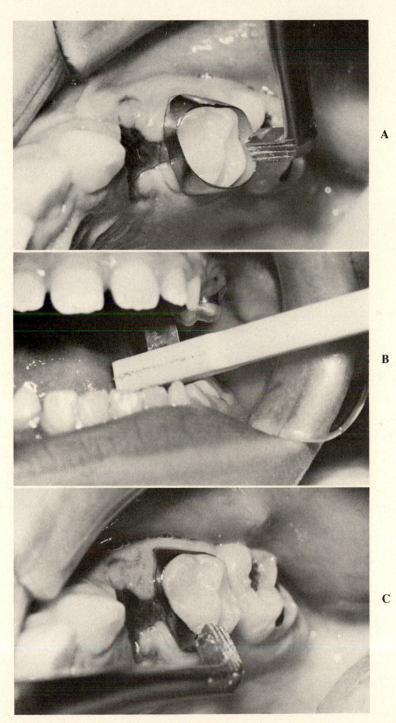

Fig. 12-5 ■ Fitting a preformed maxillary molar band (in this case, a primary second molar; the steps are the same for primary and permanent maxillary molars). **A,** The band is pressed over the height of contour with finger pressure or an instrument with a serrated tip; **B,** heavy biting force on a band seating instrument is used to seat the band, with the final pressure application to seat the band on the distolingual corner, as shown here; **C,** open margins are burnished with a hand instrument.

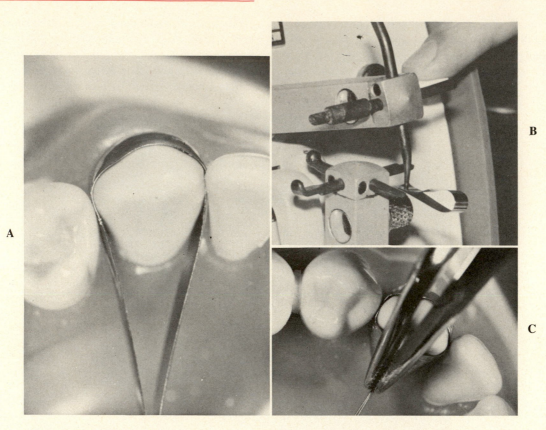

Fig. 12-6 ■ Steps in fabricating a pinched band for a mandibular canine. **A,** The strip of band material is welded into a loop. **B,** The loop of band material is carried over the tooth and contoured to the labial surface. **C,** A How plier with angulated beaks is used to pinch the lingual surface tightly.

should be supplied by the masticatory muscles of the patient, not by the arm strength of the dentist or dental assistant. Patients can bite harder and with much greater control, a fact best appreciated on the rare occasions when a patient is unable to bite bands to place.

Preformed bands are designed to be fitted in a certain sequence, and it is important that the manufacturer's instructions be followed. A typical upper molar band, for example, is designed to be placed initially by hand pressure on the mesial and distal surfaces, bringing the band down close to the height of the marginal ridges, and then to be driven to place by pressure on the mesiobuccal and distolingual corners (Fig. 12-5). Usually the final seating is with heavy biting force on the distolingual surface. Lower molar bands are designed to be seated initially with hand pressure on the proximal surfaces, and then with heavy biting force along the buccal but not the lingual margins. Maxillary premolar bands are usually seated with alternate pressure on the buccal and lingual surfaces, while mandibular premolar bands, like mandibular molars, are designed for heavy pressure on the buccal surface only.

It is easier to fabricate a pinched band for an anterior than a posterior tooth, simply because access to the lingual surface is better. The steps in pinching a canine band are shown in Fig. 12-6. In contemporary practice, this technique would rarely if ever be done, only when bonding was not possible for some specific reason.

■ Cementation

Cementing orthodontic bands is similar to cementing cast restorations, but differs in important details. The differences relate to the fact that in restorative dentistry, most if not all enamel has been removed and the cement contacts dentin, while in orthodontic treatment, the cementation is entirely to enamel.

Zinc phosphate cements are usually used for orthodontic purposes. The cements supplied for orthodontic use, however, differ from those used in restorative dentistry in that the liquid contains more free phosphoric acid. Relatively mild cements are needed for restorative purposes, because the open dentinal tubules allow free acid to irritate the pulp. A relatively acid cement is needed for orthodontic purposes,

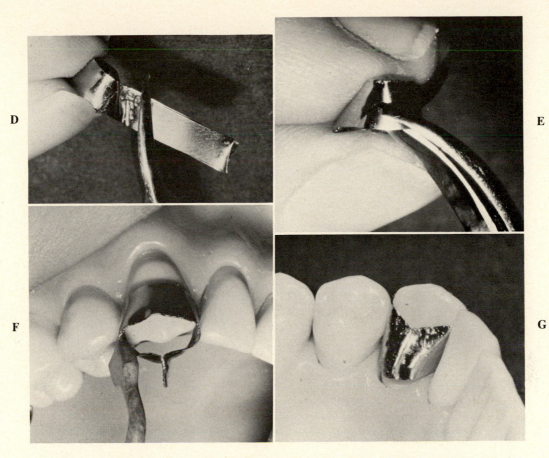

Fig. 12-6, cont'd ■ **D,** The welding tab is shortened with scissors. **E,** The gingival margin is festooned with curved scissors. **F,** The band is pressed to place over the tooth, with a 4 to 5 mm welding tab still extending lingually. This tab is folded over against the lingual surface with the band on the tooth; **G,** the welding tab is welded against the lingual surface, completing the band.

so that an acid-etch of the enamel surface, not unlike that created before bonding, is produced to aid in retention. In addition, orthodontic cement is mixed thicker than the cement for an inlay or a crown, because the escape of excess cement from the margins of a band is not the same problem that escape of cement from beneath an inlay can be, and a thicker mix provides greater strength.

Cementation of multiple bands is greatly facilitated by using a cold mixing slab. A cold slab also allows a greater amount of powder to be incorporated into the cement liquid, producing a stronger cement. Keeping the mixing slab in a freezer before use (the "frozen slab technique") is the preferred approach for cementing orthodontic bands.[2]

All interior surfaces of an orthodontic band must be coated with cement before placing the bands, so that there is no bare metal. As the band is carried to place, the occlusal surface should be covered so that cement is expressed from the gingival as well as the occlusal margins of the band (Fig. 12-7).

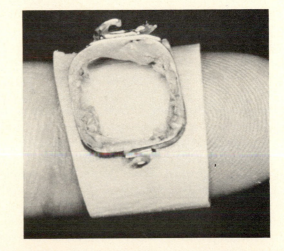

Fig. 12-7 ■ Molar band ready to cement. The cement must cover all the anterior surface of the band. Placing a piece of masking tape over the band helps to express cement gingivally when the band is carried to place, while keeping the dentist's finger cleaner.

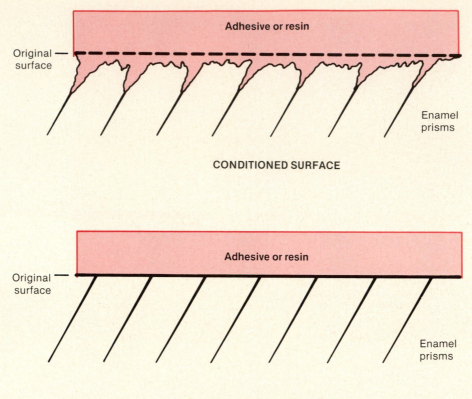

Fig. 12-8 ■ Diagrammatic representation of the effect of preparation of the enamel surface before bonding. Pretreatment with phosphoric acid creates minute irregularities in the enamel surface, allowing the bonding material to mechanically interlock with the enamel surface.

■ *Bonded Attachments*

■ The Basis of Bonding

Direct bonding of orthodontic attachments is based on the mechanical locking of an adhesive to irregularities in the enamel surface of the tooth, and to mechanical locks formed in the base of the orthodontic attachment. Successful bonding, therefore, requires careful attention to three components of the system: the tooth surface and its preparation, the design of the attachment base, and the bonding material itself.

Preparation of the tooth surface. Before bonding an orthodontic attachment, it is necessary to remove the enamel pellicle and to create irregularities in the enamel surface. This is accomplished by cleaning the enamel surface, then treating it with a chemical agent to develop the necessary surface irregularities.

The usual method of preparing the surface is by opening up pores between enamel prisms, removing a small amount of the softer interprismatic enamel so that the adhesive can penetrate into the enamel surface (Fig. 12-8). This is done by cleaning and drying the tooth surface, then treating it with an etching agent, usually 35% to 50% unbuffered phosphoric acid for 1 minute. The teeth should be cleaned before the acid etch, but this should be done gently, avoiding heavy

pumicing. It is convenient to apply the etching agent in a gel rather than a liquid form, simply because gels make it easier to confine the etch to a prescribed area and are as effective as liquids[3] (Fig. 12-9). The tooth surface must not be contaminated with saliva, which promotes immediate remineralization, until bonding is completed; otherwise, reetching is required.[4]

Rather than opening up minute irregularities extending into the enamel surface, another possible way to prepare for bonding would be to build up irregular deposits on the enamel surface and thus obtain a mechanical interlocking with the bonding agent. The loss of enamel surface when acid-etch bonds are removed is minimal, but the buildup approach would, at least in theory, eliminate any loss of enamel. At present, a system to chemically attach sulfite materials to the enamel surface in preparation for bonding is offered commercially. However, the bond between the sulfite and the enamel surface is relatively weak, resulting in frequent clinical bond failures.[5] Because the buildup material breaks cleanly away from the enamel surface, there is less cleanup at debanding, but this is no advantage if the bracket comes loose prematurely. Further progress is needed before acid etching can be replaced by enamel buildup.

Surface of attachments. The base of any bonded attachment must be manufactured so that a mechanical inter-

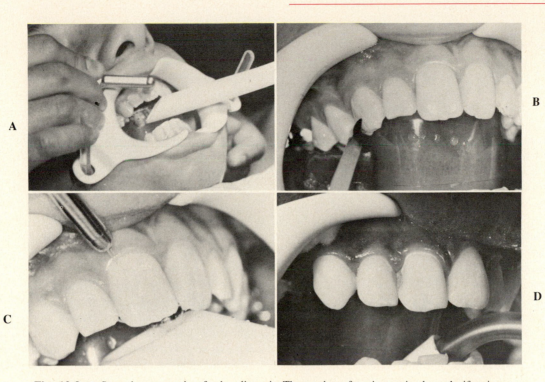

Fig. 12-9 ■ Steps in preparation for bonding. **A,** The tooth surface is pumiced gently if stain or plaque is present. This step can be omitted in patients with excellent oral hygiene. **B,** The etch material is applied to the area where the bracket will be placed. **C,** After 60 to 90 seconds, the etching material is rinsed away, and the tooth surface is dried. **D,** The chalky or frosted appearance of the enamel surface after proper etching.

lock between the bonding material and the attachment surface can be achieved. Although a number of approaches have been offered commercially, a fine mesh beneath the orthodontic attachment offers the strongest interlocking of any presently available system[6] (Fig. 12-10). In this, as in the other components of bonding systems, rapid progress during the last decade has continued. Porous metal powders on bracket bases, if commercially feasible, appear superior to mesh bases,[7] and it is likely that even better arrangements will become available in the future.

Bonding materials. A successful bonding material must meet a set of formidable criteria: it must be dimensionally stable; it must be quite fluid, so that it penetrates the enamel surface; it must have excellent inherent strength; and it must be easy to use clinically. New and significantly improved materials continue to appear regularly, and third and fourth generation materials are already available. The rapid progress in this area makes a description of materials in a text likely to be obsolete before it can be published. It is feasible, however, to place the evolution of bonding systems in perspective, highlighting how the present situation was reached and indicating the probable direction of future changes.

Although attachments were occasionally bonded to impacted teeth with black copper cement (an extremely acid version of zinc phosphate cement), bonding materials strong enough for routine clinical use did not become available until the mid 1970s. Before that, experimental bonding systems based on both epoxy resins and acrylic resins had been proposed and evaluated clinically, with some success. The greatest difficulty with the epoxy resins was their slow development of full strength, so that it was not possible to place arch wires at the same visit the bonded attachments were placed. The early resin materials suffered from their different thermal coefficient of expansion relative to enamel, which tended to weaken the bonds.

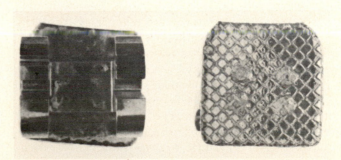

Fig. 12-10 ■ At present, a fine mesh on the back of a bracket provides the best retention for bonding.

The first really successful orthodontic bonding agents were stabilized resins whose polymerization was initiated by ultraviolet light. These second generation materials provided significantly greater bond strengths than had existed previously. The major disadvantages were the ultraviolet light itself, which even with the best control was a moderate hazard, and the fact that an indirect technique with a tray carrier was needed to position the brackets. This interfered with access of the ultraviolet light to the resin beneath the brackets and made cleanup difficult.

By the late 1970s, third generation filled or composite resins (acrylic resins containing a high percentage of an inert filler material) largely replaced the light cured resins. Compared to unfilled resins, the filled resins have greatly improved thermal expansion qualities. A small quantity of a composite resin can be mixed so that it sets rapidly and develops full strength in only a few minutes. This makes it possible to have a fresh mix of resin for each bracket, which is extremely convenient in direct bonding technique (see the following section). With direct bonding, it is easy to remove excess bonding material from the margins of each bracket before it hardens. Although filled resins are also acceptable materials for indirect placement of a number of brackets simultaneously, removing the flash around the margins of the brackets is a problem.

For indirect bonding, a fourth generation of bonding agents, in which it is unnecessary to mix the two components of the bonding material on a slab before using the material, is preferred. With these ''no mix'' materials, the composite resin can be placed on the tooth surface in unpolymerized form, while the polymerization catalyst is placed on the back of the brackets. When the tray carrying the brackets is placed against the tooth surface, the resin immediately beneath the bracket is activated and polymerizes, but excess resin around the margins of the brackets does not polymerize and can easily be scaled away when the bracket tray is removed. These no-mix materials can also be used, of course, for direct bonding of individual brackets. With rapidly setting third generation composites, the dentist has 30 to 60 seconds to remove excess material after the bracket is placed. In contrast, with the contact-catalyzed material, there is no hurry because the excess material never polymerizes.

At present, the physical properties of slab-mixed composite resins are better than the properties of no-mix contact-polymerized bonding materials.[8] It is likely that the properties of contact-polymerized bonding materials will be improved, and that these fourth generation materials will become the standard for orthodontic bonding, at least until a different fifth generation bonding agent arrives on the scene.

For many years, bonding of brackets seemed an impossible dream. It has passed from a laboratory possibility to an experimental curiosity to a routine clinical procedure in a remarkably short time, as significant improvements in all three components of the bonding systems were put together. The rapid pace of recent change makes it likely that further improvements will occur in the near future.

■ Direct Bonding Technique

Direct bonding of attachments is indicated whenever a single bracket must be changed or replaced, and it can be used as a routine clinical procedure. Preparation of the tooth surface can be either via an acid etch (preferred at present) or a sulfite buildup. Brackets and tubes with a fine mesh backing give the best results, and a composite resin with a very rapid setting time is usually used, although a no-mix material is also applicable.

The major difficulty with direct bonding is that the dentist must be able to judge the proper position for the attachment and must carry it to place rapidly and accurately. There is not much time for precise measurements of bracket position or for detailed adjustments. It is generally conceded that for this reason, direct bonding does not provide as accurate a placement of brackets as indirect bonding. On the other hand, direct bonding is generally conceded to be easier, faster (especially if only a few teeth are to be bonded), and less expensive (because the laboratory fabrication steps are eliminated). The fourth generation no-mix bonding materials have narrowed the time differential between direct and indirect bonding by making cleanup after indirect bonding easier.

Steps in the direct bonding technique are illustrated in Fig. 12-11.

■ Indirect Bonding Technique

Indirect bonding is done by placing the brackets on a model in the laboratory and using a template or tray to transfer the laboratory positioning to the teeth. An alginate impression, poured relatively rapidly, gives an accurate enough working cast for indirect bonding. Custom impression trays and silicone or rubber impressions are not necessary.

In the laboratory, a material is needed to stick the brackets to the model which will allow them to be adjusted, hold them firmly while the transfer tray is being prepared, and then be capable of total removal from the brackets, so that it does not interfere with placement of the bonding adhesive. Given the average dentist's antipathy to caramel candy, it is ironic that this is an excellent laboratory adhesive for indirect bonding. The candy adhesive is hard at room temperature but softens with moderate heat, so that brackets can be repositioned with a hot instrument at any time after they have been attached to the cast. The candy is also water soluble and so can be removed from the brackets with hot water after they have been embedded in the transfer tray. An alternative approach, the ''double-sealant technique,'' uses the bonding adhesive paste to place the brackets on the laboratory model.[9]

The transfer tray can be made from any of several materials, but is usually a quick-setting silicone rubber. It must be reasonably strong and dimensionally accurate, but elastic enough to be placed without difficulty and removed without pulling the brackets off.

Steps in the indirect bonding of a set of brackets, using a no-mix material, are shown in Figs. 12-12 and 12-13.

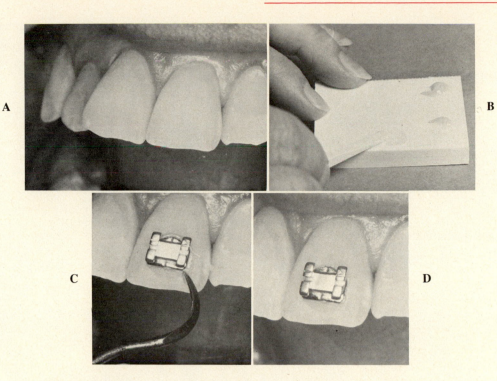

Fig. 12-11 ■ Steps in direct bonding. **A,** Teeth after preparation of the tooth surface. A liquid sealant (usually the monomer of the bonding agent) can be applied at this stage if desired. **B,** A small quantity of the bonding material is mixed so that it will set in 30 to 60 seconds. **C,** Bonding material is placed on the back of the bracket, and the bracket is pressed to place against the enamel surface, causing excess bonding material to be expressed around the edges. This is removed immediately with a scaler, before the material sets. **D,** The bonded bracket, immediately after cleanup. In this technique, a separate mix of bonding material is used for each tooth.

Visibility for direct bonding is good for canine and incisor teeth. Good direct visualization of the position of attachments is increasingly difficult as one moves posteriorly through the premolars and molars. For this reason, indirect bonding is preferred for posterior teeth and is almost mandatory if the entire arch is to be bonded. For the same reason, direct bonding of lingual attachments is difficult to the point of impossible when precise placement is required. Bonding an isolated lingual hook or button is not difficult, but precisely positioning the attachments for a lingual appliance requires indirect bonding, and even the placement of a fixed lingual retainer is done more easily with indirect technique and a transfer tray.

■ *Characteristics of Contemporary Edgewise Attachments*

■ Edgewise Brackets and Tubes in the Straight-Arch Systems

The progressive development of the edgewise applicance since its introduction in 1930 is described in the last section of Chapter 10. The most recent step, which led to the contemporary straight-arch appliance, involved the fabrication of slightly different brackets or tubes for each tooth, with the goal of minimizing the number of first, second, and third order bends in arch wires needed to produce an ideal ar-

rangement of the teeth.[10] First order bends, or in-out bends in the horizontal plane of space, were necessary in the original edgewise appliance to compensate for the differing thickness of teeth; second order or tip bends were needed to adjust the mesiodistal inclination of teeth; third order or twist bends were used to compensate for the different inclination of the labial surfaces of varying teeth, so that inadvertent torquing movements would not be produced when a rectangular arch wire was used (Fig. 12-14).

First and second order bends are important with both round or rectangular arch wires, whereas third order bends apply only to rectangular arch wires. An important concept is that unless the appliance has been modified from the original design, first, second, and third order bends are necessary to provide a passive fit of an arch wire when the teeth are ideally aligned, and are not used just to correct malaligned teeth.

In the contemporary edgewise appliance, the need for first, second, and third order bends has been reduced (but not totally eliminated) by altering the brackets placed on individual teeth, producing a custom bracket for each tooth in which a combination of varying thickness of the bracket base, inclination of the bracket slot, and torque of the slot are used to minimize wire bending for ideal arch wires. These characteristics for each tooth are called the "appliance prescription." Although the details of the prescription vary,

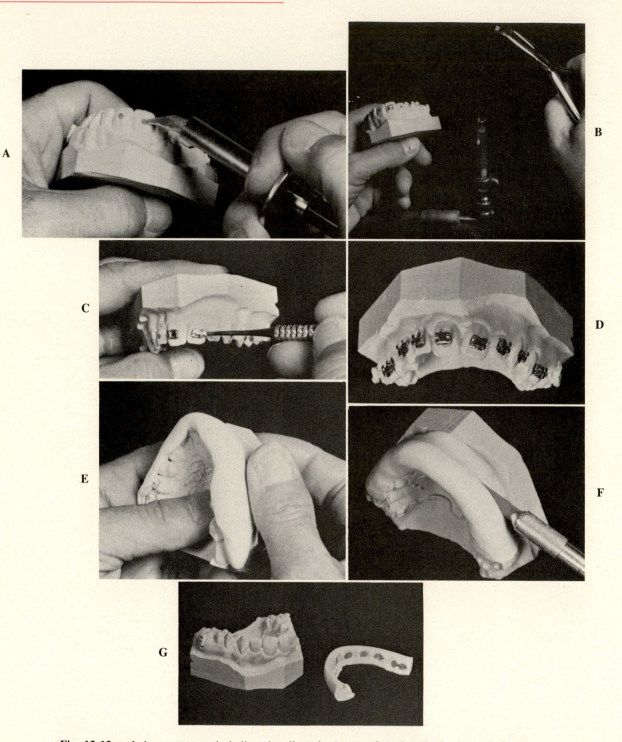

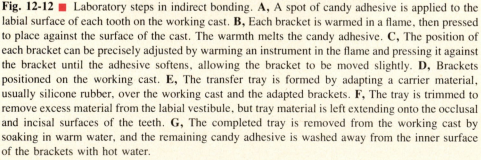

Fig. 12-12 ■ Laboratory steps in indirect bonding. **A,** A spot of candy adhesive is applied to the labial surface of each tooth on the working cast. **B,** Each bracket is warmed in a flame, then pressed to place against the surface of the cast. The warmth melts the candy adhesive. **C,** The position of each bracket can be precisely adjusted by warming an instrument in the flame and pressing it against the bracket until the adhesive softens, allowing the bracket to be moved slightly. **D,** Brackets positioned on the working cast. **E,** The transfer tray is formed by adapting a carrier material, usually silicone rubber, over the working cast and the adapted brackets. **F,** The tray is trimmed to remove excess material from the labial vestibule, but tray material is left extending onto the occlusal and incisal surfaces of the teeth. **G,** The completed tray is removed from the working cast by soaking in warm water, and the remaining candy adhesive is washed away from the inner surface of the brackets with hot water.

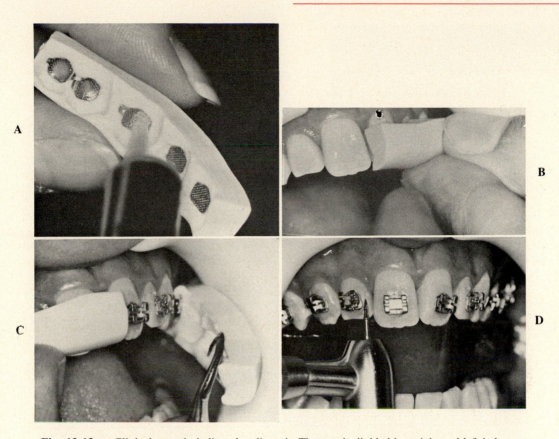

Fig. 12-13 ■ Clinical steps in indirect bonding. **A,** The tray is divided into right and left halves, if desired for easier handling. The adhesive material, if a third generation resin is used, or the paste portion of a fourth generation resin, is applied to the back of each bracket in the transfer tray. The catalyst portion of a fourth generation resin is placed on the tooth surface, so that mixing occurs when the two components contact each other when the tray is carried to the mouth. **B,** The tray or tray section is carried to place, and pressed firmly against the teeth. **C,** After the adhesive has set, the tray material is gently peeled away from the teeth. **D,** Excess bonding material is removed, with a carbide finishing bur if hardened third generation adhesive is encountered, or with a scaler if unset fourth generation material is present.

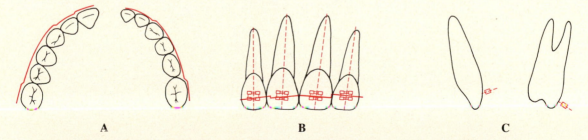

Fig. 12-14 ■ First, second, and third order bends in edgewise wires. **A,** First order bends in a maxillary (left) and mandibular (right) arch wire. Note the lateral inset required in the maxillary arch wire and the canine molar offset bends that are required in both. **B,** Second order bends in the maxillary incisor segment, to compensate for the inclination of the incisal edge of these teeth relative to the long axis of the tooth. **C,** Third order bends for the maxillary central incisors and maxillary first molars, showing the twist in the arch wire to provide a passive fit in a bracket or tube on these teeth. Twist in an arch wire provides torque in a bracket; the torque is positive for the incisor, negative for the molar.

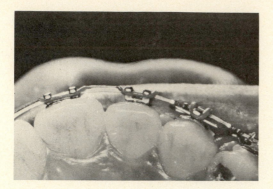

Fig. 12-15 ■ First order or in-out bends in arch wires can be minimized by varying the thickness of the bracket base. Note the thin bracket base for the canine, thick base for the lateral incisor, and intermediate thickness for the central incisor in this contemporary appliance. An elastomeric chain ties the anterior teeth together.

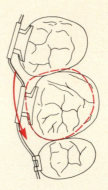

Fig. 12-16 ■ The rhomboidal surface of the upper, and to a lesser extent the lower, molars means that placing a springy arch wire through attachments that were flat against the facial surface would produce a mesiolingual rotation of these teeth, causing them to take up too much space in the arch. Compensation requires a bend in the arch wire, or placing the tube at an angle offset to the facial surface.

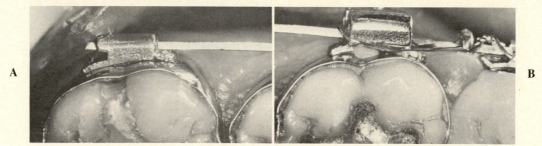

Fig. 12-17 ■ Tubes for the upper second molar **(A)** and upper first molar **(B)** in a contemporary appliance. Note the offset position of the tube so that a first order bend in the wire is unnecessary.

particularly for slot angulations and torque, the same basic approach is used in all of the commercially available "straight-arch" appliances.

Elimination of first order bends. Elimination of first order bends has been achieved largely by varying the thickness of the bracket base of individual teeth and by placing attachments for molars at an angle to the buccal surface, so that molar rotation can be controlled automatically.

The varying thickness of anterior bracket bases is shown in Fig. 12-15. Because of the prominence of the canine in each arch, its bracket base must be thin, bringing the labial surface of these teeth close to the arch wire. The difference in prominence between the maxillary lateral incisor and canine means that the bracket base for the lateral incisor, in contrast, must be quite thick, while the maxillary central incisor is intermediate. In the mandibular arch, the canine tooth is less prominent, so while a thin bracket base is used on the canine, an intermediate thickness base can be used on both lower lateral and central incisors. Bracket thickness for both maxillary and mandibular premolars is approximately equivalent to that of the canines.

Especially in the maxillary arch, control of molar rotation is important if good interdigitation of the teeth is to be

achieved. Placing a tube flat along the buccal surface of an upper molar would result in rotating it as shown in Fig. 12-16. For good occlusion, the buccal surface must sit at an angle to the line of occlusion, with the mesiobuccal cusp more prominent than the distobuccal cusp. For this reason, the tube or bracket specified for the upper molar should have at least a 10 degree offset (Fig. 12-17), as should the tube for the upper second molar.

A similar phenomenon occurs with the lower molars, but to a lesser extent. The offset for the lower first molar tubes should be about 5 to 7 degrees, half that for the upper molar. A larger offset often is useful for the lower second molar. Offsets in some typical commercially available appliances are shown in Table 12-1.

Elimination of second order bends. In the original edgewise appliance, second order bends, sometimes called artistic positioning bends, were an important part of the finishing phase of treatment (Fig. 12-14, *B*). These bends were necessary because the long axis of each tooth is inclined relative to the plane of a continuous arch wire (Fig. 12-18). Without adequate second order bends, the incisor teeth are positioned too straight up and down with the roots too close together, producing an effect seen in some orthodontically

Table 12-1 ■ Molar tube offset

	A Company straight wire	A Company Roth	Lancer Natural Arch	Ormco Vari-Simplex	Ormco Level Arch	Rocky Mountain Triple Control	Rocky Mountain Bioprogressive	Unitek Twin Torque	Unitek Level Anchorage
Maxillary first molar	10°	14°	8°,15°	15°	10°	7°	15°	7°,12°	12°
Maxillary second molar	10°	14°	7°	6°	6°	7°	15°	7°,12°	12°
Mandibular first molar	0	4°	0,8°,12°	5°	5°	0,6°	0,12°	0	12°
Mandibular second molar	0	4°	7°	6°	6°	0.6°	6°,12°	0,7°	12°

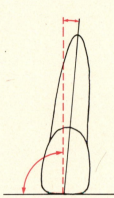

Fig. 12-18 ■ A second order bend, or an inclination of the bracket slot to produce the same effect, is necessary for the maxillary incisors because the long axes of these teeth are inclined relative to the incisal edge. The smaller angle (shown above) is the bracket angulation or the tip. (Redrawn from Andrews, L.F.: J. Clin. Orthod. **10**:179, 1976.)

treated patients and disparagingly called the "orthodontic look" (Fig. 12-19). The contemporary edgewise brackets that have a built in tip for maxillary incisor teeth routinely produce a more esthetically pleasing arrangement of the incisors than was achieved in many instances with the early fixed appliances. Bracket inclination in some commercially available appliances are shown in Table 12-2.

Distal tip of the upper first molar is also needed to obtain good interdigitation of the posterior teeth. As shown in Fig. 12-20, if the upper molar is too vertically upright, even though a proper Class I relationship apparently exists, good interdigitation cannot be achieved. Tipping the molar distally brings its distal cusps into occlusion and creates the space needed for proper relationships of the premolars.

Little if any tip is needed in the canines and premolars when an arch wire is fitted to an ideal arch. An inclination of the bracket slot for canines and premolars is often part of a straight-arch prescription, however, for two reasons: root paralleling at extraction sites, and tip of posterior teeth for anchorage.

If the bracket slots on the canine and second premolar are inclined as shown in Fig. 12-21, a straight arch wire will automatically produce a root-paralleling moment during the closure of a first premolar extraction site. The problem

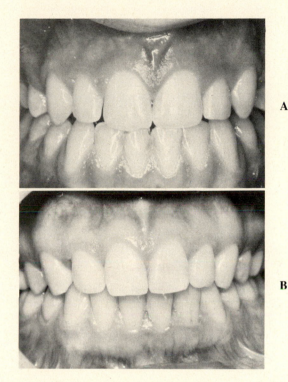

Fig. 12-19 ■ Achieving the proper inclination of the maxillary incisors is important for good esthetics. **A,** Dental appearance of a patient treated in the 1960s, with inadequate incisor torque and inclination. **B,** Dental appearance of a patient treated in 1980s with a contemporary edgewise appliance, showing improved torque and inclination.

with bracket inclinations of this type is that the desired effect can easily be overdone, so that the root apices have been brought too close together at the conclusion of orthodontic treatment. Furthermore, larger slot inclinations are required on the canines and second premolars for patients who have first premolar extractions than are appropriate for nonextraction patients. Bizarre tooth positions can result if extraction brackets are used on nonextraction patients and vice versa. Special "extraction brackets" that deviate significantly from the inclinations shown in Table 12-2 must be used with considerable caution.

A second reason for incorporating tip in posterior brackets relates to anchorage control. In the Tweed technique for

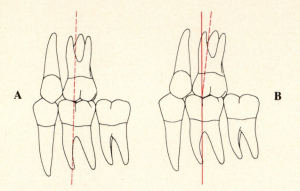

Fig. 12-20 ■ A distal inclination or tip of the maxillary first molar is important for proper posterior occlusal function. If the mesiobuccal cusp occludes in the mesial groove of the mandibular first molar, creating an apparently ideal Class I relationship, proper interdigitation of the premolars still cannot be obtained if the molar is positioned too upright **(A)**. Tipping the molar distally **(B)** allows the premolars to interdigitate properly. (Redrawn from Andrews, L.F.: Am. J. Orthod. **62:**296, 1972.)

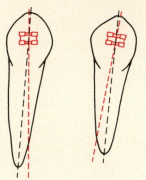

Fig. 12-21 ■ Inclination of the bracket slots on canines and premolars is not needed for normal positioning. Inclining the canine and second premolar brackets toward a first premolar extraction space, however, can be used to create an automatic root paralleling moment. Bracket inclinations of this type can produce too much root proximity at extraction sites and must be used with caution.

Table 12-2 ■ Bracket angulation (tip)

Tooth	A company Straight-wire	A company Roth Modified	Lancer Natural Arch	Ormco Alexander Vari-Simplex	Ormco Level Arch Modern	Rocky Mountain Triple Control	Rocky Mountain Bioprogressive	Unitek Twin Torque	Unitek Level Anchorage
Maxillary Central	5°	5°	5°	3°, 5°	5°	5°	0	5°	4°
Maxillary Lateral	9°	9°	9°	6°, 8°	8°	9°	8°	9°	7°
Maxillary Canine	11°	13°	11°	6°, 10°	10°, 13°	11°	5°	11°	0
Maxillary first premolar	2°	0	0	0	0	2°	0	2°	0
Maxillary second premolar	2°	0	0	0	0	2°	0	2°	0
Maxillary first molar	5°	0	5°	0	0, −10°	5°	0	0, 5°	0
Maxillary second molar	5°	0	5°	0	0, −10°	5°	0	0, 5°	−15°
Mandibular Central Lateral	2°	2°	0	0	0	2°	0	2°	2°
Mandibular Canine	5°	7°	5°	6°	6°	5°	5°	2°	−4°
Mandibular first	2°	−1°	0	0	0	2°	0	2°	−4°
Mandibular second premolar	2°	−1°	0	0	0	2°	0	2°	−6°, −4°
Mandibular first molar	2°	−1°	2°	−6°	−5°	2°	5°	0, 2°	−10°, −6°
Mandibular second molar	2°	−1°	2°	−6°	−5°	2°	5°	0, 2°	−15°, −10°

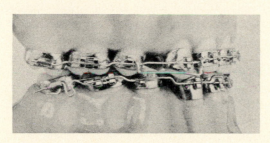

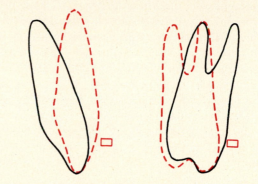

Fig. 12-22 ■ Distal tipping of the posterior teeth with second order bends in rectangular wire is used in the Tweed technique to provide increased anchorage. Brackets and molar tubes angulated to produce the same distal tipping are used in one contemporary straight-arch appliance, and distal tipping of molars for anchorage purposes is included in several other appliance prescriptions. (From Tweed, C.H.: Clinical Orthodontics, St. Louis, 1966, The C.V. Mosby Co.)

Fig. 12-23 ■ To produce the proper faciolingual position of both anterior and posterior teeth, either a rectangular arch wire must be twisted (torqued), or the bracket slot must be cut at an angle to produce the same torque effect. Otherwise, the improper inclination shown in the dotted red lines will be produced. Proper torque is necessary, not to move teeth, but to prevent undesired movement.

Table 12-3 ■ Bracket torque

Tooth	A company straight-wire	A company Roth Modified	Lancer Natural Arch	Ormco Alexander Vari-Simplex	Ormco Level Arch Modern	Rocky Mountain Triple Control	Rocky Mountain Bioprogressive	Unitek Twin Torque	Unitek Level Anchorage
Maxillary Central	7°	12°	7°	14°	14°	7°, 11°, 22°	22°	7°, 10°, 17°	15°
Maxillary Lateral	3°	8°	3°	7°	7°	3°, 7°, 14°	14°	3°, 13°	7°
Maxillary Canine	−7°	−2°	−7°	−3°	−7°, 0	−7°	7°	0, −7°	0
Maxillary first premolar	−7°	−7°	−7°	−7°	−7°	−7°	0	−7°	−7°
Maxillary second premolar	−7°	−7°	−7°	−7°	−7°	−7°	0	−7°	−7°
Maxillary first molar	−9°	−14°	−10°	−10°	−10°	−10°	0	0, −10°	−10°
Maxillary second molar	−9°	−14°	−10°	−10°	−10°	−10°	0	−10°	−10°
Mandibular central lateral	−1°	−1°	0	−5°	−1°	−1°	0	−1°	0
Mandibular Canine	−11°	−11°	−11°	−7°	−7°	−11°	7°	0, 11°	0
Mandibular first premolar	−17°	−17°	−17°	−11°	−11°	−17°	0	−17°	−11°
Mandibular second premolar	−22°	−22°	−22°	−17°	−17°	−22°	−14°	−22°	−11°
Mandibular first molar	−30°	−30°	−25°	−22°	−22°	−20°, −25°	−22°	−25°	−22°
Mandibular second molar	−33°	−30°	−25°	−27°	−27°	−25°, −30°	−32°	−20°, −25°, −30°	−22°

managing premolar extraction treatment with the original edgewise appliance, it was considered important to ''prepare anchorage.'' This was done by deliberately tipping the molar teeth distally so that they would better resist mesial displacement during space closure (Fig. 12-22). One presently available appliance (Level Anchorage, Unitek) is designed to allow the Tweed technique to be used without the necessity for the second order bends that were an important part of the original technique. In this appliance, distal tipping of the molars and premolars is a built-in feature. Interestingly, a number of the other appliance prescriptions also include some distal tipping of the molars, which is related to anchorage considerations during treatment, not to the desired final position of the molar teeth.

The same inclinations that tip the crowns distally also tend to bring the roots mesially, and careless use of an appliance with tip built into the posterior brackets can lead to loss of anchorage. If the molars are tipped somewhat distally at the end of orthodontic treatment, and the patient has vertical growth remaining (a critical point), the molars will upright into the normal position. In nongrowing patients, tipbacks in the molars do not resolve so neatly on their own. As with inclined brackets on canines and premolars, inclined attachments on molars should be used with a clear understanding of the effects that will be produced.

Elimination of third order bends. If the bracket for a rectangular arch wire is placed flat against the labial or buccal surface of any tooth, the plane of the bracket slot will twist away from the horizontal, often to a considerable extent. With the original edgewise appliance, it was necessary to place a twist in each rectangular arch wire to compensate for this (see Fig. 12-14). Failure to place third order bends meant that in the anterior region, the teeth would become too upright, while posteriorly the buccal cusps of molars would be depressed and the lingual cusps elevated (Fig. 12-23). Cutting the bracket slot into the bracket at an angle, which is called placing torque in the bracket, allows a horizontally flat rectangular archwire to be placed into the bracket slots without incorporating twist bends. The torque needed in many bracket slots is considerable. For incisors, the bracket slot must be at an angle so that the roots are lingually positioned relative to the crowns (positive torque). Canines stand relatively upright, while premolars and molars require increasing amounts of negative torque to position the roots buccally, not lingually.

The amount of torque recommended in the various appliance prescriptions varies more than any other feature of the straight-arch edgewise appliances (Table 12-3). Although a number of factors are important in establishing the appropriate torque, three are particularly germane to how much torque is used for any particular bracket: (1) the value that the developer of the appliance chose as the average normal inclination of the tooth surface (this varies considerably among individuals and therefore can be different in ''normal'' samples); (2) where on the labial surface, i.e., how far from the incisal edge, the bracket is intended to be placed (the inclination of the tooth surface varies depending on where the measurement is made, so that an appliance meant to be placed rather gingivally would have different torque values from one placed incisally); and (3) the bracket slot size (torque prescriptions for .018 slot brackets tend to be more conservative, i.e., have less torque in the brackets, than those for .022 slot appliances because .017 or .018 rectangular arch wires are routinely placed in .018 brackets, whereas .021 or .022 arch wires may never be used with .022 slot brackets thus the torque in the bracket slot tends to be more effective in the .018 appliance).

Variations in the shape and contour of individual teeth mean that any given inclination or torque built into a bracket will be correct for some teeth and incorrect for others because there is so much variation in the morphology of individual teeth. Slight errors in positioning brackets and bands also contribute to deviations from the ideal appliance prescription. For these reasons, even with the contemporary appliances, some third order bends in finishing are almost always required, and some first and second order bends are likely to be necessary.

■ Bracket Widths and Slot Sizes

Bracket width. In the original edgewise appliance, a narrow single bracket was placed in the center of the tooth, and small eyelets were soldered near the corners of the bands to provide for control of rotations (see Fig. 10-38). Even before the replacement of bands with bonded attachments made eyelets impractical for anterior teeth, two more convenient methods for obtaining rotational control had largely superceded them: the use of two brackets on the labial surface, creating a twin or Siamese bracket, and the use of wings extending from the single bracket (Fig. 12-24). Both single brackets with wings or an extended base width and twin brackets remain important in contemporary use.

Biomechanical considerations in the choice of wide (twin) or narrow (single) brackets are discussed in some detail in Chapter 10. In summary, wider brackets allow more positive control of tooth inclination (tip) and are easier to use when teeth slide along arch wires. Wider brackets inevitably reduce interbracket span, however, which makes both alignment of irregular teeth and torquing movements more difficult because arch wires become stiffer as interbracket span decreases.

There is no reason that wide brackets cannot be used for some teeth, and narrow ones for others, and just this arrangement is incorporated into some contemporary appliances (Fig. 12-24). However, one cannot evade the basic mechanical principle: the very increase in bracket width that provides better control of root position mesiodistally also reduces the springiness of arch wires. Conversely, any modification of a twin bracket that decreases interbracket span inevitably reduces control of tooth inclination. Because of this, arch wire choices will be affected throughout treatment by the width of the brackets. The effects of bracket width are discussed in detail in Chapters 15 to 17.

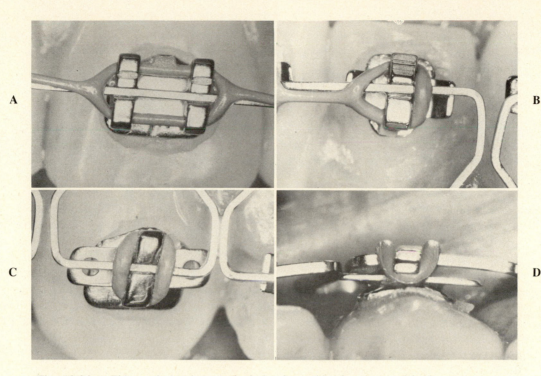

Fig. 12-24 ■ Either twin brackets or single brackets with wings are used in the contemporary edgewise appliance, and it is not unusual to find a combination of bracket types within a single contemporary appliance prescription. **A,** Twin bracket for maxillary central incisor, with the bracket in a rhomboid or "diamond" configuration to provide the desired 5 degree inclination of the bracket slot, **B,** single bracket with upswept wings (Lewis bracket) for a lower incisor. Note the elastomeric chain tie, which tends to produce rotation. The bracket wing on the right side, contacting the undersurface of the arch wire, provides an antirotation couple with a moment arm from the bracket to the end of the wing. **C,** Single bracket with flat wings (Lang bracket) on a maxillary canine. **D,** Occlusal view of Lang bracket. Note that on canines, the curvature of the arch wire tends to bring it into contact with flat wings. These wings can be bent to the precisely desired position for rotational control after the bracket is placed on the tooth.

.018 versus .022 slot. Biomechanical factors related to use of .018 as compared with .022 bracket slots are also discussed in some detail in Chapter 10. Briefly, the .022 bracket slot was originally selected to produce optimal performance with gold arch wires. It remained in use after gold was replaced by smaller stainless steel wires primarily because of its advantages in sliding teeth along the wire. With the .018 bracket, it is common to almost completely fill the slot with a rectangular arch wire, whereas with the .022 bracket, steel full-dimension arch wires are forbiddingly stiff, making finishing difficult. Either undersized steel wires or larger but more flexible titanium arch wires can be used to control this problem. Although the factors of bracket width and slot size interact strongly, slot size is even more important than bracket width in determining arch wire sizes and sequence at each stage of treatment.

■ Auxiliary Attachments

Auxiliary attachments are an integral part of the contemporary edgewise appliance. They fall into four categories:

Headgear tubes. These .045 or .051 round tubes are placed routinely on maxillary first molars, either occlusally or gingivally relative to the slot for the main arch wire (Fig. 12-25, *A*). They are used for the insertion of the inner bow of a facebow appliance (see Chapter 14) and can also accept a heavy auxiliary labial arch wire. For ease of access and better hygiene, the occlusal location is preferred.

Auxiliary edgewise tubes. The major purpose for auxiliary edgewise tubes is to allow the use of segmented arch technique, which is necessary to intrude teeth and also helpful in other situations. A rectangular auxiliary tube, placed gingivally to the plane of the main arch wire, should be present on both the upper and lower first molars. With this arrangement, the upper first molar typically has a convertible tube-bracket for the main arch wire, a gingivally positioned auxiliary rectangular tube, and an occlusally positioned headgear tube. The lower molar has a convertible tube-bracket for the main arch wire and a gingivally positioned auxiliary tube.

Auxiliary rectangular tubes on the canines are also used during closure of extraction spaces in the appliance designed by Burstone for segmented arch technique (Fig. 12-25, *B*). The auxiliary tube on the canine allows the use of springs connecting the anterior and posterior segments that are sep-

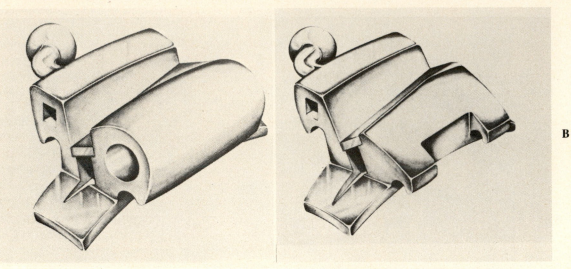

Fig. 12-25 ■ Contemporary edgewise tube-bracket attachments for first molars. **A,** Maxillary first molar attachment with convertible bracket slot, occlusal round headgear tube, and gingival auxiliary rectangular tube. (Courtesy Ormco Corporation.) **B,** Mandibular first molar attachment with convertible bracket slot and gingival auxiliary rectangular tube.

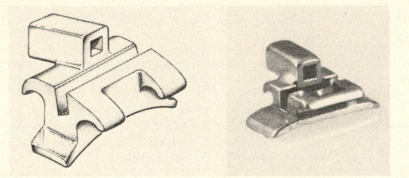

Fig. 12-26 ■ Burstone canine bracket, combining a rectangular bracket slot with a vertical tube that is used for attachment of retraction springs. (Courtesy Ormco Corporation.)

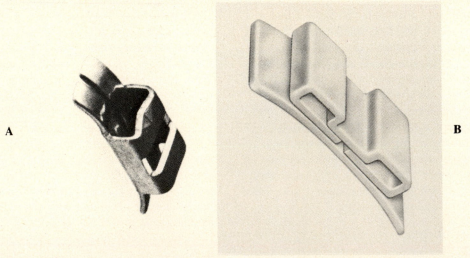

Fig. 12-27 ■ Lingual arch attachments. **A,** Horizontal lingual sheath to accept doubled-over .030 or .036 wire. (Courtesy Unitek Corporation.) **B,** double vertical lingual sheath to accept doubled-over 0.028 wire. (Courtesy Rocky Mountain Dental Company.)

arate from the base arch wire in either segment. Auxiliary tubes on the canines are only needed for space closure in special circumstances and can be added to an arch wire segment if not present as a part of the bracket (see Chapter 20). For this reason, they are not routinely used on canines in comtemporary appliance prescriptions. The auxiliary tubes for the molars are a necessity for leveling by intrusion and are strongly recommended in all patients.

Auxiliary labial hooks. Hooks for interarch elastics are routinely incorporated into the labial attachments for first and second molars in both arches (Fig. 12-26). These are used as needed for Class II, Class III, or cross-elastics (elastics that correct Class II, Class III, or crossbite relationships respectively). In addition, hooks for intraarch elastics to close extraction spaces can be added as gingival extensions from canine and premolar brackets (see Fig. 10-17). Since sliding space closure is more common with .022 edgewise, these "power arms" are used almost exclusively with the .022 system.

Lingual attachments. Some lingual attachments are needed as an adjunct for all primarily labial appliances. Buttons or cleats for lingual elastics are used routinely, and tubes or sleeves for lingual arches are often needed.

Heavy stabilizing lingual arches can serve as an important adjunct in anchorage control. They are an important part of segmented arch technique and are needed when auxiliary arch wires are used for leveling by intrusion. They can also be an important adjunct for anchorage control in space closure in premolar extraction cases, regardless of whether a totally segmented arch approach is used (see Chapter 10).

The preferred auxiliary lingual arch attachment is the horizontal lingual sheath, made to accept a doubled-over segment of .036 wire (Fig. 12-27). Twin vertical tubes are an acceptable alternative, but single vertical tubes are not recommended (see Chapter 13).

It is convenient to have a lingual cleat or button on at least one molar, to allow the use of cross elastics if necessary during treatment. In addition, lingual cleats on premolars and canines can help in controlling rotations during space closure (see Chapter 16). It is common practice to place a lingual cleat or button on banded posterior teeth, but isolated bonded lingual attachments are not recommended because of the risk that they could become detached and be swallowed by the patient. If it is necessary to use a bonded lingual attachment, tying it to the labial arch wire is a way to control this risk.

■Appliance Materials

The materials for an edgewise appliance must be precisely manufactured, so that the internal slot dimensions are accurate to at least .001 inch. The brackets and tubes supplied commercially at present are usually slightly oversized, ranging from the nominal dimension to .001 inch larger, whereas wires, though more accurate in size, tend to be slightly undersized if not produced exactly to the nominal dimension.[11] Brackets and tubes must also be quite strong to stand

up under the stresses of mastication without distorting so that slot dimensions are altered. To this point, despite a continuing search for tooth-colored attachments, it has not been possible to meet these requirements with nonmetallic materials, and the standard fixed attachments are fabricated from stainless steel.

There are two ways to produce edgewise brackets and tubes: from thin metal strip material that is stamped to shape, or by casting. Although stamped brackets and tubes were used almost routinely at one time, cast attachments are both more accurate and more durable, and clearly are superior. Most of the brackets and tubes for contemporary straight-arch appliances are now produced by casting.

There have been recurring efforts to make fixed appliances more esthetic by eliminating their metallic appearance. A major impetus to the development of bonding for orthodontic attachments was the elimination of the unsightly metal band. Tooth-colored or clear plastic brackets for anterior teeth became practical when successful systems for direct bonding were developed (Fig. 12-28). Although they were introduced with considerable enthusiasm, the brackets have suffered from three largely unresolved problems: (1) Plastic brackets tend to stain and discolor in the mouth. They look good when first placed, but their esthetic advantage decreases after a few months, particularly in patients who smoke or drink coffee. (2) The bracket materials are less dimensionally stable than metals, so that it is not possible to provide precise bracket slots. (3) Friction between the plastic bracket and metal arch wire makes it very difficult to slide teeth to a new position. For these reasons, plastic brackets with the features of the straight arch appliances are not available.

Placing a metal channel in a plastic bracket does reduce friction between the bracket and the wire without significantly compromising esthetics. This also makes it possible to incorporate at least some tip and torque, but these brackets do not compare in precision to those available as cast steel.

Developmental work has proceeded for a number of years with the goal of producing tooth-colored ceramic brackets that would be as dimensionally accurate and stable as steel. It is possible, and indeed probable, that research in this direction will eventually provide successful tooth-colored attachments. Tooth-colored arch wires will also be needed at that point, and it may eventually be possible to achieve this goal by using coatings on steel or titanium wires, or by using arch wires made from high-strength plastics.

■Preformed Archwires and Arch Form

The concept that dental arch form varies among individuals is driven home to most dentists in full denture prosthodontics, in which it is taught that the dimensions and shape of the dental arches are correlated with the dimensions and shape of the face. The same variations in arch form and dimensions, of course, exist in the natural dentition, and it is not the goal of orthodontic treatment to produce dental arches of a single ideal size and shape for everyone.

The basic principle of arch form in orthodontic treatment is that within reason, the patient's original arch form should be preserved. Most thoughtful orthodontists have assumed that this would place the teeth in a position of maximum stability, and long-term retention studies support the view that posttreatment changes are greater when arch form is altered than when it is maintained (for a recent review, see references 12 and 13). These variations in arch form, however, are not reflected in the preformed arch wires presently available, and it is important to keep in mind during orthodontic treatment that if preformed arch wires are used, their shape should be considered a starting point for the adjustments necessary for proper individualization (Fig. 12-29).

When a Class II malocclusion is present, there is a tendency for the maxillary arch to assume an excessively tapered form. In most Class II patients, it can be seen that when the lower arch is brought forward into a proper relationship, there is an incompatibility in arch form because the upper arch is too constricted across the canines and premolars (Fig. 12-30). In this circumstance, it is necessary during orthodontic treatment to change the maxillary arch form, and as a more general guideline, if the maxillary and mandibular arch forms are incompatible at the beginning of treatment, the mandibular arch form should be used as a basic guide. Obvious exceptions are encountered, however, in patients in whom the mandibular arch form has been distorted. This distortion can happen in a number of ways, the most common being lingual displacement of the mandibular incisors by habits or heavy lip pressures, and unilateral drift of teeth in response to early loss of primary canines or molars. Although some judgment is required, the arch form desired at the end of orthodontic treatment should be determined at the beginning, and the patient's occlusal relationships should be established with this in mind.

Despite wide acceptance of the idea that arch forms vary among individuals, there is a long orthodontic tradition of seeking a single ideal arch form. For many years, the Bonwill-Hawley arch form dominated orthodontic thinking. This arch form was based on establishing the anterior seg-

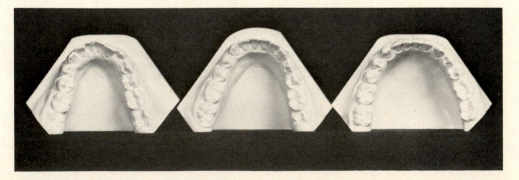

Fig. 12-28 ■ Clear or tooth-colored plastic brackets can be used on incisors to decrease the visibility of orthodontic appliances. **A,** Polycarbonate incisor brackets with an unconventional shape to minimize bracket failure; **B,** plastic brackets of conventional design with metal slots.

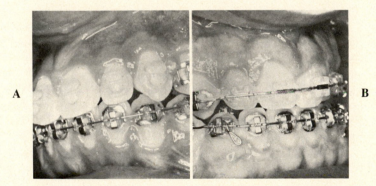

Fig. 12-29 ■ Lower casts of three untreated potential orthodontic patients. Note the difference in arch form.

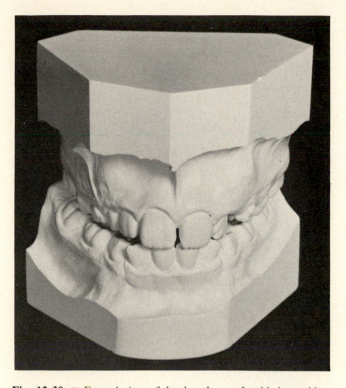

Fig. 12-30 ■ Frontal view of the dental casts for this boy with a typical Class II malocclusion, with the casts placed into a Class I molar relationship. Note that a crossbite results because of the relatively narrow upper arch. In treatment of Class II patients, this effect usually requires some change in upper arch form.

ment of the dental arch, from canine to canine, on a segment of the arc of a circle, and extending the posterior segments along a straight line. The radius of the arch varied depending on the size of the incisor teeth, so that arch dimensions differed as a function of tooth size, but arch form was constant for all individuals. The patient's original arch form was not considered. This approach can no longer be recommended.

An excellent mathematic description of the natural dental

arch form is provided by a catenary curve, which is the shape that a loop of chain would take if it were suspended from two hooks (Fig. 12-31). The length of the chain and the width between the supports determine the precise shape of the curve. When the width across the first molars is used to establish the posterior attachments, a catenary curve fits the dental arch form of the premolar-canine-incisor segment of the arch very nicely for most individuals. Exceptions include patients whose arches would fall into the prosthodontists' classifications of square or tapering arch forms. For all individuals, the fit is not as good if the catenary curve is extended posteriorly, because the dental arch normally curves slightly lingually in the second and third molar region. Most of the preformed arch wires offered by contemporary manufacturers are based on a catenary curve, with average intermolar dimensions.

Although these arch wires are a good starting point, it is apparent that even if one accepts the catenary curve as ideal, their shape should be modified if the first molar widths are unusually wide or narrow (Fig. 12-32). Modifications to accommodate for a generally more tapering or more square morphology are also appropriate, and the second molars must be "tucked in" slightly.

Another mathematic model of dental arch form, originally advocated by Brader[14] and often called Brader arch form, is based on a trifocal ellipse. The anterior segment of the trifocal ellipse closely approximates the anterior segment of a catenary curve, but the trifocal ellipse gradually constricts posteriorly in a way that the catenary curve does not (Fig. 12-33). The Brader arch form, therefore, will more closely approximate the normal position of the second and third molars. It also differs from a catenary curve in producing somewhat greater width across the premolars. In one comparative study, the ellipse came closer on the average to fitting the normal maxillary arch form, while the catenary curve came closer for the lower arch.[15]

Preformed arch wires prepared to an average Brader arch form are available commercially in a limited range of sizes, which can reduce the amount of individualization necessary.

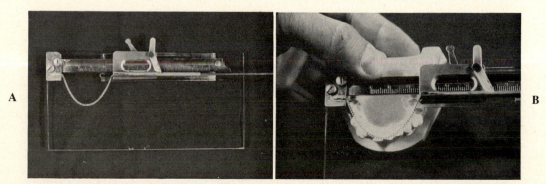

Fig. 12-31 ■ **A,** Catenary curves are formed by a loop of chain suspended from the ends, as illustrated here. The instrument is a catenometer, used for arch length measurements. **B,** The catenometer over a dental arch with severe crowding. (Courtesy Dr. James Ackerman.)

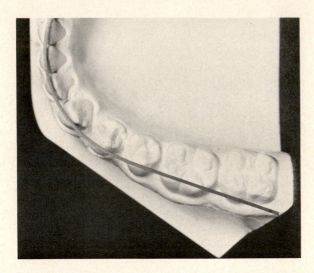

Fig. 12-32 ■ Preformed arch wire with catenary arch form, on a lower dental cast from an untreated patient. Note the good correspondence between the arch form and the line of occlusion, except for the second molar.

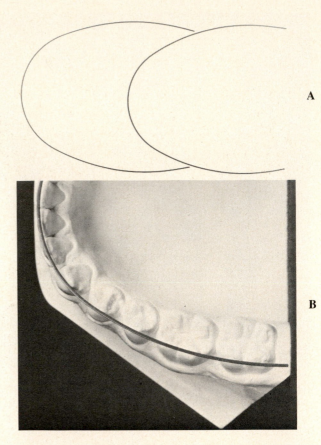

Fig. 12-33 ■ A, The Brader arch form for preformed arch wires is based on a trifocal ellipse, which slightly rounds the arch in the premolar region compared to a catenary curve and constricts it posteriorly. **B,** An arch wire formed to the Brader curve fits much better in the second molar region for this untreated patient than a catenary curve wire (compare to Fig. 12-32).

Like the catenary curve, however, the Brader arch form represents what the prosthodontists would call a midrange arch form, which will require some alteration for either the relatively square or relatively tapering normal arch form variations.

It is important to keep in mind that the adjustments placed in brackets for all of the straight-arch edgewise systems have nothing to do with arch form, which is still established by the shape of the arch wire connecting the brackets. Preformed arch wires are often listed in the catalogs as "arch blanks" and the name is appropriate, since this properly implies that a degree of individualization of the shape of the preformed arch wire will be required to accommodate the needs of patients.

■ *References*

1. Johnson, R.G.: A new method for direct bonding orthodontic attachments to porcelain teeth using a silane coupling agent: an in-vitro evaluation. St. Louis, 1980, St. Louis University, Department of Orthodontics, Master's thesis.
2. Shepherd, W.B., Leinfelder, K.F., Hershey, H.G.: Manipulation of orthodontic cements at sub-room temperatures. J. Dent. Res. **56:**B248, 1977.
3. Brannstrom, M., Nordenvall, K.J., and Malmgren, O.: The effect of various pretreatment measures of the enamel in bonding procedures. Am. J. Orthod. **74:**522-530, 1978.
4. Zachrisson, B.U.: Bonding in orthodontics. In Graber, T.M., and Swain, B.F., editors: Orthodontics: Current Principles and Techniques. St. Louis, 1985, The C.V. Mosby Co.
5. Artun, J., and Bergland, S.: Clinical trials with crystal growth conditioning as an alternative to acid-etch enamel pretreatment. Am. J. Orthod. **85:**333-340, 1984.
6. Maijer, R., and Smith, D.C.: Variables influencing the bond strength of metal orthodontic bracket bases. Am. J. Orthod. **79:**20-34, 1981.
7. Hanson, G.H.: Bonding bases coated with porous metal powder: a comparison with foil mesh. Am. J. Orthod. **83:**1-4, 1983.
8. Evans, L.B., and Powers, J.M.: Factors affecting in vitro bond strength of no-mix orthodontic cements. Am. J. Orthod. **87:**508-512, 1985.
9. Thomas, R.B.: Indirect bonding: simplicity in action. J. Clin. Orthod. **13:**93-106, 1979.
10. Andrews, F.: The straight-wire appliance. J. Clin. Orthod. **10:**99-144, 174-195, 282-303, 425-441, 507-529, 581-588, 1976.
11. Lang, R.L., Sandrik, J.C., and Klapper, L.: Rotation of rectangular wires in rectangular molar tubes. Part II. Pretorqued molar tubes. Am. J. Orthod. **81:**22-31, 1982.
12. Diggs, D.B.: The quantification of dental arch form. Seattle, 1982, University of Washington, Master's thesis.
13. Joondeph, D.B., and Riedel, R.A.: Retention. In Graber, T.M., and Swain, B.F., editors: Orthodontics: Current Principles and Techniques. St. Louis, 1984, The C.V. Mosby Co.
14. Brader, A.C.: Dental arch form related with intraoral forces: PR = C. Am. J. Orthod. **61:**541-561, 1972.
15. Neilaus, L.C.: A computerized analysis of human dental arch forms as compared to the catenary curve. Philadelphia, 1968, Temple University, Master's thesis.

TREATMENT OF ORTHODONTIC PROBLEMS IN PREADOLESCENT CHILDREN

"Preventive and interceptive orthodontics" has become a catch-all description of orthodontic treatment in children, largely devoid of meaning in an era when early treatment is usually followed by comprehensive treatment in the early permanent dentition. The problem with this description, though semantic, is not trivial: it encourages inappropriate expectations from treatment, implying that if the right treatment were done at an early age, no further treatment would be needed. "Prevention" of malocclusion is possible only in a few special circumstances. "Interceptive" treatment can be very helpful in reducing the severity of problems, but rarely is so successful that later treatment becomes unnecessary.

Despite these considerations, treatment in the mixed dentition (or occasionally in the primary dentition) can be very helpful, regardless of whether it is the only treatment the child will ever need. In the discussion that follows, treatment is described in terms of appropriate responses to specific situations, without the "preventive" or "interceptive" labels.

Orthodontic problems in children can be divided conveniently into nonskeletal (dental) and skeletal problems, treated by tooth movement and by growth modification, respectively. Treatment of nonskeletal problems is described in Chapter 13, and skeletal problems are discussed in Chapter 14. The complexity of the treatment procedures varies. Some are definitely within the scope of the general practitioner, whereas others should rarely be attempted outside specialty practice. Even the simplest treatment in children requires continuous reevaluation to be sure that the expected response is occurring. The transition of the dentition, coupled with rapid growth, means that rapid changes can and do occur. In children, appliance therapy tends to be simpler than in adults, where all changes that occur must be caused by tooth movement, but treatment planning and monitoring are more complex. Whether treatment in children involves skeletal or nonskeletal problems, the totality of changes must be considered. Although diagnosis and treatment planning are not discussed in this section, which focuses on treatment, careful analysis and planning are imperative before any treatment begins.

Chapter 13

Treatment of Nonskeletal Problems in Preadolescent Children

Treatment for potential alignment problems
    Space maintenance for missing primary teeth
    Space regaining
    Ectopic eruption
    Missing permanent teeth
    Supernumerary teeth
    Midline diastema
    Midline discrepancy from intraarch asymmetry
Crowding in the mixed dentition
    Mild crowding: adequate space predicted for the succedaneous teeth
    Moderate crowding: less than 4 mm space deficiency predicted for the succedaneous teeth
    Severe crowding: greater than 4 mm space deficiency predicted for the succedaneous teeth
Posterior crossbites
Incisor retrusion/protrusion
    Anterior crossbites
    Maxillary dental protrusion
Vertical problems
    Habits and open bites
    Deep bite
    Ankylosed primary teeth

■ *Treatment for Potential Alignment Problems*

Potential alignment problems in children are conditions that will result in crowding or displacement of permanent teeth that have not yet erupted. The goal of treatment is to prevent the potential problem from developing, by preventing drift of permanent teeth that have already erupted or by repositioning teeth that have drifted to improper positions.

■ Space Maintenance for Missing Primary Teeth

Early loss of a primary tooth presents a potential alignment problem because drift of permanent or other primary

teeth is a likely sequel. Space maintenance is appropriate only when the space available is adequate and all unerupted teeth are at the proper stage of development. If the predicted space is deficient or if succedaneous teeth are missing, space maintenance alone is inadequate. The indications and contraindications for treatment are discussed in Chapter 6, but are also noted briefly in the discussion here, which focuses on the treatment procedures.

Several treatment techniques can be used successfully for space maintenance, depending on the specific situation.

Band and loop space maintainers. The band and loop is a unilateral fixed appliance indicated for space maintenance in the posterior segments. It is used most frequently to maintain the space of a primary first molar before eruption of the permanent first molar, but it can also be used to maintain the space of either a primary first or second molar after the permanent first molar has erupted. The simple cantilever design makes it ideal for isolated unilateral space maintenance (Fig. 13-1), but the band and loop must be restricted to holding the space of one tooth because it has limited strength.

Before eruption of the permanent incisors, a pair of band and loop maintainers are recommended if a single primary molar has been lost bilaterally, instead of the lingual arch that would be used when the patient is at an older age. This is advisable because the developing succedaneous tooth buds are forming lingual to the primary incisors and often erupt lingual to their predecessors. The bilateral band and loops enable the permanent teeth to erupt without interference from a lingual arch wire. At a later time the two band and loops can be replaced with a single lingual arch if necessary.

The band portion of a band and loop can be placed on either a primary or a permanent molar. Although bonding a rigid or flexible wire across the edentulous space has been advocated as an alternative, this arrangement has not proved satisfactory clinically. It also is no longer considered advisable to solder the loop portion to a stainless steel crown because this precludes simple appliance removal and replacement. Teeth with stainless steel crowns should be banded like natural teeth.

If a primary second molar has been lost, the band can be

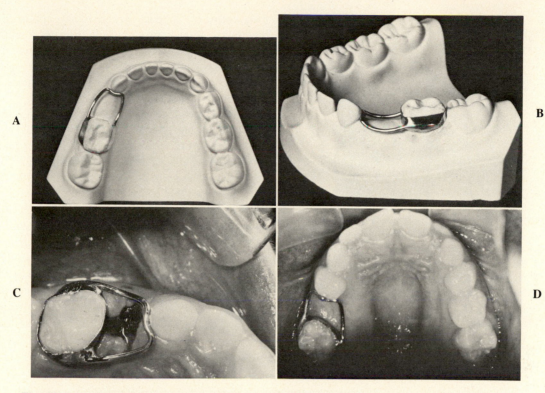

Fig. 13-1 ■ A band and loop space maintainer is generally used in the mixed dentition to save the space of a prematurely lost primary molar. It consists of a band on either a primary or permanent molar, and a wire loop to maintain space. **A,** The loop portion made from .036 inch wire is carefully contoured to the abutment tooth and **B,** the loop is also contoured to within 1.5 mm of the alveolar ridge. The solder joints must fill the angle between the band and wire to avoid food and debris accumulation. **C,** A completed band and loop maintainer, in place after extraction of a primary first molar; **D,** an occlusal rest, shown here on the primary first molar, can be added to the loop portion to prevent the banded teeth from tipping mesially.

placed on either the primary first molar or the permanent first molar. Many clinicians prefer to band the primary tooth in this situation because of the risk of decalcification around any band. A more important consideration is the eruption sequence of the succedaneous teeth. The primary first molar should not be banded if the first premolar is developing more rapidly than the second premolar, because loss of the banded abutment tooth would require replacement of the appliance, whereas loss of the abutment tooth adjacent to the loop can often be accommodated with appliance adjustment.

Ideally, the loop portion should be wide enough faciolingually to allow eruption of the permanent premolar without removing the appliance, but this arrangement is difficult to achieve. The loop should also be in close approximation to the ridge without impinging on the soft tissue, and it should not restrict any physiologic movement or adjustment of the adjacent teeth (Fig. 13-1), such as the lateral adjustment of the primary canines that accompanies eruption of the permanent incisors and provides anterior space.[1] An occlusal rest is an optional addition to the loop portion of the appliance. This addition prevents gingival tipping of the appliance and the abutment teeth, which can result in gingival irritation and space loss (Fig. 13-1). Unfortunately,

the loop provides little if any functional replacement for the missing tooth and will not prevent supereruption of teeth in the opposing arch.

Partial denture space maintainers. The partial denture is most useful for bilateral posterior space maintenance when more than one tooth has been lost per segment and the permanent incisors have not yet erupted. In these cases, because of the length of the edentulous space, band and loop space maintainers are contraindicated, and the lingual position of the unerupted permanent incisors makes the lingual arch a poor choice. The partial denture also has the advantage of replacing occlusal function. Another indication for this appliance is posterior space maintenance in conjunction with replacement of anterior teeth for esthetics (Fig. 13-2). Replacement of primary anterior teeth for esthetics is reasonable, but anterior space maintenance is unnecessary[2] because arch circumference is not lost even if the teeth drift and redistribute the space.

Excellent retention for a partial denture appliance is required for good patient compliance and usually requires several clasps. The clasps must accommodate the lateral movement of the primary canines that occurs during permanent incisor eruption. For this reason, clasps on these teeth may have to be removed or adjusted periodically.

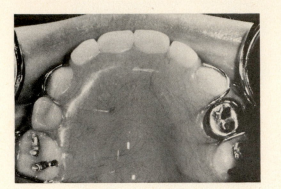

Fig. 13-2 ■ The removable partial denture is used to replace anterior teeth for esthetics and, at the same time, maintain the space of one or more prematurely lost primary molars. For this patient, the four incisors and the right primary first molar are replaced by the partial denture. Multiple clasps are necessary for good retention and both the clasps and the acrylic need frequent adjustment to prevent interference with physiologic adjustment of primary teeth during eruption of permanent teeth.

Frequently, the acrylic portion of the appliance must be modified to allow permanent teeth to erupt. A problem often encountered with partial dentures in a young child is failure to wear the appliance, which leads to space loss, or the other extreme, failure to remove it for cleaning, which can cause soft tissue irritation.

Distal shoe space maintainers. The distal shoe is the appliance of choice when a primary second molar is lost before eruption of the permanent first molar. This appliance consists of a metal or plastic guide plane along which the permanent molar erupts. The guide plane is attached to a fixed or removable retaining device (Fig. 13-3, *A* to *C*). When fixed, the distal shoe is usually retained with a band instead of a stainless steel crown so that it can be replaced by another type of space maintainer after the permanent first molar erupts. Unfortunately, this design limits the strength of the appliance and provides no functional replacement for the missing tooth. If primary first and second molars are missing, the appliance must be removable because of the length of the edentulous span, and the guide plane is in-

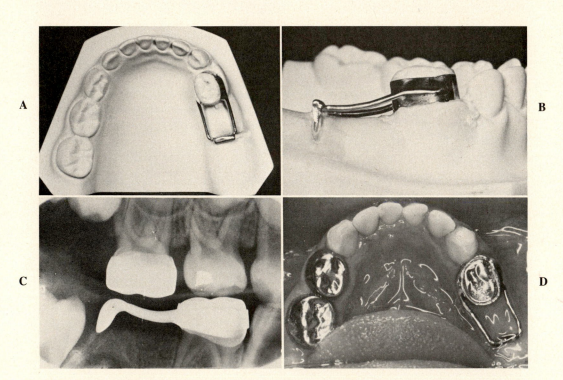

Fig. 13-3 ■ The distal shoe space maintainer is indicated when a primary second molar is lost before eruption of the permanent first molar and is usually placed at or very soon after the extraction of the primary molar. **A,** The loop portion made of .036 inch stainless steel wire and intraalveolar blade are soldered to a band so the whole appliance can be removed and replaced with another space maintainer after the permanent molar has erupted. **B,** The loop portion must be contoured closely to the ridge since the appliance cannot resist excessive occlusal forces. **C,** The blade portion must be positioned so that it extends approximately 1 mm below the mesial marginal ridge of the erupting permanent tooth to guide its eruption. This position can be measured from pretreatment radiographs and verified by a postcementation radiograph. An additional occlusal radiograph can be obtained if the faciolingual position is in doubt. **D,** This distal shoe space maintainer was placed at the time of extraction of the primary second molar.

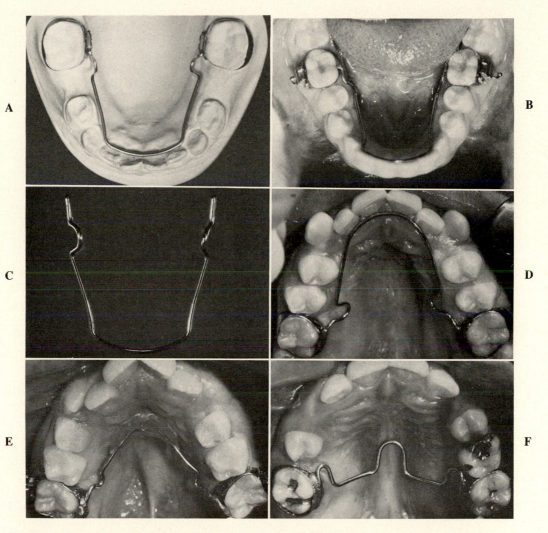

Fig. 13-4 ■ The lingual holding arch is generally used to maintain the space for the premolars after premature loss of the primary molars when the permanent incisors have erupted. **A,** The arch is made of .036 inch wire with adjustment loops mesial to the permanent first molars. **B,** This soldered lingual arch successfully maintained the space for the premolars. **C,** The ideal arch is stepped away from the premolars to allow their eruption without interference, which results in a keyhole design. The wire is also 1.5 mm away from the soft tissue at all points. **D,** A maxillary lingual arch is used when the overbite is not excessive, or **E,** a Nance arch with an acrylic button in the palatal vault is indicated if the overbite is excessive. The palatal button must be monitored since it may cause soft tissue irritation. **F,** The transpalatal arch in theory ties two molars together to prevent their rotation and drift. Several teeth should be present on at least one side of the arch to prohibit anterior drift of the posterior teeth.

corporated in a partial denture.[3] This type of appliance can provide some occlusal function.

To be effective, the guide plane must extend into the alveolar process so that it contacts the permanent first molar approximately 1 mm below the mesial marginal ridge, at or before its emergence from the bone (Fig. 13-3, *D*). An appliance of this type is tolerated well by most children, but contraindicated in patients who are at risk for subacute bacterial endocarditis since complete epithelialization around the intraalveolar portion has not been demonstrated.[4] Careful measurement and positioning are necessary to ensure that the blade will ultimately guide the permanent molar. Faulty positioning is the most common problem with this appliance.

Lingual arch space maintainers. A lingual arch is indicated for space maintainance when multiple primary posterior teeth are missing and the permanent incisors have erupted (Fig. 13-4, *A*). A conventional lingual arch, attached to bands on the primary second or permanent first molars and contacting the cingula of the maxillary or mandibular incisors, prevents anterior movement of the posterior teeth and posterior movement of the anterior teeth.

A lingual arch space maintainer is usually soldered to the molar bands but can be removable, depending on the number of adjustments anticipated and the care of the appliance expected from the patient (Fig. 13-4, *B*). Removable lingual arches, those that fit into attachments welded onto the bands, are more prone to breakage and loss. Regardless of whether it is removable, the lingual arch should be positioned to rest on the cingula of the incisors, approximately 1 to 1.5 mm off the soft tissue, and should be stepped to the lingual in the canine region to remain away from the primary molars and the unerupted premolars. This configuration results in a keyhole design that can also incorporate adjustment loops mesial to the molar abutment teeth so that the appliance can be adjusted to modify the fit or activation (Fig. 13-4, *C*).

Maxillary lingual arches of this type are not familiar to many clinicians, but are contraindicated only in patients whose bite depth allow the lower incisors to contact the arch wire on the lingual of the maxillary incisors (Fig. 13-4, *D*). When bite depth does not allow use of a conventional design, either the Nance lingual arch or a transpalatal arch can be used. The Nance arch is simply a maxillary lingual arch that does not contact the anterior teeth, but approximates the anterior palate (Fig. 13-4, *E*). The palatal portion incorporates an acrylic button that contacts the palatal tissue, which in theory provides resistance to anterior movement of the posterior teeth. The appliance is an effective space

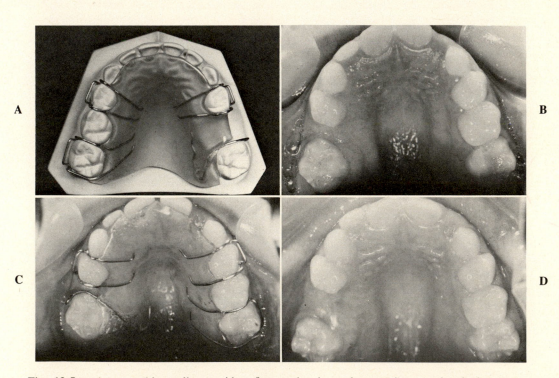

Fig. 13-5 ■ A removable appliance with a fingerspring is used to regain space by tipping a permanent first molar distally. **A,** The appliance incorporates multiple Adams' clasps and an .028 inch helical spring that is activated 1.5 mm per month. **B,** Premature loss of the primary second molar has led to mesial drift and rotation of the permanent first molar. **C,** This removable appliance can be used to regain up to 3 mm of space. **D,** After space regaining the space should be maintained with a band and loop or lingual arch.

maintainer, but soft tissue irritation can be a problem. The acrylic portion can become embedded in the soft tissue if the palatal tissue hypertrophies because of poor hygiene or if the appliance is distorted.

The transpalatal arch runs directly across the palatal vault, avoiding contact with the soft tissue (Fig. 13-4, *F*). When permanent maxillary molars move anteriorly, they rotate mesiolingually around the large lingual root. The transpalatal arch supposedly eliminates anterior molar movement by preventing this rotation. The best indication for a transpalatal arch is when one side of the arch is intact, and several primary teeth are missing on the other side. In this situation, the rigid attachment to the intact side usually provides adequate stability for space maintenance. When primary molars have been lost bilaterally, however, both permanent molars may tip mesially despite the transpalatal arch, and a conventional lingual arch or Nance arch is preferred. The most common problems with the transplanted arch are failure to adequately maintain space and failure of the appliance to remain passive. If the appliance is not passive, unexpected vertical and transverse movements of the permanent molars can occur.

Space Regaining

After premature loss of a primary tooth, space may be lost from drift of other teeth before a dentist is consulted, and repositioning the teeth to regain space rather than just space maintenance to stabilize the situation should be considered. Space regaining procedures should be limited to reestablishing 3 mm or less of space lost in a localized area. Generally, space is easier to regain in the maxillary arch than in the mandibular arch, because of the increased anchorage for removable appliances afforded by the palatal vault and the possibility for use of extraoral force (headgear). Space lost from tipping can be regained when the crown of the tooth is tipped back to its original position,

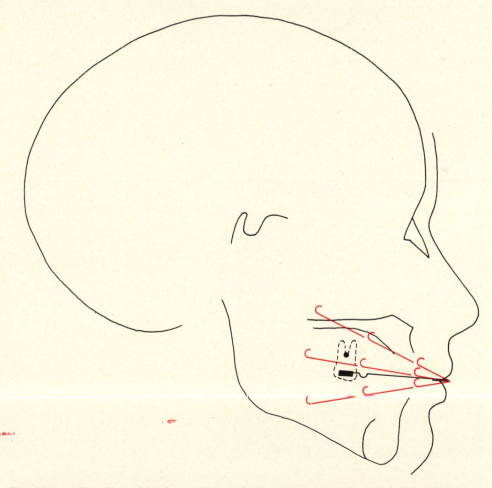

Fig. 13-6 ■ The effect of headgear on the molar is determined by the relationship of the outer bow of the facebow to the center of resistance of the tooth, located in this figure by the dot in the midroot area, and the direction of pull (head cap, neck strap, or combination anchorage). The variety of facebow options available for headgear is illustrated here. The vertical position of the outer bow can be high, straight, or low and its length can be short, medium, or long. Further details of the facebow and anchorage combinations and their resulting effects are discussed in Chapter 14.

but space lost by bodily movement requires that the tooth be bodily repositioned. This repositioning, in turn, requires more force and control for reliable movement of the crown *and* the root.

Maxillary space regaining. Permanent maxillary first molars can be tipped distally to regain space with either a fixed or removable appliance, but bodily movement requires a fixed appliance. Since the molars tend to tip forward, distal tipping for 2 to 3 mm of space regaining is often satisfactory.

A removable appliance retained with Adams' clasps and incorporating a helical finger spring adjacent to the tooth to be moved is very effective. This appliance is the ideal design for tipping one molar (Fig. 13-5). One posterior tooth can be moved up to 3 mm distally during 3 to 4 months of full time appliance wear. The spring is activated approximately 2 mm to produce 1 mm movement per month.

When space regaining by tipping is needed bilaterally or when bodily movement is required, extraoral force via a facebow to the molars is the most effective method, because the force is directed specifically to the teeth that need to be moved and reciprocal forces are not distributed on the other teeth that are in the correct positions. The force should be as nearly constant as possible, to provide effective tooth movement, and should be light because it is concentrated against two teeth. Fourteen to 16 hours or more of

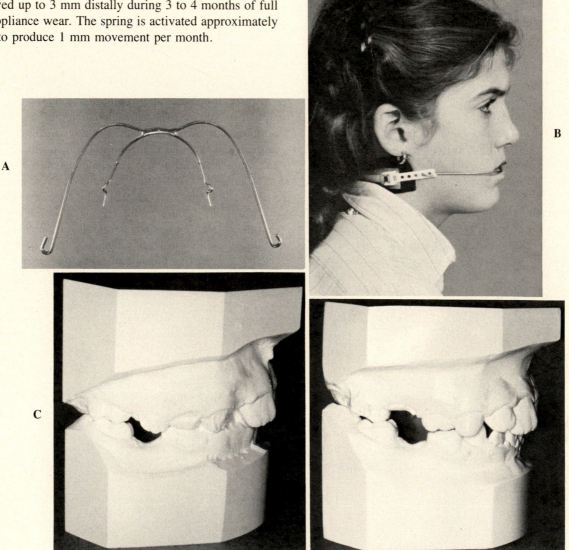

Fig. 13-7 ■ Headgear that consists of a facebow and extraoral force can be used to tip molars for space regaining. **A,** Symmetric facebow with an 0.45 inch inner bow is inserted into the tubes on the molar bands and the outer bow is attached to an extraoral strap. **B,** The long low outer bow attached to a cervical neck strap is ideal to tip molars distally for space regaining. **C,** This patient has had bilateral space loss as a result of mesial tipping of the molars. **D,** Space has been regained using a headgear and is demonstrated by the increased space and improved permanent molar relationships.

headgear wear per day, with approximately 100 to 200 gm of force per side, is appropriate.

To tip molars, the outer bow of the headgear must be positioned so that the resultant force vector passes occlusal to the center of resistance, which is near the midpoint of the root (Fig. 13-6) (see Chapter 14 for details). Tipping is accomplished best with a long outer bow on the facebow, bringing the attachment on the outer bow posteriorly nearly to the ear lobe, and with a neckstrap attachment (Fig. 13-7). For bodily movement or to move the molar roots distally, the outer bow must be positioned so that the resultant force is through or above the center of resistance. Bodily movement requires a shorter or higher outer bow and a head cap or a combination of head cap and head strap (Fig. 13-8) (see Chapter 14 for details).

It is important to remember that the direction of headgear pull relative to the crown will also determine whether the molar will be extruded, maintained at the same vertical level, or intruded as it is moved distally. Tipping the molar distally with a neckstrap attachment produces a downward as well as backward force on the molar and will extrude it. This causes no problems in most patients, particularly if the duration of extraoral force is only a few months. Tooth movement should occur at the rate of 1 mm per month, so approximately 3 months of treatment should be sufficient. Prolonged use of low-pull extraoral force should be avoided in all patients, and any use of extrusive force is contraindicated in a child who has a skeletal open bite.

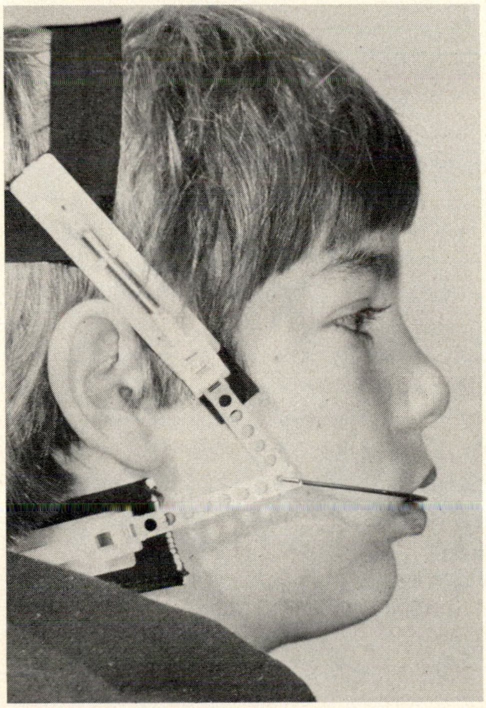

Sometimes both molars have to be moved distally, but one requires substantially more movement than the other. To accomplish this, an asymmetric facebow can be used to deliver more force to one tooth than the other (Fig. 13-9).[5] This will result in more movement on the side with the longer outer bow, but will also move that tooth toward lingual crossbite. Asymmetric headgear is neither as easy to adjust nor as comfortable to wear as symmetric headgear and requires excellent patient compliance to achieve its goal. For space regaining, it should be used only to deal with bilateral but asymmetric space loss (Fig. 13-10), not true unilateral space loss, which is treated best with a removable appliance.

Mandibular space regaining. Removable appliances can be used for space regaining in the mandibular arch as they are in the maxillary arch, but as a rule are less satisfactory because the mandibular appliance tends to distort, is prone to breakage, and may be difficult to retain. Problems with tissue irritation are frequently encountered, and patient acceptance tends to be poorer than with maxillary removable appliances.

If space has been lost on one side of the mandibular arch, the appliance of choice is a removable lingual arch, incorporating a loop that can be opened to provide the necessary

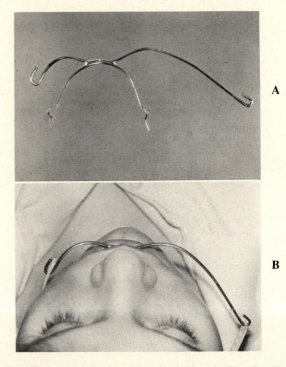

Fig. 13-9 ■ Asymmetric forces can be achieved with a headgear by using an asymmetric outer bow. **A,** The outer bow is cut short on the side that needs the smaller distal movement and is left long on the side requiring the greater distal correction. **B,** When the appliance is in place, before the neckstrap is attached, the side with the long outer bow should be approximately 4 to 5 cm from the cheek. This distance is reduced when force is applied by the strap and the outer bow rotates toward the face.

Fig. 13-8 ■ Bodily molar movement for space regaining is best achieved with a shorter and higher outer bow on the headgear than that used for tipping and should incorporate a head cap or combination head cap and neck strap as shown here.

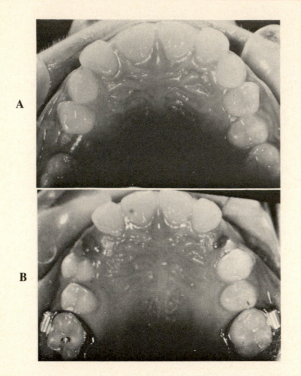

Fig. 13-10 ■ Asymmetric headgear used for space regaining. **A,** This patient has a space shortage on both sides of the maxillary arch, but more on the right side than the left because of space loss from premature loss of a primary molar. **B,** Good headgear wear resulted in space available for all succedaneous teeth.

distal force (Fig. 13-11). It is important that the lingual arch be activated so that the molar is tipped up and back, while the reaction force is expressed largely downward on the cingulum area of the lower incisors. Nevertheless, there is an inevitable tendency to tip the incisors forward also.

If space has been lost bilaterally, a lingual arch can also be used, but pitting posterior movement of both molars against the anchorage offered by the incisors means that significant forward displacement of the incisors must be expected.

An alternative fixed appliance for mandibular space regaining is the lip bumper, which is a labial appliance fitted to tubes on the molar teeth (Fig. 13-12). The idea is that the appliance presses against the lip, which creates a distal force to tip the molars posteriorly. Although some posterior movement of the molars can be observed when a lip bumper is used, the appliance also alters the equilibrium of forces against the incisors, removing any restraint from the lip against these teeth. The result is that forward movement of lower incisors occurs with a lip bumper to about the same extent as with a lingual arch. On balance, the effect of the two appliances is relatively similar.

Bilateral mandibular space regaining, in short, is difficult to accomplish with simple appliances without forcing the incisors labially. A fixed appliance with multiple banded/bonded attachments, perhaps supported by interarch elastics and extraoral force, may be required to significantly move lower molars back bilaterally.

■ Ectopic Eruption

Eruption is ectopic when a permanent tooth causes resorption of a primary tooth other than the one it is supposed to replace. When the permanent lateral incisor erupts, resorption of the primary canine is common. Less frequently, a portion of the distal root of the primary second molar is resorbed during the eruption of the permanent first molar. Potential alignment problems result if the primary tooth is lost prematurely or if the permanent tooth is blocked from erupting.

Loss of the primary canine from ectopic eruption usually indicates lack of enough space for all the permanent incisors, but occasionally may result solely from an aberrant position or orientation of the lateral incisor. When only one primary canine is lost, the lateral incisor will erupt into the primary canine space on that side and the midline will also shift in that direction. If both canines are lost, the permanent incisors may tip lingually, which reduces the arch circumference and increases the apparent crowding. In either case, space analysis, including an assessment of the anteroposterior incisor position and the facial profile, is needed to plan treatment. This evaluation will allow one to determine whether space maintenance, space regaining, or more complex treatment is indicated.

When one primary canine is lost, treatment is needed to prevent a midline shift. Depending on the overall assessment, the dentist can either remove the contralateral canine or maintain the position of the lateral incisor on the side of the canine loss, using a lingual arch with a spur. If both canines are lost, an active lingual arch for expansion, a passive lingual arch for maintenance, or no treatment may be indicated. In some children, space analysis will reveal that the crowding associated with ectopic eruption is so severe that complex treatment involving alignment of the teeth with fixed appliances, premolar extraction, or both are required.

Ectopic eruption of the permanent first molar presents an interesting problem that is usually diagnosed from routine bitewing radiographs. This painless and often unrecognized condition occurs more often in the maxilla than in the mandible. Lack of timely intervention may cause loss of the primary molar and simultaneous space loss. Because of the frequency of self correction of ectopic eruption, a period of watchful waiting is indicated when only small amounts of resorption are observed (Fig. 13-13).[6] If the blockage of eruption persists for 6 months or if resorption continues to increase, however, treatment is indicated.

Several methods can be helpful when intervention is necessary. The basic approach is to move the ectopically erupting tooth away from the tooth it is resorbing. If a limited amount of movement is needed but little or none of the permanent first molar is visible clinically, an .020 inch brass wire looped and tightened around the contact between the primary second molar and the permanent molar is suggested (Fig. 13-14). It may be necessary to anesthetize the soft tissue to place the brass wire. The brass wire should be

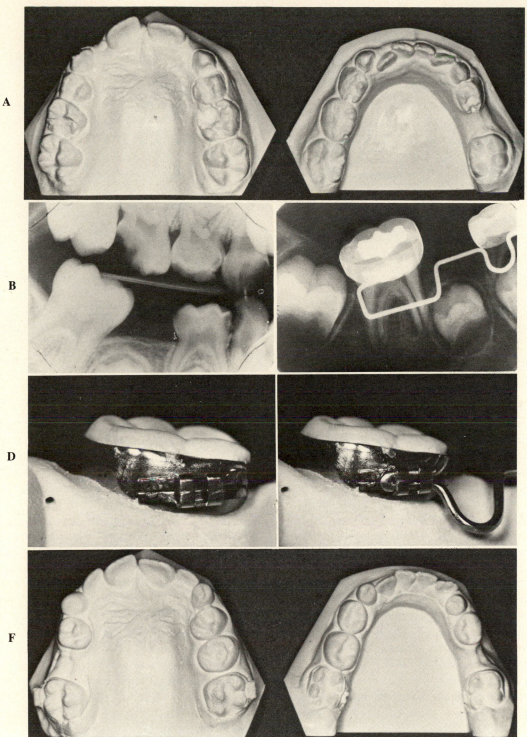

Fig. 13-11 ■ Space regaining in a child with space loss in the upper and lower arches. **A,** Casts demonstrating loss of space due to caries and early loss of a primary molar. **B,** Bitewing radiograph shows space loss due to mesial tipping of upper and lower permanent first molars. **C,** An active lingual arch, inserted from the distal in this case, was used for mandibular space regaining. **D,** When an active lingual arch is inserted from the mesial, the welded attachment on the band should be tipped up on the mesial to allow easy placement and removal. **E,** Note that when the lingual arch is fully seated, the dimple on the distal of the sheath into which it inserts serves as a lock to retain the archwire. **F,** Casts of this patient after treatment with a mandibular lingual arch and maxillary headgear, showing the space regaining that was achieved. At this point, space maintainers will be needed.

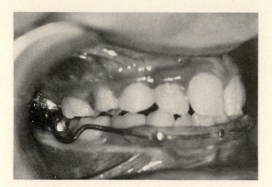

Fig. 13-12 ■ A lip bumper constructed of an .036 inch wire bow with an acrylic pad, which fits into tubes on the permanent first molars, is sometimes used to increase arch length by moving the molars distally and causing the incisors to move anteriorly. This occurs when the removable appliance stretches the lower lip and transmit force to move the molars back. This also disrupts the equilibrium between the lip and tongue and allows the anterior teeth to move facially. The result is probably equal molar and incisor change. (Courtesy Dr. M. Linebaugh.)

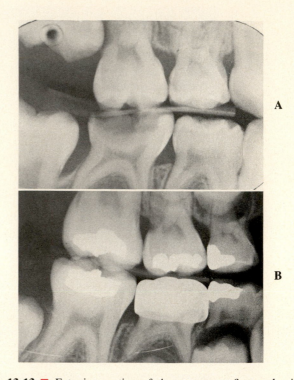

Fig. 13-13 ■ Ectopic eruption of the permanent first molar is usually diagnosed from routine bitewing radiographs. If the resorption is limited, the situation may be observed. **A,** The distal root of the primary maxillary second molar shows minor resorption from ectopic eruption. **B,** This radiograph taken approximately 18 months later illustrates that the permanent molar was able to erupt without treatment.

tightened approximately every 2 weeks. Treatment is slow but reliable.

A steel spring clip available commercially may work if only a small amount of resorption of the primary molar roots exists. These clips are difficult to place if the point of contact between the permanent and primary molar is much below the cementoenamel junction of the primary molar. Elastomeric separators should not be used for this purpose. They can become dislodged in an apical direction and cause a periodontal abscess, and if this occurs, they are hard to locate and retrieve because they are not radiopaque.

When the occlusal surface of the erupting permanent molar is accessible, a simple fixed appliance can be fabricated to move the molar distally. The appliance consists of a band on the primary molar with a soldered .028 inch helical spring attached (Fig. 13-15). A shallow preparation is made in the occlusal surface of the permanent molar, or a ledge of resin or a metal button is bonded to its occlusal surface for engagement of the spring. It is often difficult to bond to the partially erupted tooth because of contamination of the occlusal surface by saliva, which may make a surface preparation necessary.

The techniques detailed here can be extremely valuable as a means to disengage the erupting permanent tooth and retain the primary tooth. If the permanent molar has caused extensive resorption of the primary molar, there may be no choice but to extract it, and one should expect the permanent molar to continue to move mesially and shorten the arch length. Therefore, the primary tooth should be extracted only after careful consideration, since the consequences of extreme space loss can be difficult to manage. Unless the second premolar is missing and the arch length is purposefully to be reduced, or unless considerable mesial molar movement is tolerable and later premolar extraction is

planned, a distal shoe that guides the permanent tooth should be placed after the extraction. Even if this technique is used, some space has already been lost and the permanent molar will have to be repositioned distally using a space regaining appliance as previously described.

■ Missing Permanent Teeth

When permanent teeth are congenitally missing, the patient must have a thorough evaluation to determine the correct treatment, since any of the diagnostic variables of profile, incisor position, and space availability or deficiency can be crucial in treatment planning.

The most commonly missing permanent teeth are the mandibular second premolars and the maxillary lateral incisors. These two conditions pose different problems. If the patient has an ideal or an acceptable occlusion, maintaining primary second molars is a reasonable plan, since many primary molars can be retained at least until the patient reaches the early twenties if root resorption and caries have not been a problem (Fig. 13-16). There are many reports of primary posterior teeth surviving until the patient is 40 to 60 years of age. If the primary molars, which are larger than the second premolars, are retained, some reduction of their mesiodistal width is often necessary to improve the posterior interdigitation of the teeth. A limiting factor in

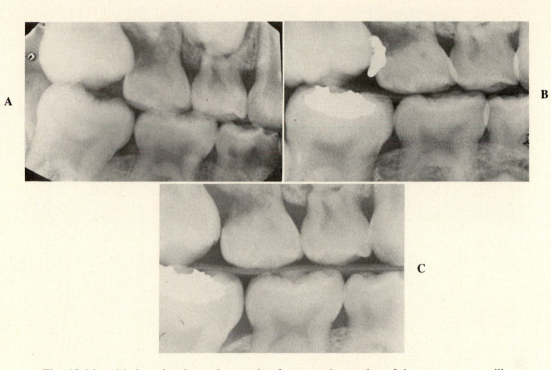

Fig. 13-14 ■ Moderately advanced resorption from ectopic eruption of the permanent maxillary first molar requires active intervention. **A,** The distal root of the primary maxillary second molar shows resorption and no self-correction. **B,** An .020 inch dead soft brass wire is looped around the contact between the teeth and tightened at approximately 2-week intervals; **C,** the permanent tooth is dislodged distally and erupts past the primary tooth that is retained.

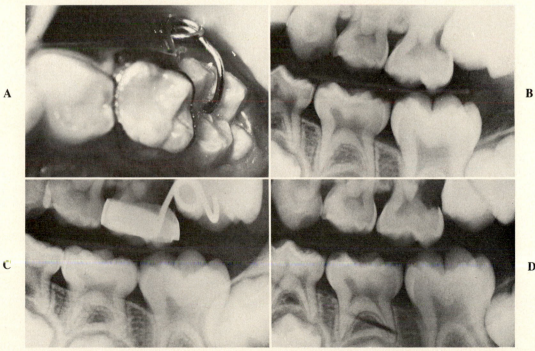

Fig. 13-15 ■ Ectopic eruption with severe resorption may require appliance therapy. **A,** If the occlusal surface of the permanent molar is accessible, the primary molar can be banded and an .028 inch spring soldered to the band. A small preparation or ledge of resin is used as a purchase point on the permanent molar. **B,** This primary maxillary second molar shows severe resorption. **C,** It is tipped distally out of the resorption defect and, **D,** once disengaged, is free to erupt.

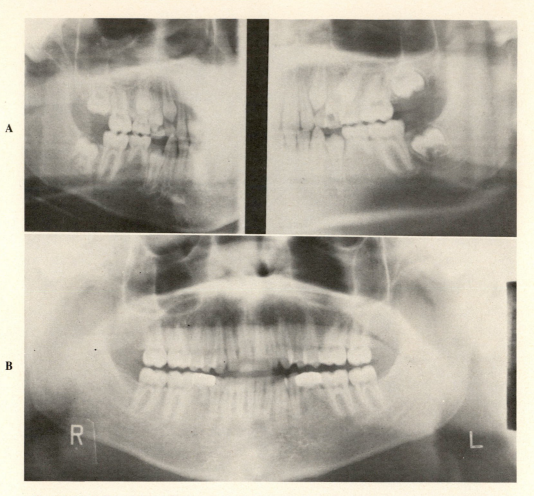

Fig. 13-16 ■ Primary mandibular second molars can be retained when the second premolars are missing. **A,** This patient has missing mandibular second premolars identified before orthodontic treatment. **B,** The primary mandibular second molars that have excellent root structure were reduced mesiodistally and restored with stainless steel crowns during the finishing stages of orthodontic treatment to provide good occlusion.

this reduction is the mesiodistal divergence of the primary molar roots. Teeth can move no closer together than their roots will allow, so a nonideal posterior occlusion may be the final compromise. It is now possible to replace the primary posterior teeth when necessary at a later time with resin bonded bridges that are much less expensive and invasive than conventional fixed bridges.

Long-term retention of primary laterals, in contrast, is almost never an acceptable plan. When the lateral incisors are missing, one of two sequelae is usually observed. In some patients, the erupting permanent canine resorbs the primary lateral incisor and spontaneously substitutes for the missing lateral incisor, which means that the primary canine has no successor (Fig. 13-17). Some of these patients are seen as adults with primary canines in place, but most primary canines are lost by the end of adolescence even if their successors have erupted mesially. Less often, the primary lateral is retained until the canine is replaced by its proper successor. The long-term prognosis of the retained primary

lateral incisors is poor, and fixed bridges will usually be required.

If permanent teeth are missing and there is evidence of developing crowding in the complete permanent dentition, the potential solutions to the problem include extraction of the primary teeth and orthodontic space closure. In some of these cases, missing permanent teeth can be treated as if they had been extracted, as a means to relieve the crowding. The mandibular second premolars and the maxillary lateral incisors, the permanent teeth most often missing, generally would not be the first teeth chosen for extraction. These patients will require comprehensive treatment during adolescence, and primary teeth should be extracted to promote drift of permanent teeth for space closure only after consultation with a specialist.

The second premolars have a tendency to form late and may be thought to be missing, only to be discovered to be forming at a subsequent visit. Good quality premolars seldom form after the child is 8 years of age. If the space,

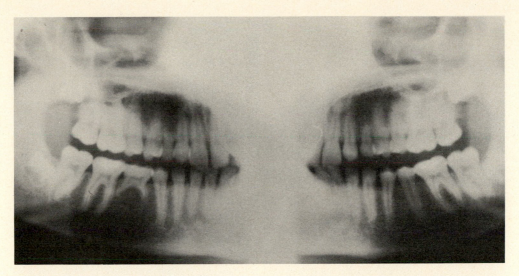

Fig. 13-17 ■ Missing permanent maxillary lateral incisors are often replaced spontaneously by permanent canines. This phenomenon occurs without intervention, but the resorption noted on the retained primary canines probably will continue to progress.

profile, and jaw relationships are good, it is possible to extract the second primary molars at age 7 to 9 and allow the first molars to drift mesially (Fig. 13-18, *A* and *B*). The mesial drift of the posterior teeth, along with some distal drift of the anterior teeth, will produce partial or even complete space closure (Fig. 13-18, *C* to *H*). Unfortunately, the amount and direction of the drift vary. Early extraction can reduce the treatment time, but comprehensive orthodontic treatment is usually needed for completion.[7]

When permanent lateral incisors are missing and space closure is desired, it helps if the primary lateral incisors are replaced by the permanent canines. When this process is occurring naturally, little immediate attention is necessary at that stage. Sometimes, the absence of lateral incisors causes a large diastema to develop between the permanent central incisors. To maximize the mesial drift of the erupting permanent canines, this diastema should be closed and retained (Fig. 13-19). Before the first premolar erupts, the primary canine should be extracted if it is not resorbing, so the premolars can migrate into the canine position and other posterior teeth can move mesially and close space (Fig. 13-20). In this situation also, comprehensive orthodontic treatment, recontouring of the anterior teeth, and resin buildups to improve esthetics are necessary to complete the treatment, but the amount of treatment and treatment length can be greatly reduced by timely removal of primary teeth.[8]

■ Supernumerary Teeth

Supernumerary teeth can disrupt both the normal eruption of the other teeth and their alignment if eruption does occur. Treatment is aimed at extraction of the supernumeraries before this occurs, or minimizing the effect if teeth have already been displaced.

The most common location for supernumerary teeth is in the anterior maxilla. These teeth are often discovered on a panoramic radiograph when the child is about 6 to 7 years of age, either during a routine examination or when disturbances of eruption are noticed. The simple cases are those in which a single supernumerary tooth is present and superficially located. If the tooth is not inverted, it will often erupt before the normal tooth and can be extracted before it interferes with the adjacent teeth.[9] In a few instances, multiple supernumerary teeth will be located superficially, and uncomplicated extractions can be performed without interfering appreciably with the normal teeth.

As a general rule, the more supernumeraries present, the more abnormal their shape and the higher their position, the harder it will be to manage the situation. Several abnormal supernumeraries are very likely to have disturbed the position and eruption timing of the normal teeth before their discovery, and tubercle teeth are unlikely to erupt (Fig. 13-21). Extractions should be done as soon as the supernumerary teeth can be removed without harming the developing normal teeth. The surgeon may wish to delay intervention until continued root development has improved the access and prognosis for extraction. This is a reasonable approach, but the earlier the supernumeraries can be removed, the more likely that the normal teeth will erupt without further treatment. Conversely, the later the extraction, the more likely that the remaining normal teeth will fail to erupt and will need surgical exposure, orthodontic traction, or both to bring them into the arch.

Some evidence indicates that changes in the overlying keratinized tissue occur in long standing edentulous regions.[10] These changes contribute to slow eruption of an incisor after the supernumerary tooth blocking it and also the overlying bone have been removed. If the delayed incisor is located superficially, it can be exposed with a simple soft tissue incision and usually will erupt rapidly (Fig. 13-22). When the tooth is more deeply positioned, the adjacent

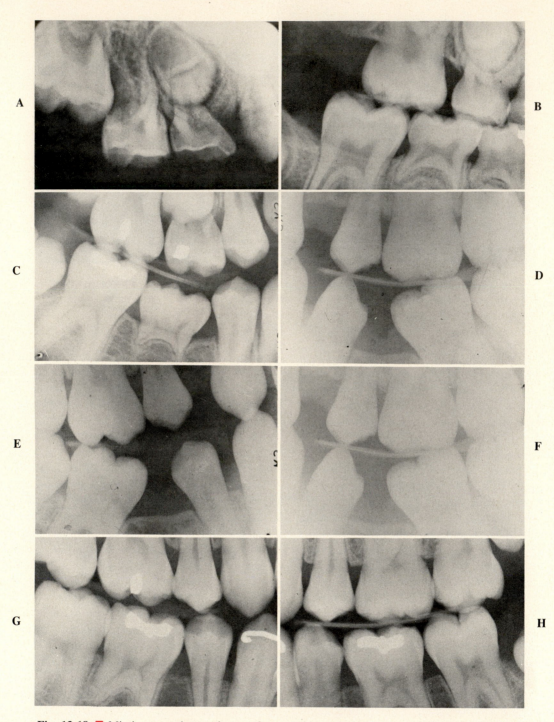

Fig. 13-18 ■ Missing second premolars can be treated by extraction of primary second molars to allow drifting of the permanent teeth and spontaneous space closure. **A,** This patient has ectopic eruption of the permanent maxillary first molar and a missing permanent maxillary second premolar. Since there was no other evidence of a malocclusion, the primary molar was extracted and **B,** the permanent molar drifted anteriorly and closed the space during eruption. This eliminates the need for a prosthesis at a later date. **C,** and **D,** Another patient has bilaterally missing permanent mandibular second premolars and the decision was made to extract the retained primary molars to allow as much spontaneous drift and space closure as possible before full appliance therapy. **E,** and **F,** There was drift of the posterior teeth anteriorly and drift of the anterior teeth distally, but the space did not completely close. This pattern of drift is highly variable and unpredictable. **G,** and **H,** The residual space was closed and the roots paralleled with full appliances.

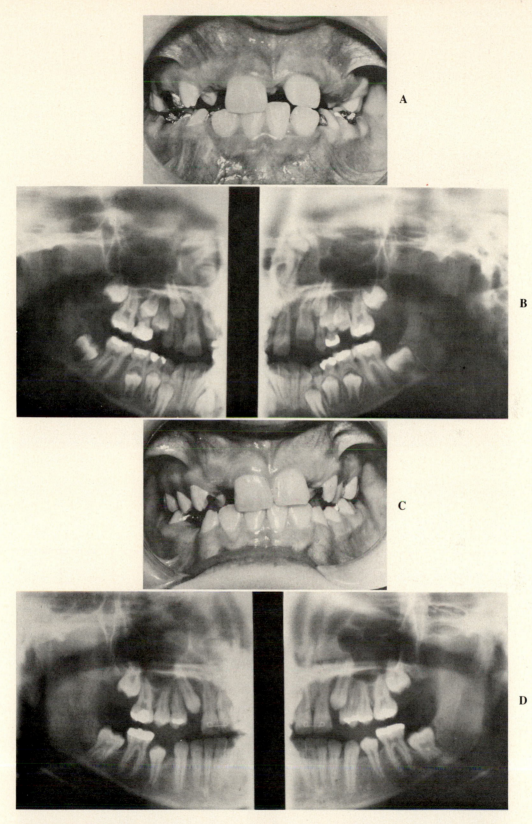

Fig. 13-19 ■ Missing permanent lateral incisors often allow a large diastema to develop between the permanent central incisors. **A,** This patient has this type of diastema and the unerupted permanent canines will be substituted for the missing lateral incisors. **B,** This radiograph shows the unerupted canines in an excellent position for substitution for the lateral incisors. **C,** The diastema has been closed to obtain maximum mesial drift of the canines. **D,** This technique enables the canines to erupt closer to their final position and eliminates unnecessary tooth movement during full appliance therapy.

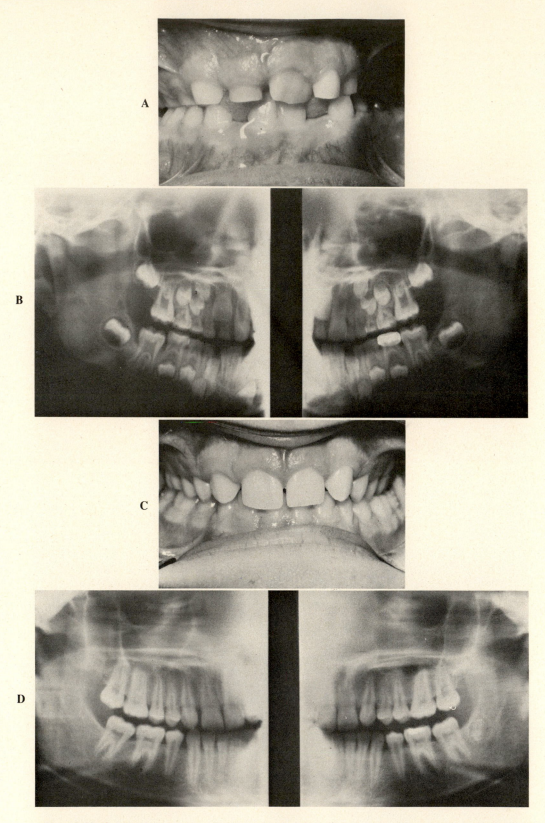

Fig. 13-20 ■ Selective removal of primary teeth when permanent maxillary lateral incisors are missing can lead to a shortened second phase of fully banded treatment. **A, B,** This patient had primary canines and first molars extracted to maximize the mesial drift of the permanent posterior teeth. **C, D,** This intervention resulted in good tooth position that will require little fixed appliance therapy to complete.

tissue can be repositioned and the crown exposed, which usually leads to normal rapid eruption. If there is further delay, traction can be applied to the exposed crown using a bonded attachment and fixed appliances (Fig. 13-23).

If it seems likely that it will be necessary to pull an unerupted tooth into the arch, because the permanent tooth has been displaced or for other reasons, an attachment should be bonded to each displaced tooth at the time it is exposed, and a wire ligature extended out of the tissue for later traction from a fixed appliance. The alternative is to loop a wire around the cervical part of the crown. Attach-

ments are sometimes difficult to bond because isolating the tooth from contamination by saliva and hemorrhage may be a problem, but usually more bone needs to be removed to pass a ligature around the cervical portion of the crown, and this approach can compromise the ultimate health of the periodontal attachment.

A fixed appliance must be placed on adjacent teeth to bring an unerupted tooth into the arch. This appliance should usually extend from molar to molar, attaching to as many other teeth as feasible. Initially, a relatively stiff archwire is needed.

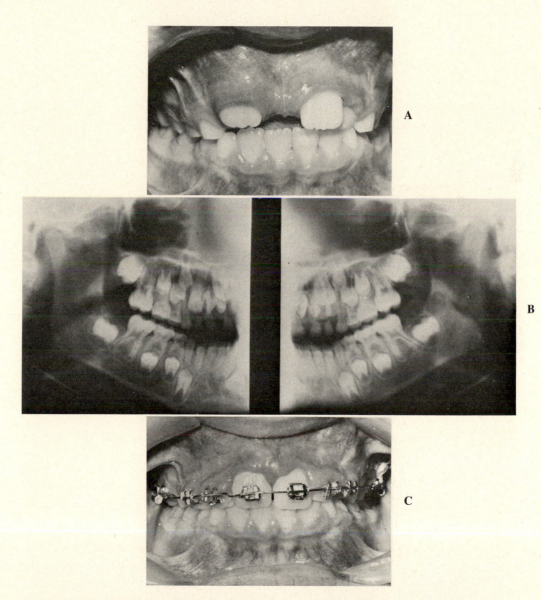

Fig. 13-21 ■ Multiple supernumerary teeth in the maxilla are often the cause of spacing and delayed eruption of anterior teeth. **A,** This patient has an exceptionally wide diastema and delayed eruption of the maxillary lateral incisors. **B,** The panoramic radiograph reveals three supernumeraries of various shapes and orientations. Conical and noninverted supernumeraries usually erupt, whereas tubercle shaped and inverted ones do not. **C,** The supernumeraries were removed, the diastema closed, and the remaining permanent teeth aligned with fixed appliances after they erupted.

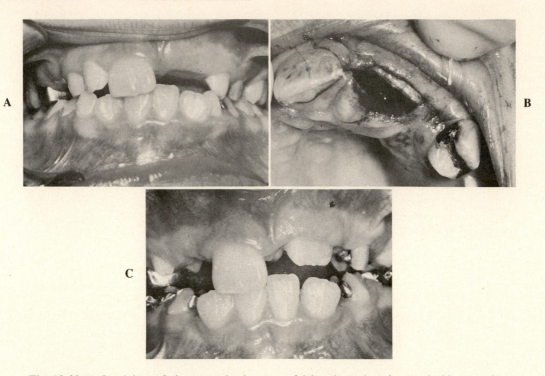

Fig. 13-22 ■ Overlying soft tissue may be the cause of delayed eruption after surgical intervention to remove primary or supernumerary teeth. **A,** This unerupted permanent maxillary left central incisor is covered by only soft tissue. **B,** Removal of a limited amount of the tissue while maintaining a band of keratinized tissue on the facial area, **C,** usually results in rapid eruption.

Before the unerupted tooth is clinically visible, the extruding force can be delivered by an elastomeric module or spring attached to the ligature extending from the tooth. Forces from elastomeric materials decay rapidly and theoretically are less desirable than those from wire springs. Despite this drawback, since a displaced permanent tooth is often high in the vestibule, the inefficient but nonbulky elastomeric modules are often less irritating than springs. Light force should be used to minimize the chance that reciprocal forces will be a problem and that adjacent teeth

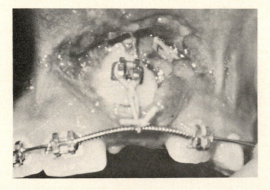

Fig. 13-23 ■ Traction delivered to a recently surgically exposed incisor. The tooth has been uncovered with an apically positioned flap and repositioned frenum. The tooth is being pulled into the line of the arch using a rubber tie to a heavy archwire while the space is held open by a coil spring.

will be intruded. Loops bent into a more resilient archwire are best used to obtain final crown and root positioning when the tooth is more occlusally located. (See Chapter 15 for further details.) Failure of the unerupted teeth to move usually indicates ankylosis, and further surgical intervention (see Chapter 15) may be needed.

■ Midline Diastema

A small maxillary midline diastema is present in many children, but is not necessarily an indication for orthodontic treatment. The unerupted canines often rest superior and distal to the lateral incisor roots, which forces the lateral and central incisor roots toward the midline while their crowns diverge distally (Fig. 13-24). This situation creates space between the incisors and is called the "ugly duckling" stage. These spaces tend to close spontaneously when the canines erupt and the incisor root and crown positions change. Until the canines erupt, it is difficult to be certain whether treatment will be necessary.

Another possible cause of a diastema is a tooth size discrepancy resulting from small upper and large lower anterior teeth. Treatment usually requires both a change in tooth size (building up small maxillary laterals with composite resin, for instance) and permanent retention[11] (see Chapter 17). Attempts to simply close the space will result in relapse because the occlusion will force the space to reopen. In this situation also, treatment should be deferred until all permanent teeth have erupted.

The major indications for closure of a midline diastema are: (1) a diastema that remains open after the permanent canines have erupted, and (2) before canine eruption, a diastema of 3 mm or more. In the former situation, there is an esthetics problem and in the latter, not only are esthetics unfavorable, but eruption of the lateral incisors or canines can be inhibited as a result of the distal position of the central incisors and a lack of space.

When the canines have erupted and the diastema is less than 2 mm, the central incisors can usually be tipped together. A maxillary removable appliance with clasps, fingersprings, and possibly an anterior bow will successfully complete this type of treatment. Use of this appliance presupposes that the incisors do not require root repositioning.

The second treatment indication for a diastema is more challenging since in few cases can more than 3 mm of incisor separation be corrected by tipping. If, by chance, a large diastema is found and the teeth are tipped apart, they can be tipped back together and retained with a removable appliance (Fig. 13-25). Sometimes the facial position of the incisors contributes more to the diastema than the mesiodistal positioning. If this is the case, a Hawley-type removable appliance with clasps and a labial bow will achieve the desired result. On the other hand, most large diastemas will require bodily repositioning of the incisors. When the situation demands only mesiodistal movement and no retraction of the incisors, the teeth can be moved along a segmental rectangular archwire that is placed in bonded brackets on the incisors (Fig. 13-26). The force to move the incisors together is provided by an elastomeric chain or, less conveniently, a coil spring.

When a wide diastema is complicated by spaced and protrusive incisors that require bodily movement, an archwire should be used with bands on posterior teeth and bonded brackets on anterior teeth. This appliance must provide a retracting and space closing force, which can be obtained from closing loops incorporated into the archwire or from a section of elastomeric chain (see Chapter 16). Bodily incisor retraction and space closure using a multiband/bond fixed appliance also place a large strain on the

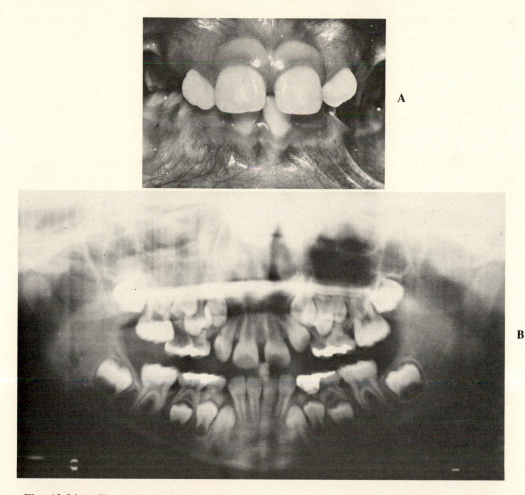

Fig. 13-24 ■ The "ugly duckling phase." **A,** Spacing of the incisors and mesial root position results from the position of the unerupted permanent canines. **B,** This panoramic radiograph shows that the canines are erupting and in close proximity to the roots of the lateral incisors. The diastemas usually close when the canines erupt.

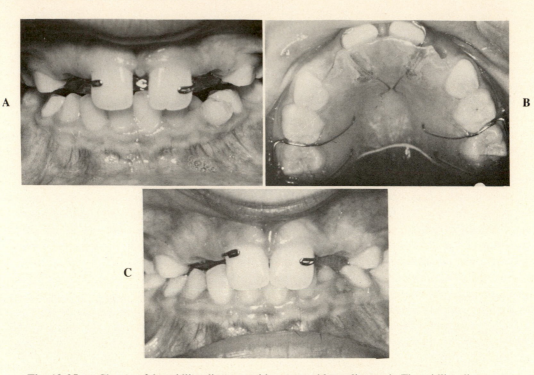

Fig. 13-25 ■ Closure of the midline diastema with a removable appliance. **A,** The midline diastema is closed with a removable appliance and fingersprings by tipping the teeth mesially. **B,** The .028 inch helical fingersprings are activated to move the incisors depending on their position and response to the force. **C,** The final position is maintained with the same appliance.

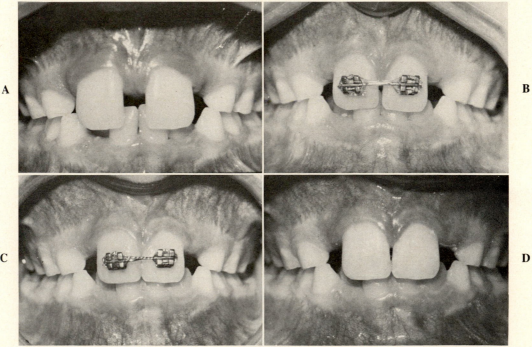

Fig. 13-26 ■ Closure of a diastema with a fixed appliance. **A,** This diastema requires closure by moving the crowns and roots of the central incisors. **B,** The bonded attachments and rectangular wire control the teeth in three planes of space while the elastomeric chain provides the force to slide the teeth along the wire. **C,** Immediately after space closure, the teeth are retained and, **D,** usually require permanent retention until adjacent permanent anterior teeth erupt (see Fig. 13-27).

posterior teeth, which tends to pull them forward. Depending on the amount of incisor retraction and space closure, a headgear, chosen with consideration for vertical facial and dental characteristics, may be necessary for supplemental anchorage support.

Any of these types of treatment will require retention. The desire to close diastemas at an early age is tempered by experience with how difficult it can be to keep the space closed. If the lateral incisors and canines have not erupted, a Hawley-type retainer will require constant modification. An alternative approach for retention if the overbite is not prohibitively deep is to bond an .0175 multistranded archwire to the linguocervical portion of the incisors (Fig. 13-27). This arrangement will provide excellent retention with less maintenance.

Another retention problem may be the presence of a large or inferiorly attached labial frenum. A frenectomy after space closure and retention may be necessary in some cases, but it is difficult to determine the potential contribution of the frenum to retention problems from its morphology alone. Therefore, a frenectomy before treatment is contraindicated, and a posttreatment frenectomy should be done only if a continued tendency of the diastema to reopen and unresolved bunching of tissue between the teeth show that it is necessary.[12]

■ Midline Discrepancy from Intraarch Asymmetry

Another potential problem that can be approached in the mixed dentition is arch asymmetry, which is usually exhibited as a shift of the dental midline to one side. This problem needs to be addressed at this time only if no permanent teeth will be extracted to provide additional space in the arch. Under these circumstances, all teeth will need a location in which to erupt. The mildest form of asymmetry is a significant but small (2 mm) midline shift. If the arch length is adequate, the incisors can be aligned and tipped back to

their optimal location using a removable appliance and fingersprings (Fig. 13-28). In some cases, disking or extraction of a primary canine or molar will be required to provide the necessary room for this correction even if space in the arch is predicted to be adequate.

If bodily drift or rotational change has accompanied the midline change, which usually occurred because of premature loss of one primary canine, the anterior teeth should be bonded and aligned with an archwire. The force to move the teeth is usually generated by a coil spring placed on the archwire (Fig. 13-29). Regardless of the type of tooth movement or the appliance used for correction, retention will be needed until the remaining permanent teeth erupt (Fig. 13-30).

■ *Crowding in the Mixed Dentition*

■ Mild Crowding: Adequate Space Predicted for the Succedaneous Teeth

In some children the space ultimately necessary to accommodate all the permanent teeth is available, but the size of the erupting incisors and the available developmental and primate spaces cause transient crowding of the permanent incisors. This crowding is usually expressed as mild faciolingual displacement or rotation of individual teeth. Stud-

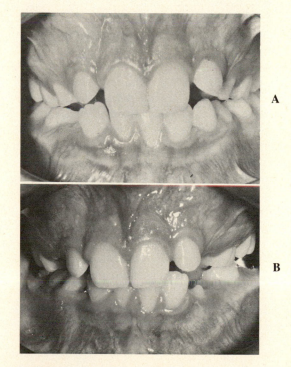

A

B

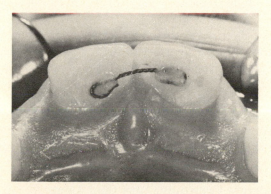

Fig. 13-27 ■ A fixed retainer to maintain diastema closure. A bonded .0175 inch multistranded wire with hooks bent into the ends is bonded to the lingual surfaces of anterior teeth to serve as a permanent retainer. This flexible wire allows physiologic mobility of the teeth and reduces bond failure but can be used only when the overbite is not excessive.

Fig. 13-28 ■ Midline shift resulting from tipping. **A,** These incisors tipped to the patient's right when the primary right canine was lost prematurely. **B,** The teeth have been tipped back to the left and overcorrected using a fingerspring and a removable appliance. They are currently maintained in this position with a lingual arch and a soldered spur.

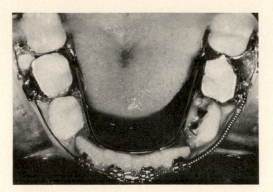

Fig. 13-29 ■ Bonded anterior teeth and banded posterior teeth with a lingual arch to reinforce anchorage are used to move the anterior teeth bodily. The coil spring generates the force to move the teeth along the archwire.

ies of children with normal occlusion indicate that when they go through the transition from the primary to the mixed dentition, up to 2 mm of incisor crowding may resolve spontaneously without treatment.[1] From this perspective, there is no need to begin treatment when less than 2 mm of incisor crowding is observed during the mixed dentition.

Another approach to managing transient crowding in the mixed dentition is based on information from postretention studies. When patients with moderate to severe crowding are examined 10 years or more after the completion of orthodontic treatment and removal of all retaining appliances, it is obvious that the irregularity and crowding eliminated during active orthodontic treatment often return in a milder form.[13]

Because of such findings, some clinicians advocate eliminating all crowding as it occurs, on the theory that if the teeth have never been crowded, they will not relapse that way. This approach requires constant attention to the dentition. It is implemented in its least invasive form by disking the interproximal enamel surfaces of the *primary* lateral incisors and canines as the anterior teeth erupt (Fig. 13-31). When the enamel thickness at the height of contour is reduced, additional space becomes available for spontaneous alignment. Minor amounts of disking do not cause patient discomfort, but maximum disking may require local anesthesia and produce some postoperative sensitivity. This sensitivity is treated best with topical fluoride after the disking. It is possible to gain as much as 3 to 4 mm of anterior space through this procedure, but since up to 2 mm of crowding may resolve spontaneously, it should probably be reserved for situations when 3 to 4 mm of anterior crowding exist.

Correction of any incisor rotations requires controlled movement to align and derotate them, using an archwire and bonded attachments on the incisors. It may be wise to defer this therapy until comprehensive treatment is begun in the early permanent dentition. If it is undertaken in the mixed dentition, the permanent first molars should be banded (and ideally reinforced with a lingual arch) to serve

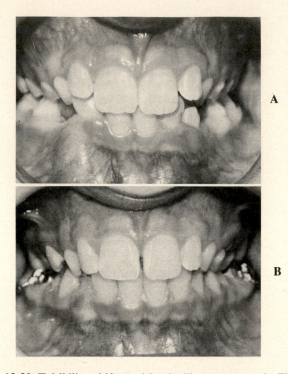

Fig. 13-30 ■ Midline shift requiring bodily movement. **A,** The midline of the mandibular arch has bodily shifted to the patient's right because of premature loss of a primary canine. **B,** The teeth were moved back to their proper position using a fixed appliance and are supported until eruption of the canines with a lingual holding arch.

as anchorage. If the archwire is not supported between the first molar and incisors, it must be relatively large for strength in the buccal segments and may have to incorporate loops for flexibility in the incisor region. If the primary first molars are also bonded, a smaller and more flexible wire can be used. After alignment has been achieved, if root position needs to be corrected, a rectangular wire is required to finish the tooth movement. It is rare that a child who needs this type of treatment in the mixed dentition does not require further treatment after all permanent teeth have erupted.

Although crowding has been alleviated in the anterior segments, it may again be evident when the lower canines and first premolars erupt, even if the total space available is adequate. This crowding occurs because the combined width of the erupting permanent canine, first premolar, and the primary second molar is greater than the total width of the permanent canine and premolars. Selective disking of the primary molar is often necessary to reduce this transitional space problem (Fig. 13-32).

■ Moderate Crowding: Less than 4 mm Space Deficiency Predicted for the Succedaneous Teeth

For these patients the first decision to be made is whether space is to be created for the unerupted permanent teeth by arch expansion or whether permanent teeth must be

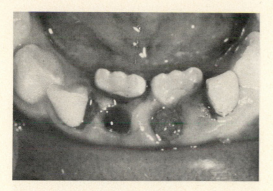

Fig. 13-31 ■ Disking of primary anterior teeth is a method to gain several millimeters of space for erupting permanent anterior teeth.

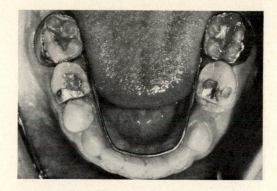

Fig. 13-32 ■ Disking primary posterior teeth in conjunction with space maintenance is an effective method to use the leeway space and all available arch length.

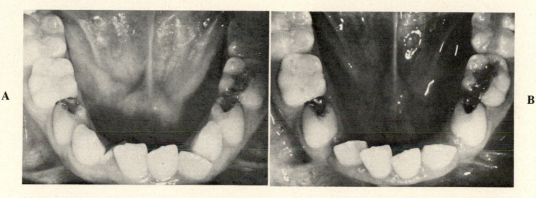

Fig. 13-33 ■ Extraction of primary canines as a method to reduce anterior irregularity. **A,** This patient has a sizable amount of anterior crowding and irregularity. **B,** The primary canines were extracted, which allowed some alignment, but the incisors have tipped lingually and further reduced the arch length.

extracted. Most patients with moderate crowding can be treated without extraction, but certainly not all. The steps discussed in Chapters 6 to 8 must be followed to develop an appropriate treatment plan.

In some of these children, the transitional anterior crowding is greater than 2 to 3 mm even though total space available is predicted to be adequate. The amount of disking required to alleviate the crowding would expose the pulps of the primary canines or cause extreme sensitivity. The option is to remove the primary canines as the crowding occurs. This creates the possibility that the permanent incisors will tip lingually, reducing the arch length even more (Fig. 13-33).

A conservative approach to this dilemma is to place a lingual arch after the extraction of the primary canines and allow the incisors to align, maintaining or slightly increasing the arch length. A word of caution is necessary here. Clinical experience indicates that faciolingual irregularity will resolve if space is available, but rotational irregularity will not resolve totally. If the incisors are rotated or demonstrate several areas of irregularity, a multiple bonded and banded appliance is indicated (Fig. 13-34). When the incisor segment is straight without anterior arch curvature, extraction

of primary canines usually leads to spacing of the incisors or maintanance of essentially the same arch form but the alignment does not improve (Fig. 13-35). In most of these children, crowding will again be evident when the canines and first premolars erupt, and selective disking or extraction of the primary second molars and continued space control with a lingual arch are necessary.

If arch expansion is to be attempted, the teeth that are to be moved, the direction, and the type of tooth movement should be established. Whether primary canines should be extracted to provide additional space for alignment of the incisors should also be addressed. Lower incisor teeth can usually be tipped 1 to 2 mm in a facial direction without much difficulty, which creates up to 4 mm of additional arch length. If the overbite is excessive and the upper and lower incisors are in contact, however, facial movement of the lower incisors will not be possible unless the upper incisors are also proclined.

When expansion by tipping the incisors facially is indicated, a removable lingual arch is the preferred appliance (Fig. 13-36). This can be accomplished by advancing the lingual arch with adjustment at the loops located mesial to the banded molars. Until the teeth have moved, the activated

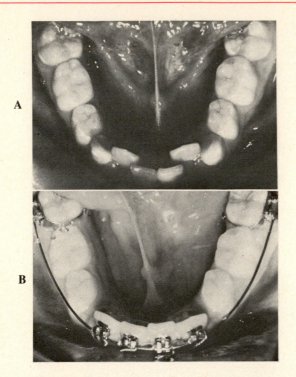

Fig. 13-34 ■ Alignment of anterior teeth with multiple attachments and an archwire. **A,** This patient has crowding and irregularity which **B,** was reduced by extraction of the primary canines and alignment using an archwire and multiple attachments.

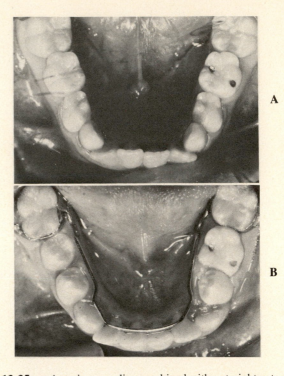

Fig. 13-35 ■ Anterior crowding combined with a straight anterior incisor segment. **A,** Straight incisor segment with lateral incisors that overlap the mesial of the primary canine, **B,** does not usually align and provide ideal arch form when the primary canines are extracted even if a lingual arch is used.

lingual arch will rest higher on the lingual surface of the incisors than is ideal and should exert an apical force to tip the teeth facially. Small amounts of activation are necessary since the wire is large and capable of delivering heavy forces. Several 1 mm activations will achieve the desired result and the appliance can then serve as a passive retainer or be replaced with a soldered lingual arch.

It is also possible to tip incisors facially with a removable appliance incorporating several clasps and fingersprings. An appliance of this type will move the teeth approximately 1 mm per month when the springs are activated 1 to 2 mm, but it requires good compliance and should be replaced with a fixed lingual arch after active tooth movement to prevent relapse.

In the previous section of this chapter, the use of bonded attachments on the anterior teeth with molar bands and an archwire was discussed as a method to align rotated or grossly irregular incisors. A similar appliance can be used to expand the arches if the overbite is not excessive. Specific archwire designs are discussed in Chapter 15. The multiple band and bond technique is usually followed with a lingual arch for retention.

Since further comprehensive treatment in the early permanent dentition will probably be required, the cost-effectiveness of elaborate mixed dentition treatment of this type must be considered carefully. If complex tooth movements are desired, however, multiple attachments are required. If

space has been maintained with a lower lingual arch so that the leeway space can be used for alignment, in many patients the maxillary molars will have to be moved distally to create approximately 1 to 2 mm of space per side and establish Class I molar relationships. In these cases, the tooth movement required generally is bodily movement, not tipping, since the whole tooth and not just the crown must be repositioned to ensure stability of the result (see Chapter 14 for details). A fixed appliance with banding of the molars and bonding of the anterior teeth and premolars is often needed to obtain a good result.

■ Severe Crowding: Greater than 4 mm Space Deficiency Predicted for the Succedaneous Teeth

Severe crowding is usually obvious even before a space analysis can be completed. Two symptoms are ectopic eruption of lateral incisors and severe crowding and irregularity of the erupting permanent incisors. After a definitive analysis of the profile and incisor position, the decision must be made to either expand the arches or extract permanent teeth (see Chapter 8). In the presence of severe crowding, limited treatment of the problem will not be sufficient; therefore, treatment with removable appliances or lingual arches to tip teeth for expansion is not indicated.

If the treatment plan is to expand the arches, one alter-

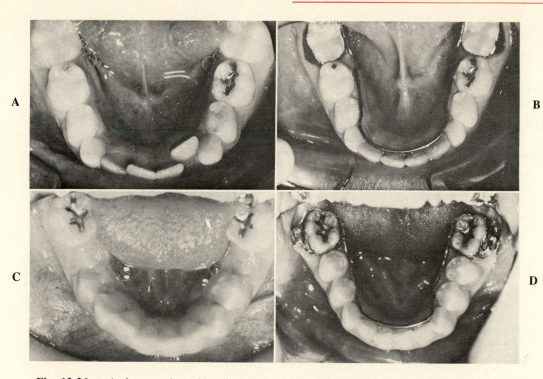

Fig. 13-36 ■ Arch expansion with a lingual arch in the early and late mixed dentition stages. **A,** In this patient anterior crowding is addressed by disking the primary canines and expansion with an active lingual arch. **B,** The removable arch can be replaced with a soldered lingual arch when tooth movement is completed. Although this patient has adequate space for the permanent teeth, other primary teeth will need disking or removal in the future. **C,** This patient has a posterior space shortage in the late mixed dentition that was treated by **D,** expanding the arch with an active removable lingual arch.

native is to use a functional appliance of the tissue-borne type such as the Frankel appliance (see Chapter 14) or any appliance design that uses lip and buccal shields to reduce the resting pressure of the lips and cheeks to facilitate dental expansion. This approach will lead to anterior movement of the incisors and buccal movement of the primary molars or premolars, which allows the teeth to align themselves along a larger arch circumference.

After additional space has been created by changing the arch dimensions, a method of retention, either with the functional appliance or a conventional retainer, should be considered. Although adequate evidence indicates that this type of expansion can be produced, its stability has not been documented.[14] It seems reasonable to assume that stability is better if the initial space discrepancy was small and initial incisor protrusion was minimal and vice versa. Appliances of this type to correct large discrepancies are rarely indicated in children with no jaw discrepancy and only dental crowding.

Another approach to arch expansion is to align the anterior teeth with bonded attachments using archwires. As described previously, the teeth can be tipped facially and buccally, increasing the available arch length. Some clinicians believe that bodily expansion of the posterior segments will lead to greater long-term stability, but this theory also lacks

adequate documentation. Expansion with both functional and fixed appliances has obvious limitations.

In many children with severe crowding, a decision can be made during the early mixed dentition that expansion is fruitless and that permanent teeth will have to be extracted. A planned sequence of tooth removal can reduce crowding and irregularity during the transition from the primary to the permanent dentition. It will also allow the teeth to erupt over the alveolus and through keratinized tissue, rather than being displaced buccally or lingually. This sequence, often termed "serial extraction" or "guidance or eruption," simply involves the timed extraction of primary and, ultimately, permanent teeth to relieve severe crowding.[15,16] This practice was advocated originally as a method to treat severe crowding with or without minimal use of appliance therapy, but is now viewed as an adjunct to later comprehensive treatment instead of a substitute for it. Although serial extraction makes later comprehensive treatment easier and often quicker, by itself it usually does not result in ideal tooth position or closure of excess space.

Serial extraction is directed toward severe dental crowding. For this reason, it is best used when no skeletal problem exists and when the space discrepancy is large, greater than 10 mm per arch. If the crowding is severe, little space will remain, which means there will be little tipping and un-

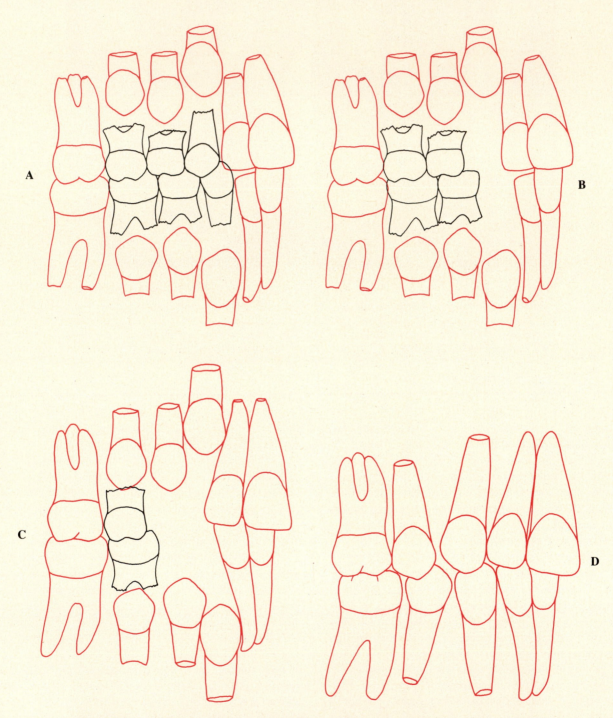

Fig. 13-37 ■ The serial extraction sequence used to relieve severe arch length discrepancies. **A,** The initial diagnosis is made when a severe space deficiency is documented and there is marked incisor crowding. **B,** The primary canines are extracted to provide space for alignment of the incisors. **C,** The primary first molars are extracted when one-half to two-thirds of the first premolar root is formed to speed the premolar eruption. **D,** When the first premolars have erupted they are extracted and the canines erupt into the remaining extraction space. The residual space is closed by drifting and tipping of the posterior teeth unless full appliance therapy is implemented.

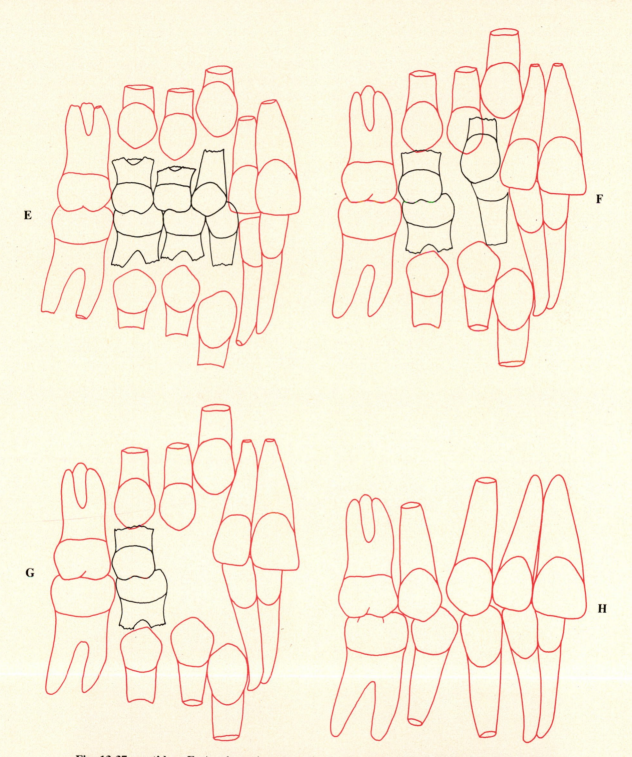

Fig. 13-37, cont'd ■ **E,** An alternative approach to serial extraction is implemented slightly later but under the same conditions and **F,** begins with extraction of the primary first molars so that there is less lingual tipping of the incisors and less tendency to develop a deep bite. Extraction of the primary first molars also encourages early eruption of the first premolars. **G,** When the first premolars have erupted, they are extracted and the canines erupt into the remaining extraction space. **H,** The residual space is closed by drifting and tipping of the posterior teeth unless full appliance therapy is implemented.

controlled movement of the teeth adjacent into the extraction sites. If the initial discrepancy is smaller, more residual space must be anticipated.

Serial extraction treatment begins in the early mixed dentition with extraction of primary incisors if necessary, followed by extraction of the primary canines to allow eruption and alignment of the permanent incisors (Fig. 13-37). As the permanent teeth align without any appliances in place, there is usually some lingual tipping of the lower incisors, and overbite often increases during this stage. Labiolingual displacments resolve better than rotational irregularity.

After extraction of the primary canines, crowding problems are usually under control for 1 to 2 years, but foresight is necessary. The goal is to influence the permanent first premolars to erupt ahead of the canines so that they can be extracted and the canines can move distally into this space. The maxillary premolars usually erupt before the canines, so the eruption sequence is rarely a problem in the upper arch. But in the lower arch, the canines usually erupt before the premolars, which causes the canines to be displaced facially. To avoid this result, the primary lower first molar should be extracted when there is ½ to ⅔ root formation on the first premolar. This technique will usually speed up the premolar eruption and cause it to enter the arch before the canine (Fig. 13-37, *C*). The result is easy access for extraction of the first premolar before the canine erupts (Fig. 13-37, *D*).

Several complications can occur. The increase in overbite mentioned previously can become a problem requiring later treatment. A variation in the extraction sequence has been

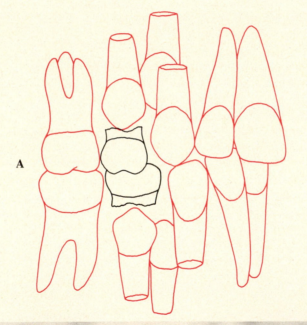

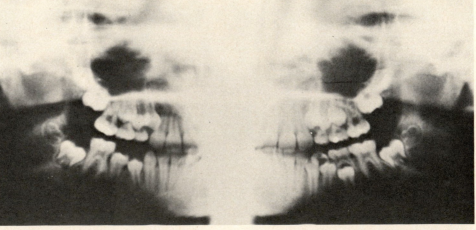

Fig. 13-38 ■ A complication of serial extraction is premature eruption of the permanent canines. **A,** When this occurs the first premolars are impacted between the canines and the second premolars. **B,** In this situation, the first premolars usually have to be surgically removed by a procedure called enucleation.

proposed in an effort to overcome this problem.[17] The mandibular primary canines are retained, and some space for anterior alignment is made available when the permanent laterals erupt by extracting the primary first molars instead. With this approach, eruption of the permanent first premolars is encouraged, and the incisors are less prone to tipping lingually (Fig. 13-37, *E* to *H*). The major goal of serial extraction is prevention of incisor crowding, however, and some crowding often persists if the primary canines are retained. In many patients with severe crowding, the primary canines are lost to ectopic eruption of the laterals and cannot be maintained.

A second complication occurs if the primary first molar is extracted early and the first premolar still does not erupt before the canine. This can lead to impaction of the premolar that requires later surgical removal (Fig. 13-38). At the time the primary first molar is removed, it may be obvious that the canine will erupt before the premolar. In this case the underlying premolar can also be extracted at the same time—a procedure termed "enucleation." If possible, however, enucleation should be avoided because the erupting premolar brings alveolar bone with it. Early enucleation leaves a bone defect that may persist.

After the first premolar has been extracted, the second primary molars should exfoliate normally. The premolar extraction space is closed partially by mesial drift of the second premolar and permanent first molar, but largely by distal eruption of the canine. If serial extraction is not followed by mechanotherapy, ideal alignment, root positioning, overbite, and space closure are usually not achieved (Fig. 13-39).

■*Posterior Crossbites*

The treatment of posterior crossbites during the mixed dentition differs markedly, depending on the underlying cause of the crossbite situation. Skeletal crossbites, resulting from a narrow maxilla or an excessively wide mandible, are discussed in Chapter 14. Dental crossbites caused by a displacement of the teeth within the dental arches often appear to be unilateral but are usually found on closer examination to result from a bilateral constriction of the maxillary arch and a shift of the mandible to one side on closure. More severe constriction may result in a bilateral crossbite without mandibular shift, and occasionally, a true unilateral posterior crossbite from an intraarch asymmetry will be noted.

Crossbites caused by a mandibular shift should be treated as soon as they are discovered and are among the few conditions recommended for treatment in the complete primary dentition. An uncorrected mandibular shift can produce undesirable growth modification, dental compensation leading to a true asymmetry at a later time, and potentially harmful functional patterns. Posterior crossbite correction in the primary dentition does appear to be stable[18] and to have some influence on permanent premolar position.[19]

There are three basic approaches to the treatment of posterior crossbites in children: equilibration to eliminate mandibular shift, expansion of a constricted maxillary arch, and repositioning of individual teeth to deal with intraarch asymmetries.

In a few cases, mostly observed in the primary dentition or the early mixed dentition, a shift into posterior crossbite will result only from interference caused by the primary canines (Fig. 13-40). These patients can be diagnosed by careful positioning of the mandible and require only limited equilibration of the primary canines to eliminate the interference and the resulting lateral shift into crossbite.

More commonly, a child with a mandibular shift has a bilateral maxillary constriction. Even a small constriction creates dental interferences that force the mandible to shift to a new position for maximal intercuspation (Fig. 13-41). A greater maxillary constriction will allow the maxillary

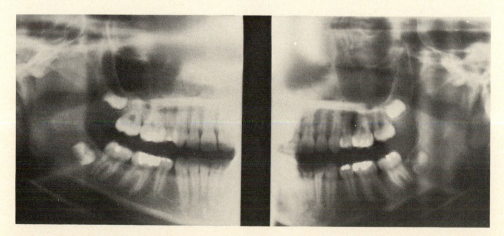

Fig. 13-39 ■ This patient had serial extraction not followed by fixed appliance treatment with an excellent result. Properly timed serial extraction usually results in incomplete space closure. Teeth drift together by tipping, which results in nonparallel roots between the canine and second premolar. The lack of root parallelism, residual space, and other irregularity can be addressed with subsequent fixed appliance therapy.

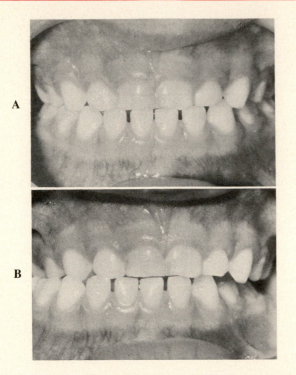

Fig. 13-40 ■ Minor canine interferences leading to a mandibular shift. **A,** Initial contact. **B,** Shift into centric occlusion. The slight lingual position of the primary canines can lead to occlusal interferences and an apparent posterior crossbite. This etiology of posterior crossbite is infrequent and is best treated by occlusal adjustment of the primary canines.

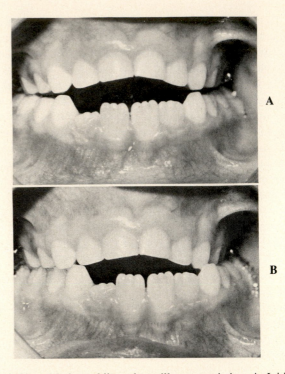

Fig. 13-41 ■ Moderate bilateral maxillary constriction. **A,** Initial contact. **B,** Shift into occlusion. Moderate bilateral maxillary constriction often leads to posterior interferences upon closure and a lateral shift of the mandible into an apparent posterior crossbite. This problem is best treated by bilateral maxillary expansion.

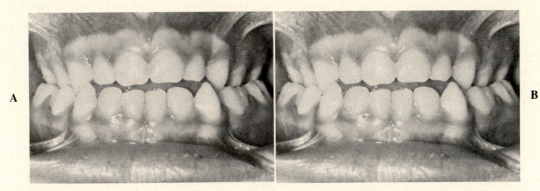

Fig. 13-42 ■ Marked bilateral maxillary constriction. **A,** Initial contact. **B,** Full occlusion (no shift). A marked bilateral maxillary constriction often produces no interferences upon closure and the patient has a bilateral posterior crossbite in centric relation. This problem is best treated by bilateral maxillary expansion.

teeth to fit inside the mandibular teeth and will not be accompanied by a mandibular shift (Fig. 13-42). Both of these types of crossbite should be corrected in the primary dentition if they are discovered then, unless the permanent first molars are expected to erupt within less than 6 months. In that situation, it is better to allow the permanent molars to erupt so that correction can include these teeth if necessary.

The preferred appliance for correction of maxillary dental constriction is an adjustable lingual arch that requires little patient cooperation. Both the W-arch and the quad helix are reliable and easy to use. The W-arch is a fixed appliance constructed of .036 inch wire soldered to molar bands (Fig. 13-43). To avoid soft tissue irritation, the lingual arch should be constructed so that it rests 1 to 1.5 mm off the palatal soft tissue. This appliance will move both primary and permanent teeth and may accelerate the rate of normal expansion of the midpalatal suture, particularly in a young child. Therefore correction may result from a combination of skel-

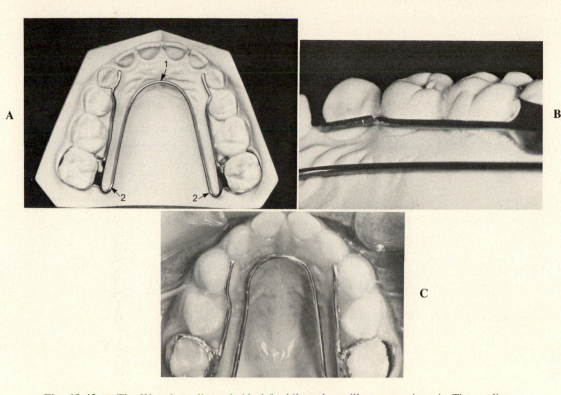

Fig. 13-43 ■ The W-arch appliance is ideal for bilateral maxillary expansion. **A,** The appliance is fabricated from .036 inch wire and soldered to the bands. The lingual wire should contact the teeth involved in the crossbite and extend not more than 1 to 2 mm distal to the banded molars to eliminate soft tissue irritation. Activation at point *1* produces posterior expansion and activation at point *2* produces anterior expansion. **B,** The lingual wire should remain 1 to 1.5 mm away from the marginal gingiva and the palatal tissue. **C,** This W-arch is being used to correct a bilateral constriction in the primary dentition.

etal and dental change even if only dental change is required. This is of no consequence and will require no difference in either treatment or retention techniques.

The W-arch is activated simply by opening the apices of the W and is easily adjusted to provide more anterior than posterior expansion, or vice versa, if this is desired. Bending the anterior palatal portion of the wire increases the posterior arch width, and bending the wire bilaterally near the solder joint at the molar bands increases the anterior arch width (Fig. 13-43). The appliance delivers proper force levels when opened 3 to 4 mm wider than the passive width and should be adjusted to this dimension before being inserted.

Expansion should continue at the rate of 2 mm/month (1 mm tooth movement on each side) until the crossbite is slightly overcorrected. In other words, the lingual cusps of the maxillary teeth should occlude on the lingual inclines of the buccal cusps of the mandibular molars at the end of active treatment (Fig. 13-44). Intraoral appliance adjustment is possible but may lead to unexpected changes. For this reason, removal and recementation are recommended at each active treatment visit. Most posterior crossbites require 2 to 3 months of active treatment and 3 months of retention (during which the W-arch is left passively in place)

for stability.

A variant of this appliance uses cemented bands with attachments that allow the active arch to be removed and activated without removing the bands (Fig. 13-45). Although this technique is attractive in principle, it is difficult to activate the appliance in the desired direction and have it remain passive in all other dimensions. Unwanted and unexpected intrusion and extrusion of teeth are common with this technique and it is more prone to appliance breakage.

The quad helix is a more flexible version of the W-arch.[20] It is constructed with .038 inch wire and helices that increase the range and springiness of the appliance. The helices in the anterior palate are bulky, which can effectively serve as a reminder to aid in stopping a finger habit (Fig. 13-46). The combination of a posterior crossbite and a finger sucking habit is the best indication for this appliance. The extra wire incorporated in this appliance gives it slightly greater range of action than the W-arch, but the forces are equivalent. Appropriate forces are produced when the appliance is widened by 3 to 8 mm. This adjustment can be performed either intra- or extraorally, but care must be exercised with intraoral adjustments. Overcorrection, attention to soft tissue irritation, and 3 months of retention are also recommended with this appliance.

Another method to treat posterior crossbite is the use of a split-plate type of removable appliance incorporating a wire spring or jackscrew for force generation. This approach is less successful than the expansion lingual arches. Removable appliances rely on patient compliance for success, and the fact that the appliance is retained by clasps limits the force that can be used, since the appliance can be displaced easily.

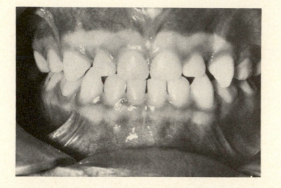

Fig. 13-44 ■ A posterior crossbite should be overcorrected until the maxillary posterior lingual cusps occlude with the lingual inclines of the mandibular buccal cusps, as shown here, and then retained. After retention, slight lingual movement of the maxillary teeth results in a stable result.

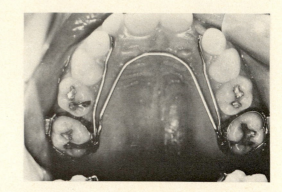

Fig. 13-45 ■ The W-arch can be made removable by fabricating it with attachments on the molar teeth. This appliance design is inviting but is difficult to manage and more prone to appliance breakage.

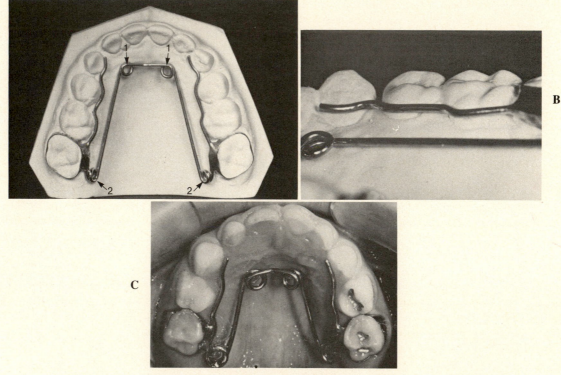

Fig. 13-46 ■ The quad helix used to correct bilateral maxillary constriction. **A,** The appliance is fabricated from .038 inch wire and soldered to the bands. The lingual wire should contact the teeth involved in the crossbite and extend no more than 1 to 2 mm distal to the banded molars to eliminate soft tissue irritation. Activation at point *1* produces posterior expansion, while activation at point *2* produces anterior expansion. **B,** The lingual wire should remain 1 to 1.5 mm away from the marginal gingiva and palatal tissue. **C,** This quad helix is being used to correct a bilateral maxillary constriction in the primary dentition.

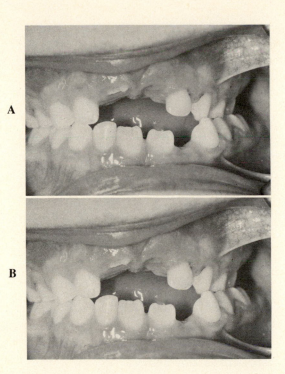

Some children do have true unilateral crossbites, usually from unilateral maxillary constriction. This condition is diagnosed by discovering a unilateral crossbite in centric relation and in maximum intercuspation without a mandibular shift (Fig. 13-47). In these cases the ideal treatment would be to move selected teeth on the constricted side of the upper arch. The easiest way to accomplish this movement is to arrange an orthodontic appliance so that there are more teeth in the anchorage unit than in the unit where teeth are

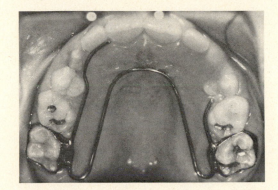

Fig. 13-47 ■ True unilateral maxillary posterior constriction. **A,** Initial contact. **B,** Full occlusion. True unilateral constriction has a unilateral posterior crossbite in centric relation and in centric occlusion, without a lateral shift. This problem is best treated with unilateral posterior expansion.

Fig. 13-48 ■ An unequal W-arch used to correct a true unilateral maxillary constriction. The side of the arch to be expanded has fewer teeth against the lingual wire than the anchorage unit. Even with this arrangement, both sides can be expected to show some expansion movement.

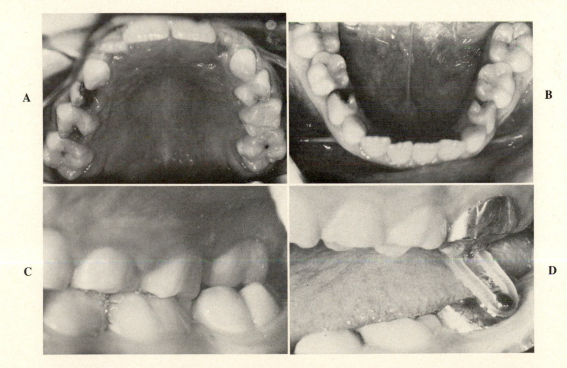

Fig. 13-49 ■ Cross elastics are indicated for crossbite correction when maxillary and mandibular teeth need to be moved. **A,** This patient has the permanent maxillary left first molar displaced lingually and **B,** the permanent mandibular left first molar displaced facially. **C,** This results in a posterior crossbite between these teeth. **D,** The cross elastic is placed between the buttons welded on the bands. The elastic should be worn full time and changed frequently.

expected to move. To a limited extent, this goal can be achieved by using different length arms on a W-arch or quad helix (Fig. 13-48), but some bilateral expansion must be expected. An alternative method is to use a mandibular lingual arch to stabilize the lower teeth and attach cross elastics to the maxillary teeth that are at fault. This type of arrangement is more complicated and requires cooperation by the patient to be successful, but is more unilateral in its effect.

All of the previously described appliances are aimed at correction of teeth in the maxillary arch, which is usually where the problem is located. If teeth in both arches contribute to the problem, cross elastics between banded or bonded attachments in both arches can be helpful (Fig. 13-49) to reposition both upper and lower teeth. Cross elastic treatment requires cooperation, since the patient has to wear the elastics full time and replace them at least once a day. The vector of the elastic pull encourages the teeth to move vertically as well as faciolingually, which will elongate the posterior teeth and reduce the overbite. Therefore, cross elastics should be used with caution in children with increased lower face height or limited overbite. Crossbites treated with elastics should be overcorrected and the bands left in place immediately after active treatment. If there is relapse, the elastics can be reinstated without rebanding or rebonding. When the occlusion is stable after several weeks without elastic force, the attachments can be removed. The most common problem with this form of crossbite correction is lack of cooperation by the child.

■ *Incisor Retrusion/Protrusion*

■ Anterior Crossbites

Anterior crossbites of dental origin are encountered relatively frequently in the primary and early mixed dentitions. If the etiology is truly dental and space is available, the problem should be corrected when it is encountered. Appliance therapy in the primary dentition is feasible if the child is old enough to tolerate an appliance. In very young children, delaying treatment until the child is more mature is recommended. If the primary anterior teeth are mobile or have considerable root resorption and would exfoliate immediately after correction, extraction of the primary incisors is the treatment of choice.

The most common etiology of nonskeletal anterior crossbites is lack of space for the permanent incisors, and it is important that a treatment plan focus on management of the total space situation in addition to the crossbite. Since the permanent tooth buds form lingual to the primary teeth, a shortage of space may force the permanent maxillary incisor teeth to remain lingual to the line of the arch and erupt into crossbite. If the developing crossbite is discovered before eruption is complete and overbite has been established, the adjacent primary teeth can be extracted to provide the necessary space (Fig. 13-50). Primary teeth should be extracted

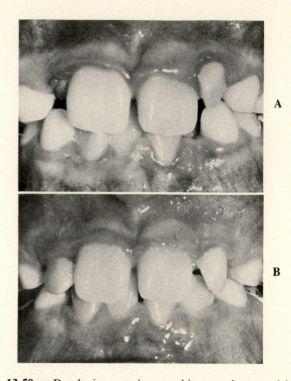

Fig. 13-50 ■ Developing anterior crossbites can be treated by extracting adjacent primary teeth if space is not available for the erupting permanent teeth. **A,** The permanent maxillary right lateral incisor is beginning to erupt lingual to the other anterior teeth. **B,** Extraction of both primary maxillary canines has allowed spontaneous correction of the crossbite.

bilaterally to prevent the midline from migrating to the side of a unilateral extraction, where extra room is available.

Anterior crossbites diagnosed after the incisors have erupted require appliance therapy for correction. The first concern is that adequate space is available so that tooth movement can be completed, which usually requires bilateral disking or extraction of the adjacent primary teeth. The diagnostic evaluation should determine whether tipping would provide appropriate correction (which is usually the case) or whether bodily movement is necessary to correct the crossbite. If teeth are tipped when bodily movement is required, stability of the result is questionable.

The best method for tipping maxillary and mandibular anterior teeth is a removable appliance using fingersprings for facial movement of maxillary incisors (Fig. 13-51), or (less frequently) an active labial bow for lingual movement of mandibular incisors. Two maxillary anterior teeth can be moved facially with one .022 inch double helical cantilever spring. Z-springs (Fig. 13-52) are another possibility, but these deliver excessively heavy forces and lack range of action. The removable appliance should have multiple clasps for retention, but a labial bow on this appliance is usually contraindicated because it would interfere with facial movement of the incisors and would add little or no retention.

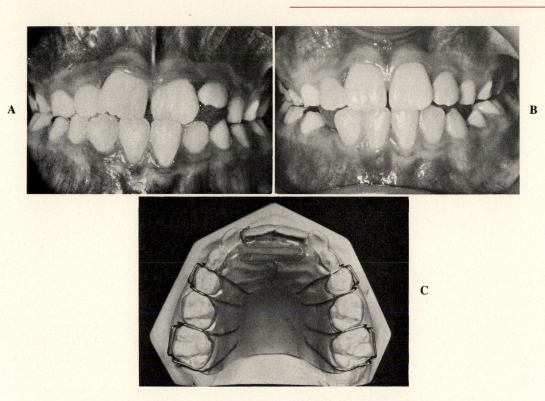

Fig. 13-51 ■ Anterior crossbite correction with a removable appliance to tip teeth. **A,** The permanent maxillary left central incisor has erupted into crossbite and **B,** has been corrected with a removable appliance. **C,** This appliance is used to tip both central incisors facially with an .022 inch double helical fingerspring activated 1.5 to 2 mm per month. Note that acrylic baseplate material extends over the spring to maintain its vertical position (see Chapter 11). The appliance is retained with multiple Adams' clasps.

An anterior or posterior biteplane to reduce the overbite while the crossbite is being corrected is unnecessary in children unless the overbite is excessively deep. A reasonable approach is to place the appliance without a biteplane and attempt tooth movement. If, after 2 months, the teeth in the opposing arch are moving in the same direction as the teeth to which the force is being applied, a biteplane is indicated and can be added to the appliance. Since teeth are not in occlusion except during swallowing and parafunctional habits, a biteplane should be needed only in a child with a clenching or grinding habit. Using a biteplane risks the chance that teeth not in contact with the appliance or the opposing arch will erupt excessively.

A maxillary lingual fingerspring can be activated 1.5 to 2.0 mm per month and will produce approximately 1 mm of tooth movement in that time. Greater activation will slow tooth movement because of excessive force, and lesser activation will prolong treatment unnecessarily. The appliance requires nearly full time wear to be effective and efficient. The offending teeth should be slightly overcorrected and retained until overbite is adequate to retain the corrected tooth positions. One or two months of retention with a passive appliance is usually sufficient, but if overbite is inadequate, the appliance should be continued as a passive retainer until incisor eruption has established an overbite.

The most common problems associated with these simple removable appliances are lack of patient cooperation, poor design leading to lack of retention, and improper activation.

Teeth can also be tipped out of anterior crossbite using fixed appliances, either with or without attachments placed

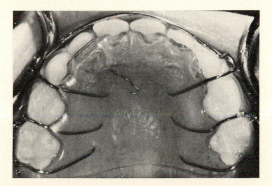

Fig. 13-52 ■ A Z-spring is sometimes used for anterior crossbite correction with a removable appliance, but is not recommended since it delivers heavy forces and has a limited range of action. Note that the labial bow is nearly in contact with the tooth being moved. In this situation the labial bow, which must be adjusted carefully, prevents excessive labial movement and then has a fail-safe action, but offers little retention.

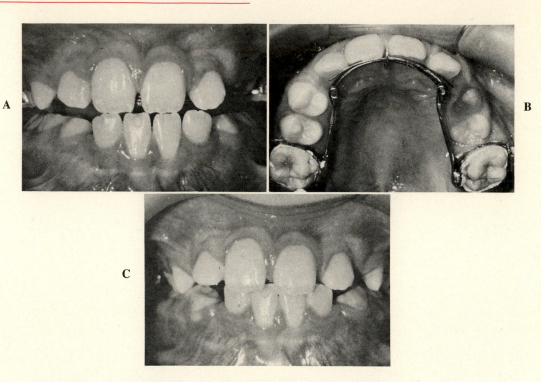

Fig. 13-53 ■ A fixed lingual arch with fingersprings used for anterior crossbite correction. **A,** An anterior crossbite caused by lingual position of the maxillary incisors can be corrected using, **B,** an .036 inch lingual arch with soldered 0.022 inch fingersprings. A guide wire can be placed between the incisors as shown here to keep the springs from moving incisally. **C,** After correction, the appliance can be modified to serve as a retainer by soldering the free ends of the springs to the lingual arch.

on individual teeth. This technique reduces some of the need for patient compliance, but will not overcome the resistance of a determined and destructive child. Fixed appliances also have a greater range of action and are more continuous in force application than removable appliances.

One of the simplest fixed appliances for this purpose is a maxillary lingual arch with fingersprings (sometimes referred to as whip springs). This appliance is indicated for a very young child or a preadolescent with whom compliance problems are anticipated. It consists of an .036 inch maxillary lingual arch to which .022 inch springs are soldered (Fig. 13-53). The springs are usually soldered on the opposite side of the arch from the tooth to be corrected, in order to increase the length of the spring, and are most effective if they are approximately 15 mm long. This length provides exceptional flexibility and range, but occasionally a spur is needed to serve as a guide wire to keep the wires from slipping over the incisal edge of the incisors. When these springs are activated properly at each monthly visit (advancing the spring about 3 mm), they produce tooth movement at the optimal rate of 1 mm/month. Overcorrection and retention are recommended with this appliance. The greatest problems with it are a lack of care for the appliance by the patient, which can distort or break the appliance, and poor oral hygiene that leads to decalcification and decay.

Another fixed appliance method to tip the maxillary incisors forward is the use of posterior bands and anterior bonded attachments with a round archwire. This may be the best choice for a somewhat older mixed dentition patient with crowding, rotations, and more permanent teeth in crossbite (Fig. 13-54). In these children, adjacent primary teeth may not be available for disking and permanent teeth need to be moved facially to increase the circumference of the arch. With generalized crowding and irregularity, a flexible wire can be used to solve both problems. If only selected teeth are at fault, a stiffer archwire with loops bent for local flexibility and tooth movement would be more appropriate. When the teeth have been moved to their ideal position, they should be stabilized for 1 to 2 months before debonding. Retention should not be necessary if there is adequate overbite after the crossbite is corrected. The greatest problem with this technique is appliance breakage.

A similar technique can be used for teeth in crossbite that need bodily movement to obtain posttreatment stability. After banding the molars and bonding the anterior teeth with edgewise appliances, an initial flexible or multilooped archwire can be used for alignment, followed by a rectangular archwire that will control the root position of the incisors (see Chapters 15 to 18 for details). Controlling the teeth in three planes of space is much more difficult than simply tipping them and requires careful planning and ex-

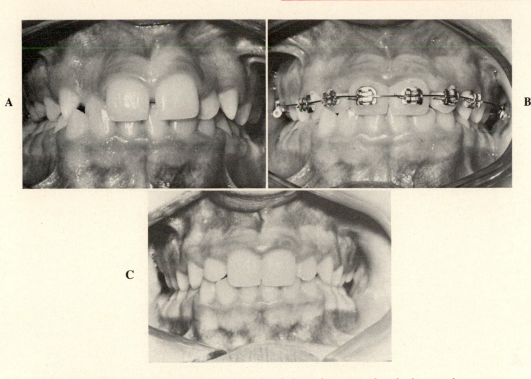

Fig. 13-54 ■ Fixed appliance treatment with bonded attachments and archwires used to correct anterior crossbite and alignment problems. **A,** The maxillary right lateral incisor is in crossbite and the other maxillary anterior teeth are malaligned. **B,** The anterior teeth are bonded and the permanent first molars banded so that an archwire can be used to efficiently correct the rotation and faciolingual displacements. **C,** The patient shows a stable correction after retention and appliance removal.

cellent clinical technique. As with any anterior crossbite correction, these teeth should be stabilized for 1 to 2 months after tooth movement, and can then be released without further retention if the overbite is sufficient. Patient care for the appliance is the most critical factor during treatment.

■ Maxillary Dental Protrusion

Treatment for maxillary dental protrusion during the early mixed dentition is indicated only when the maxillary incisors protrude with spaces between them and are esthetically objectionable or are in danger of traumatic injury. When this condition occurs in a child who has no skeletal discrepancies, it is often a sequel to prolonged thumbsucking. If there is adequate vertical clearance and space within the arch, the maxillary incisors can be tipped lingually with a removable or a fixed appliance. With either appliance, the anchorage may have to be reinforced with the use of a headgear to the molars. If the overbite is enough to bring the upper and lower incisors into vertical contact, however, the upper incisors cannot be retracted until the overbite is corrected. In properly selected patients this can be corrected with a biteplane (see below).

A Hawley-type removable appliance (see Chapter 11) utilizing multiple clasps and an .028 inch labial bow can be very effective in tipping the incisors lingually (Fig. 13-55). The labial bow is activated 1.5 to 2.0 mm and will achieve approximately 1 mm of retraction per month. One and one-half millimeters of acrylic must be removed lingual to the maxillary incisors to allow tooth movement into this area and to accommodate the soft tissue that often piles up on the side of a tooth to which it is moving. The acrylic and the labial bow should both be adjusted and evaluated at each appointment.

A fixed appliance consisting of banded molars, bonded incisors, and archwires can also be used to retract flared and spaced maxillary incisors. The force to retract the incisors can be provided by a closing loop in the archwire (Fig. 13-56) or a straight archwire and an elastomeric chain. If all teeth in the arch are included in the appliance, better control is provided. If only some of the teeth are included, care must be taken not to force the teeth that are not banded or bonded out of alignment. Closing loops should be activated approximately 1 mm per side per month, and the incisors will be retracted a similar amount.

If the protruding incisors are to be retracted bodily, which is rarely the case when they have flared forward in a preadolescent child, control of root position demands the use of a rectangular archwire bent to include closing loops. The archwire can be activated approximately 1 mm per side per month and a similar amount of movement will be achieved. Reinforcement of posterior anchorage will be required.

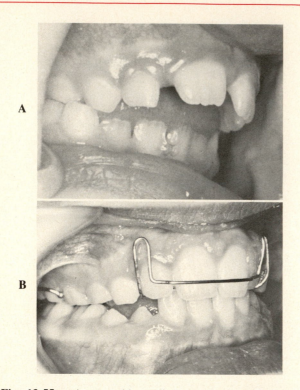

Fig. 13-55 ■ A removable appliance used to retract protrusive incisors that require lingual tipping when space and overbite permit. **A,** This patient has protrusive incisors and spacing caused by a prolonged thumb habit. **B,** A removable appliance is used to tip the incisors lingually by activating the .028 inch labial bow 1 to 1.5 mm and relieving the acrylic lingual to the incisors at each appointment.

■ Vertical Problems

■ Habits and Open Bites

Most children engage in some form of nonnutritive sucking. The effect of this habit on the hard and soft tissues depends on its frequency and duration (see Chapter 8). Although it is possible to deform the alveolus and dentition during the primary dentition years with an intense habit, most clinicians agree that intervention is usually not indicated until approximately 5 years of age. As long as the sucking stops before the eruption of the permanent incisors, most of the dental changes resolve spontaneously. By that time, the majority of children spontaneously stop the sucking habit, another group still suck but want to stop, and yet another small group do not want to stop. If a child does not want to quit sucking, habit therapy, especially appliance therapy, is not indicated.

As the time of eruption of the permanent incisors approaches, the simplest approach to habit therapy is a straightforward discussion between the child and the dentist that expresses concern and includes an explanation by the dentist. This "adult" approach (and restraint from intervention by the parents) is often enough to terminate the habit. If this approach fails, a reward system can be implemented that provides a small tangible reward daily for

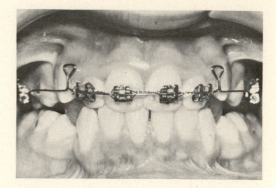

Fig. 13-56 ■ This closing loop archwire was used to retract protrusive maxillary incisors and close space. Each loop was activated approximately 1 mm per month and the posterior anchorage was reinforced with a headgear.

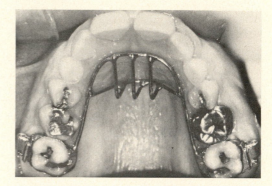

Fig. 13-57 ■ A cemented habit crib made of .038 to .040 inch wire can be used as a reminder along with an explanation to interrupt a fingersucking habit. The appliance can be cemented to either primary or permanent molars and should be extended anteriorly to interfere with the finger position during sucking. The amount of overbite will also help determine the appliance position.

not engaging in the habit. In some cases, a large reward must be negotiated for complete cessation of the habit.

A more complicated method involves reminding the child that the thumb is in the mouth and removing the pleasure of sucking. This can be achieved by placing a cotton glove on the hand or a Band-aid on the thumb or finger, to discourage the habit. This approach will often interrupt the passive sucker who engages in the habit during sleep, reading, or television watching. A maxillary lingual arch, especially the quad helix design, can have the same reminder effect when it is used for maxillary expansion.

If the previous methods have not succeeded in terminating the habit, the child who wants to stop sucking can be fitted with a cemented reminder appliance to actively impede sucking (Fig. 13-57). This consists of a maxillary lingual arch and a crib constructed of soldered wire so that it is difficult to insert the thumb into the mouth. This appliance is bulky but not sharp. Heavy wire (.038 to .040 inch) should be used to eliminate any flexibility. A removable appliance

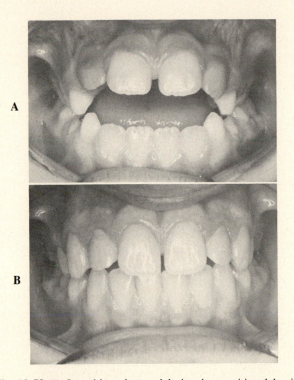

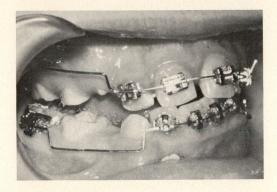

Fig. 13-59 ■ A utility arch can be used to intrude, tip, or reposition either maxillary or mandibular incisors, but with limited posterior anchorage, posterior teeth can be expected to move as well. The archwire is stepped away from the occlusal plane to eliminate distortion from interference with food during chewing.

Fig. 13-58 ■ Open bites observed during the transitional dentition years often close spontaneously. **A,** This patient had good skeletal relationships and an open bite during the early mixed dentition years. **B,** Four years later, without appliance therapy, the open bite has spontaneously closed. (Courtesy Dr. R. Scholz.)

is contraindicated since lack of compliance is part of the problem. The purpose of the therapy must be explained so the patient realizes that the appliance serves as a reminder and not as punishment.[21] If this is understood by the child as a "helping hand," the treatment will be successful and psychologic problems will not result. When sucking apparently ceases, the appliance should be retained in place for approximately 3 months to ensure the habit has truly stopped.

The open bites associated with sucking in children with normal jaw relationships often resolve after sucking stops and the remaining permanent teeth erupt. An appliance to laterally expand a constricted maxillary arch or retract flared and spaced incisors may be needed, but the open bite should require no further treatment in child with good skeletal proportions (Fig. 13-58).[22] Open bites that persist almost always have a significant skeletal component (see Chapter 14).

■ Deep Bite

Before treating a deep bite, it is necessary to establish its cause. The problem may result from reduced lower face height and lack of eruption of the posterior teeth, or from

overeruption of the anterior teeth. The possible treatments attack the cause of the problem and are mutually exclusive.

Removable biteplane appliances to reduce the overbite can be used for patients who have less than normal eruption of the posterior teeth (which is usually associated with reduced face height). An anterior biteplane is incorporated into a removable appliance so that the mandibular incisors occlude with the acrylic plane lingual to the maxillary incisors. This approach prevents the posterior teeth from occluding and encourages their eruption, which may take several months. The appliance must be worn on a full time basis during this phase of treatment. The posterior eruption is hard to regulate and once the proper vertical dimension has been established, the bite plane must continue to be worn or the anterior teeth will erupt and the deep bite will return. This type of treatment, which normally is better deferred until the early permanent dentition, is discussed in detail in Chapter 15.

A more challenging approach to deep bite is necessary when the maxillary or mandibular anterior teeth have erupted excessively. For these patients the task is to stop the eruption (relatively intrude) or actually intrude the incisors. This type of tooth movement requires light continuous forces and careful management of the posterior teeth that provides anchorage. It is often better to defer this treatment until the early permanent dentition, using an intrusion arch during the first stage of comprehensive fixed appliance therapy (see Chapter 15 for details).

A utility arch that incorporates molar and incisor teeth can be used during the mixed dentition to intrude, tip, or reposition both molars and incisors (Fig. 13-59). This appliance is versatile and effective in reducing overbite by relative intrusion but it can be difficult to control and often produces unwanted reciprocal movements. Molar extrusion should be expected with any incisor change. Molar rotation often occurs and the archwire may become imbedded in the buccal mucosa. Like many effective orthodontic appliances,

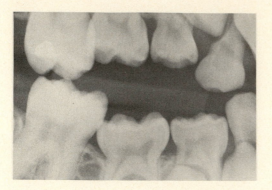

Fig. 13-60 ■ This radiograph demonstrates both anterior and posterior teeth tipping over adjacent ankylosed primary molars. The ankylosed teeth should be removed if tipping and space loss are occurring.

the utility arch is deceptively simple and must be used with considerable care.

■ Ankylosed Primary Teeth

Appropriate management of an ankylosed primary tooth consists of maintaining it until an interference with eruption or drift of other teeth begins to occur, then extracting it and placing a space maintainer or other space management appliance if needed. Ankylosed primary teeth can be maintained in the dental arch for a considerable length of time, often until the time of normal exfoliation, provided they are monitored carefully.

Ankylosed primary teeth are usually resorbed in the normal manner,[23] but occasionally they are not exfoliated on schedule and are retained by attachment between the tooth and hard tissue in the cervical region. This can delay the erupting tooth or deflect it from the normal erupting path.

Another problem that can arise during retention of ankylosed primary molars is mesial tipping of the first permanent molars if the discrepancy between the marginal ridges increases by a significant amount (Fig. 13-60). When the teeth tip, the arch circumference will decrease. If the tipping is recognized before it has progressed too far, the ankylosed primary molar can be restored with a stainless steel crown to maintain the space. If the tipping has progressed and space has been lost, the primary tooth should be removed and the teeth repositioned to regain space.

Supereruption of the opposing teeth can also be a problem. If supereruption has not proceeded too far, the solution again is to restore the ankylosed tooth with a stainless steel crown. This remedy is only temporary. When significant vertical facial growth and eruption occur, the ankylosed tooth will again be out of occlusion.

If the rate of eruption is rapid or the ankylosis has been long-standing, a large vertical discrepancy can develop. In these cases, periodontal or alveolar defects may develop adjacent to the ankylosed teeth and the ankylosed teeth should be extracted (Fig. 13-61). If the defects are severe and there are no successors to the ankylosed teeth, the defects can cause long-term periodontal problems. If the ankylosed teeth do have permanent successors, the alveolar process will be carried to a new and higher level by the erupting permanent teeth, but bone adjacent to the extraction site can still be compromised. It is advisable to have an experienced clinician remove these teeth, one who has high regard for the soft and hard tissue.

When an ankylosed tooth is extracted prematurely, the space should be maintained by the techniques previously described. If occlusal discrepancies have developed, the use of partial dentures may be possible only after extensive occlusal adjustments. Unless opposing permanent teeth have supererupted, the vertical irregularity will be resolved during the establishment of the occlusal plane in the permanent dentition.

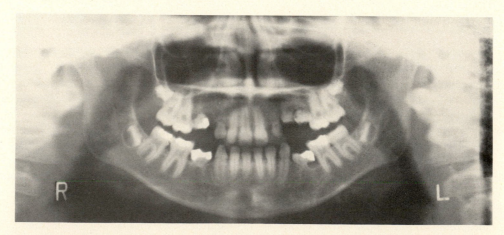

Fig. 13-61 ■ Ankylosed primary teeth should be removed if the vertical discrepancy is so large that periodontal defects such as those adjacent to the primary molars in this patient are developing.

■ *References*

1. Moorrees, C.F.A.: The dentition of the growing child: a longitudinal study of dental development between 3 and 18 years of age. Cambridge, 1959, Harvard University Press.

2. Owen, D.: The incidence and nature of space closure following the premature extraction of deciduous teeth: a literature survey. Am. J. Orthod. **59:**37-49, 1971.

3. Drinkard, C., and Oldenburg, T.: Appliances for guiding first permanent molar eruption. In McDonald, R., Hurt, W., Gilmore, H., and Middleton, R., editors: Current therapy in dentistry, vol. 7. St. Louis, 1980, The C.V. Mosby Co., pp. 446-456.

4. Mayhew, M., Dilley, G., Dilley, D., et al.: Tissue response to intragingival appliances in monkeys. Pediatr. Dent. **6:**148-152, 1984.

5. Hershey, H., Houghton, C., and Burstone, C.: Unilateral facebows: a theoretical and laboratory analysis. Am. J. Orthod. **79:**229-249, 1981.

6. Pulver, F.: The etiology and prevalence of ectopic eruption of the maxillary first permanent molar. J. Dent. Child. **35:**138-146, 1968.

7. Joondeph, D., and McNeill, R.: Congenitally absent second premolars: an interceptive approach. Am. J. Orthod. **59:**50-66, 1971.

8. Fields, H.W.: Bonded resins in orthodontics. Pediatr. Dent. **4:**51-60, 1982.

9. Primosch, R.: Anterior supernumerary teeth—assessment and surgical intervention in children. Pediatr. Dent. **3:**204-215, 1981.

10. DiBase, D.: Mucous membrane and delayed eruption. Trans. Br. Soc. Study Orthod. **56:**149-158, 1969-70.

11. Fields, H.W.: Orthodontic-restorative treatment for relative mandibular anterior excess tooth-size problems. Am. J. Orthod. **79:**176-183, 1981.

12. Edwards, J.: The diastema, the frenum and the frenectomy: a clinical study. Am. J. Orthod. **71:**489-508, 1977.

13. Riedel, R.: Post pubertal occlusal changes. In McNamara, J., editor: The biology of occlusal development. Monograph No. 7, Craniofacial Growth Series, Ann Arbor, 1977, University of Michigan, Center for Human Growth and Development.

14. Owen, A.: Morphologic changes in the sagittal dimension using the Frankel appliance. Am. J. Orthod. **80:**573-603, 1981.

15. Kjellgren, B.: Serial extraction as a corrective procedure in dental orthopedic therapy. Trans. Eur. Ortho. Soc., pp. 134-160, 1947-48.

16. Hotz, R.: Guidance of eruption versus serial extraction. Am. J. Orthod. **58:**1-20, 1970.

17. Dewel, B.: A critical analysis of serial extraction in orthodontic treatment. Am. J. Orthod. **45:**424-455, 1959.

18. Schroder, I., and Schroder, U.: Early treatment of unilateral posterior skeletal crossbite in the primary dentition (Abstract no. 828, J. Dent. Res. **60:**516, 1981.

19. Kutin, G., and Hawes, R.: Posterior cross-bites in the deciduous and mixed dentitions. Am. J. Orthod. **56:**491-504, 1969.

20. Chaconas, S., and deAlbay-Levy, J.: Orthopedic and orthodontic applications of the quad-helix appliance. Am. J. Orthod. **72:**422-428, 1977.

21. Haryett, R., Hansen, R., Davidson, P., et al.: Chronic thumbsucking: the psychological effects and the relative effectiveness of the various methods of treatment. Am. J. Orthod. **53:**559-585, 1967.

22. Worms, F., Meskin, L., and Isaacson, R.: Openbite. Am. J. Orthod. **59:**589-595, 1971.

23. Steigman, S., Koyoumdjisky-Kaye, F., and Matrai, Y.: Relationship of submerged deciduous molars to root resorption and development of permanent successors. J. Dent. Res. **53:**88-93, 1974.

Chapter 14

Treatment of Skeletal Problems in Preadolescent Children

■ *Principles of Growth Modification Treatment*

Whenever a jaw discrepancy exists, the ideal solution is to correct it by modifying growth, so that the skeletal problem literally disappears as the child grows. As noted in Chapter 8, the alternatives are camouflage, which consists of treatment to move teeth so that the patient has good occlusion despite the continuing jaw discrepancy, or surgery to reposition the jaws.

The period of rapid growth during the mixed dentition just before puberty is the ideal time for growth modification. Camouflage should rarely be the major focus of treatment in preadolescent children and, if attempted, should be deferred until all the primary teeth have exfoliated. A few children with very severe skeletal discrepancies will require surgical intervention before puberty, conditions discussed in more detail in Chapter 21. Except in these rare instances, however, orthognathic surgery should not be planned during the mixed dentition. Growth modification is the preferred treatment of this stage of development and these treatment procedures are the focus of this chapter. The goal of a first phase of treatment for a skeletal problem is to reduce or eliminate the problem so that once the permanent teeth erupt, any remaining dental problems can be addressed during an uncomplicated second phase of treatment.

■ The Mechanism of Growth Modification

There are three theoretic possibilities for growth modification:

1. An absolute increase or decrease in size of the jaws. In this case treatment would result in small or deficient skeletal structures becoming larger than they would have been without treatment, or in large or excessive skeletal structures decreasing in size or at least not experiencing the further growth that otherwise would have occurred, so that they end up smaller than they would have been. Examples of this would be causing additional growth of a small mandible in a Class II patient, or stopping the growth of a large lower jaw in a Class III patient, so that normal jaw proportions were the result.

2. Changes in the spatial relationships of the jaws, without decreasing or increasing the size of the skeletal structures. This approach could be viewed as a change in jaw orientation. The growth would be redirected so that it was expressed in a different direction, even if the ultimate size did not change. An example of this would be redirecting the growth of the mandible more downward and less forward in a child with a Class III problem because of excessive mandibular growth. The redirection of growth would produce both a reduction in the Class III relationship and a lengthening of the face, which would be desirable in a child with a short face initially, but undesirable in one with a long face.

3. Acceleration of desirable growth, especially the mandible in mandibular-deficient children, even though the ultimate size and shape of the mandible are not significantly altered. In other words, the mandible might not end up larger than it would ultimately have become without treatment, but it would attain the final size sooner. This approach would shorten treatment time and facilitate correction from redirecting maxillary growth and dentoalveolar changes.

Although the last two of these theoretic possibilities can be shown to occur,[1,2] some doubt still exists about absolute inhibition of growth,[3] and considerable doubt about true growth stimulation leading to an absolute increase in jaw

354

size in humans.[4,5] There are two problems in demonstrating absolute size changes. First, comparing what happened as a result of treatment to what would have happened without treatment in the same patient requires growth prediction, an inexact science at best. Second and more important, the data in humans indicate that if changes can really be found in the absolute size of jaws between treated and untreated groups of patients, the differences are quite small,[6,7] so small that even if statistically significant, they are probably clinically insignificant. Studies of experimental animals show that the changes do occur at the cellular level when pressure or tension is applied to the jaws,[8,9] and similar changes most likely occur in humans. Over a long enough period of time, these changes could lead to absolute size differences. However, it is not necessary to invoke changes in absolute size to understand the clinical efficacy of growth modification treatment in humans.

A redirection of growth, changing vertical and horizontal jaw positions to alter facial proportions, definitely does occur in many patients.[10] This change can be seen for both the maxilla and the mandible. Downward rotation of the mandible in response to pressure against the chin is the classic example, but pressure or tension against the maxilla can alter the proportions of downward and forward growth that would otherwise have been expressed. Although it is difficult to demonstrate growth stimulation in the form of a change in absolute size, there is little doubt that growth stimulation in the form of acceleration of mandibular growth occurs frequently as a response to functional appliances that position the mandible forward.[8,11] Acceleration is also observed when forward traction is placed against the maxilla in young children.[12] Most of the changes that occur during growth modification treatment can be explained by a combination of redirection of growth and changes in its timing. Appliances to produce these effects are clinically useful, regardless of whether they produce changes in absolute size.

■ The Timing of Growth Modification

Irrespective of the type of appliance used or the type of growth effect, if growth is to be modified, the patient has to be growing.[13] Because of the rapid growth exhibited by children during the primary dentition years, it would seem that treatment of jaw discrepancies by growth modification should be successful at a very early age. The rationale for treatment at ages 4 to 6 would be that because of the rapid rate of growth, significant amounts of skeletal discrepancy could be overcome in a short time. This treatment approach relies on the premise that once jaw discrepancies are corrected, proper function will cause them to continue to grow in harmony without future treatment.

If this were the case, very early treatment would be advocated for many skeletal discrepancies. Unfortunately, most anteroposterior and vertical problems treated during the primary dentition years relapse because of continued growth in the original disproportionate pattern. If children are treated very early, they usually need further treatment during the mixed dentition and again in the early permanent dentition to maintain the correction. For this reason, growth modification therapy for commonly occurring skeletal discrepancies is best deferred until growth modification will be more stable.

The opposite point of view would be to say, as many orthodontists did until recently, that since treatment in the permanent dentition would be required anyway, there is no point in starting treatment until then. Certainly, a second phase of treatment is often necessary after successful growth modification to correct any remaining dental problems. If eruption of the permanent teeth precedes the adolescent growth spurt, growth modification and definitive treatment can be combined and only one phase of treatment is necessary. For most children, however, growth modification of significant skeletal problems must begin in the mixed dentition, because there simply is not enough growth remaining if treatment is delayed until the dental transition is completed. This is true for nearly all girls and the great majority of boys.

A typical treatment plan for jaw discrepancies, therefore, does call for two stages of treatment. The mixed dentition stage that focuses on correcting the skeletal problem should begin 1 to 3 years before the peak of the adolescent growth spurt. The general guideline is that the more severe the skeletal problem, the earlier the treatment should begin. A second phase of comprehensive fixed appliance treatment in the early permanent dentition should be anticipated from the beginning. Treatment planning principles, and their application to these patients, are discussed in detail in Chapters 9 and 10.

■ *Appliances for Growth Modification*

■ Extraoral Appliances

Extraoral force in the form of headgear and chin cups, very similar to those used today, was used by the pioneer orthodontists of the late 1800s. Both Kingsley and Angle described and used astonishingly modern-appearing appliances of this sort, apparently with reasonable success.[14,15] As orthodontics progressed in the early twentieth century, however, extraoral appliances and mixed dentition treatment were abandoned, not because they were ineffective, but because they were considered an unnecessary complication. By 1920, Angle and his followers were convinced that Class II and III elastics not only moved teeth but also caused significant skeletal changes, stimulating the growth of one jaw while restraining the other. If intraoral elastics could produce a true stimulation of mandibular growth while simultaneously restraining the maxilla, there would be no need to ask a patient to wear an extraoral appliance, nor would there be any reason to begin treatment until the permanent teeth were available.

The first cephalometric evaluations of the effects of orthodontic treatment, which became available in the 1940s,

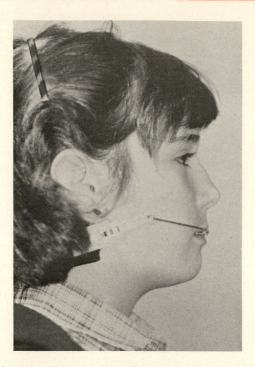

Fig. 14-1 ■ A Kloehn-type headgear appliance. This appliance uses a cervical neck strap and a facebow to produce distal force on the maxillary teeth and maxilla, which is aimed at altering maxillary size and position.

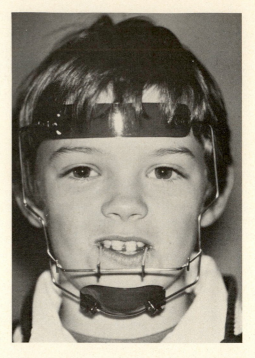

Fig. 14-2 ■ A Delaire-type facemask. This appliance is used to produce an anterior (protraction) force on the maxillary teeth and maxilla for children who have a small or distally positioned maxilla.

did not support the concept that significant skeletal changes occurred in response to intraoral forces. A 1936 paper by Oppenheim revived the idea that headgear would serve as a valuable adjunct to treatment.[16] However, it was not until Silas Kloehn's impressive results with headgear treatment of Class II malocclusion became widely known after World War II that extraoral force to the maxilla again became an important part of American orthodontics.[17] Cephalometric studies of patients treated with Kloehn-type headgear (Fig. 14-1), which utilized a neck strap and relatively light (300 to 400 gm) force, showed that skeletal change in the form of a reorientation of jaw relationships did occur.[18] Rapid developments in headgear treatment followed in the 1950s and 1960s. It became apparent that greater skeletal changes might be produced by beginning treatment before all permanent teeth erupted, and that it was necessary to control the magnitude, direction, and duration of the extraoral forces to achieve specific effects.[19] Experience soon revealed that although greater skeletal effects might be produced by higher levels of force than Kloehn had advocated, this procedure required an upward direction of pull from a head cap to prevent excessive downward movement of the maxilla and a consequent downward and backward rotation of the mandible. The use of headgear to control the maxilla and the maxillary teeth in all three planes of space is described in some detail in the following sections of this chapter, relating to specific problems.

Neither chin cups to restrain mandibular growth nor facemasks to pull the maxilla forward were an important part of the orthodontics of the early twentieth century, but neither was as totally abandoned as headgear. Both approaches were used occasionally, primarily as desperation measures in severe Class III problems, and neither was considered effective. With the demonstration in the 1960s of skeletal changes from headgear force to the maxilla, interest in chin cups revived. Primate experiments suggested that force against the mandibular condyles could produce an inhibition of growth,[20] but unlike the favorable responses noted with headgear, most clinicians did not observe significant clinical changes from chin cups, and this approach remains of equivocal value in contemporary treatment.

Until the 1970s, facemasks to bring the maxilla forward were dismissed as ineffectual (Fig. 14-2). The French surgeon Delaire, working primarily with cleft palate children, demonstrated that the maxilla can be moved forward if the protracting forces on the maxilla are used at early ages.[12] Facemask therapy is an area of continuing innovations in treatment at present, and it may yet offer a more satisfactory way of treating maxillary deficiency problems than has been the case in the past.

Specific configurations of each of these types of extraoral appliances and their application to specific problems are presented in the following section.

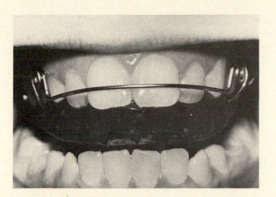

Fig. 14-3 ■ Functional appliances like this bionator cause the mandible to function in a predetermined position. This posture stretches the soft tissue and muscles, and the resulting forces are transmitted to the teeth and skeletal structures.

■ Functional Appliances

A functional appliance by definition is one that changes the posture of the mandible, holding it open or open and forward (Fig. 14-3). Stretch of the muscles and soft tissues creates pressures transmitted to the dental and skeletal structures, moving teeth and modifying growth. The monobloc developed by Robin in the early 1900s is generally considered the forerunner of all functional appliances, but the activator developed in Norway by Andresen in the 1920s was the first functional appliance to be widely accepted.[21] Andresen's activator became the basis of the ''Norwegian system'' of treatment. Both the appliance system and its theoretic underpinnings were improved and extended elsewhere in Europe, particularly by the German school led by Haupl, who believed that the only stable tooth movement was produced by natural forces and that alterations in function produced by these appliances would give stable corrections of malocclusion.

This philosophic approach was diametrically opposite to that espoused by Angle and his followers in the United States, who emphasized fixed appliances to precisely position the teeth. These opposing beliefs contributed to the great differences between European and American orthodontics at midcentury.

Functional appliances were introduced into American orthodontics in the 1950s, largely in the beginning through the influence of Harvold, and later from personal contact by a number of American orthodontists with their European counterparts. (Fixed appliances spread to Europe at the same time in the same way.) A major boost to functional appliance treatment in the United States came from the publication of animal experiments in the 1970s showing skeletal changes produced by posturing the mandible to a new position and holding out the possibility that true stimulation of mandibular growth could be achieved.[8,22] At this point, although some of the enthusiasm for functional appliance treatment caused by the favorable animal experiments has faded in the light of less impressive clinical results,[4,5] functional appliances have achieved a major place in contemporary growth modification treatment.

Although functional appliances are not interchangeable with fixed appliances because they cannot produce detailed tooth movement, there are unique applications for this type of treatment, especially as the first stage of two-stage treatment. Functional appliances can restrain maxillary growth in the same way (though perhaps not to the same extent) as headgear.[23] In addition, the amount and direction of dental eruption can be regulated to influence the vertical and anteroposterior skeletal and dental relationships[24]; teeth can be tipped to new positions; and evidence shows that mandibular growth can be accelerated and perhaps even stimulated to attain a slightly larger absolute size. All of these effects can be useful in the treatment of jaw discrepancy problems.

Conventionally designed functional appliances. The many types of functional appliances differ considerably in appearance and often bear the developer's name. The eponyms can be confusing and often imply regional and personal differences that impede communication among clinicians and between laboratory personnel and clinicians.

In general, functional appliances can be grouped into three major categories: tooth-borne and passive; tooth-borne and active; or tissue-borne and passive:

    Tooth-borne passive
        Andresen activator
        Woodside and Harvold activator
        Bionator
        Herbst appliance
    Tooth-borne active
        Modified activator (many named types)
        Expansion activator
        Orthopedic corrector
        Stockli headgear activator
    Tissue-borne
        Frankel appliance

Unfortunately, this categorization does not totally describe the effects and purposes of each appliance. In this section, some of the more common appliances will be classified, briefly described, and illustrated. In the following section, we will approach functional appliances from a different perspective, emphasizing their components, and will show that analyzing them on a components basis offers a better approach to predicting and planning treatment effects.

Tooth-borne passive appliances. These appliances have no intrinsic force-generating capacity from springs or screws and depend only on soft tissue stretch and muscular activity to produce treatment effects.

THE ANDRESEN ACTIVATOR. The original functional appliance design (Fig. 14-4) of Andresen falls into this category. Haupl modified the original design, and his activator was the major appliance in German orthodontics for many years. This activator fits loosely, advances the mandible several millimeters for Class II correction, and uses moderate opening of vertical dimension with the appliance in place.

WOODSIDE AND HARVOLD ACTIVATORS (Fig. 14-5). These originally had an increased vertical opening to help maintain the appliance in the mouth during sleep by stretching the soft tissue. Presently, this appliance is constructed with a moderate opening and incorporates displacing springs to increase muscle activity by forcing the patient to more actively maintain the appliance in position.

In addition to the effects on jaw growth, these essentially passive appliances can tip anterior teeth and control eruption of teeth to alter vertical dental relationships. They can also be trimmed to provide dental arch expansion, so despite the simple design, dental relationships in all three planes of space can be changed with an activator.

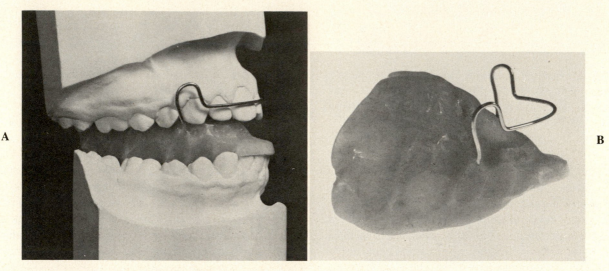

Fig. 14-4 ■ The Andresen-type activator is a tooth-borne passive appliance that was the first widely used functional appliance. **A,** The appliance opens the bite and the mandible is advanced for Class II correction. This particular design incorporates a labial bow for control of maxillary anterior teeth and an acrylic cap over the lower incisors. **B,** The facets cut in the acrylic help direct eruption of the posterior teeth, mesially in the lower arch and distally and buccally in the upper. Both the lingual flange and the acrylic cap on the incisors help to position the mandible.

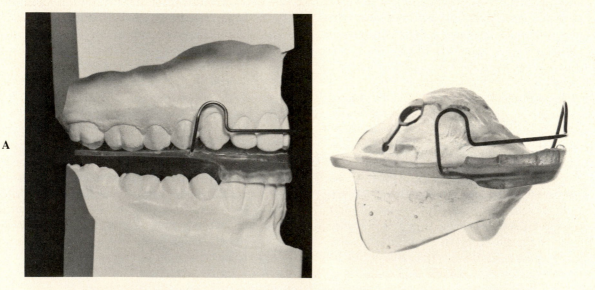

Fig. 14-5 ■ **A,** This Woodside-type activator has a modest vertical opening and the mandible is advanced so that the incisors are in an edge-to-edge relationship for Class II correction. The maxillary posterior teeth are prevented from erupting by the acrylic stop while the mandibular posterior teeth are free to erupt upward and forward. **B,** This type of appliance is also typified by a deep lingual flange extension and a displacement spring on the upper first molar, which requires the patient to actively maintain the appliance in the proper position. The Harvold and Woodside-type activators originally exaggerated the vertical opening of the mandible to accentuate soft tissue forces.

THE BIONATOR (Fig. 14-6). Originated by Balters and sometimes still bearing his name, the bionator is another major member of the passive tooth-borne group (unless addition of an expansion screw puts it into the active category). The best short description of a bionator is that it is a cut-down activator. The reduced bulk of the appliance and its ability to reposition the mandible and modify dental eruption have been important in its ready acceptance by both parents and clinicians. Like the activator, vertical control is present, and the bionator can be used for Class II, Class III, deep bite, and open bite problems.

THE HERBST APPLIANCE. This device, developed in the early 1920s and reintroduced recently by Pancherz[11] is the only fixed functional appliance. The maxillary and mandibular arches are splinted with cemented or bonded frameworks. Jaw position is controlled by a pin and tube apparatus that runs between the arches (Fig. 14-7). The appliance requires little patient compliance. The appliance produces a highly variable mixture of skeletal and dental changes.

Tooth-borne active appliances. These are largely modifications of activator and bionator designs that include expansion screws or springs to provide intrinsic forces for transverse and anteroposterior changes (expansion activator,

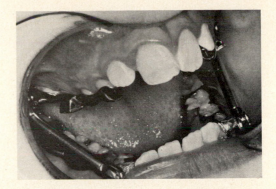

Fig. 14-7 ■ The Herbst appliance is the only fixed functional appliance. The maxillary and mandibular splints are cemented or bonded to the teeth. The upper and lower splints are joined by the pin and tube apparatus that dictates the mandibular position.

orthopedic corrector, and a number of named activators) (Fig. 14-8).

In the correction of a Class II malocclusion, some transverse expansion of the upper arch is nearly always needed, as observed by having the patient hold the lower jaw forward in a Class I position; a crossbite tendency is usually apparent. The springs or screws in active functional appliances were added to the basic design in some instances to provide this expansion, but in many appliances an additional goal is further expansion of the upper and lower arches to correct crowding. Tooth movement is usually undesirable in preadolescent children, particularly anteroposterior movement of upper and lower incisors to camouflage jaw discrepancies. Every millimeter of incisor tipping is a millimeter of potential skeletal correction that has been lost. This means that active springs for camouflage should be avoided. Springs and screws for expansion to correct crowding can produce unstable results (see Chapter 11) and should also be used cautiously.

Active elements in tooth-borne functional appliances, in short, may detract from the overall effectiveness of growth modification treatment and are recommended only for special treatment needs. Headgear tubes and torquing springs are added to the Stockli headgear activator (Fig. 14-9) so that extraoral force is available to supplement the Class II correction and to reduce the tipping effect on maxillary anterior teeth. This appliance is a notable exception among the active functional appliances in that the active components are designed to decrease dental and increase skeletal effects.[25]

Tissue borne-appliances. The Frankel appliance is the only tissue-borne appliance, and even the Frankel has some contact with the teeth (Fig. 14-10). Much of the appliance is located in the vestibule, however, and it alters both mandibular posture and the contour of facial soft tissue. Despite its minimal contact with the dentition, the appliance can be used to enhance dental eruption, to utilize the anteroposterior drift to alter dental relationships, and to generate arch expansion in addition to its effects on jaw growth.

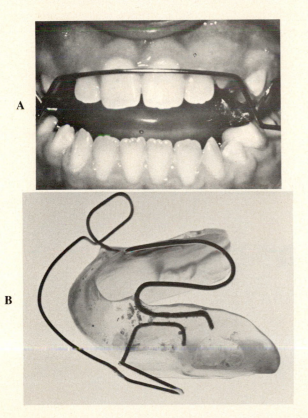

Fig. 14-6 ■ The Balters-type bionator is another of the tooth-borne passive appliances. **A,** This appliance uses a lingual flange to regulate the posture of the mandible and usually incorporates a buccinator wraparound or labial bow. **B,** The design, which removes much of the bulk of the activator, can include posterior facets or acrylic occlusal stops to control amount and direction of eruption.

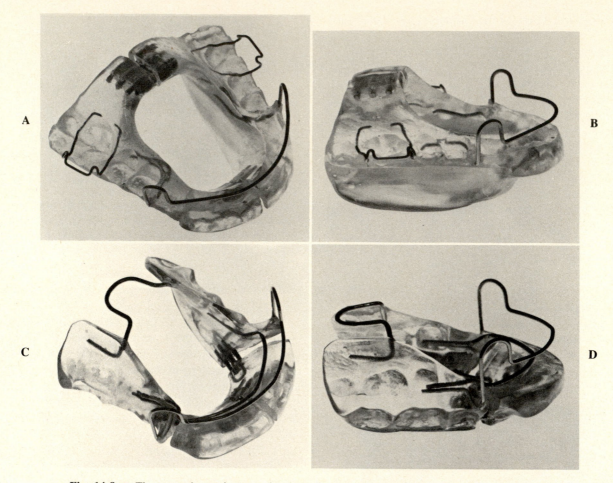

Fig. 14-8 ■ The expansion activator and orthopedic corrector are examples of active tooth-borne appliances. **A,** The expansion activator resembles the classic activator design with the addition of anterior and posterior expansion screws to facilitate transverse expansion. This modification also requires posterior clasps to aid in retention. **B,** The lingual flange length is usually modest and the posterior occlusal stops can be modified to direct eruption. **C,** The orthopedic corrector is closer in design to the bionator but it incorporates expansion screws for transverse expansion and anteroposterior changes. **D,** The lingual flange is modest and the posterior acrylic can be modified to control eruption.

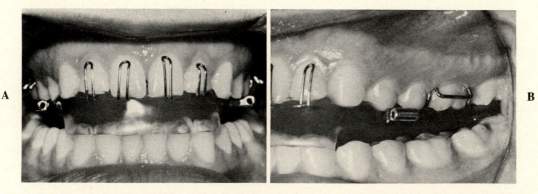

Fig. 14-9 ■ The Stockli-type activator is a tooth-borne active appliance that attempts to reduce undesirable dental changes with the addition of high-pull headgear and torquing springs. **A,** The vertical anterior torquing springs are designed to reduce lingual tipping of the maxillary incisors while, **B,** a facebow placed in the tubes augments horizontal restriction of maxillary growth and controls descent of the maxilla. The acrylic prohibits posterior maxillary eruption and allows mandibular eruption, and the clasps add retention.

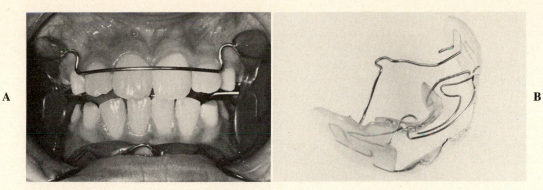

Fig. 14-10 ■ The Frankel appliance is the only tissue-borne functional appliance. The mandible can be either positioned in centric relation for Class III correction or advanced as shown here for Class II correction **(A). B,** The large buccal shields and lip pads reduce soft tissue pressure on the dentition; the lingual pad dictates the mandibular position. The appliance looks bulky, but for the most part is restricted to the buccal vestibule and interferes less with speech than most other designs of functional appliances.

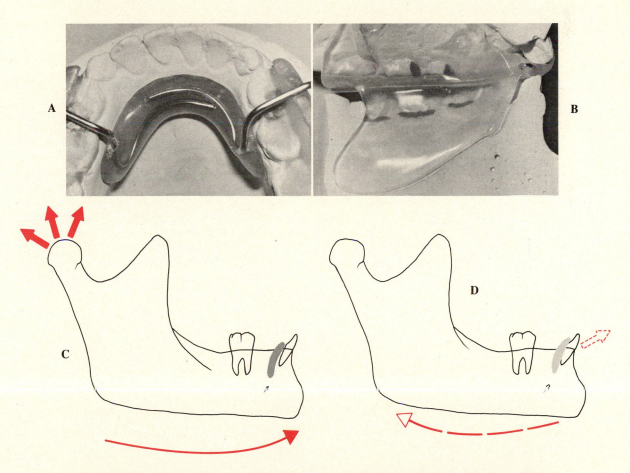

Fig. 14-11 ■ The lingual pad or flange determines the anteroposterior and vertical mandibular posture for most functional appliances. **A,** The small lingual pad from a Frankel appliance; **B,** the extensive lingual flange from a modified activator; **C,** these lingual components not only position the mandible forward but, **D,** also exert a protrusive effect on the mandibular incisors when the mandible attempts to return to its original position and the pad or flange contacts the lingual of the incisors.

Functional appliance components. Each functional appliance, no matter whose name it carries, is simply a melding of wire and acrylic components. If one understands the different component parts of these appliances and how the components translate into treatment effects, it is possible to plan functional appliance treatment by combining the appropriate components to deal with specific aspects of the child's problems. This approach demands more knowledge and thought during treatment planning and appliance design, but should lead to more appropriate treatment for the patients. This can be described as the components approach to functional appliance therapy.

The following components are listed in categories as functional, active, or miscellaneous components. The functional components generate forces by altering posture of the mandible, changing soft tissue pressures against the teeth, or both. The active components can generate intrinsic forces.

Functional components

LINGUAL PAD OR FLANGES. In all functional appliances, lingual pads or flanges, large or small, provide the stimulus to posture the mandible to a new position (Fig. 14-11). Contact of the lingual component against the mandibular alveolar mucosa causes the child to position the mandible forward. This approach may have several effects. First, if the mandible if protruded, growth at the condyle may be accelerated. Second, the lingual pads can be used to increase the vertical dimension beyond the normal resting vertical position, creating a space into which tooth eruption can be allowed or prevented as desired. Third, when the mandible attempts to return to the normal resting posture, a labially directed force will be applied to the mandibular incisors if the appliance contacts these teeth. For this reason, the lingual pads or flanges are usually relieved behind the lower incisors.

LIP PADS. These acrylic pads are positioned in the vestibule and remove lip pressure from the teeth (Fig. 14-12). These also force the lip musculature to be stretched to function and obtain a seal, presumably improving the tonicity of the lips.

BUCCAL SHIELDS, CUSPID WIRES, AND BUCCINATOR BOWS. These components are used to remove the buccal soft tissue from contact with the dentition (Fig. 14-13). The effect is to disrupt the tongue-cheek equilibrium, and this in turn leads to facial movement of the teeth and arch expansion. Some advocates claim that buccal shields placed high in the vestibule stretch the periosteum, promote deposition of bone, and even open the midpalatal suture. Regardless of the mechanism, the result is that arch width increases in the area where the shield is relieving the buccal tissue pressure.

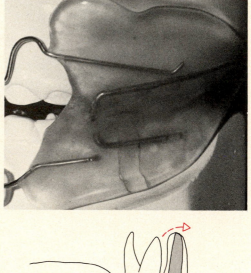

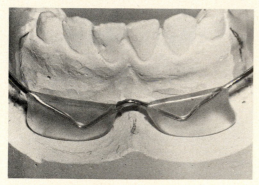

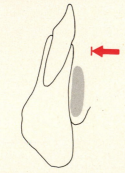

Fig. 14-12 ■ Lip pads hold the lips away from teeth and force the lips to stretch to obtain an oral seal. The lip pad is positioned low in the vestibule, and must have the proper inclination to avoid soft tissue irritation.

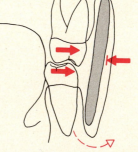

Fig. 14-13 ■ The buccal shield holds the soft tissue away from the dentition and facilitates posterior dental expansion by disrupting the tongue-cheek equilibrium. **A,** The buccal shield is usually placed away from the teeth and alveolus in the arch where expansion is needed. **B,** The potential for periosteal stretching to facilitate deposition of bone when the shields are appropriately extended is noted here with a dashed arrow.

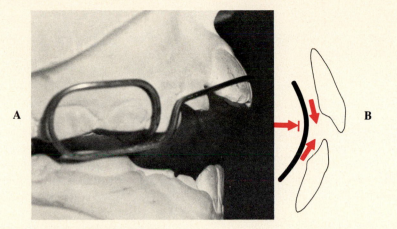

Fig. 14-14 ■ The lingual shield restricts the resting tongue from a position between the teeth. **A,** The acrylic shield is placed behind the anterior teeth and, **B,** encourages the anterior teeth to erupt into the space previously occupied by the tongue.

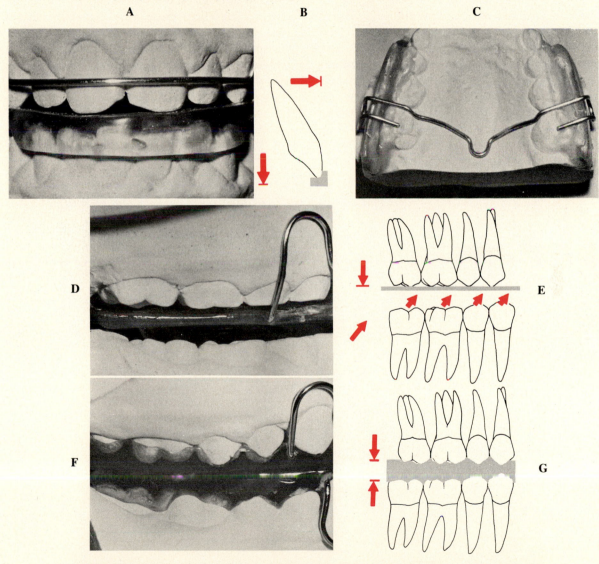

Fig. 14-15 ■ Incisal and occlusal stops control eruption of anterior and posterior teeth, respectively. **A,** The acrylic above and below the incisal edges prohibits eruption of these incisors; **B,** these stops can extend to the facial surface and control the anteroposterior incisor position; **C,** posterior stops can be constructed of wire or **D,** acrylic; **E,** this positioning of occlusal stops inhibits maxillary eruption but allows mandibular eruption; **F,** the complete acrylic posterior bite block, **G,** eliminates both maxillary and mandibular eruption and is extremely useful in controlling vertical facial dimensions.

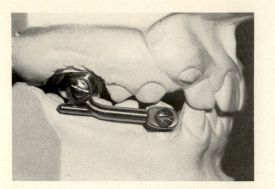

Fig. 14-16 ■ The sliding pin and tube apparatus is a component of the Herbst appliance and dictates the mandibular position.

A combination of lip pads and buccal shields will result in an increase in arch circumference as well. The acrylic buccal shield is more effective in producing buccal expansion than wires to hold the cheeks away from the teeth.

LINGUAL SHIELDS. These serve the same purpose as buccal shields in that they remove the resting tongue from between the teeth (Fig. 14-14). This has the effect of enhancing tooth eruption, since there are reduced antagonistic forces when the patient wears the appliance, especially during sleep.

OCCLUSAL OR INCISAL STOPS (INCLUDING BITE BLOCKS). When acrylic or wire is placed in contact with a tooth and the vertical dimension is opened past the normal postural position, the stretch of the soft tissue will exert an intrusive force on the teeth (Fig. 14-15). Intrusion usually does not occur, probably because the force is not constant, but if the patient wears the appliance most of the time, neither does eruption. This component provides a way to control the vertical position of the dentition and can be used on anterior or posterior teeth.

SLIDING PIN AND TUBE. These components found only in the Herbst appliance also force the mandible to be positioned forward, not by directing the mandible to a new position with pressure against the mucosa, but by holding the teeth (Fig. 14-16). This approach has the advantage that the postural change is permanent (at least until the dentist removes the appliance) and the disadvantage that pressure against the teeth, which produces compensatory incisor movements, cannot be avoided.

FACETS OR FLUTES. The acrylic is shaped to contact the teeth so that their eruption is guided (Fig. 14-17). Nearly

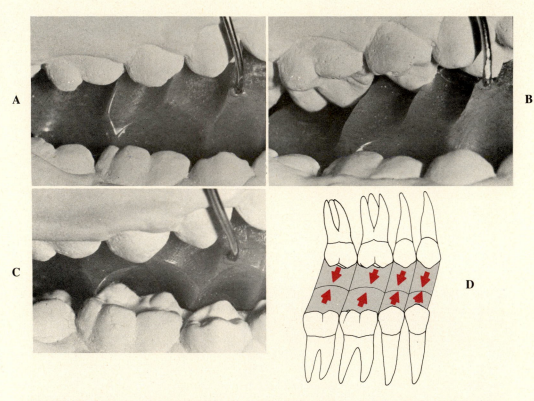

Fig. 14-17 ■ Facets or flutes carved in the acrylic can be used to control posterior tooth position. **A,** For this Class II patient, the facets are inclined to the facial to expand both the maxillary and mandibular arches; **B,** the maxillary acrylic contacts the mesial, but not the distal surface of the teeth to force distal drift during eruption; **C,** the mandibular facets contact the distal surface of the teeth, but not the mesial, to encourage mesial drift during eruption; **D,** these opposite directions of eruption will facilitate dental correction of the Class II malocclusion.

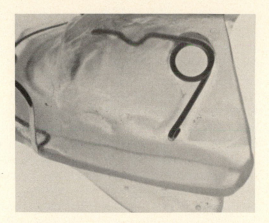

Fig. 14-18 ■ Displacing springs press against the mesial surface of the maxillary permanent first molar and tend to dislodge the appliance. This movement causes the patient to use muscular forces to maintain the appliance in the correct position in the mouth.

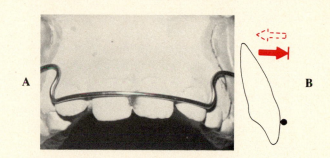

Fig. 14-19 ■ The labial bow can be either active or passive depending on whether it contacts the anterior teeth. **A,** Even if it does not touch the anterior teeth, displacement of the appliance can bring the bow into contact with the teeth and cause a lingual tipping force; **B,** the labial bow may produce distal movement, but certainly prohibits facial movement of the incisors.

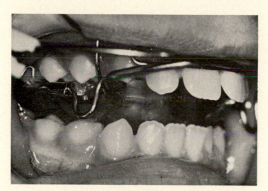

Fig. 14-20 ■ Headgear tubes can be incorporated into any tooth-borne appliance so that additional distal and vertical force can be applied with a facebow and headcap.

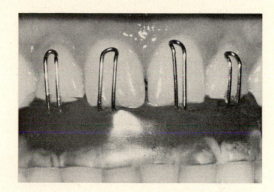

Fig. 14-21 ■ Torquing springs are designed to apply a moment to the incisor crowns and produce bodily incisor movement, or at least overcome some of the lingual incisor tipping common with functional appliances.

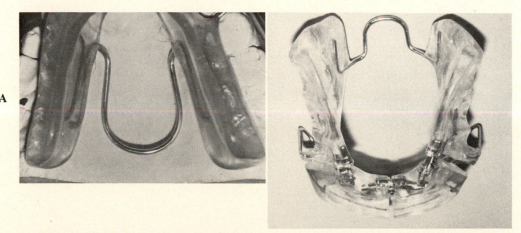

Fig. 14-22 ■ Expansion springs and screws are active methods to increase the transverse arch dimension. **A,** Either a spring activated gradually by the dentist or, **B,** a jackscrew activated by the patient can be incorporated into functional appliances.

always, a ramp is created to influence eruption into a wider dimension, and the facet can also be used to direct the teeth mesially or distally. Movement of the appliance as the patient wears it can create transient forces against the teeth that may actively move teeth.

DISPLACING SPRINGS. These springs tend to dislodge the appliance and force the patient to use muscular force to maintain the appliance in the proper position (Fig. 14-18).

Active components

LABIAL BOW. The labial bow may not always contact the teeth. Even when the labial bow does not touch the teeth when the appliance is seated in position, it often contacts them during movement of the appliance. When it does contact the incisors, it will tend to tip them lingually regardless of whether it is activated to have a spring effect, because force is transmitted to the teeth as the appliance is repositioned in the mouth during relaxation toward normal resting posture (Fig. 14-19). At a minimum, this contact will prevent the teeth from moving facially, but some retraction is likely to occur.

HEADGEAR TUBES. If a distal or vertical extraoral force is desired, a facebow can be fitted into the tubes and a headgear worn in conjunction with a tooth-borne functional appliance (Fig. 14-20).

TORQUING SPRINGS. These springs contact the incisors in the cervical third and are aimed at counteracting the tipping movement often produced by a labial bow (Fig. 14-21).

EXPANSION SCREWS AND SPRINGS. These components can be used to actively increase the transverse dimension of the arches or modify the anteroposterior dimension of the appliance (Fig. 14-22). They do not work through conventional functional approaches, but generate tooth moving forces within the appliances. The effect of these active components is discussed in more detail in Chapter 13.

Miscellaneous components

CLASPS. An assortment of clasps can be used to help retain the appliance in position in the mouth (Fig. 14-23). Some clinicians argue that by having the appliance firmly seated

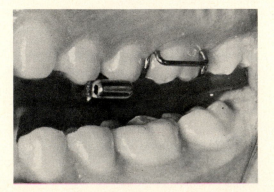

Fig. 14-23 ■ To increase retention of the appliance, clasps are often added to functional appliances when active components are used. If clasps are used to help the patient adapt to the appliance, they can later be removed or deactivated. Note that this appliance also incorporates a headgear tube.

in the mouth, jaw activity to maintain the appliance is reduced and functional changes are minimized. On the other hand, clasps enable the first time wearer to readily adapt to the appliance, and soft tissue stretch probably contributes as much to the "functional" effect as muscular contraction. Clasps can be used initially and then removed if desired when the patient has learned to wear the appliance.

NOTCHING. This is not a component in the conventional sense, but allows the wire components to seat positively against the dentition as they fit into notches cut in the enamel of some primary teeth. Notching is strongly recommended by Frankel to anchor the appliance against the maxillary arch, thereby minimizing the incisor tipping from the labial bow. It is not needed when the acrylic components of tooth-borne appliances contact the teeth.

WIRE AND ACRYLIC CONNECTORS. These components serve to tie the other components together and give the appliance rigidity and structural integrity.

■ ■ ■

In the maturation of any technology, an early stage of minor variations associated with particular names is succeeded by a later stage in which the principles underlying the system have been understood and variations are characterized by their function, not by who first proposed them. The process is by no means unique to dentistry or orthodontics, but can be seen clearly in the evolution of fixed appliances. This evolution is now occurring with functional appliances, and it represents significant progress. The components approach to functional appliances allows a clinician to design an appliance for the specific problems of an individual patient.

Custom-designed appliances can and should be used for children with all the types of jaw discrepancies, so that the therapy is focused on that patient's specific problems. Appliance designs for asymmetry problems are particularly likely to end up quite different from any conventional design (see section 6 of this chapter below), but subtle variations in the appliance for common Class II problems can enhance treatment. The use of a laboratory prescription form keyed to the components approach (Fig. 14-24) makes it feasible to design a functional appliance to meet the patient's needs. In the following discussion, comments about functional appliances for specific jaw discrepancy situations are made in terms of components, with occasional reference to named appliances.

■ *Treatment for Class II Jaw Relationships*

The careful diagnostic approach advocated in the earlier chapters must be used to identify the cause of a Class II problem. It is not appropriate to begin treatment of a skeletal problem in a child without cephalometric analysis. The four commonly observed skeletal relationships that cause Class

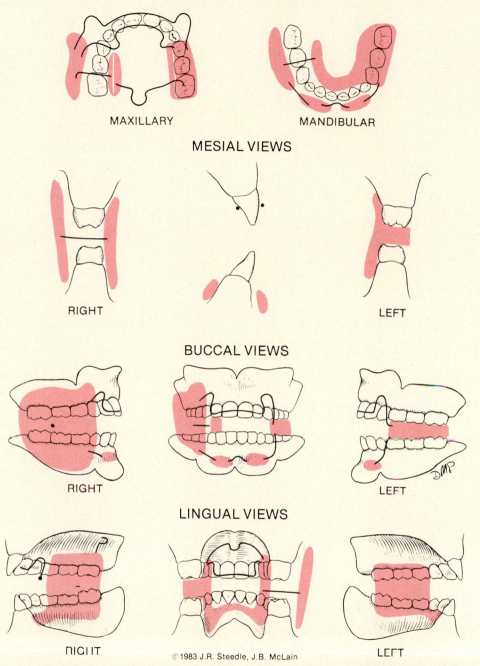

OCCLUSAL VIEWS

MAXILLARY   MANDIBULAR

MESIAL VIEWS

RIGHT   LEFT

BUCCAL VIEWS

RIGHT   LEFT

LINGUAL VIEWS

RIGHT   LEFT

©1983 J.R. Steedle, J.B. McLain

Fig. 14-24 ■ This laboratory prescription form, on which the doctor draws what is wanted, is designed to be used with the components approach to functional appliances. The form allows the practitioner to choose the appliance components necessary to treat the malocclusion and modify and position them for maximum treatment effects. The example drawn here illustrates a posterior bite block on the left to limit eruption, combined with buccal and lingual shields on the right to encourage eruption while incorporating lip pads, a labial bow, and a lingual pad. The resulting appliance may not resemble any conventional appliance or any other components-approach appliance, but it addresses the patient's problems. (Courtesy Drs. J.R. Steedle and J.B. McLain.)

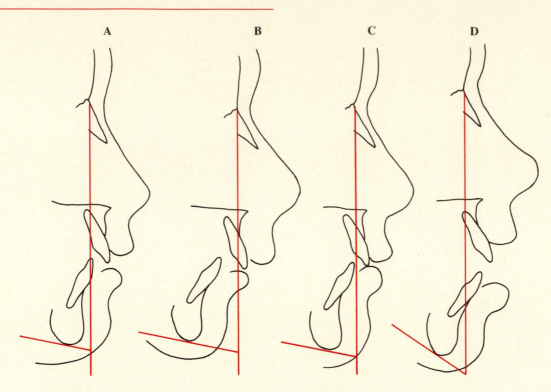

Fig. 14-25 ■ Combinations of skeletal components that can lead to a Class II malocclusion: **A,** maxillary protrusion with a normal mandible; **B,** mandibular retrusion with a normal maxilla; **C,** a combination of maxillary protrusion and mandibular retrusion; or **D,** downward and distal rotation of the mandible.

II jaw relationships are maxillary protrusion with normal mandibular position, mandibular retrusion with normal maxillary position, a combination of maxillary protrusion and mandibular retrusion, and downward rotation of the mandible, which is really a vertical problem although it produces a Class II relationship (Fig. 14-25). Treatment should be directed at the individual patient's particular problem area. Dental displacements, of course, may also be present and must be considered in planning treatment.

■ Maxillary Protrusion

Maxillary protrusion may be the result of a large maxilla or a normal maxilla that is anteriorly positioned relative to the cranial base. In either case, the goal is to restrict forward growth of the maxilla while the mandible grows into a more prominent and normal relationship with it (Fig. 14-26).

Extraoral force for maxillary protrusion. In a preadolescent child, extraoral force is almost always applied to the first molars via a facebow and a strap on the head or neck for anchorage. This direct approach to children with maxillary skeletal protrusion has been documented in numerous studies to produce a maxillary skeletal change.[26] To be effective for this purpose, headgear should be worn at least 12 to 14 hours per day with a force of 12 to 16 ounces (350 to 450 gm) per side. When teeth are used as the point of force application, some dental as well as skeletal effects must be expected. For this reason, relatively heavy but in-

termittent forces are applied to make use of the "hyalinization effect" that limits tooth movement and transmits the force to the skeletal structure. If moderate forces are continued for many hours per day, increasing amounts of dental changes will occur. Extremely heavy forces (greater than 1000 gm) are unnecessarily traumatic to the teeth and their supporting structures.

The direction of force must be compatible with the vertical relationships observed in the patient. A distal and inferior direction of headgear force will restrict forward maxillary growth but will allow or accentuate growth in a downward direction. If the mandible rotates in a clockwise direction and makes the lower face longer, this will nullify most of the forward mandibular growth that reduces the Class II relationship (Fig. 14-27). On the other hand, distal and superior headgear force will limit vertical maxillary development and should not be used on a patient who has a short face in conjunction with a Class II jaw relationship.

In theory, the movement of skeletal components can be controlled in the same way as a single tooth is controlled, by managing forces and moments relative to the center of resistance of the jaw (Fig. 14-28). In practice, it is difficult to analyze exactly where the center of resistance and center of rotation of the maxilla might be, but it is apparent that the line of force should be above the teeth. This is the major reason for including an upward direction of pull for most children who have headgear force to the maxilla.

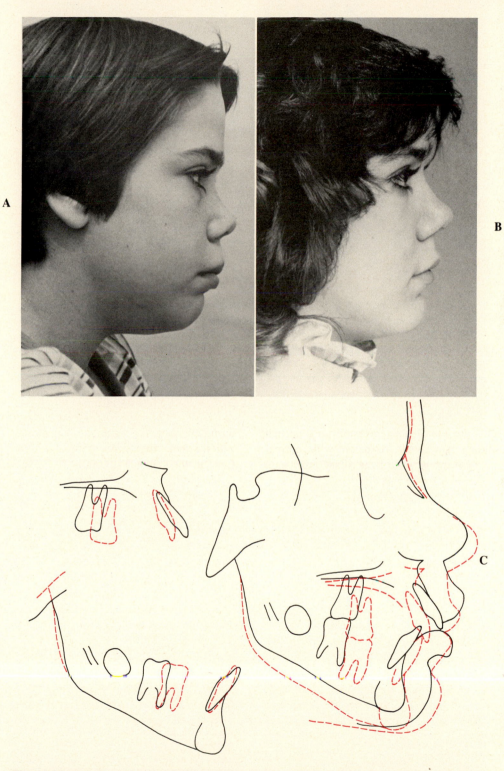

Fig. 14-26 ■ A Class II malocclusion resulting from maxillary skeletal protrusion, treated with a headgear and premolar extractions. **A,** This child has a convex profile and full lips before treatment. **B,** After treatment the face is less convex and the lip protrusion is reduced. **C,** The cranial base superimposition shows that the lips were retracted, the maxilla was directed inferiorly in response to the headgear, and the mandible grew inferiorly and forward. In the maxillary and mandibular superimpositions, the incisors were retracted and the molars moved forward.

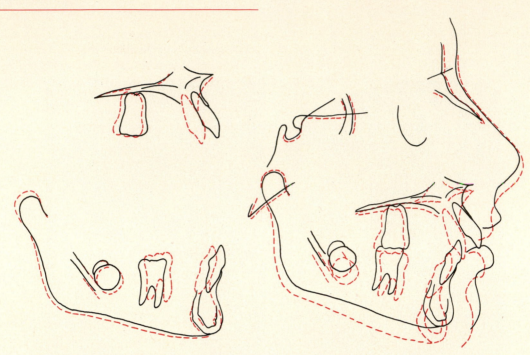

Fig. 14-27 ■ This child had a poor response to headgear treatment for a Class II malocclusion. The cranial base superimposition indicates that the lips were retracted and the maxilla did not grow anteriorly. The maxilla superimposition shows that the incisors were retracted and the molar movement and eruption were limited. All these effects were beneficial for Class II correction, but the mandible rotated inferiorly and backward because of the inferior movement of the maxilla and eruption of the lower molar. As a result, the profile is more convex than when treatment began and the Class II malocclusion is uncorrected.

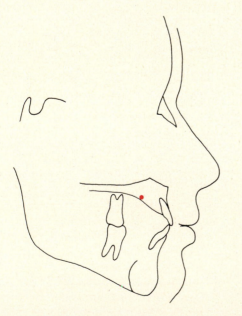

Fig. 14-28 ■ Although the center of resistance of the maxilla is difficult to estimate, a location above the roots of the premolar teeth has been proposed. If this theory is true, it is difficult to direct forces through the center of resistance by traditional force delivery systems.

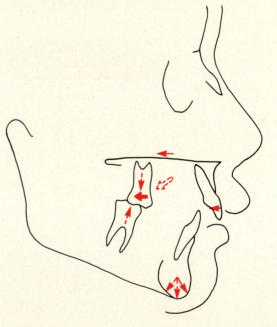

Fig. 14-29 ■ Headgear treatment can have several side effects that complicate correction of Class II malocclusions. If the child wears the appliance, maxillary skeletal and dental forward movement will be restricted or the maxilla and the teeth will be retracted. Although this retraction helps in correction of the Class II malocclusion, the mandible can be directed forward, inferiorly, or rotated clockwise to a more retrusive position. Inferior maxillary skeletal movement or maxillary and mandibular molar eruption, all shown in dashed arrows, can reduce or totally negate the beneficial treatment effects.

Headgear also has several side effects (Fig. 14-29). Since the forces are delivered to the maxilla via the teeth, there is some retraction of the maxillary dentition. In a child who exhibits dental protrusion as well as skeletal protrusion, this is a benefit, but in others whose dentitions are well related to the underlying skeletal structures, this effect can be deleterious. Extrusion or intrusion of teeth also can significantly alter overall treatment effects and result in clockwise and counterclockwise mandibular rotation.

There are two practical clinical problems to be solved during headgear selection. First, headgear anchorage location must be chosen that will provide a correct vertical component of force to the skeletal and dental structures. A high pull head cap (Fig. 14-30, *A*) will place a superior and

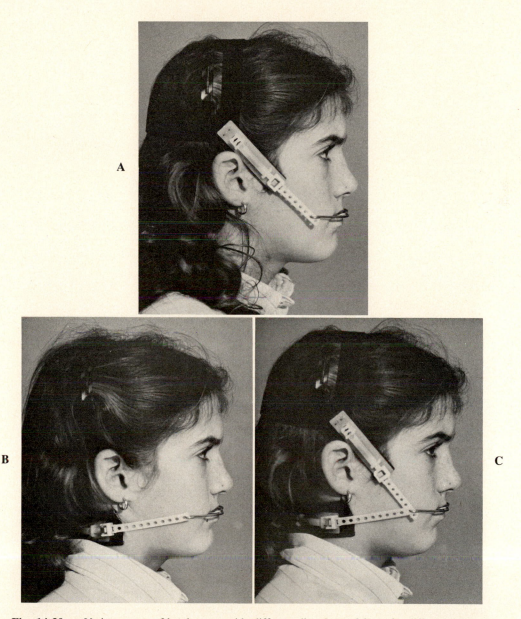

Fig. 14-30 ■ Various types of headgear provide different directions of force for different clinical situations. **A,** High-pull headgear consists of a head cap connected to a facebow. The appliance places a distal and upward force on the maxillary teeth and maxilla. **B,** Cervical headgear is made up of a neck strap connected to a facebow. This appliance produces a distal and downward force against the maxillary teeth and the maxilla. **C,** The combination headgear is a marriage of the high-pull and cervical headgears with both connected to a facebow. When the force is equal from each headgear, a distal and slightly upward force is placed on the maxillary teeth and maxilla. Varying the proportions of the total force derived from the head cap and neck strap allows the resultant force vector to be altered.

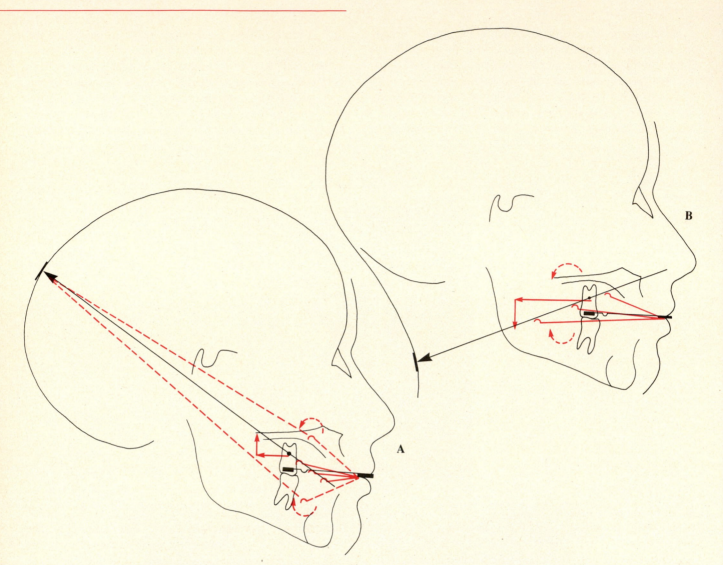

Fig. 14-31 ■ These diagrams illustrate effects on the maxillary permanent first molar from three commonly used types of facebow attachments. In each diagram, the inner bow is shown in black, various outer bow possibilities in red or dotted red. **A,** High pull headgear using a headcap. To produce bodily movement of the molar (no tipping), the line of force (black arrow) must pass through the center of resistance. This will produce both backward and upward movement of the molar. Note that the line of force is affected by the length and position of the outer bow, so that a longer outer bow bent up or a shorter one bent down could produce the same line of force. If bow length or position produces a line of force above or below the center of resistance (dotted red), the tooth will tip because of the moment that is produced. **B,** Cervical head gear using a neck strap. Again, bodily movement is produced by an outer bow length and position that places the line of force through the center of resistance, but with a lower direction of pull, the tooth is extruded as well as moved backward. Note that the outer bow of a facebow used with cervical traction nearly always is longer than the outer bow used with a high pull headcap. If the line of force is above or below the center of resistance, the tooth will tip, as indicated by the dotted arrows. **C,** Combination head gear using both a headcap and a neck strap. The resultant force vector (black) determines the movement of the molar, which in this example will be back and slightly up. With the resultant line through the center of resistance, the moments created by the headcap and neck strap cancel. Again, if the resultant force vector is above or below the center of resistance, the tooth will tip.

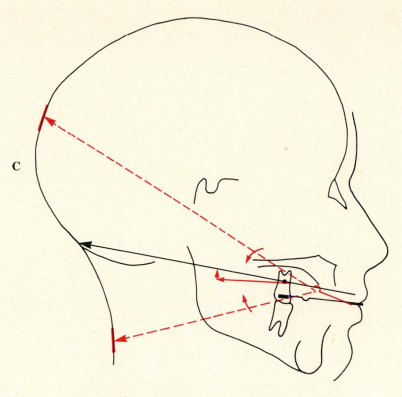

C

Fig. 14-31, cont'd ■ For legend see opposite page.

distal force on the teeth and maxilla. A cervical neck strap (Fig. 14-30, *B*) will place an inferior and distal force on the teeth and skeletal structures. When the head cap and neck strap are combined (Fig. 14-30, *C*), the force direction can be varied by altering the proportion of the total force provided by each component. If each delivers equal forces, the resultant force is slightly upward and distal for both teeth and maxilla.

The second decision is whether bodily movement of the first molars, distal root movement, or distal crown tipping is desired. Since the center of resistance for a molar is estimated to be in the midroot region, force vectors above this point will result in distal root movement. Forces through the center of resistance will cause bodily movement and vectors below this point will cause distal crown tipping. The length and position of the outer headgear bow relative to the center of resistance will determine the molar movement when combined with any of the forms of anchorage (headcap, neckstrap, or combination). The various combinations of force direction (anchorage), length of outer bow, and position of outer bow are diagrammatically illustrated in Fig. 14-31.

For headgear treatment in a preadolescent child, molar bands with headgear tubes in addition to other attachments that may be necessary later in treatment are fitted and cemented (see Chapter 12 for details). Preformed facebows

are supplied in a variety of inner bow sizes, and usually also have an adjustment loop as part of the inner bow. The inner bow should fit closely around the upper arch without contacting the teeth except at the molar tubes (within 3 to 4 mm of the teeth at all points) (Fig. 14-32). The correct size can be selected by fitting the bow against the maxillary cast. It is then placed into the tube on one side for an examination of how it fits relative to the other tube and the teeth. By adjusting the loops to expand or contract the inner bow and by bending the short portion of the bow that fits into the molar tubes, it is possible to make the bow passive, allow clearance from the teeth, and have the bow rest comfortably between the lips.

As a Class II molar relationship is corrected, the relative forward movement of the lower arch will produce a crossbite tendency unless the upper arch width is expanded. This must be taken into account from the beginning of treatment. The inner bow should be expanded by 2 mm symmetrically so that when it is placed in one tube, it rests just outside the other tube. The patient will need to squeeze the inner bow as it is inserted to make it fit the tubes, but this will provide the appropriate molar expansion.

The outer bow should rest several millimeters from the cheeks (Fig. 14-33). It must be cut to the proper length and have a hook formed at the end (Fig. 14-34). The length and the vertical position of the outer bow are selected relative

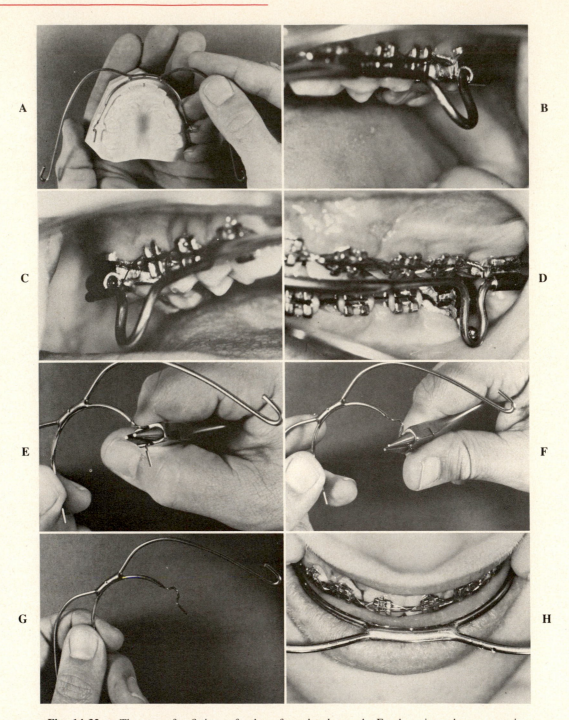

Fig. 14-32 ■ The steps for fitting a facebow for a headgear. **A,** Facebow inner bows come in graduated sizes. A simple method for selecting the appropriate size is to fit the bow to the pretreatment maxillary cast. **B,** After the bow is placed in one molar headgear tube, **C,** it is adjusted to be passive and aligned with the tube on the other molar band. It should be easy to insert and remove at this point. **D,** Often the adjustment loops mesial to the maxillary first molar need to be opened or closed to move the inner bow farther from or closer to the anterior teeth. **E,** Similarly, the inner bow must often be stepped away from the teeth in the buccal segments. This can be accomplished by bending the adjustment loop lingually and, **F,** the portion of the bow that inserts in the molar tube back to its original position. **G,** When the inner bow is then expanded, there is no interference with the buccal teeth. **H,** These adjustments should result in the inner bow being several millimeters from the teeth and, **I,** resting passively between the lips. Vertical adjustments can be made at the molar adjustment loops. **J,** The inner bow must be expanded by 1 to 2 mm to keep the posterior teeth out of crossbite as anteroposterior changes are made.

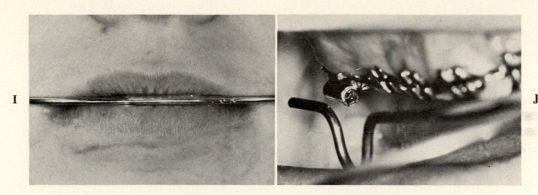

Fig. 14-32, cont'd ■ For legend see opposite page.

to the center of resistance to achieve the correct force direction (see Fig. 14-31). For example, if a cervical neck strap is to be used, either a medium-length high or long straight outer bow will provide distal root movement along with extrusion. With a cervical neck strap, a high short or low medium length outer bow will produce distal crown tipping along with distal and extrusive molar movement.

The appropriate head cap, neck strap, or combination of the two is fit by selecting the appropriate size. A spring mechanism to provide the force is strongly recommended. This is adjusted with the patient sitting up or standing, not reclining in the dental chair, until the desired force level is achieved (Fig. 14-35, *A* and *B*). It is usually a good idea to start with a low force level to acclimate the patient to the headgear and then gradually increase the force at subsequent appointments. Even if the correct force level is set at the first appointment, the forces will drop when the straps stretch slightly and contour to the patient. Once the forces are correct, the bow position must be rechecked since the pull of the straps often alters the previous bow position so that it needs adjustment.

The child should place and remove the headgear under supervision several times, to be certain that he or she understands how to manipulate it and to assure proper adjustment. Most headgear is worn after school and during sleep. It is definitely not indicated for vigorous activity, bicycle riding, or general roughhousing. Children should be informed that if anyone grabs the outer bow, they should grab the bow with their hands also. This will prevent breakage and injury. It is important for the headgear straps to be equipped with a safety release mechanism (Fig. 14-35, *C* to *E*) to prevent the bow from springing back at the child and injuring him if it is grabbed and pulled by a playmate. Severe injuries, including loss of sight, have occurred from headgear accidents of this type.

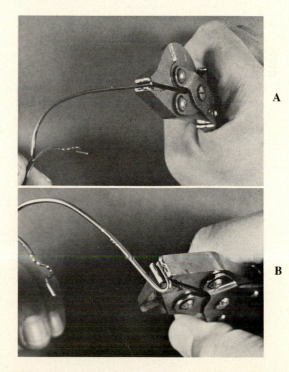

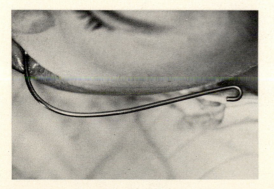

Fig. 14-33 ■ The outer bow should rest several millimeters from the soft tissue of the cheek. This adjustment must be checked both before and after the straps for the head cap or neck strap are attached.

Fig. 14-34 ■ The length of the outer bow is critical to the desired dental changes. **A,** After the correct length is chosen and the outer bow cut with a plier, **B,** a hook is bent at the end with a heavy plier.

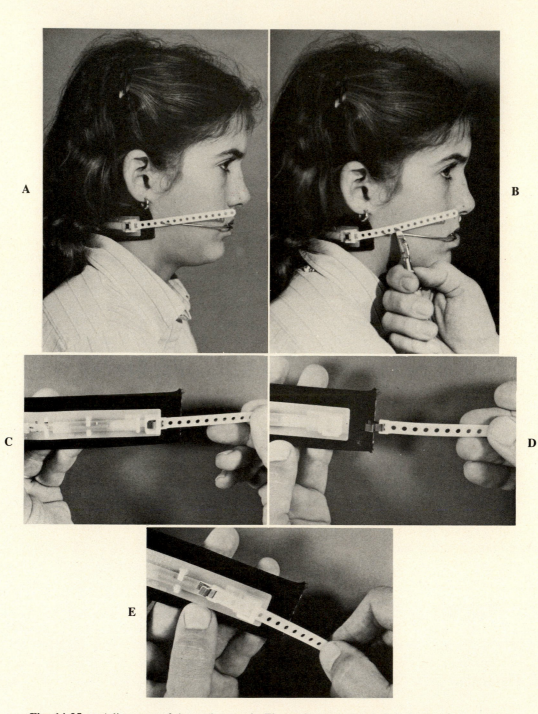

Fig. 14-35 ■ Adjustment of the neckstrap. **A,** The neckstrap is attached to the facebow and the proper force obtained from the spring mechanism by moving the hook to adjacent holes on the neckstrap. **B,** When the force is correct, the plastic connector is cut so that one extra hole is present in front of the correct hole. This provides a tab for the patient to grasp when placing the headgear. **C,** The spring mechanism delivers a predetermined force when the plastic connector is moved forward and aligned with a calibration mark. **D,** If the connector is stretched farther, such as it might be if someone grabbed the facebow and pulled on it, the plastic connector strap will release, preventing the bow from springing back into the patient's face. **E,** The connector can be threaded through the back of the mechanism to reassemble it after operation of the safety release.

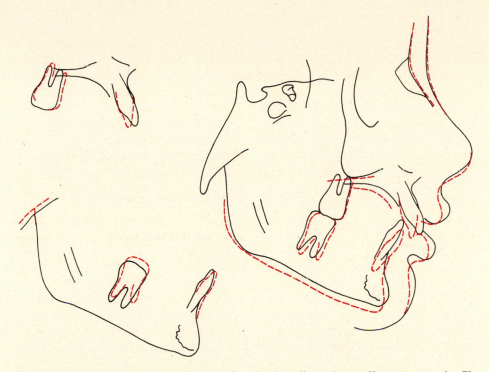

Fig. 14-36 ■ This child was treated with a functional appliance in an effort to correct the Class II malocclusion by changing the skeletal relationships. Note that the major skeletal change seen in the cranial base superimposition is the restriction of forward change of the maxilla. This "headgear effect" is observed in most functional appliance treatment that anteriorly positions the mandible to stimulate mandibular growth. Note also the differential eruption of the lower molars and forward movement of the lower teeth.

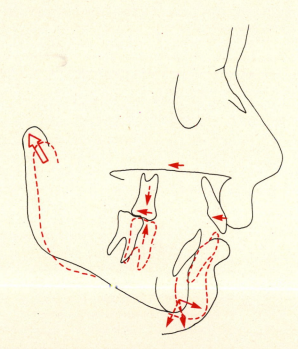

Fig. 14-37 ■ The side effects of functional appliance therapy for correction of a Class II skeletal malocclusion are illustrated here. The most desirable and variable effect is for the mandible to increase in length as shown by the open arrow. The "headgear effect" restrains the maxilla and the maxillary teeth, and mandibular repositioning often creates forces against the lower teeth that cause anterior movement of the mandibular dentition. The direction in which mandibular growth is expressed, forward, inferiorly, or clockwise, is most related to the eruption of the molars. If the molars erupt more than the ramus grows in height (dashed arrows), the forward mandibular change will be negated and the Class II malocclusion will not improve.

Functional appliances for maxillary protrusion. Although they are not commonly advocated for children with maxillary skeletal protrusion, functional appliances used to correct Class II problems nearly always have a "headgear effect" (Fig. 14-36). After the mandible has been positioned forward into the appliance, the stretched soft tissues pull the mandible back toward its normal retruded position. These distally directed forces are transmitted through the appliance to the maxillary dental and skeletal components. This results in restriction of maxillary anterior growth, to the extent that it is often difficult to distinguish between the effects of headgear and functional appliances on the maxilla.

To be effective, functional appliances should be worn approximately 16 to 18 hours per day, which means that there will be a nearly continuous force on the skeletal and dental structures. This force results in other effects that may not always facilitate treatment (Fig. 14-37). As with headgear, the distal force against the teeth tends to retract the maxillary dentition. This movement can be greater with a functional appliance than with headgear, depending on how the relationship between the labial bow and the anterior teeth is handled. Unlike headgear, most functional appliances exert a protrusive effect on the mandibular dentition because the appliance contacts the lower teeth and some of the reaction force from forward posturing of the mandible is transmitted to them. This "Class II elastics effect" can be quite helpful in children who have maxillary dental protrusion and mandibular dental retrusion in conjunction with a Class II skeletal problem. The same effect is deleterious, however, in patients who exhibit maxillary dental retrusion or mandibular dental protrusion. Mandibular dental protrusion usually contraindicates functional appliance treatment.

Functional appliances can also exert a treatment effect on the eruption of posterior teeth. If upper posterior teeth are prohibited from erupting and moving forward in a Class II malocclusion while lower posterior teeth are erupting up and forward, the resulting rotation of the occlusal plane contributes to correction of the Class II dental relationship. This is another treatment effect of most functional appliance

treatment for Class II problems (Fig. 14-38).[27] Excessive posterior eruption should be controlled so that forward growth of the mandible relative to the maxilla can be maximized. If there is a tendency toward excessive vertical facial development and limited overbite, further posterior eruption must be prevented by incorporating posterior stops or a bite block into the appliance design. Procedures in the clinical management of functional appliances are presented in the following section.

■ Mandibular Deficiency

Many children with a skeletal Class II relationship have a component of mandibular retrusion caused by either a small mandible or a normal mandible in a posterior position. One possibility is to hold the maxilla and, relatively speaking, let the mandible catch up (Fig. 14-39). This type of treatment corrects the Class II malocclusion but tends to fit the maxilla to the mandible and not to its ideal position. Some evidence indicates that patients who wear headgear to the maxilla exhibit more mandibular growth than untreated Class II patients, but the average extra growth, although statistically significant, is not of a magnitude that would be clinically significant.[7] Therefore, when headgear is used for mandibular deficient children, the most probable mechanism of treatment and the one that has been documented in the literature is that the mandible expresses its regular growth and catches up with the maxilla, which has been prevented from growing forward as it normally would.

A more obvious treatment for mandibular skeletal deficiency, clearly the treatment of choice if possible, is enhancement of mandibular skeletal growth (Fig. 14-40). It would be ideal if an appliance could be placed that would reliably increase mandibular growth. All of the previously mentioned functional appliances, whether tooth-borne or tissue-borne, purport to address skeletal mandibular retrusion by enhancement of mandibular growth. In theory, this growth occurs in response to the movement of the mandibular condyle out of the fossa and may be mediated by the reduced pressure on the condylar tissue or by the altered muscle tension on the condyle.

Animal studies have documented that an increase in cellular activity does take place when the mandible is positioned forward.[8,9] These studies documented small changes that were nonetheless significant in the animal model. It is more difficult to demonstrate the same types of changes in humans, because histologic examination of the condylar tissues is not possible. The response must be detected by cephalometric radiographic analysis. Given the inaccuracy of radiographic patient positioning and point locating techniques, a larger change must occur for the skeletal change to be as statistically significant as in histologic studies. (Since changes that cannot be detected clinically, even if statistically significant, are hard to call clinically significant, this factor does not seem to be an overwhelming bias.)

Another problem in the human studies of functional appliances is the variability of response among patients. This

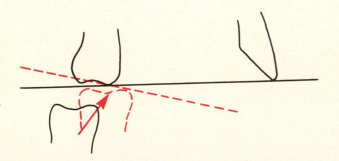

Fig. 14-38 ■ To facilitate Class II correction, the mesial and vertical eruption of the mandibular molar can be used advantageously. The upward and forward movement will improve the molar relationship and establish the posterior occlusal plane at a higher level.

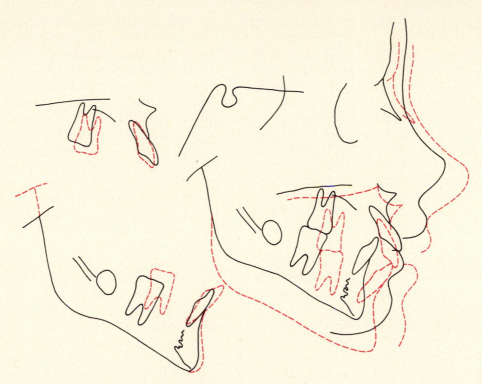

Fig. 14-39 ■ Headgear is sometimes used to treat children with a mandibular skeletal deficiency. Although there is some indication that mandibular growth may be stimulated by headgear treatment, most studies find the amount to be clinically insignificant. The cranial base superimposition for this patient, treated with headgear and Class II elastics, shows that during treatment, the maxilla moved mostly inferiorly, while the mandible moved down and forward. Fortunately, the large amount of molar eruption was balanced by growth of the ramus.

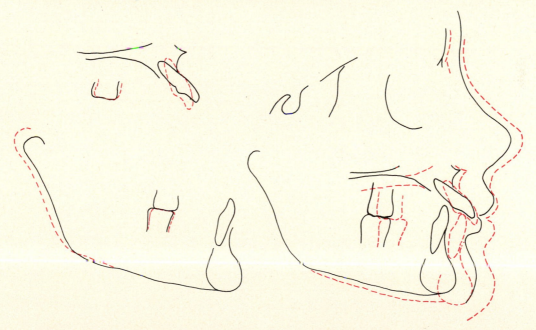

Fig. 14-40 ■ This child illustrates an excellent response to functional appliance therapy for a Class II malocclusion resulting from a mandibular deficiency. The cranial base superimposition indicates that the maxilla continued to develop in a downward and forward direction. The mandible grew almost directly forward and reduced both the Class II malocclusion and the mandibular deficiency. The maxillary and mandibular superimpositions show only lingual tipping of the maxillary incisors, which decreased the overjet. The lack of eruption of the molars contributed to the strongly forward expression of mandibular growth.

large variability has led to difficulty in detecting consistent treatment benefits.[28]

Nevertheless, most well constructed studies have found little anteroposterior difference in mandibular response between headgear and functional appliance treatment.[7] When differences between groups of patients have been detected, there is a small increment of mandibular growth in favor of the functional appliance group, so small that is is difficult to be sure it is clinically significant. On the other hand, some children treated with functional appliances exhibit much more mandibular growth than would be expected without treatment. It is probably fair to say that functional appliances aimed at stimulating mandibular growth produce a highly variable response, but the growth acceleration that sometimes occurs can be very useful.

Functional appliances intended to correct mandibular retrusion have the same dental side effects mentioned in the discussion of maxillary protrusion and inevitably have a skeletal effect on the maxilla also. Their tendency to tip the mandibular anterior teeth facially and retract the maxillary anterior teeth may not always be advantageous for correction of the overall Class II malocclusion. Most of the named appliances also allow mandibular molars to erupt and move in a mesial direction. This effect encourages a dental correction of the Class II malocclusion and increases the lower facial height of these patients. This result is beneficial for children who have decreased or normal lower face heights, but detrimental in those who have excessive lower face height (Fig. 14-41). These children must have the conventional appliances modified to reduce or inhibit eruption of lower posterior teeth to control mandibular rotation. In other words, functional appliance therapy for the Class II mandibular retrusive patient with increased lower face height must be managed very carefully if treatment benefits are to be realized, even in an optimally growing patient.

After the decision has been made to use a functional appliance and the treatment goals are outlined, the first step is to make impressions of the upper and lower arches and register the desired mandibular position, the "working bite." The impression technique depends on the appliance components that will be used. An accurate representation of the area where the lingual pads or flanges will be placed is mandatory. If buccal shields or lip pads are to be used, it is important not to overextend the impressions so that tissue is displaced, because this makes it difficult or impossible to accurately locate the appliance components in the vestibule.

The working bite is obtained with multiple layers of a wax hard enough to maintain its integrity after cooling to room temperature. The patient's preliminary record casts can be used to trim the wax to a size that will register all posterior teeth while not covering the anterior teeth (Fig. 14-42). With the anterior teeth exposed, the position of the mandible can easily be judged while the bite is being taken.

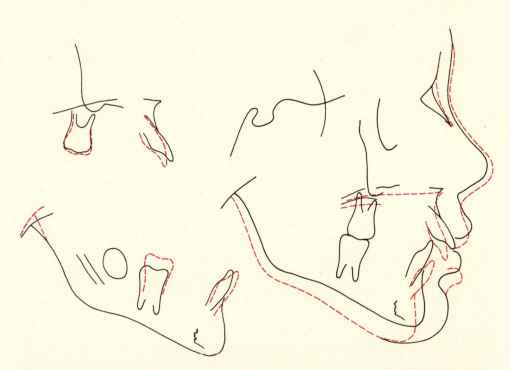

Fig. 14-41 ■ These tracings demonstrate a poor vertical response to Class II functional appliance treatment. Before treatment the child had a tendency toward increased lower face height and a convex profile. The cranial base superimposition indicates that the mandible rotated inferiorly and backward because of excessive eruption of the lower molar, which further increased the lower face height and facial convexity.

Care must be exercised not to produce any soft tissue interference with the wax, which will deflect the mandible or interfere with closure.

A working bite for a Class II patient is obtained by advancing the mandible forward to move the condyle from the fossa. Most clinicians recommend a 4 to 6 mm advancement, but always one that is comfortable for the patient and does not move the incisors past an edge-to-edge incisor relationship. Unless an asymmetry is to be corrected, the mandible should be advanced symmetrically so that the midline relationships do not change appreciably.

When the mandible is advanced, the bite must also be opened. There must be enough space for the laboratory technician to place wire and acrylic between the teeth to either connect major parts of the appliance or construct occlusal and incisor stops, and incisor interferences may require some additional opening. The minimal posterior opening is 3 to 4 mm. If dental changes from differential eruption are not a major part of the desired treatment response, wire occlusal stops (as in the Frankel appliance) can be used at this minimal opening. Interocclusal stops or facets to guide eruption, as in most activators and bionators, usually require 4 to 5 mm of posterior separation to be effective. If eruption of upper and lower posterior teeth is

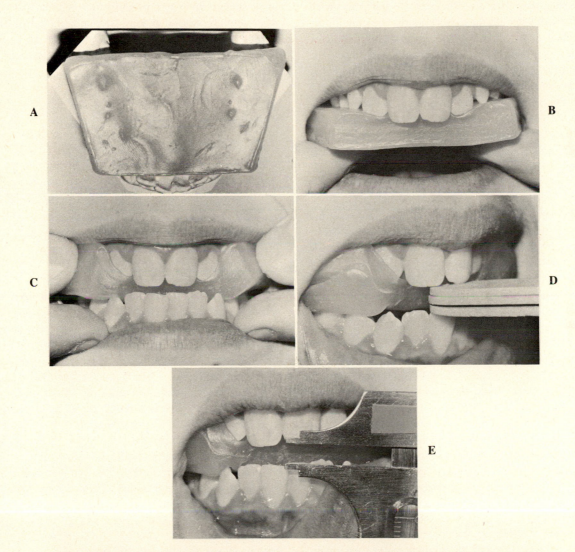

Fig. 14-42 ■ Steps for obtaining a "working bite" for functional appliance construction. **A,** Multiple layers of hard wax are luted together and cut to the size of the mandibular arch. Care must be taken not to cover the anterior teeth or extend the wax to areas of soft tissue interference. **B,** The softened wax is seated on the maxillary posterior teeth and pressed to place to ensure good indexing of the teeth. **C,** The mandible is guided to the correct anteroposterior and vertical position by observation of the midline relationships and the incisal separation. **D,** Either stacked tongue blades or, **E,** a Boley gauge can be used to control the amount of closure and help the patient reproduce the correct bite. The wax is then cooled with air and removed for inspection. Definite registration of both maxillary and mandibular teeth is required for proper appliance construction.

to be limited as in a child with a long face pattern, the working bite should be taken with the patient open 2 to 3 mm past the resting vertical dimension, so that the soft tissue stretch against the bite blocks will produce a continuous force opposing eruption.

While the wax is being softened in hot water, the child can practice the working bite position of the mandible. To produce the working bite, the technique is as follows (Fig. 14-42): first, firmly seat the softened wax on the maxillary arch so all teeth are indexed. Next, have the child position the mandible forward to the correct position and begin to close, paying careful attention to reproducing the previous midline relationship. Some children can easily reproduce working bites after only a few practice tries, but others need help. It is possible to aid these patients by constructing an index to guide them. This is most easily accomplished by using a stack of tongue blades with notches carved into the top and bottom blade (Fig. 14-42, *D*). This guide will stop the bite closure at the predeterminined jaw separation and determine the anteroposterior mandibular position at the same time. Other children can be directed very simply with the use of a Boley gauge held near the teeth and "coaching" (Fig. 14-42, *E*). When the correct bite has been obtained, the wax should be cooled and removed from the mouth. The bite should be examined for adequate dental registration and rechecked for accuracy.

The prescription for the laboratory should emphasize the desired components, which is accomplished best by a drawing. A prescription form that makes it easier to use the components approach is shown in Fig. 14-24.

When the functional appliance is returned from the laboratory, it should be checked for correct construction and fit on the working cast. The best technique for delivery is to adjust the appliance and work with the child to master insertion and removal before any discussion with the parent. This approach enables the child to be the full focus of attention initially and forestalls the effect of comments by the parents like "How could she possibly get that big thing in her mouth?"

With any functional appliance, a break-in period is helpful. Having the child wear the appliance only a short time per day to begin with, and increasing this time gradually over the first few weeks, improves compliance later. The child should be informed that speaking may be difficult for a while, but that comfort and speaking facility will increase. A good appointment schedule is to see the child at 1 week if problems are developing, but certainly at 2 weeks for inspection of the tissues and the appliance and to evaluate compliance. If a sore spot develops, the child should be encourage to wear the appliance a few hours each day for 2 days before the appointment, so the source of the problem can be determined accurately. Usually smoothing of the acrylic components can be accomplished quickly. Gross adjustments should be avoided, because appliance fit and purpose can be greatly altered. For example, heavy reduc-

tion of the lingual flange will allow the patient to position the mandible in a more posterior position.

Most components that occupy the vestibular area have a high potential for irritation if overextended or oriented improperly to the soft and hard tissue. It is not unusual to have to trim back buccal shields, but this should not be overdone. Lip pads facial to the lower incisors may have to be adjusted and contoured during treatment to eliminate gingival irritation.

Since the mandibular advancement is limited to a modest 4 to 6 mm and many children require more anteroposterior correction, a new appliance may be needed after 6 to 12 months of wear and a favorable response. It is a good idea to reevaluate appliance progress at 6 months after delivery with new records or at least a cephalometric headfilm. If changes have not occurred in that time, either compliance is poor or the design is improper. In either case, a new treatment plan is needed.

■ *Treatment for Class III Jaw Relationships*

Class III skeletal relationships result from a normal maxilla and mandibular skeletal protrusion, maxillary retrusion and a normal mandible, or a combination of maxillary skeletal retrusion and mandibular skeletal protrusion (Fig. 14-43). The treatment of choice, insofar as possible, is to correct the faulty skeletal component.

■ Maxillary Retrusion

For children with skeletal maxillary retrusion, the preferred treatment is to move the maxilla into a more anterior position, which also increases its size as bone is added at the posterior sutures. This is most possible in young children (see Chapter 10). In children under age 8, this treatment can be accomplished with a facemask that obtains anchorage from the forehead and chin and exerts force on the maxilla via elastics that attach to a maxillary splint, producing both tooth movement and displacement of the maxilla (Fig. 14-44). In older children (above 9 years of age), the same treatment produces more dental movement and usually very little skeletal change. Pulling the maxillary teeth forward simply produces dental compensation for the skeletal malocclusion and does not provide the ideal result.

Extraoral force to move the maxilla forward is best for children in the 6- to 8-year-old age group who have erupted permanent central incisors and first molars. To resist tooth movement as much as possible, the maxillary teeth should be splinted together into a single unit. Although it is possible to use a heavy wire crib with attachments on the primary molars and whatever permanent teeth are available, an acrylic occlusal splint usually gives better results. If necessary, the splint can be bonded in place, but this causes hygiene problems and should be avoided if possible. Multiple clasps

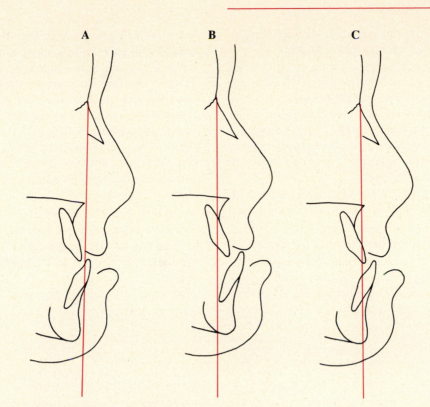

Fig. 14-43 ■ Combinations of skeletal structures that can lead to a Class III malocclusion: **A,**
maxillary retrusion with a normal mandible; **B,** mandibular protrusion with a normal maxilla; **C,**
a combination of maxillary retrusion and mandibular protrusion.

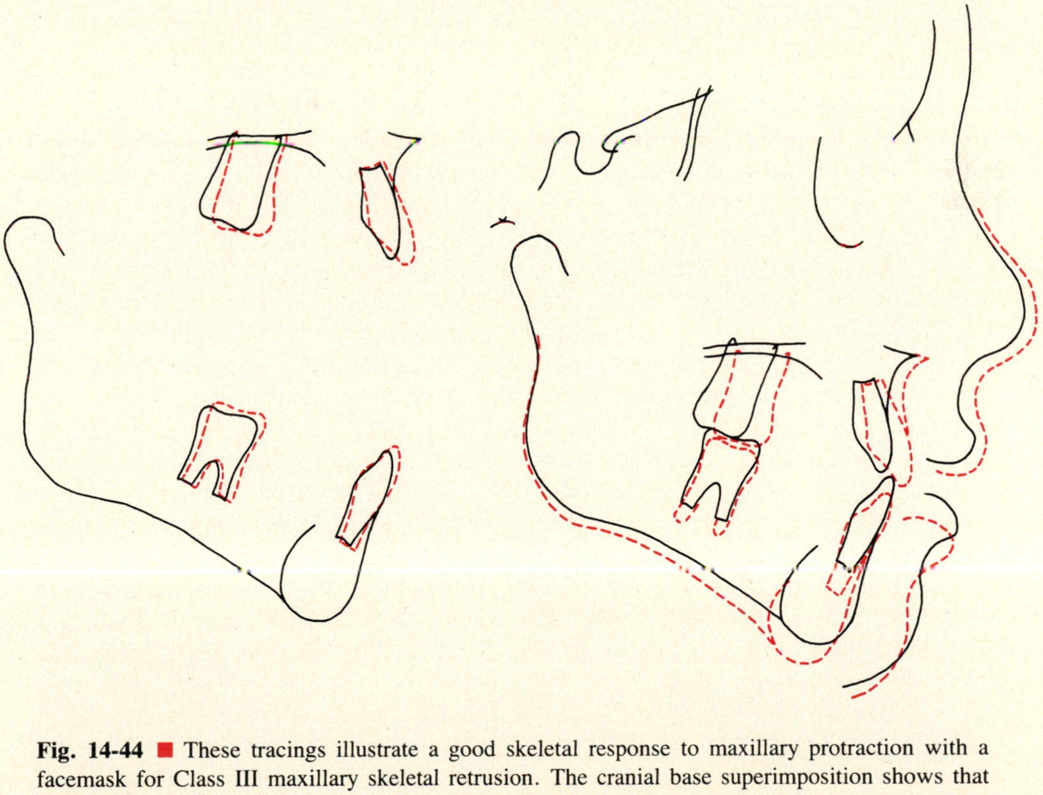

Fig. 14-44 ■ These tracings illustrate a good skeletal response to maxillary protraction with a
facemask for Class III maxillary skeletal retrusion. The cranial base superimposition shows that
the maxilla was moved forward during the treatment period, whereas the maxillary superimposition
shows that the maxillary teeth moved forward a lesser amount. In young growing children, the
magnitude of the skeletal change is usually greater than the dental change.

combined with acrylic that extends over the incisal edges usually provide adequate retention (Fig. 14-45).

Contouring an adjustable facemask for a comfortable fit in the forehead is not difficult for most children (Fig. 14-46), but may be challenging for the patient who wears eyeglasses. The plastic forehead and chin pads occasionally require relining with acrylic for an ideal fit or with an adhesive backed protective pad to reduce soft tissue irritation. For most young children, however, a facemask is as well accepted as conventional headgear.

Approximately 12 ounces of force per side is applied for 14 hours per day. The elastics should be fastened to the splint in the canine primary first molar area to reduce the tendency for the maxilla to rotate as it comes forward. Most children with maxillary deficiency are deficient vertically as well as anteroposteriorly, which means that a slight downward direction of pull is usually desirable. Lowering the maxilla increases face height and rotates the mandible downward and backward, which also contributes to correct the skeletal Class III relationship. A downward pull would be contraindicated, however, if face height were already large.

Another treatment sometimes advocated for maxillary skeletal retrusion is a functional appliance made with the mandible positioned posteriorly and rotated open (Fig. 14-

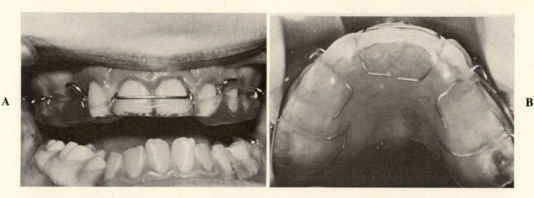

Fig. 14-45 ■ A maxillary removable splint is often used to make the upper arch a single unit for maxillary protraction. **A,** The splint incorporates hooks in the canine-premolar region for attachment of elastics and, **B,** should cover the anterior and posterior teeth and occlusal surfaces for best retention. Multiple clasps also aid in retention.

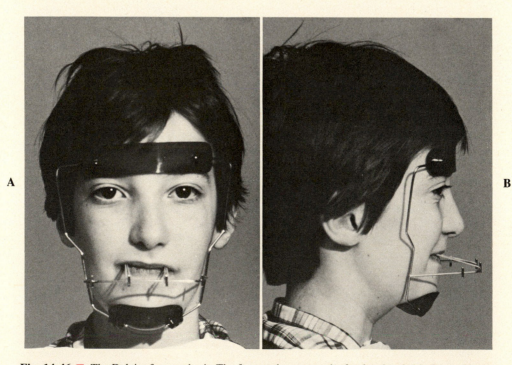

Fig. 14-46 ■ The Delaire facemask. **A,** The facemask contacts the forehead and chin for anchorage and should be adjusted several millimeters away from the other soft tissues. **B,** Adjustment of the wire framework will produce the desired fit and direction of pull on the maxilla when the elastics are placed from the mask to splint.

47). In theory, lip pads, as used in the Frankel appliance, stretch periosteum in a way that pulls the maxilla forward. Clinical experience suggests that variable results are obtained,[34] and often there is little evidence of a true forward movement of the upper jaw (Fig. 14-48).

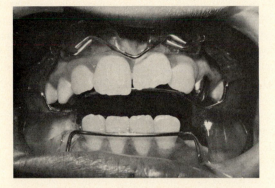

Fig. 14-47 ■ The Frankel III appliance stretches the soft tissue adjacent to the maxilla, attempting to stimulate forward growth of the maxilla by stretching the periosteum, and does not advance the mandible. The vertical opening is used to enhance downward and forward eruption of maxillary posterior teeth.

Most functional appliances for treatment of Class III malocclusion make no pretense of increasing the size of the maxilla or moving the maxilla in a more anterior position, but correct the malocclusion by facially tipping the maxillary anterior teeth and retracting the mandibular anterior teeth.[4] This tooth movement helps in the development of a normal overbite and overjet, but has no effect on the skeletal malocclusion. Class III functional appliances also routinely allow the maxillary molars to erupt and move mesially while holding the lower molars in place vertically and anteroposteriorly. The rotation of the occlusal plane and the tooth movement contribute to the change from a Class III to a Class I molar relationship (Fig. 14-49). If the functional appliance rotates the chin down and back (see following), the Class III relationship will improve, but again with no effect on the maxilla. In short, functional appliance treatment, except for the use of upper lip pads, has no effect on maxillary retrusion, and lip pads are limited in their effectiveness.

To produce the working bite for a Class III functional appliance, the steps in preparation of the wax, practice for the patient, and the use of a guide to determine the correct

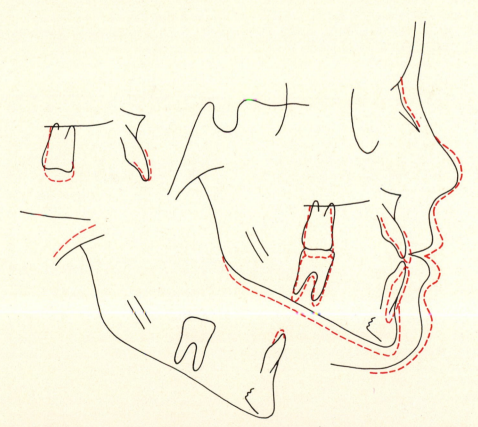

Fig. 14-48 ■ These tracings demonstrate no maxillary skeletal growth stimulation or mandibular growth restriction in response to Class III functional appliance therapy, although the anterior dental relationships have improved by tipping the anterior teeth. Note the differential eruption of the upper molar, which also contributes to correction of the occlusal relationships.

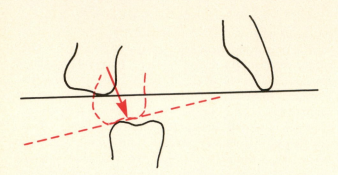

Fig. 14-49 ■ To facilitate Class III correction, the mesial and vertical eruption of the maxillary molar can be emphasized. This will improve the molar relationships and establish the posterior occlusal plane at a lower level.

vertical position are identical to the procedure for Class II patients. However, the working bite itself is significantly different: the mandible is rotated open on its hinge axis but is not advanced. This type of bite is easier for the dentist to direct since light force can be placed on the chin point to retrude the mandible and seat the condyles in the fossa. How far the mandible is rotated open depends on the type of appliance and the need to interpose bite blocks and occlusal stops between the teeth to limit eruption. Less vertical opening would be needed for an appliance with lip pads to try to encourage forward movement of the maxilla than for one that encourages eruption and deliberately rotates the mandible significantly back. Appliance adjustments and instructions are similar to those for Class II appliances except that the maxillary anterior lip pads often cause soft tissue irritation and must be observed carefully.

■ Mandibular Protrusion

Children who have Class III malocclusion because of excessive growth of the mandible are extremely difficult to treat. The treatment of choice would be to reduce the size of the mandible or at least prevent it from increasing in size, but there is little or no evidence to substantiate the idea that appliances can reduce mandibular growth. Many of these patients ultimately need surgery if they have severe problems.

For growth modification treatment of mandibular prognathism, both functional appliances and chin cups have been used before and throughout the adolescent growth spurt. Class III functional appliances for excessive mandibular growth are designed to rotate the mandible down and back and to produce proper occlusal relationships by allowing the upper posterior teeth to erupt down and forward while restraining eruption of mandibular teeth. This approach does not really restrain mandibular growth, but does change the direction in which it is expressed (Fig. 14-48). This type of treatment is appropriate with normal or reduced lower anterior face height but is definitely contraindicated for a child who has excessive lower face height from the beginning. These appliances also tip the mandibular incisors lin-

gually and the maxillary incisors facially, introducing an element of dental camouflage for the skeletal discrepancy. The sum total of these changes can produce an acceptable result in a child who has a Class I skeletal pattern and a mild skeletal discrepancy, or a pseudo–Class III problem because of an anterior shift, but there is simply no way to correct severe mandibular prognathism with this approach to treatment.

Another treatment that has been used for decades to treat mandibular skeletal protrusion is a chin cup attached to a head cap for anchorage. In theory, extraoral force directed against the mandibular condyle would restrain growth at that location, but most studies have found little difference in mandibular dimensions between treated and untreated subjects.[29] What chin cup therapy does accomplish is lingual tipping of the lower incisors as a result of the pressure of the appliance on the lower lip and dentition, and a change in the direction of mandibular growth, rotating the chin down and back (Fig. 14-50). Children who have increased lower anterior face height and are treated with chin cups may end up with skeletal open bites after treatment. The effects, in other words, are rather similar to those obtained with Class III functional appliances, and the two approaches are approximately equally effective.

A hard chin cup can be custom fitted from acrylic, using an impression of the chin; a commercial metal or plastic cup can be used if it fits well enough; or a soft cup can be made from a football helmet chin strap. Any of these can irritate the soft tissue of the chin and may require a protective liner or talcum powder for comfort. The more the chin cup or strap migrates up toward the lower lip during appliance wear, the more lingual movement of the lower incisors will be produced. Soft cups tend to produce more tooth movement than hard ones.

The head cap that includes the spring mechanism can be the same one used for high pull headgear. It is adjusted in the same manner as the headgear so as to direct a force of approximately 16 to 24 ounces per side through the head of the condyle, or a somewhat lighter force below the condyle.

■ *Treatment for Vertical and Transverse Problems*

■ Vertical Excess

Children with excessive face height (skeletal open bite or long face syndrome) generally have a normal upper face and normal maxilla. This problem has been described as vertical maxillary excess but recent data indicate that before adolescence, most of the anatomic discrepancies from normal are located below the palatal plane.[30] These children usually exhibit an anterior open bite, and they nearly always have some excessive eruption of posterior teeth. Most have a short mandibular ramus, which accounts for the steep mandibular plane and the large discrepancy between pos-

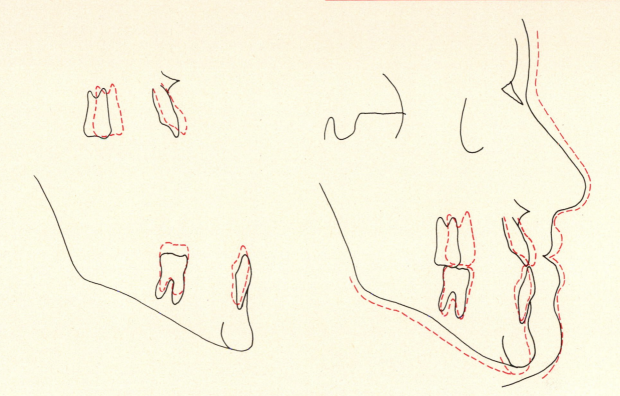

Fig. 14-50 ■ These tracings illustrate a typical response to chin cup treatment. The cranial base superimposition shows that the mandible rotated inferiorly and backward to a less prominent position and that the maxillary incisors moved facially as the mandibular incisors tipped lingually in response to the pressure of the chin cup. This treatment reduces mandibular protrusion and increases lower anterior face height.

terior and anterior face height. The ideal treatment for these patients would be to control all subsequent growth so that the mandible would rotate in a counterclockwise direction, upward and forward (Fig. 14-51). Unfortunately, vertical facial growth extends into the adolescent and postadolescent years, which means that even if growth can be modified successfully in the mixed dentition, active retention is likely to be necessary for a number of years.

One approach to vertical excess problems is to maintain the vertical position of the maxilla and inhibit eruption of the maxillary posterior teeth. This can be attempted with high-pull headgear to the posterior teeth, worn 14 hours a day with a force greater than 12 ounces per side (Fig. 14-52). If the headgear involves a conventional facebow to the first molar, delivery and adjustment of the headgear are identical to the high-pull headgear described previously for Class II problems.

An alternative headgear approach for children with excessive vertical development is the addition of an anterior plate to the inner bow (Cervera headgear, Fig. 14-53) or the use of an acrylic occlusal splint attached to the face-bow.[31] This allows vertical force to be directed against all the maxillary teeth, not just the molars. An appliance of this type would be most useful in a child with excessive vertical development of the entire maxillary arch and too much exposure of the maxillary incisors from beneath the

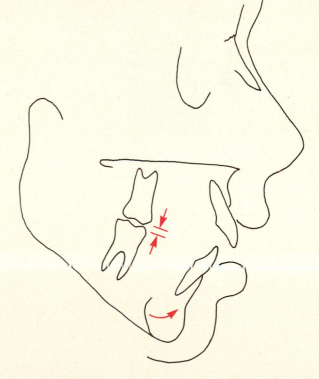

Fig. 14-51 ■ Children with excessive lower face height can be treated successfully by restricting posterior eruption, which allows mandibular growth to be expressed in an anterior direction as the mandible rotates counterclockwise.

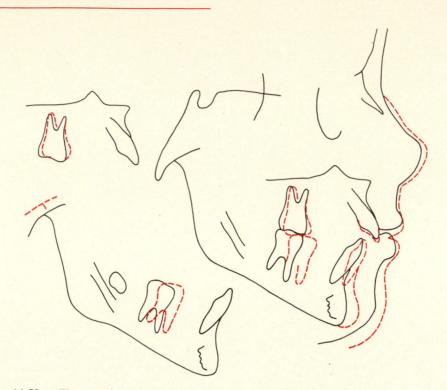

Fig. 14-52 ■ These tracings show an excellent response to high-pull headgear for a child with excessive lower face height. The cranial base superimposition demonstrates that the maxilla and the maxillary teeth did not move inferiorly and as a result the mandible moved forward and not inferiorly. The lower molar drifted forward into the leeway space.

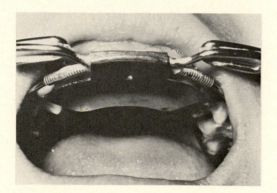

Fig. 14-53 ■ A bite plate, as in this Cervera headgear, or acrylic splint can be added to the inner bow of a high-pull headgear so that forces are directed against more teeth than just the molars, and vertical maxillary control is increased.

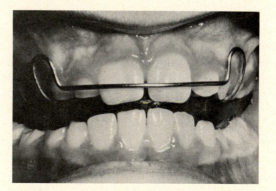

Fig. 14-54 ■ The bite blocks incorporated in this functional appliance are used to control vertical changes by limiting the eruption of all posterior teeth with bite blocks. The anterior teeth are free to erupt and will contribute to closing anterior open bites.

lip. To achieve both skeletal and dental correction, the patient must be compliant throughout what can be a very long treatment period.

Unfortunately, even though extraoral force can inhibit vertical maxillary growth and eruption of the maxillary teeth, the headgear allows mandibular dental eruption to proceed. If these teeth erupt freely, there may be no redirection of growth and favorable counterclockwise rotation of the mandible. In addition, headgear treatment by itself

will not be successful in reducing the amount of anterior open bite if it is present.

A better alternative is the use of a functional appliance that includes posterior bite blocks (Fig. 14-54). The purpose is to inhibit eruption of posterior teeth and vertical descent of the maxilla. The appliance can be designed with or without positioning the mandible anteriorly, depending on how much mandibular deficiency is present. Regardless of whether it is brought forward in the working bite, the man-

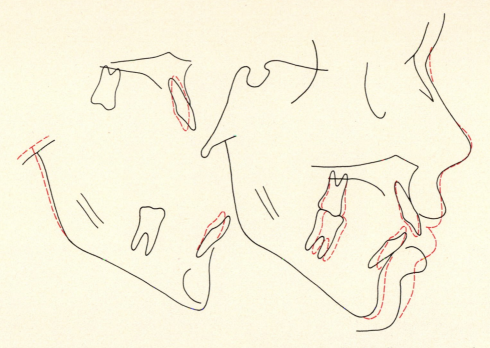

Fig. 14-55 ■ These tracings demonstrate a good response to functional appliance treatment designed to control vertical development with posterior bite blocks in a child with excessive lower face height. The superimpositions indicate that no posterior eruption occurred and all mandibular growth was directed anteriorly. Face height was maintained and anterior eruption closed the open bite.

dible must be opened past the normal resting vertical dimension. When it is held in this position by the appliance, the stretch of the soft tissues (including but not limited to the muscles) exerts a vertical intrusive force on the posterior teeth. In children with anterior open bites the anterior teeth are allowed to erupt, which reduces the open bite, while in the less common long face problems without open bite, all teeth are held by the bite blocks. Since there is no compensatory posterior eruption, all mandibular growth will be directly anteriorly.

In the short term, this type of functional appliance treatment is effective in controlling vertical facial growth and closing anterior open bites (Fig. 14-55). The long time period of vertical growth means that if a functional appliance is used for the first phase of treatment, posterior bite blocks or other components to control vertical growth and eruption will be needed during fixed appliance therapy (Fig. 14-56) and probably into retention, because fixed appliances do not control eruption well.

As an interesting sidelight, the same principle of inhibiting eruption of posterior teeth can be used during functional appliance treatment of children with anteroposterior mandibular deficiency, in an effort to take maximal advantage of mandibular growth by having it expressed in an anterior direction. A child treated in this manner may exhibit a posterior open bite after anteroposterior correction when the appliance is not in place (Fig. 14-57). The posterior bite

block, which is usually constructed of acrylic, can be relieved at that point so that slow eruption of posterior teeth back into occlusion can occur. This type of treatment places into sharp focus the interaction between the anteroposterior and vertical planes of space that must be addressed during growth modification treatment.

■ Vertical Deficiency

Some children exhibit skeletal vertical deficiencies or short faces, usually in conjunction with an anterior deep

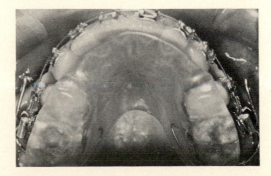

Fig. 14-56 ■ During fixed appliance treatment, posterior eruption can be controlled by using a removable posterior bite block that opens the bite and causes an intrusive force to be placed on teeth in contact with the block. The appliance is retained by clasps over the headgear tubes.

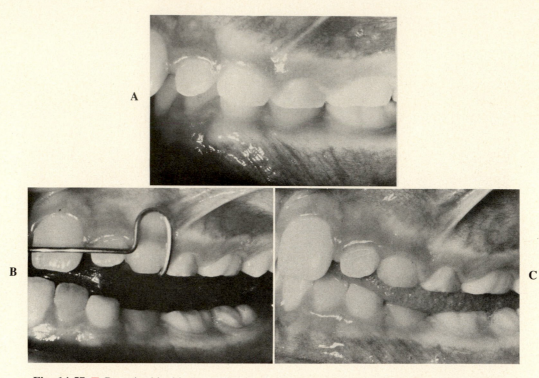

Fig. 14-57 ■ Posterior bite blocks can be used with any appliance that advances the mandible in an effort to limit posterior eruption and take maximum advantage of growth in an anteroposterior direction. **A,** The pretreatment occlusal relationships; **B,** when the mandible is advanced, the acrylic prevents posterior eruption. **C,** After a phase of appliance therapy that resulted in anteroposterior changes, there is a posterior open bite that can be closed by adjusting the acrylic bite blocks.

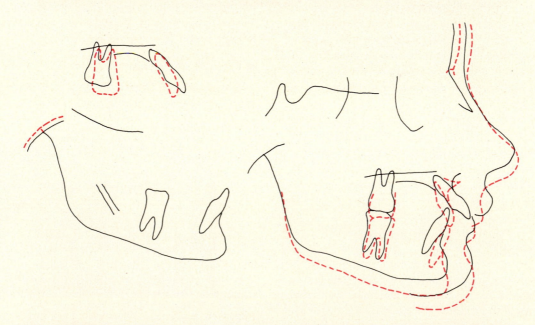

Fig. 14-58 ■ These tracings show increased vertical development in a child who initially had decreased lower anterior face height. This result was accomplished by increasing the maxillary molar eruption with a cervical pull headgear, which resulted in downward movement of the mandible.

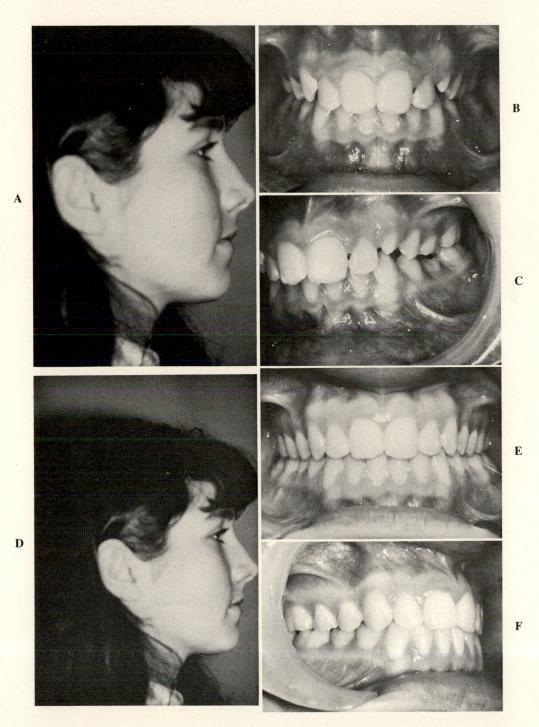

Fig. 14-59 ■ Illustration of treatment to increase vertical development in a child who initially had a Class II malocclusion and slightly decreased lower anterior face height. This result was accomplished by using a functional appliance. **A,** Before treatment the facial profile is convex with equal contributions of maxillary protrusion and mandibular retrusion. **B,** The overbite is increased, **C,** as is the overjet, and the molar and canine relationships are Class II. **D,** The posttreatment facial profile is less convex and the vertical facial proportions are well balanced. **E, F,** The overbite has been reduced and the molar and canine relationships are Class I.   *Continued.*

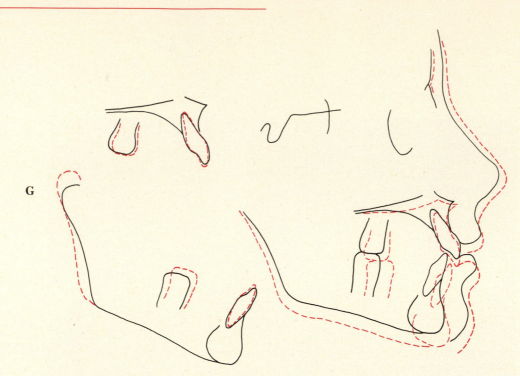

Fig. 14-59, cont'd ■ **G,** The tracings indicate that the correction was accomplished by limiting anterior movement of the maxilla while the mandible grew downward and forward. The maxillary and mandibular superimpositions show little incisor change, in conjunction with eruption of the lower molar, which increased the vertical facial development and aided in the Class II dental correction.

bite and a Class II division 2 malocclusion. The reduced lower anterior face height is often accompanied by long and protrusive lips, which would be appropriate if the face height were normal. Children who have vertical deficiencies can be identified at an early age. They have normal maxillas (except for those with a history of cleft palate surgery, who fall into a totally different category), but decreased eruption of maxillary and mandibular teeth. They have low mandibular plane angles and a tendency toward a long mandibular ramus. Growth is expressed in an anterior direction, with a

tendency toward counterclockwise rotation of the mandible. The challenge in correcting these problems is to increase the dental eruption, especially in the posterior area, and to influence the mandible to rotate in a clockwise direction without decreasing chin prominence too much.

There are two ways to increase face height in a vertically deficient child. One is with cervical headgear, taking advantage of the extrusive tendency of extraoral force directed below the center of resistance of the teeth and the maxilla (Fig. 14-58). The other is to use a functional appliance that

Fig. 14-60 ■ Pretreatment alignment for functional appliance patients. **A,** Crowded and lingually positioned maxillary incisors can prevent the mandible from advancing into an appropriate working bite; **B,** patient after alignment and labial positioning of the incisors, with the mandible postured forward as it would be in the functional appliance bite registration.

allows free eruption of the posterior teeth. Since most short face children also have a Class II malocclusion, it can be significant whether the eruption that occurs during treatment is primarily of the upper or the lower molars. Cervical headgear produces more eruption of the upper molars, while with a functional appliance eruption can be manipulated so that the increased vertical height can be gained with eruption of either the upper or the lower molar. Class II correction, however, is easier if the lower molar erupts more than the upper, which means that, all other factors being equal, the functional appliance would be preferred (Fig. 14-59).

Some children who have a short face, mandibular deficiency, and a Class II division 2 incisor pattern have such deep overbite and upright or retrusive maxillary incisors that it is not possible to advance the mandible for correct positioning in the functional appliance. For these children, alignment and forward positioning of the upper incisors should be accomplished as the first phase of treatment (Fig. 14-60). This approach will create overjet and a Class II division 1 malocclusion. At this point an appropriate working bite can be obtained with the mandible positioned anteriorly and inferiorly to correct the horizontal and vertical deficiency.

Most patients who are growing respond to a functional appliance with enhanced eruption, but increased mandibular growth is more variable. Some short face children show extremely rapid mandibular growth when the incisor interferences are removed. Unfortunately, this phenomenon does not always occur. The functional appliance delivery and adjustment are similar to that already discussed under mandibular retrusion.

■ Maxillary Constriction

Skeletal maxillary constriction is distinguished by a narrow palatal vault. It can be corrected by opening the midpalatal suture, which widens the roof of the mouth and the floor of the nose. Growth at this suture is an important mechanism for normal widening of the arch, which continues in most children until the late teens, then ceases. Opening the midpalatal suture to increase the width of the maxilla is relatively easy in preadolescent children. With increasing age, the suture becomes more and more tightly interdigitated, and opening it eventually becomes very difficult, but in most individuals, it remains possible to obtain significant increments in maxillary width up to age 15 to 18.

Sutural expansion is accomplished by placing a relatively heavy force directed across the suture to move the halves of the maxilla apart. A fixed appliance is required because the necessary force magnitude is large enough to displace removable appliances. As many teeth as possible should be included in the anchorage unit.

As mentioned earlier (see Chapter 8), several forms of palatal expansion have been advocated. Rapid palatal expansion (RPE) involves the use of a heavy force directed across the midpalatal suture to open it by forcing the halves of the maxilla away from one another. Force of 5 to 7 pounds

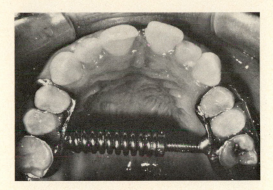

Fig. 14-61 ■ This rapid palatal expander uses a screw device together with a spring to deliver the forces to the maxilla. The spring produces more constant force levels than are obtained with a nonflexible system.

is usually advocated, for an active treatment period of 2 to 4 weeks. The appliance is activated by the patient making one or two quarter-turns of a screw type device each day. This amounts to 0.25 or 0.5 mm of activation daily. When a screw is the only activating device, the force is transmitted immediately to the teeth and then to the suture. Sometimes a large coil spring is incorporated along with the screw, which modulates the amount of force, depending on the length and stiffness of the spring (Fig. 14-61).

Regardless of the method of force application, the suture is separated faster than bone can be deposited along its margins, and a void is formed. The expansion proceeds faster and to a greater extent at the anterior portion of the palate, probably because of the buttressing effect of the other maxillary structures in the posterior regions. A large diastema usually appears between the central incisors as the bones separate in this area (Fig. 14-62). The diastema closes spontaneously during the next few weeks because of the pull of the supracrestal gingival fibers. Also both the maxillary bones and the posterior teeth tip slightly. This tipping leads to interferences between the lingual cusps of the maxillary molars and the lower posterior teeth and causes at least a transitional opening of the bite. Expansion is usually continued until the maxillary lingual cusps occlude with the lingual inclines of the buccal cusps of the mandibular molars.

When expansion has been completed, a 3-month period of retention with the appliance in place is recommended. Theoretically, during this time bone fills in the space that was created between the left and right halves of the maxilla. Some skeletal relapse begins to occur almost immediately, even though the teeth are held in position. The net treatment effect, therefore, is a combination of skeletal and dental effects (see Chapter 8). After the 3-month retention period, the fixed appliance should be removed, but a removable retainer that covers the palate is often needed as further insurance against early relapse (Fig. 14-63).

As discussed in Chapter 8, it now appears that slower activation of the expansion appliance, producing 2 pounds

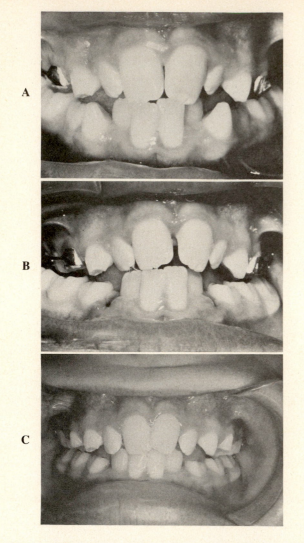

A

B

C

Fig. 14-62 ■ Spacing of the maxillary central incisors during rapid palatal expansion. **A,** When the appliance is placed and treatment begins, there is only a tiny diastema; **B,** after 1 week of expansion, the teeth have moved laterally with the skeletal structures; **C,** after retention, the gingival fibers have pulled the incisors together and closed the diastema.

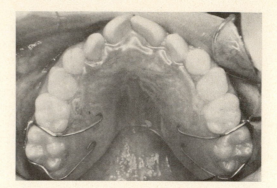

Fig. 14-63 ■ An acrylic palatal plate is useful to control relapse after the fixed appliance removal following rapid palatal expansion.

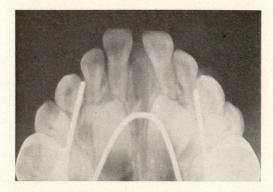

Fig. 14-64 ■ This occlusal radiograph taken during the primary dentition years illustrates sutural opening in response to the W-arch appliance.

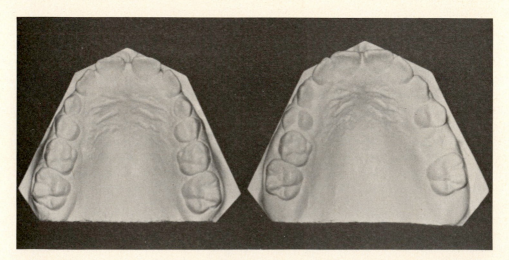

Fig. 14-65 ■ The pretreatment cast on the left and the progress cast on the right demonstrate the increase in transverse dimension that usually occurs in response to Frankel appliance therapy, as a result of the alteration of the cheek-tongue equilibrium.

of pressure in a mixed dentition child over a 10 to 12 week period, may provide the same ultimate result with less trauma to the teeth and bones. This form of treatment opens the suture at a slower rate that is closer to the speed of bone formation. Obviously more dental change takes place during the phase of active treatment, but the ultimate change may be very similar to that obtained in rapid palatal expansion, i.e., approximately equal amounts of skeletal and dental expansion. It appears that simply turning the screw more slowly in a typical fixed expansion appliance is effective. Alternatively, a spring to produce 2 pounds of force can be used.[32]

Less force is necessary to open the suture in younger children, and some skeletal expansion can be achieved in the primary and early mixed dentitions with expansion lingual arches[33] (see Chapter 11). These W-arch and quad helix appliances generally deliver less than 2 pounds of force, but have been demonstrated to open the midpalatal suture in very young patients (Fig. 14-64). The effect is similar to what slow palatal expansion with a jackscrew device achieves in the older age group.

Most functional appliances incorporate some components to expand the maxillary arch, either intrinsic force-generating mechanisms like springs and jackscrews, or buccal shields to relieve buccal soft tissue pressure. Treatment changes in transverse arch dimension and arch circumference have been documented[2] (Fig. 14-65), and it is possible that some opening of the midpalatal suture can also be obtained in this way, especially in young children. Unfortunately, the long-term stability of these changes has not been documented.

■ *Treatment for Facial Asymmetry*

Although most people have some facial asymmetry, asymmetric development of the jaws severe enough to cause a problem is relatively rare. Severe asymmetry in preadolescent children usually arises either from congenital anomalies such as facial clefts or as a result of injury, typically early fracture of the mandible.

The components approach to functional appliances can be particularly helpful in dealing with asymmetry problems,

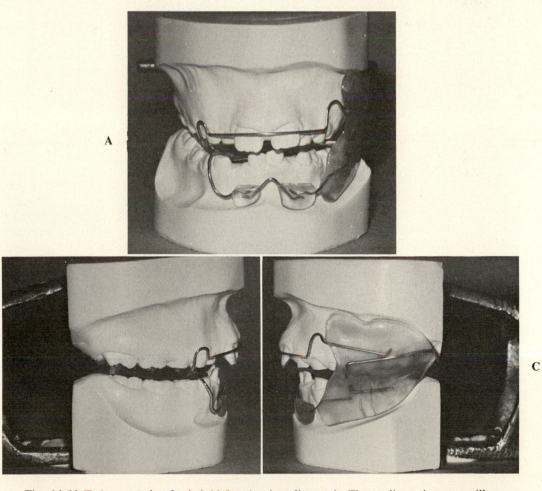

Fig. 14-66 ■ An example of a hybrid functional appliance. **A,** The appliance has a maxillary labial bow and mandibular lip pads; **B,** the right side has a posterior bite block, while, **C,** the left side has a buccal shield and unblocked mandibular posterior teeth. This appliance has the effect of leveling a transversely canted occlusal plane.

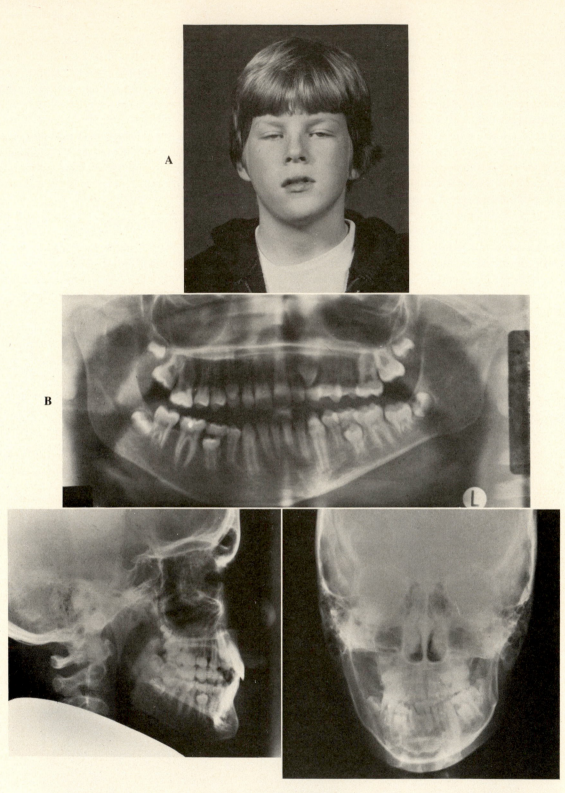

Fig. 14-67 ■ Eleven-year-old boy with severe facial asymmetry resulting from an osteochondroma of the right condyle, treated by condylectomy and reconstruction with a rib graft, then growth guidance with a hybrid functional appliance. **A,** Initial facial appearance; **B,** panoramic film showing enlarged right condyle; **C,** lateral cephalometric film; **D,** posteroanterior cephalometric film. Note the severe cant to the occlusal plane, with greater eruption of maxillary teeth on the right side. The right condyle was removed surgically, and the area was reconstructed with a rib graft; but there was no maxillary surgery. Leveling the maxilla was a primary objective of postsurgical treatment.

because skeletal asymmetry usually involves all three planes of space and differential control of eruption becomes important. Functional appliances with strikingly different components on the two sides of the arch, as for example an appliance combining buccal shields and free eruption on one side with bite blocks to prevent eruption on the other, are often called hybrid functional appliances (Fig. 14-66). In reality, they are simply an obvious expression of the use of various components to achieve specific purposes.

It may be possible to control and modify asymmetric growth with a hybrid functional appliance alone, if the problem is moderately severe. One indication for surgical intervention before adolescence, however, is a severe and progressive facial asymmetry. This condition is most likely to arise from partial ankylosis leading to a deficiency in growth on one side, but may also occur because of an osteochondroma at one condyle with a resultant overgrowth

on that side. In both these circumstances, treatment with a hybrid functional appliance will be needed after surgery to correct the primary growth problem (Fig. 14-67).

Although there is no such thing as a standard appliance for problems of this type, the principle of treatment is the same as with standard functional appliances. A construction bite is taken, bringing the jaw to the midline, or as close to the midline as it can be moved, and the appliance components are used to guide eruption of the teeth while differential growth at the condyles corrects the asymmetry. For these patients, well-designed functional appliances have advantages over both extraoral force and fixed appliances because of their ability to differentially influence development of the teeth and jaws in all three planes of space. Because of the complexity of treatment planning and the probability that surgery will also be needed, these patients are usually better managed through a major medical center.

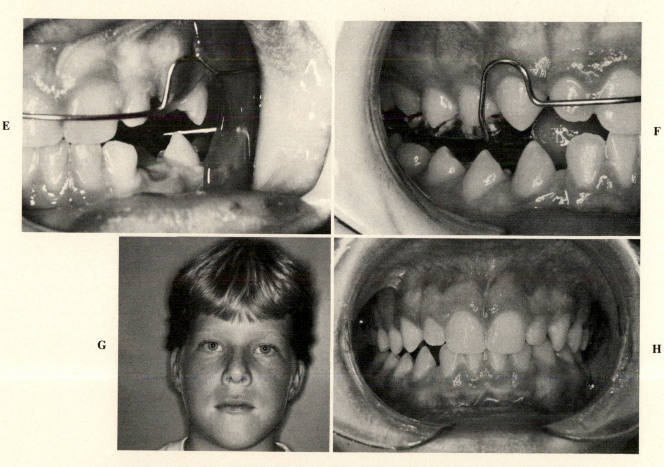

Fig. 14-67, cont'd ■ **E,** Hybrid functional appliance in place, showing buccal and lingual shields on the left side, allowing maxillary vertical development; **F,** hybrid appliance toward the end of treatment, showing bite blocks on the right side, now trimmed to allow eruption of the right lower but not upper teeth; **G,** Facial appearance fifteen months after surgery, with the asymmetry corrected; **H,** dental occlusion; at this time functional appliance treatment was discontinued.

■ *References*

1. Bookstein, F.L.: Measuring treatment effects on craniofacial growth. In McNamara, J., Ribbens, K., and Howe, R., editors: Clinical alteration of the growing face. Monograph No. 4, Craniofacial Growth Series. Ann Arbor, 1975, University of Michigan, Center for Human Growth and Development.
2. Owen, A.H.: Morphologic changes in the sagittal dimension using the Frankel appliance. Am. J. Orthod. **80:**573-603, 1981.
3. Poulton, D.R.: A three year survey of Class II malocclusions with and without headgear therapy. Angle Orthod. **34:**181-183, 1967.
4. Robertson, N.R.G.: An examination of treatment changes in children treated with the functional regulator of Frankel. Am. J. Orthod. **83:**299-309, 1983.
5. Weislander, L, and Lagerstrom, L.: The effects of activator treatment on Class II malocclusions. Am. J. Orthod. **75:**20-26, 1979.
6. Jakobsson, S.: Cephalometric evaluation of treatment effect on Class II maloccusion. Am. J. Orthod. **53:**446-457, 1967.
7. Baumrind, S., Dorn, E., Molthen, R., et al.: Changes in facial dimensions associated with the use of forces to retract the maxilla. Am. J. Orthod. **80:**17-30, 1981.
8. McNamara, J., and Carlson, D.: Quantitative analysis of temporomandibular joint adaptations to protrusive function, Am. J. Orthod. **76:**593-611, 1979.
9. Petrovic, A., Stutzman, J., and Oudet, C.: Control processes in the postnatal growth of the mandibular condylar cartilage. In McNamara, J., editor: Determinants of mandibular form and growth. Monograph No. 4, Craniofacial Growth Series, Ann Arbor, 1975, University of Michigan, Center for Human Growth and Development.
10. Baumrind, S., and Korn, E.: Patterns of change in mandibular and facial shape associated with the use of forces to retract the maxilla. Am. J. Orthod. **80:**31-47, 1981.
11. Pancherz, H.: Treatment of Class II malocclusion by jumping the bite with the Herbst appliance. Am. J. Orthod. **76:**423-442, 1979.
12. Delaire, J.: La croissance maxillaire: deductions therapeutiques. Trans. Europ. Orthod. Soc. 81-102, 1972.
13. Ahlgren, J., and Laurin, C. Late results of activator treatment: a cephalometric study. Br. J. Orthod. **3:**181-187, 1976.
14. Kingsley, N.W.: Treatise on oral deformities. New York, 1880, Appleton and Co.
15. Angle, E.H.: Treatment of malocclusion of the teeth and fractures of the maxillae, Angle's system. Philadelphia, 1900, S.S. White.
16. Oppenheim, A.: Biologic orthodontic therapy and reality. Angle Orthod. **6:**69-79, 1936.
17. Kloehn, S.: Guiding alveolar growth and eruption of the teeth to reduce treatment time and produce a more balanced denture and face. Am. J. Orthod. **17:**10-33, 1947.
18. Weislander, L.: The effects of orthodontic treatment on the concurrent development of the craniofacial complex. Am. J. Orthod. **49:**15-27, 1963.
19. Armstrong, M.M.: Controlling the magnitude, direction and duration of extraoral force. Am. J. Orthod. **59:**217-243, 1971.
20. Janzen, E., and Bluher, J. The cephalometric, anatomic and histologic changes in Macaca mulatta after application of a continuous-acting retraction force on the mandible. Am. J. Orthod. **51:**823-855, 1965.
21. Andresen, V.: The Norwegian system of functional gnatho-orthopedics. Acta Gnathol. **1:**5-36, 1936.
22. Stockli, P.W., and Willert, H.G.: Tissue reaction in the temporomandibular joint resulting from anterior displacement of the mandible in the monkey. Am. J. Orthod. **60:**142-155, 1971.
23. Harvold., E., and Vargervik, K.: Morphogenetic response to activator treatment. Am. J. Orthod. **60:**478-490, 1971.
24. Frankel, R.: The treatment of Class II division 1 malocclusion with functional correctors. Am. J. Orthod. **55:**265-275, 1969.
26. Weislander, L.: The effect of force on craniofacial development. Am. J. Orthod. **65:**531-538, 1974.
27. Woodside, D.: The activator. In Saltzmann, J.A.: Orthodontics in daily practice. Philadelphia, 1974, J.B. Lippincott.
28. Gianelly, A., Arena, S. and Bernstein, L.: A comparison of Class II treatment changes noted with the light wire, edgewise, and Frankel appliances. Am. J. Orthod. **86:**269-276, 1984.
29. Sakamoto, T., Iwase, I., Uka, A., et al.: A roentgenocephalometric study of skeletal changes during and after chin cap treatment. Am. J. Orthod. **85:**341-350, 1984.
30. Fields, H., Proffit, W., Nixon, W., et al.: Facial pattern differences in long-faced children and adults. Am. J. Orthod. **85:**217-223, 1984.
31. Fotis, V., Melsen, B., Williaims, S., et al.: Vertical control as an important ingredient in the treatment of severe sagittal discrepancies. Am. J. Orthod. **86:**224-232, 1984.
32. Hicks, E.: Slow maxillary expansion: a clinical study of the skeletal versus the dental response to low magnitude force. Am. J. Orthod. **73:**121-141, 1978.
33. Bell, R., and Lecompte, E.: The effects of maxillary expansion using a quad helix appliance during the deciduous and mixed detentions. Am. J. Orthod. **79:**152-161, 1981.
34. McNamara, J.A., and Huge, S.A.: The functional regulator (FR-3) of Frankel. Am. J. Orthod. **88:**409-424, 1985.

COMPREHENSIVE ORTHODONTIC TREATMENT IN THE EARLY PERMANENT DENTITION

Comprehensive orthodontic treatment implies an effort to make the patient's occlusion as ideal as possible, repositioning all or nearly all the teeth in the process. From this perspective, the mixed dentition treatment described in Chapters 13 and 14 is not comprehensive, despite its importance, because the final position of all the permanent teeth is not affected. A second phase of comprehensive treatment after the permanent teeth erupt, during which the details of occlusal relationships are established, is usually needed for children with moderate or severe malocclusion even if significant improvement occurred during a first phase of treatment in the mixed dentition.

The ideal time for comprehensive treatment is during adolescence, when the succedaneous teeth have just erupted, some vertical and anteroposterior growth of the jaws remains, and the social adjustment to orthodontic treatment is no great problem. Not all adolescent patients require comprehensive treatment, of course, and limited treatment to overcome specific problems can certainly be done at any age. Comprehensive treatment is also possible for adults, but it poses some special problems. These are discussed in Chapter 20.

Comprehensive orthodontic treatment usually requires a complete fixed appliance. In the chapters that follow, the use of a contemporary edgewise appliance that incorporates offsets, angulation, and torque in the brackets (one of the family of "straight arch" appliances) is assumed during much of the discussion. Three major stages of treatment are used to conveniently divide comprehensive treatment into sequential steps for discussion in Chapters 15 to 17. In each of these chapters, the different archwires and archwire sequences for sliding versus loop mechanics and .022 versus .018 slots are emphasized. A brief description of treatment with the Begg appliance is included at appropriate points.

Whatever the orthodontic technique, treatment must be discontinued gradually, using some sort of retention appliance for a time, and this important subject is covered in the last chapter of this section.

Chapter 15

The First Stage of Comprehensive Treatment: Alignment and Leveling

The idea of dividing treatment into stages, which makes it easier to discuss technique, is particularly associated with the Begg technique. The three major stages discussed in this and the following two chapters are those traditionally used to describe the stages of Begg treatment,[1] but that division is reasonably applicable to edgewise treatment as well. Not every patient will require the steps of each treatment stage, but whatever the technique, it is likely that both the archwires used and the way that they are utilized will be changed at the various stages. In theory at least, there is more to be done in the finishing stage with the Begg appliance, particularly torquing of incisors and root uprighting of canines and premolars, than if a contemporary edgewise appliance is used. Nevertheless, the considerations are the same, and at least some appliance adjustment is needed to finish comprehensive treatment with even the most cleverly preadjusted edgewise appliance.

The three major stages of comprehensive treatment are: (1) alignment and leveling, (2) correction of molar relationship and space closure, and (3) finishing. The latter two stages are covered in Chapters 15 and 16, respectively.

■ Goals of the First Stage of Treatment

Treatment for any patient should be undertaken only after a thorough analysis of the patient's problems, the preparation of a treatment plan to maximize benefit for that patient, and the development of a sequence of orthodontic treatment steps (mechanotherapy) to produce the desired result. The procedure outlined in Chapters 6 and 7, culminating in an outline of the steps in treatment, is recommended.

In almost all patients with malocclusion, at least some teeth are initially malaligned. The great majority also have excessive overbite, resulting from some combination of an excessive curve of Spee in the lower arch and an absent or reverse curve of Spee in the upper arch. The goals of the first phase of treatment are to bring the teeth into alignment and correct the overbite by leveling out the arches. In this form, however, neither goal is stated clearly enough. For proper alignment, it is necessary not only to bring malposed teeth into the arch, but also to control the anteroposterior position of incisors, the width of the arches posteriorly, and the form of the dental arches. Similarly, in leveling the arch, it is necessary to control whether the leveling occurs by elongation of posterior teeth, intrusion of incisors, or some specific combination of the two (see Chapters 7 and 10 for more detail).

The form of the dental arches obviously varies between individuals. Although the orthodontist has some latitude in changing arch form, and indeed must do so in at least one arch if the upper and lower arch forms are not compatible initially, more stable results are achieved when the patient's original arch form is preserved during orthodontic treatment (see Chapter 12 for a discussion of arch form and archwire shape). The light resilient archwires used in the first stage of treatment need not be shaped to the patient's arch form as carefully as the heavier archwires used later in treatment, but from the beginning, the archwires should reflect each individual's arch form. If preformed archwires are used, their shape should be adjusted with this in mind.

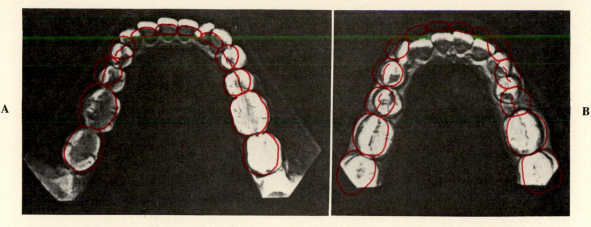

Fig. 15-1 ■ Goals of the first stage of treatment can be visualized on a print (from an ordinary office copying machine) of the dental arches. **A,** Expansion of the arch in a 12-year-old girl, to provide space for a blocked out second premolar. Some anterior movement of the incisors will occur, but this can be partially prevented by including a component of lateral expansion. **B,** Alignment of crowded incisors with premolar extraction in a young adult. With the incisors aligned in the same anteroposterior position, about half the extraction space on each side will remain. This view does not show space required for leveling, which must not be overlooked in planning (see Chapter 6).

Because the orthodontic mechanotherapy will be different depending on exactly how alignment and leveling are to be accomplished, it is extremely important that the desired position of the teeth at the end of each stage of treatment be clearly visualized before that stage is begun (Fig. 15-1). The best mechanotherapy for alignment will result in incisors that are far too protrusive, for instance, if the extractions necessary to prevent protrusion were not part of the plan. Similarly, unless leveling by intrusion is planned when it is needed, the appropriate mechanics are not likely to be selected.

In this and the subsequent chapters, it is expected that the appropriate goals for an individual patient have been clearly stated, and the discussion here concerns only the treatment techniques necessary to achieve those goals. Orthodontic treatment without specific goals can be an excellent illustration of the old adage, ''If you don't know where you're going, it doesn't matter which road you take.''

■ *Alignment*

■ Principles in the Choice of Alignment Arches

In nearly every patient with malaligned teeth, the root apices are closer to the normal position than the crowns, simply because malalignment develops as the eruption paths of teeth are deflected. Putting it another way, a tooth bud occasionally develops in the wrong place, but (barring surgery that displaces all tissues in the area, as sometimes happens in cleft palate repairs) the root apices are likely to be reasonably well aligned even though the crowns have been displaced as the teeth erupted. To bring teeth into alignment, a combination of labiolingual and mesiodistal tipping along an archwire is needed, but root movement

usually is not. Several important consequences for orthodontic mechanotherapy follow from this:

1. Initial archwires for alignment should provide light, continuous forces, to produce the most efficient tipping tooth movements. Heavy forces, in contrast, are to be avoided.

2. The archwires should be able to move freely within the brackets. For mesiodistal sliding along an archwire and reasonably free tipping, at least .002 inch clearance between the archwire and the bracket is needed, and .004 inch clearance is desirable. This means that the largest initial archwire that should be used with an .018 edgewise bracket is .016, while .014 would be more satisfactory. With the .022 edgewise bracket, an .018 archwire would be close to ideal from a bracket clearance point of view.

3. Rectangular archwires, particularly those with a tight fit within the bracket slot so that the position of the root apex could be affected, normally should be avoided. The principle is that it is better to tip crowns to position during initial alignment, rather than displacing the root apices; the corollary is that although highly resilient rectangular archwires such as .017 × .025 nickel-titanium could be used in the alignment stage, this is unwise because the rectangular archwire will create unnecessary and undesirable root movement during alignment (Fig. 15-2). Round wires for alignment are preferred.

Like orthodontic archwires at any stage of treatment, the wires for initial alignment purposes require a combination of excellent strength, excellent springiness, and a long range of action. The variables in selecting appropriate archwires for alignment are the archwire material, its diameter, and the distance between attachments (interbracket span). These factors have been discussed in Chapter 10 but are briefly reviewed here. Considering them in turn:

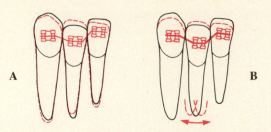

Fig. 15-2 ■ A tightly fitting resilient rectangular archwire for alignment is almost always undesirable because it produces back-and-forth movement of the root apices as the teeth move into alignment. This occurs because the moments generated by the archwire change as the geometry of the system changes with alterations in tooth position. **A,** Diagrammatic representation of the alignment of a malposed lateral incisor with a round wire and clearance in the bracket slot. With minimal moments created within the bracket slot, there is little displacement of the root apex. **B,** With a resilient rectangular archwire, back-and-forth movement of the apex occurs before the tooth ends up in essentially the same place as with a round wire.

Archwire material. The titanium-based archwires, both nickel-titanium (any of the NiTi wires) and beta-titanium (TMA), offer a better combination of strength and springiness than do steel wires. The NiTi wires, however, are both springier and stronger in small cross-section than TMA. For this reason, NiTi wires are particularly useful in the first stage of treatment. If steel is used at this stage, either multistranded wires or loops to increase springiness (see following) are needed. TMA rarely is the best choice for an initial archwire.

Size of wire. As wire size increases, strength increases rapidly, while springiness decreases even more rapidly. For alignment, therefore, one would like to choose the smallest archwire that has adequate strength. When multiple strands of the same diameter wire are used, strength is added while springiness is relatively unaffected.

Distance between attachments. As the distance increases between the points of attachment of a beam, strength decreases rapidly while springiness increases even more rapidly. The width of brackets is an important factor: the wider the individual brackets, the smaller the interbracket span. A powerful means of gaining increased springiness and range of action, without sacrificing too much strength, is to bend a loop into an archwire between two teeth, thus increasing the distance along the archwire between attachments.

Four archwire segments with equivalent springiness are displayed in Fig. 15-3. The loop designs for the .014 and .016 steel wires were deliberately configured to produce this response. Note that with the addition of more wire to produce a typical vertical loop (the average vertical loop is 5 to 6 mm high), the spring properties of .016 steel would be somewhat better than NiTi or multistranded steel, whereas .014 steel would be markedly superior.

Based on this information, what combinations of bracket

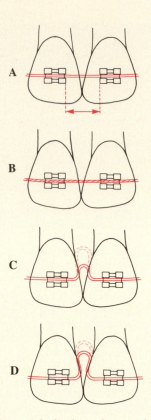

Fig. 15-3 ■ Four equivalently springy archwire segments: **A,** .016 nickel-titanium; **B,** .0175 (3 × .008) twist steel; **C,** .014 steel; **D,** .016 steel. The small amount of wire added in the loops to give equivalent springiness in .014 and .016 steel (solid red) may be surprising. With the addition of more wire to produce the size of loops normally used (dashed red), spring properties of these solid wires can be superior to nickel-titanium or braided steel wires, particularly with .014 steel.

widths, bracket slot size, and archwire characteristics would be logical choices for initial alignment? As the analysis in Chapter 10 illustrates, it is most logical to use narrow brackets with the .018 edgewise system, because in the later stages of treatment the rectangular steel archwires that fill the slot are more effective with larger interbracket spans, and sliding teeth along the archwire is relatively unimportant. With the .022 edgewise system, wider brackets are logical, since the larger slot dimension provides the clearance needed for sliding but makes it difficult to obtain close engagement of rectangular archwires for space closure with loops. Accordingly, the selection of initial archwires for the two major systems seen in clinical practice, .018 slot with narrow brackets, and .022 slot with wider brackets, is described in the following section.

■ Alignment Arches for .018 Edgewise

The principle that there should be .002 inch clearance for initial wires means that an .016 diameter wire is the largest that should be considered for initial alignment in the .018 slot system. The three major possibilities for alignment arches are multistranded steel wires, nickel-titanium wires,

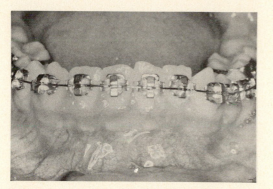

Fig. 15-4 ■ An .016 NiTi wire used for initial alignment in a patient with single .018 slot brackets. Note that the wire, held by elastomeric ligatures, is not totally seated at first in the bracket slot for the left lateral incisor. The elasticity of the system will bring this tooth into place, while correcting minor rotations.

and single-stranded steel wires with loops. Considering each in turn:

Multistranded steel wires. Despite its excellent properties, .0175 multistranded wire (3 × .008) is too large for effective use in .018 brackets. The difficulty of sliding teeth along an .0175 wire in .018 brackets is compounded by the irregular surface of the twisted strands, which increases friction between the wire and the bracket. An .015 twist wire (3 × .007) gives adequate clearance, but its physical properties are markedly inferior, and so this size of twist wire can also be eliminated as impractical.

Nickel-titanium. In contrast, .016 nickel-titanium has outstanding properties of springiness and range and also has good strength. The original martensitic NiTi wire (Nitinol) has very little formability, which means that the wire distorts only a small distance beyond its elastic limit before it breaks. A newer formulation of martensitic NiTi (Titanal) does provide good formability, with other physical properties very similar to Nitinol. In clinical practice, .016 Nitinol wires

do have a tendency to break, whereas an arch wire of a different material, though stressed beyond its failure point so that it would no longer be active, would remain intact but permanently distorted. The fact that Nitinol breaks in this circumstance is not a sign that it has less strength than its competitors, only that the consequences of exceeding its strength are more immediately obvious.

The nonlinear (superelastic) responses characteristic of the new austenitic NiTi wires (Ni-Ti, Sentinol) (see Chapter 10) make them difficult to compare to other materials, but in the .016 size, these wires do not deliver as much force as martensitic NiTi. An approximation is that .016 superelastic NiTi would be equivalent to .015 martensitic NiTi (Nitinol, Titanal). The slightly lighter forces from the newer material are an advantage in most circumstances. A .014 nickel-titanium wire can also be used as an initial wire, with some advantage because of its greater clearance in the bracket slot. Because of its reduced strength, however, .014 NiTi would be recommended only with relatively wide brackets and a consequently reduced interbracket span. The .016 NiTi wire is superior when single brackets are used. The inherently slick surface of NiTi probably contributes to the overall effectiveness of .016 NiTi in a .018 slot bracket, (Fig. 15-4).

Steel wires with loops. Another excellent choice in .018 brackets is .014 steel wire, incorporating loops as necessary. An .014 steel archwire with loops has two significant advantages over .016 with loops: (1) the greater clearance in the bracket slot allows easier sliding, and (2) the smaller diameter of the wire makes it possible to use fewer and simpler loops than would be needed with an .016 archwire. Elaborate loops that incorporate a great deal of wire are both time-consuming to fabricate and potentially troublesome in clinical use. With .014 initial archwires, three basic loop designs, as illustrated in Fig. 15-5, suffice for almost all purposes. It is important that the loops not be too long occlusogingivally. Keeping the height of loops between 5

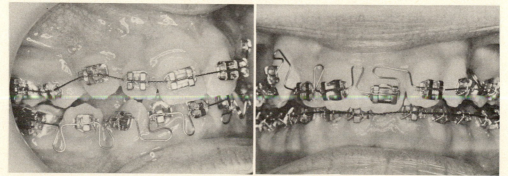

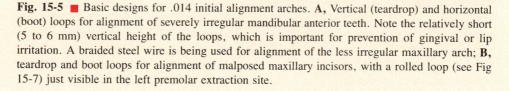

Fig. 15-5 ■ Basic designs for .014 initial alignment arches. **A,** Vertical (teardrop) and horizontal (boot) loops for alignment of severely irregular mandibular anterior teeth. Note the relatively short (5 to 6 mm) vertical height of the loops, which is important for prevention of gingival or lip irritation. A braided steel wire is being used for alignment of the less irregular maxillary arch; **B,** teardrop and boot loops for alignment of malposed maxillary incisors, with a rolled loop (see Fig 15-7) just visible in the left premolar extraction site.

and 6 mm makes them short enough to avoid almost all problems with impingement on the gingiva or irritation of the lips. Loops with a greater vertical height are much more likely to be troublesome.

■ ■ ■

The decision on whether to use .016 NiTi or .014 steel usually depends on how severely the teeth are malaligned. The greater range of action of an .014 archwire with loops (see Fig. 15-3) means that fewer reactivations are needed to complete the alignment process, and this must be balanced against the extra clinical time required to make and insert a loop archwire. For most patients, an .016 Nitinol initial archwire is satisfactory for alignment. For those with severe malalignment, however, an .014 loop archwire is so much more efficient that the extra time to make the loop archwire initially can be more than regained in reduced treatment time and shorter appointments later. In addition, loops to provide greater flexibility where it is needed help prevent the distortion of arch form that can occur with a stiffer alignment arch. The superelastic properties of the new austenitic NiTi wires probably will decrease the number of patients for whom the extra time to bend loops in steel wire is warranted.

In patients with severe crowding of anterior teeth, extraction of a premolar on each side is usually indicated, and it is necessary to retract the canines into the extraction sites while aligning the incisors. In extremely severe crowding, it is better to retract the canines independently before placing attachments on the incisors. This can be done either with segmental retraction loops (Fig. 15-6), or by sliding the canines along an archwire (which produces more stress on the posterior anchorage). In moderately severe crowding, it is possible to simultaneously tip the canines distally and align the incisors, using a loop archwire of the design shown in Fig. 15-7. The principle is that described by Stoner[2] as a "drag loop." The loop in the extraction site is activated slightly, producing a gentle space-closing force. As the activated distal loop closes, the loop mesial to the canine opens, allowing the canine to tip back independently while the incisors are being aligned.

■ Alignment with .022 Edgewise

In .022 edgewise, twin brackets are typically used on all teeth. The reduced interbracket span makes archwires stiffer and also means that loops, if they are used, must be located more precisely. The same choice of wires is available as for .018 edgewise.

Multistranded wires. With an .022 bracket slot, there is optimal clearance for an .0175 twist archwire, and this is an excellent choice as an initial alignment archwire. Although .0195 twist also can be used, this wire is undesirably stiffer, and the combination of its irregular surface and small clearance prevents sliding as freely as might be desired. Another form of multistranded wire has a central core wire with multiple smaller wires wound around it. The spring

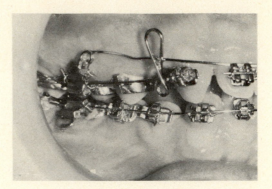

Fig. 15-6 ■ Segmental retraction of the maxillary right canine, in conjunction with an auxiliary depressing arch to the maxillary incisors. Independent retraction of the canine in this way is most applicable when the canine is severely displaced mesially or when the anchorage control strategy (see Chapter 16) calls for canine retraction as a first stage procedure.

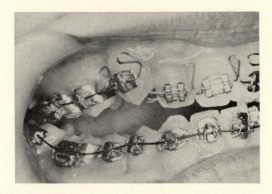

Fig. 15-7 ■ The use of a rolled or drag loop in the extraction site, to independently tip the canine distally into the extraction site while the incisors are being aligned. If the loop in the extraction site is gently activated by pulling the posterior end of the wire 1 to 1.5 mm through the molar tube and bending it up, a force is generated to tip the canine distally, as the wire segment passing through the canine is prevented from sliding distally by the loop configuration to the mesial. As the canine tips distally, however, the mesial loop opens up, and there is essentially no retraction of the incisors.

properties of the best-known example (Respond, American Ormco) are such that .0195 Respond is quite similar to .0175 twist, which means that .0195 Respond is the better choice if for some reason a larger diameter wire is desired.

Nickel-titanium wires. Both .016 and .018 NiTi can be used as initial archwires with .022 slot edgewise, but even in NiTi, .018 wires are undesirably stiff. With .016 NiTi, the .006 inch clearance within the bracket, though large, is not enough to cause clinical problems. Since the stiffness of .0175 twist and .016 NiTi wires is quite similar, it makes good economic sense to use the twist wire with the .022 appliance except in patients with the most severe malalignment, for whom the greater range and strength of NiTi are useful.

Steel wires with loops. With .022 slot, the major indication for loop arches are independent retraction of the ca-

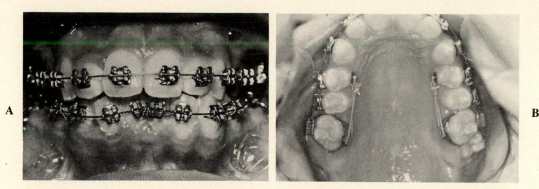

Fig. 15-8 ■ The .0175 twist wire used in the .022 edgewise appliance for initial alignment. **A,** Frontal view. Note that the twist archwire is not fully engaged in the mandibular central incisor brackets. An .016 steel wire is used here in the upper arch. **B,** Occlusal view of the maxillary arch of a different patient. Elastomeric ties to lingual attachments are being used to facilitate correction of rotations. Note that only one of the twin brackets of the more irregular left premolars is tied.

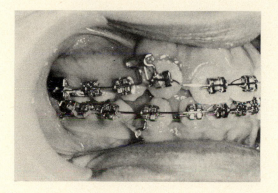

Fig. 15-9 ■ Independent retraction of the mandibular canine, sliding it posteriorly along the archwire (.016 steel) with an elastomeric ligature. The attachment to the ''power arm'' that extends gingivally from the bracket reduces the tendency for the canine to tip.

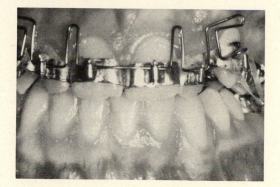

Fig. 15-10 ■ Alignment loops in .016 wire, in a patient wearing the Begg appliance in the upper arch.

nines before aligning very severely crowded incisors (Fig. 15-5) and severe localized crowding so that greater flexibility is needed in one area. One logical approach with .022 twin brackets is to use .0175 twist for most patients (Fig. 15-8) and to use .016 NiTi for those who have more severe irregularities, sliding the canines distally along the NiTi wire with elastic ties to the posterior teeth while the anterior teeth are being aligned (Fig. 15-9). Loops then would be reserved for the few patients in whom they were needed to prevent distortion of arch form.

■ Alignment with Begg Technique

The narrow brackets used in Begg technique provide the maximum possible interbracket span without placing loops in archwires. It was originally common practice with this appliance to use loops in .016 arch wires to facilitate initial alignment (Fig. 15-10). Indeed, loops for alignment were introduced into American edgewise orthodontics from the early Begg appliance. The long posterior span of archwires used in the Begg technique makes it difficult to use a highly

flexible titanium-based archwire at the initial stage without losing control of molar position (see leveling, following). Although alignment loops are used less in current Begg therapy than they were previously, this remains a valuable adjunct to Begg treatment.

■ Special Problems in Alignment

■ Crossbite Correction

It is important to correct posterior crossbites and mild anterior crossbites in the first stage of treatment. Severe anterior crossbites, in contrast, are usually not corrected until the second stage of conventional treatment, or might remain pending surgical correction. For both posterior and anterior crossbites, it is obviously important to make the appropriate distinctions between skeletal and dental problems, and to quantitate the severity of the problem. The appropriate diagnostic steps are discussed in Chapters 6 and 7. The assumption here is that appropriate treatment has been selected, and the discussion is solely about implementing a treatment plan based on differential diagnosis.

Transverse maxillary expansion by opening the midpalatal suture. It is relatively easy to widen the maxilla by opening the midpalatal suture before and during adolescence, but this becomes progressively more difficult as patients become older. The chances of successful opening of the suture are nearly 100% before age 15, but begin to decline thereafter because of the increased interdigitation of the sutures that must respond.[3]

Patients who are candidates for opening the midpalatal suture often have severe crowding and will require extraction of premolars for alignment. In these patients, however, separation of the suture should be the first step in treatment, before either extraction or alignment. The first premolar teeth are needed as anchorage for the lateral expansion and can serve for that purpose even if they are to be extracted later, and the additional space provided by the lateral expansion facilitates alignment.

Occasionally, transverse maxillary expansion can provide

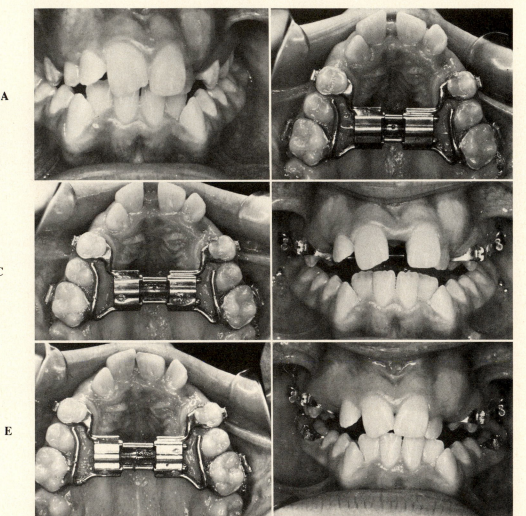

Fig. 15-11 ■ Maxillary expansion with a jackscrew appliance to open the midpalatal suture. **A,** Maxillary constriction and crowding before treatment; **B,** jackscrew appliance in place, soldered to bands on the maxillary first molars and first premolars, with an arm contacting the second premolars. At this point, the appliance has been opened approximately 3 mm. Note the separation between the maxillary central incisors. **C,** Occlusal view after 10 days of separation. Note the wide central diastema. **D,** Labial view after 10 days of separation. A tendency toward anterior open bite is created by contact of the maxillary lingual and mandibular buccal molar cusps. **E,** Occlusal view 3 months after separation was begun and 10 weeks after the screw was stabilized by tying it with brass wire. Note the spontaneous closure of the diastema, which occurs because of the elastic rebound of the gingival fibers. **F,** Labial view at 3 months. Overcorrection of the posterior crossbite is being maintained by the stabilized appliance.

enough additional space to make extraction unnecessary, but rarely is it wise to use sutural expansion as a means of dealing with an alignment problem in an individual who already has normal maxillary width (see Chapter 8). Opening the midpalatal suture should be used primarily as a means of correcting a skeletal crossbite, increasing a narrow maxillary width to a normal dimension.

The basic mechanism for separation of the midpalatal suture is a jackscrew built into a fixed appliance that is rigidly attached to as many posterior teeth as possible. The appliance can be made so that it has plastic palate-covering shelves or can consist solely of a metal framework that does not contact the palatal tissue (Fig. 15-11). In theory, the flanges extending into the palate should cause a more bodily repositioning of the alveolar processes, but in fact, there seems to be little or no difference in response to the two types of appliances. In addition, the palate-covering appliance remains in contact with the soft tissue for an extended period and is quite likely to cause tissue irritation. For this reason, an appliance that does not contact the palate is preferred.

Separation of the midpalatal suture can be produced by either rapid or slow expansion, and the same type of palate separating appliance can be used for either approach (see Chapter 14). Whether the expansion is done rapidly or slowly, the fixed appliance remains in place for approximately the same length of time, because a shorter period of stabilization is sufficient with slow expansion. With rapid expansion, the expansion itself is carried out in approximately 2 weeks, but the screw should then be stabilized and the appliances maintained in place for 3 months of retention. With slow expansion, approximately 2½ months are needed to obtain the expansion, and the appliance can be removed in another 2 months.

Some degree of relapse can be expected after palatal expansion because of the elasticity of the palatal soft tissue. Therefore, it is wise to overcorrect the crossbite initially (Fig. 15-11). Even if 2 to 4 months of stabilization with the palate-separating device have been provided, additional retention of the crossbite correction is needed when the fixed appliance is removed. A palate-covering removable retainer is satisfactory but may be somewhat awkward in combination with fixed appliances to align the teeth as the first stage of treatment proceeds. An alternative is a heavy labial archwire placed in the headgear tubes (Fig. 15-12), which will maintain the lateral expansion while light resilient archwires are being used to align the teeth.

Correction of dental crossbites. Three approaches to correction of less severe dental crossbites are feasible: a heavy labial expansion arch, as shown in Fig. 15-12, an expansion lingual arch, or cross elastics. Removable appliances, though theoretically possible, are not compatible with comprehensive treatment and should be reserved for mixed dentition or adjunctive treatment.

The inner bow of a facebow is also, of course, a heavy labial arch, and expansion of this inner bow is a convenient way to expand the upper molars. This expansion is nearly always needed for patients with a Class II molar relationship, whose upper arch is too narrow to accomodate the mandibular arch when it comes forward into the correct relationship. The inner bow is simply adjusted at each appointment to be sure that it is slightly wider than the headgear tubes and must be compressed by the patient when inserting the facebow. If the distal force of a headgear is not desired, a heavy labial auxiliary can provide the expansion effect alone.

A transpalatal lingual arch for expansion must have some springiness and range of action, which means that it must contain some sort of loop or loops to provide flexibility. As a general principle, the more flexible a lingual arch is, the less it adds to anchorage stability, which can be an important consideration in adolescent and adult patients. If anchorage is of no concern, a highly flexible lingual arch, like the quad helix design discussed in Chapter 11, is an excellent choice. When the lingual arch is needed for both expansion

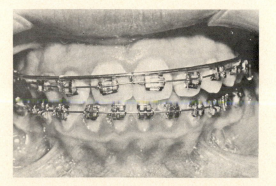

Fig. 15-12 ■ A heavy labial archwire (usually .036 or .040 steel) placed in the headgear tubes on first molars can be used to maintain arch width after palatal suture opening while the teeth are being aligned. This is more compatible with fixed-appliance treatment than a removable retainer and does not depend on patient cooperation.

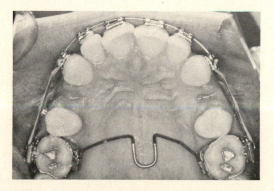

Fig. 15-13 ■ An expansion lingual arch of this type, rather than the more flexible expansion arches shown in Chapter 14, is often used for small amounts of expansion in the first stage of comprehensive treatment because it also contributes to stabilization of the posterior segments, augmenting the posterior anchorage.

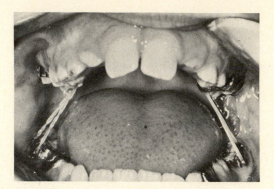

Fig. 15-14 ■ Cross elastics from the lingual of the upper molars to the buccal of the lower molars. Cross elastics are an effective way of correcting transverse dental relationships, but must be used with an awareness of their extrusive tendency.

and anchorage, however, it is better to use a straight transpalatal arch with an adjustment loop as shown in Fig. 15-13. Even the smallest adjustment loop decreases the rigidity needed for maximum anchorage, and there is no reason to place any type of loop unless crossbite correction is part of the treatment plan.

The third possibility for crossbite correction is the use of cross elastics, typically running from the lingual of the upper molar to the buccal of the lower molar (Fig. 15-14). These elastics are effective, but their strong extrusive component must be kept in mind. As a general rule, adolescent patients can tolerate a short period of cross elastic wear to correct a simple crossbite, because any extrusion is compensated by vertical growth of the ramus, but crosselastics should be used with great caution, if at all, in adults. As any posterior crossbite is corrected, interference of the cusps increases posterior vertical dimension and thereby tends to rock the mandible downward and backward, even if cross elastics are avoided. The cross elastics simply accentuate this tendency.

If teeth are tightly locked into a crossbite relationship, it may be necessary to use a biteplane to separate them vertically, so that a crossbite can be corrected. In children and young adolescents, this is rarely needed. The necessary vertical clearance is achieved by mandibular repositioning of the type that accompanies growth anyway. In older adolescents and adults, however, a biteplane may be helpful.

■ Impacted or Unerupted Teeth

Bringing an impacted or unerupted tooth into the arch creates a set of special problems during alignment, primarily because an unerupted tooth is usually a long way from the line of occlusion. The most frequent problem of this type is an impacted maxillary canine or canines, but it is occasionally necessary to bring other unerupted teeth into the arch, and the same techniques apply for incisors, canines, and premolars. Impacted lower second molars pose a different problem and are discussed separately following.

The problems in dealing with an unerupted tooth can be

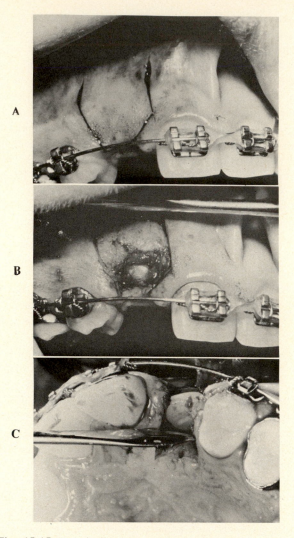

Fig. 15-15 ■ Apically root positioned flap for exposure of an unerupted canine. **A,** Initial incision lines; **B,** crown exposed with apical repositioning of the labial tissue; **C,** lingual exposure of the same tooth.

divided into three categories: (1) surgical exposure, (2) attachment to the tooth, and (3) orthodontic mechanics to bring the tooth into the arch.

Surgical exposure. It is important for a tooth to erupt through the attached gingiva, not through alveolar mucosa, and this must be considered when flaps for exposure of a labially positioned tooth are planned. If the unerupted tooth is in the mandibular arch or on the labial side of the maxillary alveolar process, a flap should be reflected from the crest of the alveolus and sutured so that attached gingiva has been transferred to the region where the crown is exposed (Fig. 15-15). If this is not done, and the tooth is brought through alveolar mucosa, it is quite likely that tissue will strip away from the crown, leaving both an unsightly and periodontally compromised gingival margin.[4] If the unerupted tooth is on the palatal side, similar

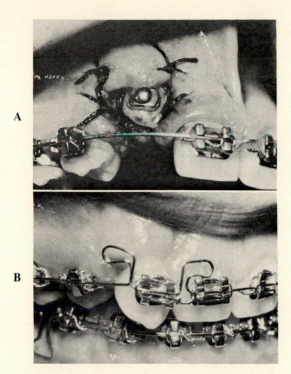

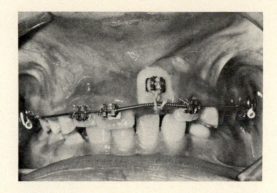

Fig. 15-17 ■ An elastomeric thread tied to the bracket placed on an unerupted tooth when it is exposed surgically is often used initially to pull it toward occlusion, as in this maxillary central incisor.

Fig. 15-16 ■ **A,** Attachment bonded to the labial surface of the crown of an unerupted canine (same patient as Fig 15-15), with the apically repositioned flap sutured in place. An elastomeric attachment from the archwire to the bonded button will be used initially to bring the canine toward the line of occlusion. Later, the button will be replaced with a bonded bracket. **B,** Tooth in position, after placement of a normal bonded bracket and boot loops to complete the repositioning.

problems with the heavy palatal mucosa are unlikely, and flap design is less critical.

Occasionally, a tooth will obligingly erupt into its correct position after obstacles to eruption have been removed by surgical exposure, but this is rarely the case after root formation is complete. Even a tooth that is aimed in the right direction usually requires orthodontic force to bring it into position after surgical exposure.

Method of attachment. The least desirable way to obtain attachment is for the surgeon to place a wire ligature around the crown of the impacted tooth, but occasionally no alternative is practical. This inevitably results in loss of periodontal attachment, because bone destroyed when the wire is passed around the tooth does not regenerate when it is removed.

Before the availability of direct bonding, a pin was sometimes placed in a hole prepared into the crown of an unerupted tooth, and in special circumstances, this remains a possible alternative. The best contemporary approach, however, is simply to expose an area on the crown of the tooth and directly bond an attachment of some type to that surface (Fig. 15-16). In many instances, a button or hook is better than a standard bracket because it is smaller. A wire or elastomeric ligature can then be looped around the bonded

attachment before the flap is repositioned and sutured into place.

Mechanical approaches for aligning unerupted teeth. Orthodontic traction to pull an unerupted tooth toward the line of the arch should begin as soon as possible after surgery. Ideally, a fixed orthodontic appliance should already be in place before the unerupted tooth is exposed, so that orthodontic force can be applied immediately. If this is not practical, active orthodontic movement should begin no later than 2 or 3 weeks postsurgically.

An unerupted tooth is usually so far from the line of occlusion that is impossible to tie even the most flexible continuous wire against it. One possible approach is to tie from the impacted tooth to a relatively heavy base archwire, using an elastomeric material (Fig. 15-17). A second alternative is to use a special alignment spring, either soldered to a heavy base archwire or bent into a light archwire (Fig. 15-18). Compared to tying with an elastic material, this technique has the advantage of a considerably longer range and a more constant force magnitude. When the unerupted tooth has been brought relatively close to the line of occlusion and a standard bracket can be bonded in the proper position, loops in a continuous archwire can be used to complete the alignment. A box loop (Fig. 15-19), usually formed in .014 wire, is preferred for this purpose.

Ankylosis of an unerupted tooth is always a potential problem. If an area of fusion to the adjacent bone develops, orthodontic movement of the unerupted tooth becomes impossible, and displacement of the anchor teeth will occur. Occasionally, an unerupted tooth will start to move and then will become ankylosed, apparently held by only a small area of fusion. It can sometimes be freed to continue movement by being anesthetized and lightly luxated, breaking the area of ankylosis. If this procedure is done, it is critically important to apply orthodontic force immediately after the luxation, since it is only a matter of time until the tooth reankyloses. Nevertheless, this approach can sometimes allow a tooth to be brought into the arch, which otherwise would be imposible to move.

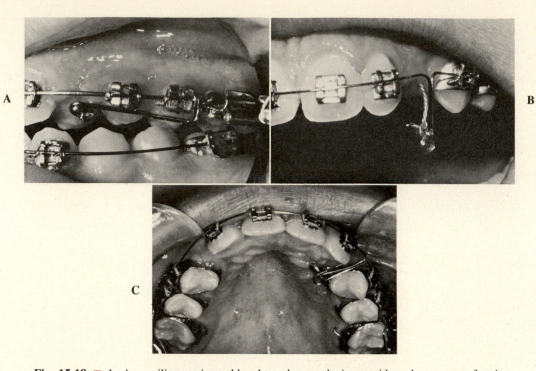

Fig. 15-18 ■ **A,** An auxiliary spring soldered to a base archwire provides a long range of action to bring an unerupted canine facially and occlusally. This is more efficient than elastomeric ties. **B,** A vertical spring bent into an .014 steel archwire to bring down an impacted maxillary canine, before activation; **C,** same spring activated by rotating the loop 90 degrees. A stop against the molars, so that the wire cannot just spin in the molar tubes, is essential. This method is also very effective, providing excellent force characteristics with a long range of action.

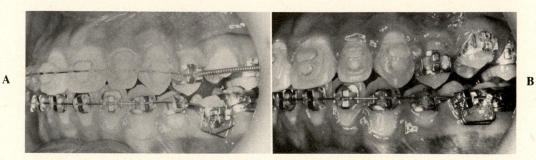

Fig. 15-19 ■ Box loop in .014 wire to elevate a mandibular second premolar into occlusion. **A,** Loop at initial placement; **B,** 8 weeks later.

Unlike impaction of most other teeth, which is an obvious problem from the beginning of treatment, impaction of lower second molars usually develops during orthodontic treatment (Fig. 15-20). This occurs when the mesial marginal ridge of the second molar catches against the distal surface of the first molar, so that the second molar progressively tips mesially instead of erupting. Moving the first molar posteriorly during the mixed dentition increases the chance that the second molar will become impacted, and this possibility must be taken into account when procedures to increase mandibular arch length are employed.

Correction of an impacted second molar requires that the tooth be moved posteriorly and uprighted. In most cases, if the mesial marginal ridge can be unlocked, the tooth will erupt on its own. When the second molar is not severely tipped, the simplest solution is to place a separator between the two teeth (Fig. 15-21). Another possibility for a more severe problem is to solder an auxiliary spring to an archwire mesial to the first molar and extend it posteriorly into the embrasure between the first and second molars. The long arms of an auxiliary spring of this type gives excellent flexibility and range of action, but also makes it difficult to

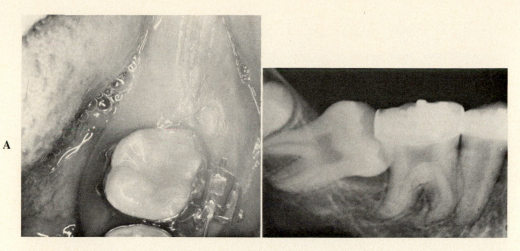

Fig. 15-20 ■ Impacted mandibular second molar in a 14-year-old patient. **A,** Occlusal view; **B,** radiographic view. The clinically exposed cusp is the distobuccal cusp, not the mesiobuccal cusp one would expect to see in this location.

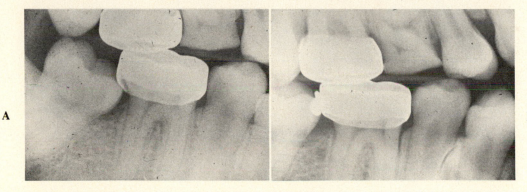

Fig. 15-21 ■ Brass wire separator used to de-impact a mandibular second molar. **A,** Second molar trapped beneath distal bulge of first molar; **B,** uprighting obtained with separator. Separating springs can be used in the same way. Separators are effective only if the tooth is minimally tipped.

keep the spring in place and may lead to substantial soft tissue irritation. A better alternative is to surgically expose the second molar, bond a tube to the buccal surface, and then use an auxiliary spring into this tube to upright the second molar (Fig. 15-22).

An auxiliary spring, soldered to a heavy archwire or extending from the first molar auxiliary tube, is often useful to bring both upper and lower second molars into alignment when they erupt late in orthodontic treatment (Fig. 15-23). This allows the use of a flexible wire in the posterior part of the arch, while a heavier and more rigid wire is in place anteriorly.

■ Diastema Closure

A maxillary midline diastema is often complicated by the insertion of the labial frenum into a notch in the alveolar bone, so that a band of heavy fibrous tissue lies between the central incisors. When this is the case, a stable correction of the distema almost always requires surgery to remove the interdental fibrous tissue and reposition the frenum. The

frenectomy must be carried out in a way that will produce a good esthetic result and must be properly coordinated with orthodontic treatment.

It is an error to surgically remove the frenum and then delay orthodontic treatment in the hope that the diastema will close spontaneously. If the frenum is removed while there is still a space between the central incisors, scar tissue forms between the teeth as healing progresses, and a long delay may result in a space that is more difficult to close than it was previously.

It is better to align the teeth before frenectomy. Sliding them together along an archwire is usually better than using a closing loop, because a loop with any vertical height will touch and irritate the frenum. If the diastema is relatively small, it is usually possible to bring the central incisors completely together before surgery (Fig. 15-24). If the space is large and the frenal attachment is thick, it may not be possible to completely close the space before surgical intervention. The space should be closed at least partially, and the orthodontic movement to bring the teeth together

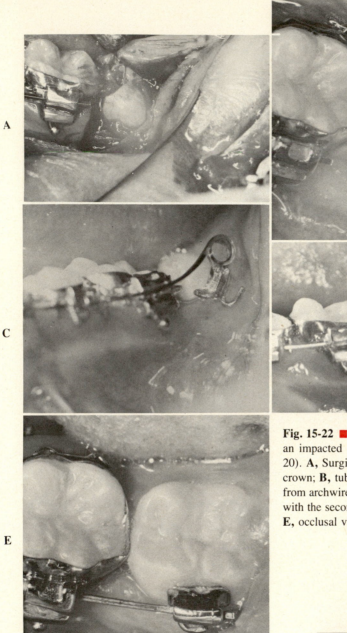

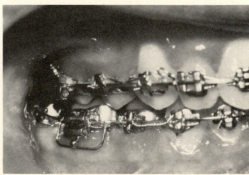

Fig. 15-22 ■ Use of a bonded tube and auxiliary spring to upright an impacted mandibular second molar (same patient as Fig 15-20). **A,** Surgical exposure of a portion of the facial surface of the crown; **B,** tube bonded on the distobuccal cusp; **C,** helical spring from archwire inserted into buccal tube; **D,** uprighting completed, with the second molar in position for normal banding or bonding; **E,** occlusal view after uprighting.

should be resumed immediately after the frenectomy, so that the teeth are brought together quickly after the procedure. When this is done, healing occurs with the teeth together, and the inevitable postsurgical scar tissue stabilizes the teeth in their correct position instead of creating obstacles to final closure of the space.

The key to successful surgery is removal of the interdental fibrous tissue. It is unnecessary, and in fact undesirable, to excise a large portion of the frenum itself. Instead, a simple incision is used to allow access to the interdental area, the

Fig. 15-23 ■ When a second molar is banded relatively late in treatment, a spring soldered to the main archwire and extending beneath the first molar tube as shown here provides excellent flexibility to align the second molar while allowing a heavy archwire to remain in place anteriorly to maintain arch form.

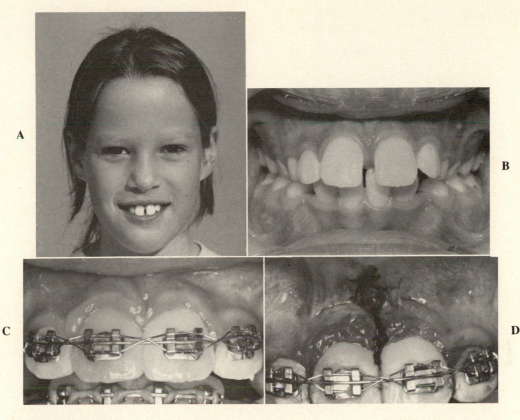

Fig. 15-24 ■ Management of a maxillary midline diastema. **A,** Facial appearance, showing the protuding maxillary incisors caught on the lower lip; **B,** intraoral view before treatment; **C,** teeth aligned and held tightly together with a figure-8 wire ligature, before frenectomy; **D,** appearance immediately after frenectomy, using the conservative technique advocated by Edwards in which a simple incision is used to allow access to the interdental area, the fibrous connection to the bone is removed, and the frenal attachment is sutured at a higher level.

fibrous connection to the bone is removed, and the frenum is then sutured at a higher level.[5]

A maxillary midline diastema tends to recur, no matter how carefully the space was managed initially. A bonded fixed retainer (see Chapter 18) is recommended.

■ Leveling

The archwire design for leveling depends on whether there is a need for absolute intrusion of incisors, or whether relative intrusion is satisfactory. This important point is discussed in detail in Chapter 7, and the biomechanical considerations in obtaining intrusion are described in Chapters 9 and 10. The discussion following assumes that an appropriate decision about the type of leveling has been made and focuses on the rather different techniques for leveling by relative intrusion (which is really differential elongation of premolars, for the most part) as contrasted to leveling by absolute intrusion of incisors (see Fig. 7-3).

■ Leveling by Extrusion (Relative Intrusion)

This type of leveling can be accomplished with continuous archwires, simply by placing an exaggerated curve of Spee in the maxillary archwire and a reverse curve of Spee in the mandibular archwire (Fig. 15-25). For most patients, it is necessary to replace the initial highly resilient alignment arch with a slightly stiffer one to complete the leveling. As with the alignment archwire, the choice of wires for this purpose depends on which type of edgewise appliance is being used.

The .018 slot, narrow brackets. In a patient with both malaligned teeth and excessive overbite, the initial .016 nickel-titanium or .014 steel loop archwire should be bent to level as well as align, that is, the upper arch should contain an exaggerated curve of Spee, while the lower has a reverse curve. When preliminary alignment is completed, the second archwire is almost always .016 steel, again with an exaggerated or reverse curve. In most instances, this approach is sufficient to complete the leveling.

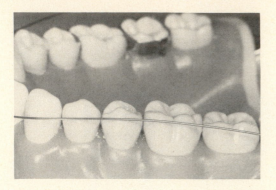

Fig. 15-25 ■ A reverse curve of Spee in the lower archwire, illustrated here alongside the lower arch with which it would be used, is a satisfactory method if vertical growth will occur to compensate for the extrusion that occurs in the premolar region.

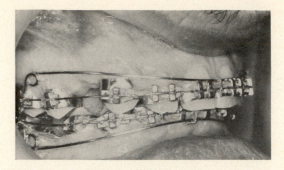

Fig. 15-26 ■ An auxiliary leveling arch extending from the auxiliary tubes on the first molars and tied beneath the base arch anteriorly can be used to augment the leveling ability of light round continuous archwires. The principal indication for use of an auxiliary with a continuous round leveling arch is to supplement an .016 archwire in .018 edgewise brackets.

In some patients, particularly in nonextraction treatment of older patients who have little if any remaining growth, an archwire heavier than .016 is needed to complete the leveling of the lower arch (the upper arch is rarely a problem with .016 alone if true intrusion is not required). Rather than use an .018 archwire, it is usually preferable to add an auxiliary leveling arch. This arch inserts into the auxiliary tube on the molar and is tied anteriorly beneath the .016 base arch (Fig. 15-26). This will result in efficient completion of the leveling, augmenting the curve in the base arch.

It is sometimes said, as an argument in favor of the .022 appliance, that the wires available for use with the .018 slot appliance are not large enough to accomplish all necessary tooth movements. One of the few situations in which that may be true is in final leveling with continuous archwires, which may require either a continuous .018 archwire or the auxiliary wire suggested previously.

The .022 slot, wider brackets. For a typical patient using the .022 appliance, initial alignment with an .0175 twist or .016 Nitinol wire is usually followed by an .016 steel wire with a reverse or accentuated curve, and then by an .018 round wire to complete the leveling. This arch wire sequence is nearly always adequate for completion of leveling, and it is rare that .020 wire or an auxiliary archwire is required.

■ Leveling by Intrusion

Leveling by intrusion requires a mechanical arrangement other than a continuous archwire attached to each tooth. The key to successful intrusion is light continuous force directed toward the tooth apex. It is necessary to avoid pitting intrusion of one tooth against extrusion of its neighbor, since in that circumstance, extrusion will dominate. This can be accomplished in two ways: (1) with continuous archwires that bypass the premolar (and frequently the canine) teeth, and (2) with segmented base archwires, so that there is no connection along the arch between the anterior and posterior segments, and an auxiliary depressing arch.

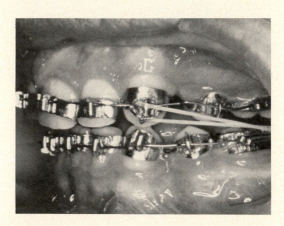

Fig. 15-27 ■ Illustration of .016 archwires for leveling near the end of the first stage of Begg technique. An "anchor bend" is placed mesial to the first molar, and the archwire is lightly ligated or clipped as it passes the second premolar, rather than being pinned into the bracket on these teeth.

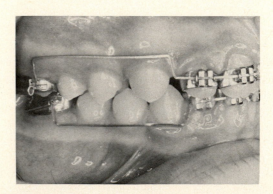

Fig. 15-28 ■ Utility arches for leveling, showing the long span from molars to incisors.

Bypass arches. This approach to intrusion is most useful for patients who will have some growth, i.e., who are in either the mixed or early permanent dentitions. Three different mechanical arrangements are commonly used, each based on the same mechanical principle: uprighting and distal tipping of the molars are pitted against intrusion of the incisors.

A classic version of this approach to leveling is seen in the first stage of Begg technique, in which the premolar teeth are bypassed and only a loose tie is made to the canine. An .016 resilient steel archwire is fabricated as shown in Fig. 15-27, using an "anchor bend" anterior to the first molar. The long span of the archwire anterior to the anchor bend provides a gentle intrusive force on the incisors, while the reaction force on the molar tends to upright it and tip it distally. Light Class II elastic forces are used while this arch-wire is in place. The result is stabilization of the lower molar against the distal tipping, at the cost of an increase in the extrusion of the molar. Hence there is a need for some vertical growth while this treatment is being carried out, to prevent downward and backward rotation of the mandible. The light archwire, however, does intrude the lower incisors. The upper incisors are being pulled downward by the Class II elastic, which counterbalances the intrusion these teeth otherwise might experience.

Exactly the same effect can be produced in exactly the same way using the edgewise appliance, if the premolars and canines are bypassed. Mulligan has advocated just this approach to the fabrication of a leveling archwire, using an .016 wire with an anchor bend very similar to the initial archwire in the Begg technique.[6]

A more flexible variation of the same basic idea is developed in Rickett's utility arch[7] (Fig. 15-28). The utility arch is characterized by step-down bends between the first molar and the lateral incisors, so that the arch wire is less likely to be distorted by the forces of occlusion. It is fabricated of .016 × .016 wire, used in .018 brackets. In most cases, the rectangular wire is placed into the brackets with slight labial root torque to control the inclination of the teeth as the incisors move labially while they intrude.

Successful use of any of these bypass arches for leveling requires that the forces be kept light. This is accomplished in two ways: by selecting a small diameter archwire, and by using a long span between the first molar and the incisors. Wire heavier than .016 steel should not be used, and Ricketts recommends a relatively soft .016 × .016 chrome-cobalt wire as utility arches to prevent heavy forces from being developed. Overactivation of the vertical bends can cause loss of control of the molars in all three planes of space.

The .016 wires typically used in bypass arches, though resilient, are too stiff for efficient alignment of severely malposed incisors, even if loops are bent into the wire between adjacent teeth. Small rotations or displacements can be corrected simply by tying to an .016 wire and gradually bringing the wire into the bracket slot, particularly if the brackets are narrow so that interbracket span is adequate.

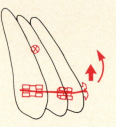

Fig. 15-29 ■ When the incisor segment is viewed from a lateral perspective, the center of resistance can be seen to be lingual to the point at which an archwire attaches to the crown. For this reason, the incisors tend to tip forward when an intrusive force is placed at the central incisor brackets. This tendency toward labial tipping can be controlled either by applying a force to tip the incisors distally as they are being intruded, cancelling the mesial tipping, or by applying the intrusive force more posteriorly, as by attaching an intrusion arch to stabilized anterior segment more distally, in the vicinity of the lateral rather than the central incisors, for instance (see Fig. 15-34).

Where significant malpositions exist, hower, it is better to correct the alignment with a resilient wire, perhaps using only a resilient anterior segment, before proceeding with a round or rectangular bypass arch.

In contrast to leveling with continuous fully engaged archwires, the size of the edgewise bracket slot is largely irrelevant when bypass arches for leveling are used. Whether the slot size is .018 or .022, the bypass arch should not be stiffer than .016 steel wire. If preliminary alignment is needed before the bypass arch for leveling is placed, of course, slot size would be a factor and the alignment archwires recommended previously as appropriate for each bracket slot would be the best choices.

Two weaknesses of the bypass arch systems previously described limit the amount of true intrusion that can be obtained. The first is that, except for some applications of the utility arch, only the first molar is available as posterior anchorage. This means that significant extrusion of that tooth may occur. In actively growing patients with a good facial pattern, this is not a major problem, but in nongrowing patients or those with a poor facial pattern in whom molar extrusion should be avoided, the lack of posterior anchorage can compromise the ability to intrude incisors. High-pull headgear to the upper molars can be added with any of the bypass arch systems to improve upper posterior anchorage, and with a utility arch setup, the second molar and second premolar can be incorporated into the posterior segment for better anchorage control.

The second weakness is that the intrusive force against the incisors is applied anterior to the center of resistance, and therefore the incisors tend to tip forward as they intrude (Fig. 15-29). Without an extraction space, forward movement of the incisors is an inevitable consequence of leveling, but often in extraction cases, this result is undesirable. The anchor bend at the molar in the Begg approach creates a space-closing effect that somewhat restrains forward incisor

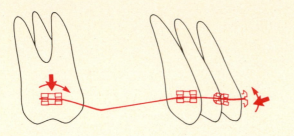

Fig. 15-30 ■ Diagrammatic representation of forces from a leveling archwire that bypasses the premolars, with an anchor bend mesial to the molars. A force system is created that elongates the molars and intrudes the incisors. The wire tends to slide posteriorly through the molar tube, tipping the incisors distally at the expense of bodily mesial movement of the molars. An archwire of this design is used in the first stage of Begg treatment but can also be used in edgewise systems. A long span from the molars to the incisors is essential.

movement (Fig. 15-30), but this also tends to bring the molar forward, straining the posterior anchorage. A utility arch can be activated to keep the incisors from moving forward and has the additional benefit of a rectangular cross-section anteriorly so that tipping can be controlled, but the result is still a strain on posterior anchorage. The segmented arch approach to leveling developed by Burstone, which overcomes these limitations, is recommended for maximum control of the anterior and posterior segments of the dental arch.

Segmented archwires for leveling. The segmented arch approach depends upon establishing stabilized posterior segments and controlling the point of force application against an anterior segment. This technique requires auxiliary rectangular tubes on first molars, in addition to the regular bracket or tube. After preliminary alignment if needed, a full dimension rectangular archwire is placed in the bracket slots of teeth in the buccal segment, which typically consists of the second premolar, first molar, and second molar. This connects these teeth into a solid unit. In addition, a heavy

lingual arch (.036 steel) is used to connect the right and left posterior segments, further stabilizing them against undesired movement (Fig. 15-31). A resilient anterior segmental wire is used to align the incisors, while the posterior segments are being stabilized.

For intrusion an auxiliary depressing arch placed in the auxiliary tube on the first molar is used to apply intrusive force against the anterior segment. This arch should be made of rectangular wire that will not twist in the auxiliary tube. Burstone recommends .018 × .025 steel wire with a 2½-turn helix (Fig. 15-32), or .019 × .025 beta-titanium wire without a helix.[8] This depressing arch is adjusted so that it lies gingival to the incisor teeth when passive and applies a light force (approximately 15 gm per tooth) when it is brought up beneath the brackets of the incisors. It is tied underneath the incisor brackets, but not into the bracket slots, which are occupied by the anterior segment wire.

An auxiliary depressing arch can be placed while a light resilient anterior segment is being used to align malposed incisors, but it is usually better to wait to add the depressing arch until incisor alignment has been achieved and a heavier anterior segment wire has been installed. A braided rectangular steel wire or a rectangular TMA wire is usually the best choice for the anterior segment while active intrusion with an auxiliary depressing arch is being carried out.

Two strategies can be used with segmented arches to prevent forward movement of the incisors as they are intruded. The first is the same as with bypass arches: a space-closing force can be created by tying the depressing arch back against the posterior segments (see Fig. 15-32). Even with stabilized posterior segments, this produces some strain on posterior anchorage.

The second and usually preferable strategy is to vary the point of force application against the incisor segment. If the anterior segment is considered a single unit (which is reasonable when a stiff archwire connects the teeth within the segment), the center of resistance is located as shown in Fig. 15-29. Tying the depressing arch distal to the midline, between the central and lateral incisors, or distal to the

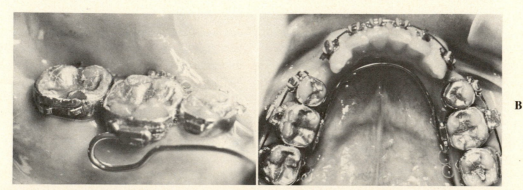

A   B

Fig. 15-31 ■ Mandibular stabilizing lingual arch in .036 steel wire, used for anchorage control in segmented arch leveling. **A,** Distal insertion into the horizontal tube on the first molar; **B,** the wire must clear the anterior segment, lying lingually and gingivally to these teeth.

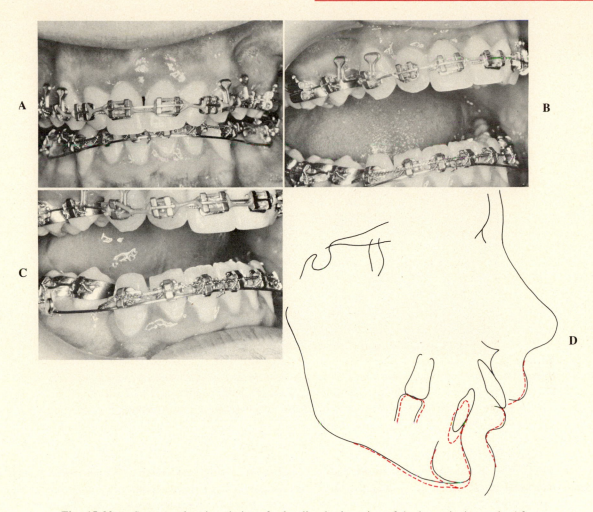

Fig. 15-32 ■ Segmented arch technique for leveling by intrusion of the lower incisors. **A,** After preliminary alignment, an anterior segment of .017 × .025 braided steel wire has been placed in the mandibular anterior segment. Posterior segments are stabilized, and an .017 × .025 steel depressing arch is placed in auxiliary tubes on the first molars and tied beneath the incisor brackets anteriorly; **B,** lateral view of appliance at initial activation; **C,** lateral view, 8 weeks later; **D,** cephalometric superimposition showing the amount of intrusion obtained in 3 months.

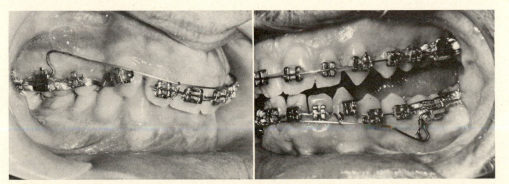

Fig. 15-33 ■ **A,** Auxiliary depressing arch to intrude severely overerupted maxillary incisors, made from TMA wire. Note the point of attachment of the depressing arch to the anterior segment. Tying between the lateral and central incisors moves the point of force application more posteriorly, closer to the center of resistance of the anterior segment. **B,** Auxiliary depressing arch to intrude the mandibular anterior segment. In this instance, the depressing arch is tied to the anterior segment distal to the laterals, carrying the point of attachement farther posteriorly to prevent labial tipping during intrusion.

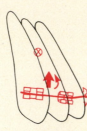

Fig. 15-34 ■ Tying an auxiliary depressing arch distal to
the midline, as shown in Fig. 15-33, moves the line of force
more posteriorly and therefore closer to the center of resistance of the anterior segment, diminishing or eliminating
the moment that causes tipping.

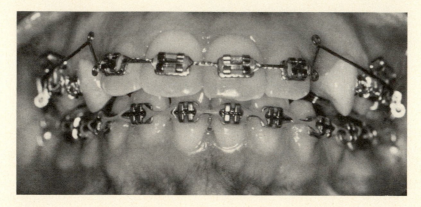

Fig. 15-35 ■ Utility arch inserted in auxiliary tube on molars, to intrude maxillary incisors while
alignment loops are used in the buccal segments. The loops in this utility arch can be activated to
exert a distal or space closing effect, providing a force to counteract the labial tipping of incisors
that otherwise would occur.

laterals (Fig. 15-33), also brings the point of force application more posteriorly so that the force is applied more
nearly through the center of resistance (Fig. 15-34). This
prevents anterior tipping of the incisor segment without
causing anchorage strain.

Even with the control of posterior anchorage obtained by
placing rectangular stabilizing segments and an anchorage
lingual arch, the reaction to intrusion of incisors is extrusion
and distal tipping of the posterior segments. With careful
attention to appropriate technique with the segmented arch
approach, it is possible to produce approximately four times
as much incisor intrusion as molar extrusion in nongrowing
adults. Although successful intrusion can be obtained with
round bypass arches, the ratio of anterior intrusion to posterior extrusion is much less favorable. A utility arch can
be used in conjunction with stabilized posterior segments,
simply by placing the utility arch into an auxiliary tube on
the first molar (an arrangement recommended by Ricketts
for older patients). With this alteration (Fig. 15-35), the
ratio of intrusion to extrusion improves. For adults, however,
to control anterior tipping, it is advantageous to tie the
depressing arch beneath a separate base archwire anteriorly,
rather than tying directly into the incisor brackets as is
usually done with a utility arch.

At the conclusion of the first stage of treatment, the arches
should be level, and teeth should be aligned to the point
that rectangular steel archwires can be placed without generating excessive forces. The duration of the first stage,
obviously, will be determined by the severity of both the
horizontal and vertical components of the initial malocclusion. For some patients, only a single initial archwire will
be required, while for others, several months may be needed
for alignment, and several more months for segmental leveling, before the next stage can begin. As a principle of
treatment, it is important not to move to the second stage
of treatment until both leveling and alignment are adequate.

■ *References*

1. Begg, P.R., and Kesling, P.C.: Begg orthodontic theory and
   technique. Philadelpia, 1977, W.B. Saunders.
2. Stoner, M.M.: Wire: clinical considerations. In Graber, T.M.,
   and Swain, B.F., editors: Current orthodontic concepts and
   techniques, ed. 2, Philadelphia, 1975, W.B.Saunders.
3. Haas, A.J.: The treatment of maxillary deficiency by opening
   the midpalatal suture. Angle Orthod. **35:**200-217, 1965.
4. Vanarsdall, R.L., and Corn, H.: Soft-tissue management of
   labially positioned unerupted teeth. Am. J. Orthod. **72:**53-64,
   1977.
5. Edwards, J.G.: The diastema, the frenum, the frenectomy: a
   clinical study. Am. J. Orth. **71:**489-508, 1977.
6. Mulligan, T.F.: Common sense mechanics. 6. Clinical application of the diving board concept. J. Clin. Orthod. **14:**98-103,
   1980.
7. Ricketts, R.W., et al.: Bioprogressive Therapy. Denver, 1979,
   Rocky Mountain Orthodontics.
8. Burstone, C.J.: Deep overbite correction by intrusion. Am. J.
   Orthod. **72:**1-22, 1977.

Chapter 16

The Second Stage of Comprehensive Treatment: Correction of Molar Relationship and Space Closure

At the beginning of the second stage of treatment, the teeth should be well aligned, and any excessive or reverse curve of Spee should have been eliminated. The objectives of this stage of treatment are correction of molar and buccal segment relationships to provide normal occlusion in the anteroposterior plane of space and the closure of extraction spaces or residual spaces in the arches.

■ Correction of Molar Relationship

Correction of the molar relationship nearly always involves moving from a Class II or partially Class II relationship to Class I, although occasionally the treatment will be aimed at a Class III problem. Excluding surgical repositioning of the jaws, which is especially likely to be required in Class III correction, there are three major possibilities for correcting the molar relationship: (1) differential growth of the jaws, guided by extraoral force or a functional appliance, (2) differential anteroposterior movement of the upper and lower posterior teeth as extraction spaces are closed, and (3) differential anteroposterior movement of the teeth under the influence of Class II or Class III elastics. These approaches are not mutually exclusive, and in fact some combination of the three is almost always used in the treatment of an individual patient.

■ Correction of Molar Relationship by Differential Growth

The use of extraoral force or functional appliances to influence jaw growth is discussed in some detail in Chapter 14. The different timing of skeletal growth in males and females must be kept in mind when this approach is used.

During adolescence, the mandible tends to grow forward more than the maxilla, providing an opportunity to improve a skeletal Class II jaw relationship. Girls mature considerably earlier than boys and are often beyond the peak of the adolescent growth spurt before the full permanent dentition is available and comprehensive orthodontic treatment can begin. Boys, who mature more slowly and have a more prolonged period of adolescent growth, are much more likely to have a clinically useful amount of anteroposterior growth during comprehensive treatment.

Whether extraoral force or a functional appliance is used to modify growth in Class II patients, a favorable response includes both restraint of maxillary growth and differential mandibular growth. Extraoral force is more compatible with the fixed appliances needed for comprehensive treatment than are functional appliances, and functional appliance therapy alone is unlikely to provide a satisfactory result in the early permanent dentition. In skeletally immature patients with a permanent dentition, there is nothing wrong with using a first phase of functional appliance treatment even though the permanent teeth have erupted, and then using a fixed appliance to obtain detailed occlusal results, but it is likely that the functional appliance therapy will have to be modified or discontinued when the fixed appliance treatment begins. Headgear therapy can be continued quite nicely.

An ideal patient for use of extraoral force in the early permanent dentition is a 12- to 14-year-old boy with a Class II problem, whose skeletal maturity is somewhat behind his stage of dental development, but who has good growth potential (Fig. 16-1). Boys at age 13, it must be remembered, are on the average at the same stage of maturation as girls at 11, and significant skeletal growth is almost always continuing. On the other hand, girls at age 13 are, on the average, at the same developmental stage as boys at 15, and by this time, clinically useful changes in jaw relationship from growth guidance are unlikely.

Although correction of molar relationship is a major goal of the second rather than the first stage of treatment, extraoral force should be applied against the first molars from the beginning in any patient for whom molar correction by differential growth is desired. There is no reason to wait for alignment and leveling to be completed, especially since every passing day decreases the probability of a favorable growth response. The extraoral force can also help control anchorage during alignment.

Although the main purpose of extraoral force is growth modification, some tooth movement in all three planes of space inevitably accompanies it. When there is good vertical growth and the maxillary molars are allowed to elongate, the maxillary teeth erupt downward and backward, and spaces may open up in the maxillary arch. Even though the extraoral force is applied against the first molar, it is unusual

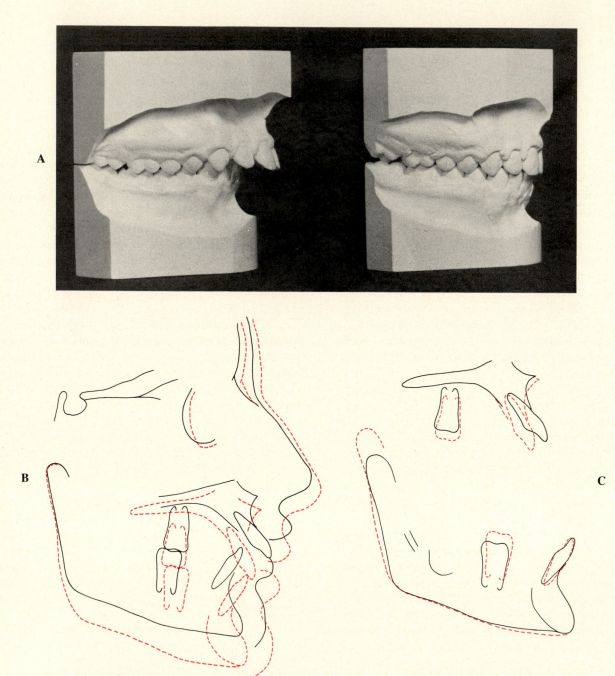

Fig. 16-1 ■ Class II correction in a 13 year-old boy, using extraoral force to the maxilla. **A,** Dental casts before and after treatment; **B, C,** cephalometric superimposition showing treatment changes. Note the large amount of vertical growth, which allowed the maxilla and maxillary dentition to be displaced distally as they moved vertically, while the mandible grew downward and forward. Overbite was corrected by relative intrusion, i.e., the lower incisors were held at the same vertical level while the molars erupted.

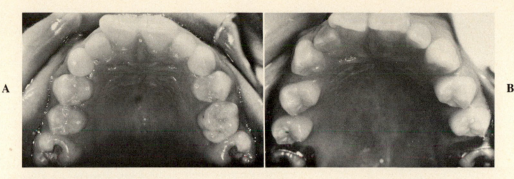

Fig. 16-2 ■ Space tends to open up within the maxillary arch when extraoral force to the upper first molars is used and the patient grows well. **A,** Occlusal view before treatment; **B,** same patient after 12 months of treatment with only a headgear. When a complete fixed appliance is placed at this stage, one of the first steps is consolidation of the space distal to the canines.

for space to develop between the first molar and second premolar. Instead, the second and to a lesser degree, the first premolars follow the molars. The result is often a space distal to the canines, along with a partial reduction of overjet as the jaw relationship improves (Fig. 16-2).

When this result occurs, the preferred approach is to consolidate space within the maxillary arch at a single location, using elastic ties to bring the canines and incisors into an anterior segment and the molar and premolars into a posterior segment. When the molar relationship has been corrected, the residual overjet is then reduced by retracting the incisors in this nonextraction patient in exactly the same way as in a patient who had a first premolar extraction space (see following). Extraoral force should be continued until an intact maxillary arch has been achieved. Discontinuing it when only the molar relationship has been corrected is unwise, both because the maximum skeletal effect probably has not been obtained at that point, and because the retraction of the incisor teeth requires posterior anchorage, which can be reinforced by the headgear.

■ Differential Anteroposterior Tooth Movement, Using Extraction Spaces

There are two reasons for extracting teeth in orthodontics, as discussed in detail in Chapter 7: (1) to provide space to align crowded incisors without creating excessive protrusion, and (2) to allow the camouflage of moderate Class II or Class III jaw relationships when correction by growth modification is not possible. The more extraction space required for alignment, the less there is available for differential movement in camouflage, and vice versa. An important part of treatment planning is deciding which teeth to extract and how the extraction spaces are to be closed (by retraction of incisor teeth, mesial movement of posterior teeth, or some combination). These decisions determine the orthodontic mechanics.

In this chapter, it will be assumed that appropriate decisions have been made, and the orthodontic mechanotherapy necessary to produce different types of tooth movement for molar correction will be described.

Class II correction by distal movement of maxillary posterior teeth: upper second molar extraction. The concept of "distal driving" of the maxillary posterior teeth has a long orthodontic history. Despite the belief of many practitioners that their usual correction of a Class II molar relationship was obtained by moving the upper molars back, the early cephalometric studies showed that this was not the case. It is now clear that significant distal positioning of the upper posterior teeth occurs only in the relatively few patients who have a great deal of vertical growth and elongation of the maxillary teeth (see Fig. 16-1). Without this, it is difficult to produce more than 2 mm of distal movement of the upper molars even with excellent cooperation in wearing headgear, unless the upper second molars are extracted. With second molar extraction and good headgear cooperation, the maxillary dental arch can be moved posteriorly (Fig. 16-3).

Extraction of upper second molars to camouflage a skel-

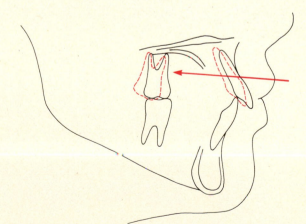

Fig. 16-3 ■ After extraction of maxillary second molars, extraoral force can successfully move the maxillary dentition posteriorly, as this cephalometric superimposition shows. To achieve this effect, the extraoral force must be applied nearly full time, to promote efficient tooth movement. (Retraced from Armstrong, M.M.: Am. J. Orthod. **59:**217-243, 1971.)

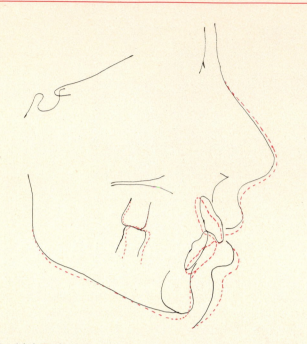

Fig. 16-4 ■ Cephalometric superimposition showing the response to Class II elastics in a girl in whom this was the major method for correcting a Class II malocclusion. The forward and downward movement of the lower incisors is apparent. Note that with rectangular archwires, some torque of the upper incisor was obtained. The rotational effects often associated with Class II elastics were less apparent for this patient than is sometimes the case, but the forward displacement of the lower teeth is apparent.

etal Class II relationship should be considered only when specific indications are present (see Chapter 8). The key to success is headgear force of moderate intensity with long duration. Skeletal effects in rapidly growing patients can be achieved with fewer hours per day of headgear wear than are necessary to successfully move teeth. The patient must wear the headgear full time or nearly so to move the maxillary teeth posteriorly. The force magnitude should be large enough to simultaneously reposition all the maxillary teeth, which means that with an archwire tying the teeth together, the force should be approximately 300 gm on each side.

Force from Class II elastics can also be used to position the upper molars distally. If an intact lower arch is pitted against an intact upper arch, even with upper second molars extracted, there will be considerably more mesial movement of the lower than distal movement of the upper teeth (Fig. 16-4). For this reason, if Class II elastics are used to drive upper molars distally, it is preferable at first to apply the elastic force against the first molars alone, via sliding jigs as illustrated in Fig. 16-5. The upper archwire is reduced in size posteriorly to allow freer sliding and the lower arch is stabilized with a full dimension rectangular archwire. This procedure is important not only to impede forward tipping of the mandibular teeth but also to maintain transverse control of the lower arch. Class II elastics tend to widen the lower molars, to the point that they can produce a molar crossbite. A heavy rectangular archwire, slightly constricted across the molars, is needed to prevent this complication.

Once the upper molar has been moved distally into a correct relationship, the jig is altered and force applied against the second premolars. As a final step, Class II elastic force is continued as the space between the first and second premolars is closed. With this approach, the elastic force against the lower arch should not exceed 100 gm per side. Even though this force is distributed over all the lower teeth, some mesial movement of the lower arch is an inevitable side effect.

Class II camouflage by extraction of upper first premolars. Like upper second molar extraction, extraction of upper first premolars is a deceptively attractive solution to Class II problems and should be adopted only when its specific indications exist (Chapter 8). With this approach, the objective during orthodontic treatment is to maintain the existing Class II molar relationship, closing the first premolar extraction space entirely by retracting the protruding

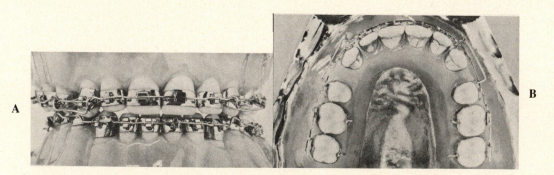

Fig. 16-5 ■ Sliding jigs to transfer Class II elastic force to the posterior segment of the maxillary arch. **A,** Anterior view; **B,** occlusal view. In typical use, a jig is used to transfer Class II elastic force to the first molar, then is shortened to apply the Class II force to the second premolar, as shown here. To achieve a horizontal component, the Class II elastic must attach anteriorly, so the anterior part of the jig is placed mesial to the canine, and the posterior part against the tooth to which pressure should be applied. (From Tweed, C.H.: Clinical orthodontics. St. Louis, 1966, The C.V. Mosby Co.)

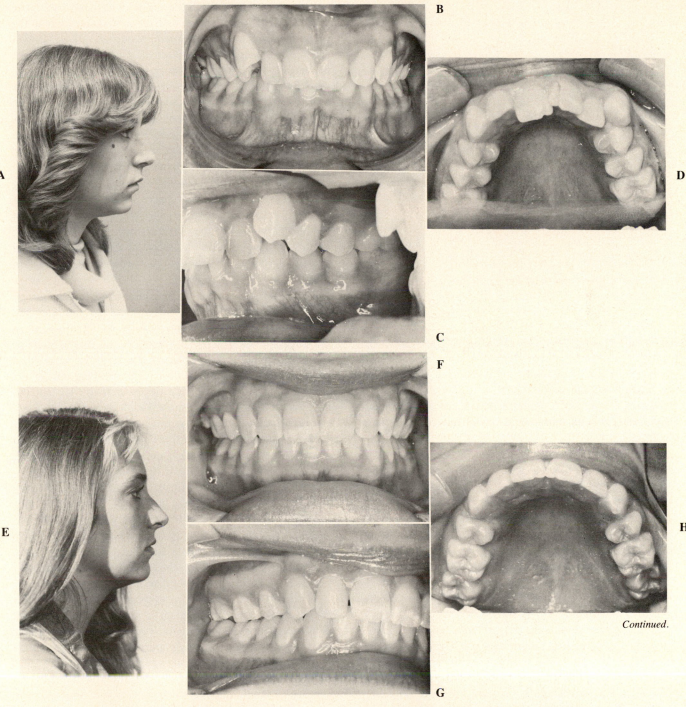

Fig. 16-6 ■ Records of a patient who was treated with extraction of upper first premolars for camouflage of a Class II malocclusion. **A,** Pretreatment profile photograph; **B** to **D,** pretreatment intraoral photographs; **E,** posttreatment profile; **F** to **H,** posttreatment intraoral photograph; **I,** *(next page),* cephalometric superimposition. For this patient, retraction of the maxillary incisors was accomplished with good anchorage control achieved with the use of a transpalatal stabilizing arch and headgear at night, and the esthetic change was quite acceptable.

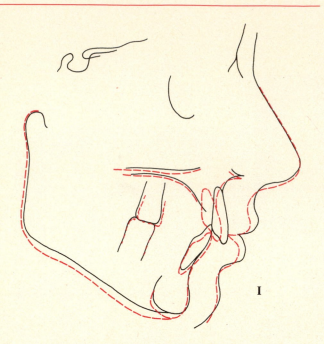

I

Fig. 16-6, cont'd ■ For legend see p. 423.

incisor teeth (Fig. 16-6). Maxillary posterior anchorage must be reinforced, but one method, Class II elastics from the lower arch, is specifically contraindicated. The remaining possibilities are extraoral force to the first molars, a stabilizing lingual arch, or retraction of the maxillary anterior segment with extraoral force directly against these teeth.

If retraction springs or closing loops between the maxillary anterior and posterior segments are used, reinforcing the posterior anchorage with both a lingual arch and extraoral force is possible and usually desirable. The advantage of retracting the anterior teeth with springs is that an optimal force system can be placed against the anterior teeth; the disadvantage is that this force system will also tend to displace the maxillary posterior teeth forward.

Excellent reinforcement of posterior anchorage can be obtained with extraoral force, if it is applied consistently and for long durations. The more constant the headgear wear, the less a stabilizing lingual arch will be needed. Conversely, a stabilizing lingual arch augments the posterior anchorage full time, while headgear is likely to be worn a good bit less. All the strategies described in Chapter 10 for reducing strain on anchorage (avoiding friction, retracting canines individually, etc.) are appropriate with upper first premolar extraction and can be brought into use.

Retracting the protruding maxillary anterior teeth with extraoral force (Fig. 16-7) totally avoids strain on the posterior teeth and is extremely attractive from that point of view. This technique has two major disadvantages: (1) The force system applied to the anterior teeth is far from ideal. When extraoral force is applied directly to the anterior segment, it is difficult to keep it from being undesirably heavy,

but the force intermittently falls to zero when the headgear is removed. (2) There is significant friction, not only where teeth slide along the archwire but also within the headgear mechanism itself. This factor makes it difficult to control the amount of force, and more friction on one side than the other may lead to an asymmetric response.

Excellent patient cooperation is essential. Only if the headgear is worn nearly full time will efficient tooth movement be obtained, and although it is possible to obtain this level of cooperation, it is unwise to rely on it routinely. Patients for this approach should be selected carefully.

Extraction of maxillary and mandibular premolars. Correction of Class II buccal segment relationships with extraction of all four first premolars implies that the mandibular posterior segments will be moved anteriorly nearly the width of the extraction space. At the same time, the protruding maxillary anterior teeth will be retracted without forward movement of the maxillary buccal segments. This, in turn, implies (though it does not absolutely require) that Class II elastics will be used to assist in closing the extraction sites.

The Begg technique is a classic illustration of the use of Class II elastics to produce differential movement of the arch segments while correcting the molar relationship. In the Begg approach, at the beginning of the second stage of treatment, light interarch elastics are added to help close space, while Class II elastics are continued (Fig. 16-8). An anchor bend is placed in the upper archwire so that the maxillary anterior teeth are tipped back in part by the force system associated with the arch wire itself (see Fig. 15-30).

In the lower arch, the anchor bend is used to control the amount of mesial tipping of the molars. The Class II elastics reinforce and accentuate the differential tooth movements along the archwires (Fig. 16-9). Friction as the archwires slide through the molar tubes during space closure is minimized by the considerable freedom between the .016 base arch and the .025 round tube through which it slides. It is extremely important that only light forces be used, so that optimal force levels are reached where tipping is desired while forces for bodily movement remain suboptimal.

A similar mechanical arrangement, of course, can be produced with the edgewise appliance. A round wire in an edgewise bracket allows tipping of the incisors in essentially the same way as with the Begg approach, but the mesiodistal width of the canine brackets tends to keep the canine teeth more upright, thereby increasing the strain on posterior anchorage. For this reason, when a Begg-like sliding space closure in both arches is used with the edgewise appliance, reinforcement of maxillary anchorage with headgear is a good idea, and somewhat heavier Class II elastic force is needed.

It is also possible with the edgewise appliance to structure anchorage so that space closure by retraction of the maxillary anterior teeth and protraction of the mandibular posterior segments occurs without the use of Class II elastics. The best control is achieved with segmented arch tech-

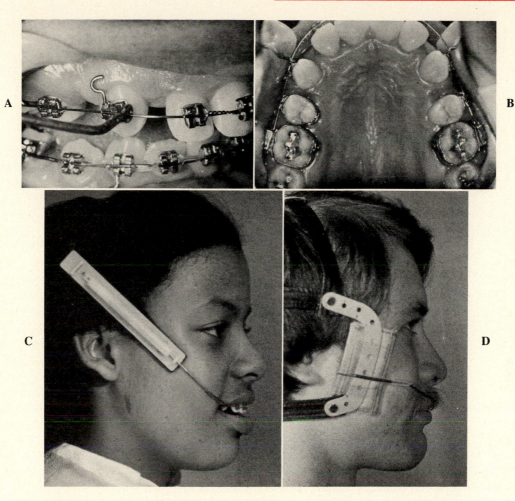

Fig. 16-7 ■ Retraction of the maxillary canines with a J-hook headgear. **A,** The headgear hooks over the archwire mesial to the canine bracket and pushes distally against the bracket. Approximately 200 gm of force on each side should be used; **B,** an occlusal view shows the distal translation of both canines. Note that the response at this stage is greater on one side than the other, which is not uncommon with headgear applied directly to the archwire for tooth movement; **C,** high-pull head cap with J-hook for canine retraction; **D,** an alternative head cap, providing a more directly posterior force.

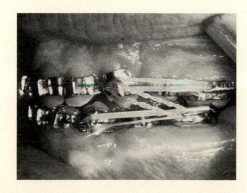

Fig. 16-8 ■ The second stage of Begg treatment, in which intraarch elastics are used simultaneously with Class II elastics for space closure and correction of molar relationship. This pattern of elastic force is continued until the extraction spaces are closed.

nique, using space-closing springs in each arch fabricated specifically for the type of space closure desired (see Closure of Extraction Spaces, this chapter).

When differential space closure without interarch elastics is desired, a more common approach with the edgewise appliance is to extract maxillary first but mandibular second premolars, thus altering the anchorage value of the two segments (Fig. 16-10). With this approach, routine space-closing mechanics will move the lower molars forward more than the upper, particularly if maxillary posterior anchorage is reinforced with a stabilizing lingual arch or headgear. This upper first–lower second premolar extraction pattern greatly simplifies the mechanics needed for differential space closure with continuous-arch edgewise technique.

■ Molar Correction with Interarch Elastics

Molar correction with Class II elastics, without extraction spaces as previously described, is produced largely by me-

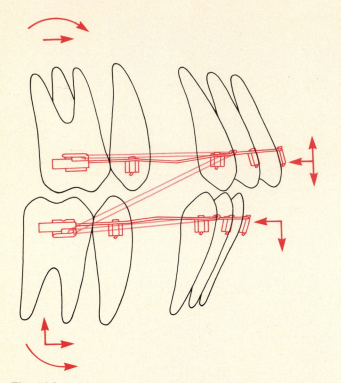

Fig. 16-9 ■ Diagrammatic representation of forces encountered in the second stage of Begg treatment, in which base archwires (red) with anchor bends are combined with intraarch and Class II elastics (pink). The anchor bends produce bodily forward movement of the molars and allow lingual tipping of the incisors, which receive no moments. These bends also depress the incisors and elongate the molars, which is counteracted by the Class II elastics for the upper arch but accentuated by the elastics for the lower.

sial movement of the mandibular arch, with a small amount of distal positioning of the maxillary arch. The amount of force varies with the amount of tipping allowed in the mandibular arch. Unless tipping is desired, which is rarely the case, Class II elastics should be used only with a well-fitting rectangular wire in the lower arch that is somewhat constricted posteriorly. Large amounts of force must be used (approximately 300 gm per side) to displace one arch relative to the other when both are stabilized with rectangular wires in edgewise brackets. Incorporating the lower second molars in the appliance and attaching the elastics to a mesial hook on this tooth increase the anchorage and give a more horizontal direction of pull than hooking the elastic to the first molar.

It is important to keep in mind that with or without extraction, Class II elastics produce not only anteroposterior and transverse effects but also a vertical force (Fig. 16-11). This force elongates the mandibular molars and the maxillary incisors, rotating the occlusal plane up posteriorly and down anteriorly. If the molars extrude more than the ramus grows vertically, the mandible itself will be rotated downward. Class II elastics are therefore contraindicated in nongrowing patients who cannot tolerate some downward and backward rotation of the mandible. The rotation of the occlusal plane, in and of itself, facilitates the desired correction of the posterior occlusion (Fig. 16-12), but even if elongation of the lower molars can be tolerated because of good growth, the corresponding extrusion of the maxillary incisors can be unsightly.

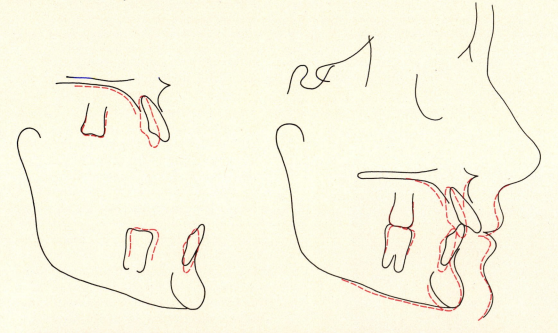

Fig. 16-10 ■ Cephalometric superimposition showing the result of treatment with extraction of upper first and lower second premolars. Even with second premolar extraction, some retraction of the mandibular incisors may occur, but most of the space closure will be by mesial movement of the lower molar. This adult patient experienced no growth, and a slight downward and backward rotation of the mandible occurred.

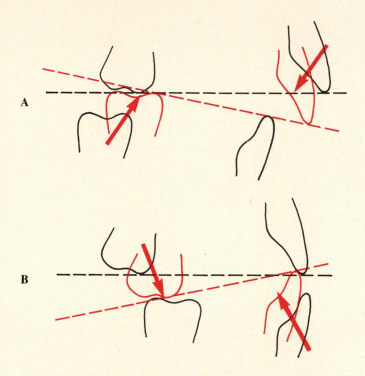

Fig. 16-11 ■ Rotation of the mandibular plane with Class II (**A**) or Class III (**B**) elastics. The rotational pattern helps correct the molar relationship, but can be deleterious in some patients because it may cause undesirable rotation of the mandible or produce undesirable tooth-lip relationships. (Redrawn from Woodside, D.G. In Salzmann, J.A. *Orthodontics in Daily Practice*. Philadelphia, 1974, J.B. Lippincott Co.)

Class II elastics, in short, may produce occlusal relationships that look good on dental casts but are less satisfactory when viewed from the perspective of skeletal relationships and facial esthetics (see Fig. 16-4).

Because of their vertical effects, prolonged use of Class II elastics, particularly with heavy forces, is rarely indicated. Using Class II elastics for 3 or 4 months at the completion of treatment of a Class II patient, to obtain good posterior interdigitation, is often acceptable. Applying heavy Class II force for 9 to 12 months as the major method for correcting a Class II malocclusion is rarely good treatment.

Class III elastics also have a significant extrusive component, tending to elongate the upper molars and the lower incisors (Fig. 16-13). Elongating the molars enough to rotate the mandible downward and backward is disastrous in Class II treatment, but within limits can help treatment of a Class III problem. If it is desired to use Class III elastics to assist in retracting mandibular incisors (see further discussion following), high-pull headgear to the upper molars worn simultaneously with the elastics can control the amount of elongation of the upper molars. Elongation of the lower incisors, however, can still be anticipated.

■ *Closure of Extraction Spaces*

To obtain the desired result in closing spaces within the arch, it is essential that the amount of incisor retraction

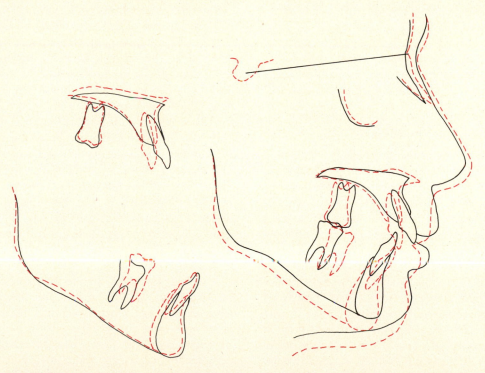

Fig. 16-12 ■ Cephalometric superimposition showing the effects of Class II elastics in the correction of this malocclusion. Note the elevation of the lower molar, extrusion and distal tipping of the upper incisor, rotation of the occlusal plane, and downward and backward rotation of the mandible.

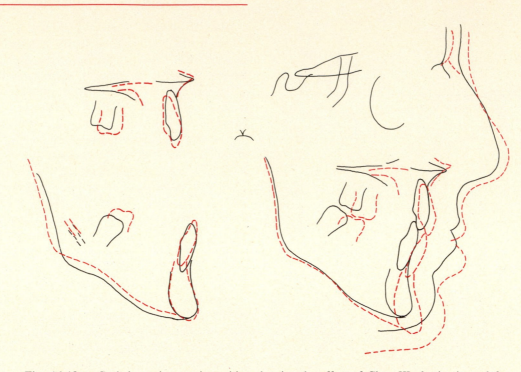

Fig. 16-13 ■ Cephalometric superimposition showing the effect of Class III elastics in a cleft palate patient with considerably more mandibular than maxillary growth. Note that the maxillary molar has been elongated as it was brought forward, causing the mandibular growth to be expressed more downward and less forward than otherwise would have been the case.

versus molar-premolar protraction be controlled. Indications for extraction have been discussed in Chapters 6 and 7, and the biomechanical concepts related to control of posterior anchorage and the amount of incisor retraction are described in Chapter 10. In this section, the focus is on contemporary mechanotherapy for space closure with the .018 and .022 edgewise appliances.

■ Moderate Anchorage Situations

Most patients fall into the moderate anchorage category, meaning that after alignment of the incisors has been completed, it is desired to close the remainder of the premolar extraction space with a 50:50 or 60:40 ratio of anterior retraction to posterior protraction. The different wire sizes in .018 and .022 edgewise appliances require a different approach to mechanotherapy.

Moderate anchorage treatment with .018 edgewise: closing loops. Although either sliding or loop mechanics can be used, the .018 appliance with single brackets on canines and premolars is ideally suited for use of closing loops in continuous archwires. Appropriate closing loops in a continuous archwire will produce approximately 60:40 closure of the extraction space if only the second premolar and first molar are included in the anchorage unit and some uprighting of the incisors is allowed. Greater retraction will be obtained if the second molar is part of the anchorage unit, less if incisor torque is required.

The spring characteristics of a closing loop, a critical part of its design, are largely determined by two major factors: the size of the archwire, and the distance between points of attachment. This distance in turn is largely determined by the amount of wire incorporated into the loop but is affected also by the distance between brackets. Closing loop archwires should be fabricated from rectangular wire to prevent the wire from rolling in the bracket slots. Closing loops with equivalent properties can be produced from different sizes of wire, by increasing the amount of wire incorporated into the loop as the size of the wire increases, and vice versa. Wires of smaller cross-sectional area allow the use of simpler loop designs. The first principle of closing loop design is that the simplest possible loop is preferred because more complex configurations are less comfortable for patients, more difficult to fabricate clinically, and more prone to breakage or distortion.

A second principle is that, to the greatest extent possible, the loop should be "fail safe." This means that, although a reasonable range of action is desired from each activation, tooth movement should stop after a prescribed range of movement even if the patient does not return for a scheduled adjustment. Too long a range of action, with too much flexibility, could produce disastrous effects if a distorted spring were combined with a series of broken appointments. The ideal loop design, therefore, would produce a continuous, controlled force designed to produce tooth movement

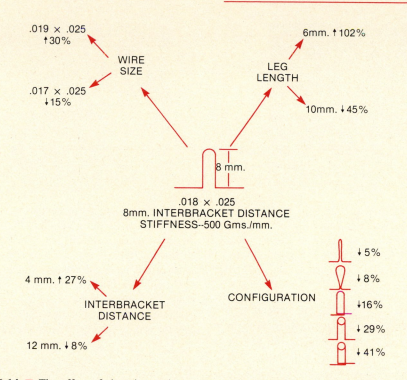

Fig. 16-14 ■ The effect of changing various aspects of a closing loop in an arch wire. Note that an 8 mm vertical loop in .018 × .025 wire produces twice as much force as the desired 250 gm/mm. The major possibilities for producing clinically satisfactory loops are incorporating additional wire by changing leg length, interbracket distance, and/or loop configuration, or reducing the wire size (redrawn from Booth).

at a rate of approximately 1 mm per month, but would not include more than 2 mm of range, so that movement would stop if the patient missed a second consecutive monthly appointment.

Fig. 16-14, taken from the work of Booth,[1] illustrates the effects on the spring characteristics of a vertical closing loop from changing wire size, the design of the loop, and the interbracket span (the combination of these latter two parameters, of course, determines the amount of wire in the loop). Note that, as expected, changing the size of the wire produces the largest changes in characteristics but the amount of wire incorporated in the loop is also important.

For closure of a first premolar extraction space without tipping, pitting the canine and two incisors against the posterior segment, the ideal retraction force would be approximately 250 gm (100 gm for the canine, 75 gm each for the lateral and central incisors). Obviously, this force could vary depending on the size of the teeth and whether the incisors could be allowed to tip slightly or would require total bodily movement. A closing loop should produce this amount of force at about 1.5 mm activation and should retain a significant fraction of this force level at least down to 0.5 mm.

From Fig. 16-14, it can be seen that based on these criteria, most of the commonly used steel wires produce far too much force when a simple vertical loop is used. Even .017 × .025 wire is too stiff unless additional wire is incorporated, changing the configuration as shown in the low-

er right part of Fig. 16-14. A 10 mm vertical loop in .016 × .022 wire produces force characteristics that reasonably approximate those desired.

To close an extraction space while producing bodily tooth movement, a closing loop must generate not only a closing force, but also appropriate moments to bring the root apices together at the extraction site. As discussed in Chapter 10, a moment-to-force ratio of approximately 10:1 is needed, meaning that a canine tooth being retracted with a 100 gm force must also receive a 1000 gm mm moment. If the bracket is 1 mm wide, a vertical force of 1000 gm must be produced by the archwire at each side of the bracket.

This factor limits the amount of wire than can be incorporated to make a closing loop springier, because if the loop becomes too flexible, it will be unable to generate the necessary moments even though the retraction force characteristics are satisfactory. Loop design is also influenced. Placing some of the wire within the closing loop in a horizontal rather than vertical direction improves its ability to deliver the moments needed to prevent tipping. Both because of this effect and because a vertically tall loop can impinge upon soft tissue, using a closing loop only 7 mm tall while incorporating 10 to 12 mm of wire—a delta or T-shaped loop—is preferred (Fig. 16-15).

All other factors being equal, a loop is more effective when it is closed rather than opened during its activation. On the other hand, a loop designed to be opened can be

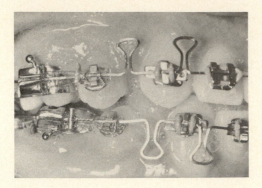

Fig. 16-15 ■ Delta-shaped closing loops in .016 × .022 wire. The loop mesial to the canine serves as an attachment for an elastic, or as an auxiliary to close any space mesial to the canine, while the loop in the extraction site provides the active space closure.

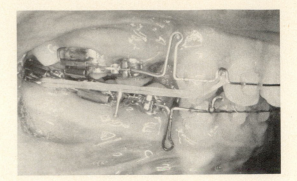

Fig. 16-16 ■ Eight millimeter closing loops in .016 × .022 wire used with Class II elastics in this patient. Note that the maxillary loop has been activated by pulling the wire through the maxillary tube and bending it up. In the mandibular arch, the loop is not active at this time, and the approximation of the legs to create a rigid archwire is apparent. The lower arch wire has a tieback mesial to the first molar, so that this loop can be activated by tying a ligature from the posterior teeth to the wire rather than by bending over the end of the wire distal to the molar tube.

made so that when it closes completely, the vertical legs come into contact, effectively preventing further movement and producing the desired fail-safe effect (Fig. 16-16). A loop activated by closing, in contrast, must have its vertical legs overlap. This creates a transverse step, and the archwire does not develop the same rigidity when it is deactivated. The smaller and more flexible the wire from which a closing loop arch is made, the more important it is that the wire become rigid when the loop is deactivated.

Based on these design considerations, it becomes apparent that one excellent closing loop for .018 edgewise is a delta-shaped loop in .016 × .022 wire activated by opening (Fig. 16-15). An .016 × .022 wire fits tightly enough in an .018 × .025 bracket to give good control of root position. The spring characteristics are excellent, and contact of the vertical legs when the loop is deactivated limits movement between adjustments and makes the archwire more rigid. It is important to activate the upper horizontal portion of a delta or T-loop so that the vertical legs are pressed

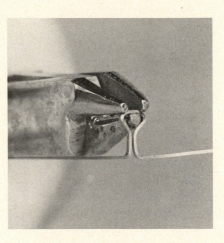

Fig. 16-17 ■ A three-prong plier can be used to bring the vertical legs of a closing loop together if they are separated. The legs should touch lightly before activation of the loop by opening it.

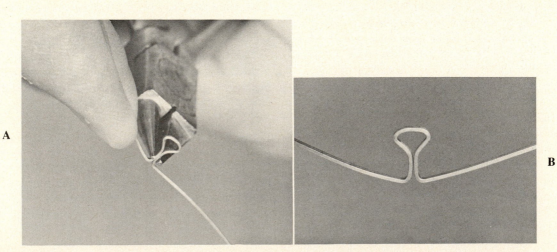

Fig. 16-18 ■ Gable bends for a closing loop archwire. **A,** Gable bends are placed by bending the wire at the base of the loop; **B,** appropriate gable for an .016 × .022 closing loop.

lightly together when the loop is not activated (Fig. 16-17). This also ensures that the loop will still be active until the legs come into contact.

A second important adjustment of a closing loop archwire is placing a gable bend at the extraction site. This adjustment is necessary to generate the root-paralleling moments. With .016 × .022 wire and a loop of the delta design shown in Fig. 16-15, a gable bend of approximately 20 degrees on each side is needed (Fig. 16-18). With the same loop in .017 × .025 wire, a smaller gable bend would generate the same moment. With an .016 × .022 closing loop, it is ordinarily necessary to remove the archwire and reactivate the gable bends after 3 to 4 mm of space closure, but is is not necessary to do this at each appointment.

A final factor in the design of a closing loop archwire is the location of the loop. Mechanically, it would be ideal to place the loop in the exact center of the extraction space, but a loop placed in the center of the initial extraction site becomes displaced distally as the space closes, and this is undesirable. The preferred location, therefore, is at the spot that will be the center of the embrasure when the space is closed (Fig. 16-19). This means that, in a first premolar extraction situation, the closing loop should be placed about 5 mm distal to the center of the canine tooth.

A closing loop archwire is activated by pulling the posterior part of the archwire distally through the molar tubes, which activates the closing loop the desired amount (1.0 to 1.5 mm), and then fastening the wire in that position. The wire slides through the brackets and tubes only when it is being activated. After that, as the closing loop returns to its original configuration, the teeth move with the archwire, not along it (Fig. 16-19). There are two ways to hold the

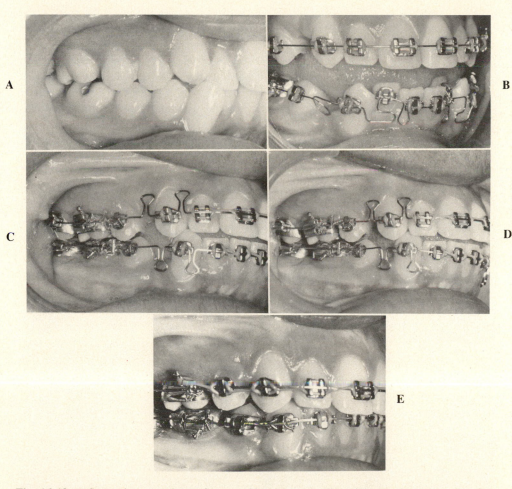

Fig. 16-19 ■ Stages in space closure for a specific patient. **A,** The original malocclusion; **B,** .014 loop arches for preliminary alignment. Note the independent distal tipping of the mandibular canines into the premolar extraction space; **C,** .016 × .022 closing loops at initial activation. Note the soldered tiebacks for activation. **D,** Closing loops later during space closure; **E,** spaces closed and finishing archwire in place.

archwire in its activated position. The simplest is by bending the end of the archwire gingivally behind the last molar tube. The alternative is to place an attachment on the posterior part of the archwire, usually a soldered tieback as shown in Figs. 16-15 and 16-19, so that a ligature can be used to tie the wire in its activated position.

As a general rule, if it is anticipated that a closing loop archwire will not have to be removed for adjustment (the distance to be closed is 4 mm or less), bending the posterior end of the wire is satisfactory. It can be quite difficult to remove an archwire that has been activated by bending over the end, however, and it saves time in the long run to use tiebacks for closing loops that will have to be removed and readjusted.

Specific recommendations for closing loop archwires with the .018 appliance and narrow brackets are:

1. .016 × .022 wire, delta or T-shaped loops, 7 mm vertical height, additional wire incorporated in the loop to make it equivalent to 12 mm vertical height
2. Gable bends of 40 to 45 degrees total
3. Loop placement 4 to 5 mm distal to the center of the canine tooth, at the center of the space between the canine and second premolar with the extraction site closed

These recommendations certainly are not the only clinically effective possibilities. The principle should be that if a heavier wire (.017 × .025, for instance) is used, the loop design should be altered to incorporate additional wire for better force-deflection characteristics. Also, the gable angulations should be adjusted according to both the springiness of the loop and the width of the brackets. With twin brackets on the canines, for instance, the reduced interbracket span would make any loop somewhat stiffer, and both this and the longer moment arm across the bracket would dictate a smaller gable angle.

Moderate anchorage space closure with .022 edgewise. As a general rule, space closure in moderate anchorage situations with the .022 edgewise appliance is done in two steps, first retracting the canines, usually sliding them along the archwire, and second, retracting the four incisors, usually with a closing loop. This two-step space closure will produce an approximately 60:40 closure of the extraction space, varying somewhat depending on whether second molars are included in posterior anchorage and incisor torque requirement.

An .019 × .025 wire is the largest on which sliding retraction of a canine should be attempted (because clearance in the bracket slot is needed), and .018 × .025 wire can also be used. An archwire with a posterior stop, usually in front of the first molar tube, is needed. This stop has the effect of incorporating all the teeth except the canine into the anchorage unit. The canine retraction can then be carried out with a coil spring, a spring soldered to the base archwire, an intraarch latex elastic, or an elastomeric material (Fig. 16-20). As a general rule, wire springs are preferred because of their more constant force characteristics. Elastics produce variable and intermittent forces, and elastomerics produce rapidly decaying interrupted forces.

In addition to its convenience and straightforward design,

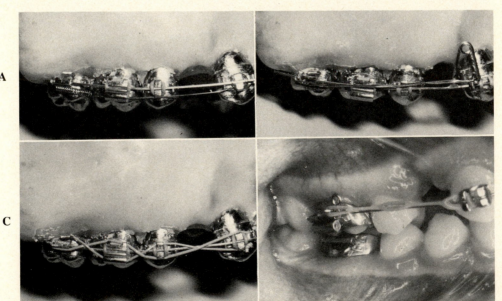

Fig. 16-20 ■ Methods for sliding canine retraction in .022 edgewise appliance. **A,** Use of a coil spring (Pletcher spring) to pull the canine back; **B,** soldered spring (Hice spring) for sliding retraction; **C,** elastomeric thread in a figure-of-eight tie; **D,** elastomeric chain from the molar to the canine.

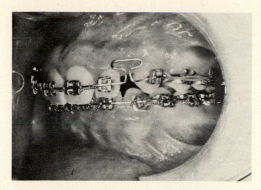

Fig. 16-21 ■ T-shaped loop in .018 × .025 wire, typically used with the .022 edgewise appliance to retract the four incisors after independent retraction of the canine.

this type of sliding space closure has the important advantage that it fails safe in two ways: (1) The moments necessary for root paralleling are generated automatically by the twin brackets normally used. Unless the archwire itself bends, there is no danger that the teeth will tip excessively. (2) The rigid attachment of the canine to the continuous ideal archwire removes the danger that this tooth will be moved far outside its intended path if the patient does not return for scheduled adjustments. For this reason, a long range of action on the retraction springs is not dangerous, as long as the force is not excessive. The ideal force to slide a canine distally is approximately 200 gm, about half of which is used to overcome friction (see Chapter 10).

The second stage in the two-stage retraction is usually accomplished with a closing loop, although it is possible to close the space now located mesial to the canines by again sliding the archwire through the posterior brackets. For this stage of incisor retraction, the smallest rectangular steel

archwire capable of engaging within the .022 × .028 bracket is desirable, and an .018 × .025 steel wire with a T-loop serves this purpose reasonably well (Fig. 16-21). Although an .019 × .025 steel wire can also be used, the better force-deflection characteristics of .018 × .025 wire make it the preferred choice. A third alternative is a closing loop in .019 × .025 beta-titanium wire, which provides even better properties than .018 × .025 steel.

Although the two-step procedure is predictable and has excellent fail-safe characteristics, which explains why it remains frequently used, it takes longer to close space in two steps than one.

It is possible to use a closing loop archwire for one-step (en masse) closure in the .022 edgewise system as described previously for .018 edgewise. In this case, an overlap design in .019 × .025 or a T-loop in .018 × .025 wire can be considered. The stiffer wires place a greater strain on anchorage than would be encountered with .018 slot and lighter wires. If en masse space closure is desired with the .022 appliance, a segmented arch technique offers advantages.

The segmented arch approach to space closure is based on incorporating the anterior teeth into a single segment, and both the right and left posterior teeth also into a single segment, with the two sides connected by a stabilizing lingual arch (Fig. 16-22). A retraction spring is used to connect these stable bases, and the activation of the spring is varied to produce the desired pattern of space closure (Figs. 16-23 and 16-24). Because the spring is separate from the wire sections that engage the bracket slots, a wire size and design that produce optimal properties can be used. An auxiliary rectangular tube, usually positioned vertically, is needed on the canine bracket or on the anterior wire segment to provide an attachment for the retraction springs (see Chapter 12). The posterior end of each spring fits into the auxiliary tube

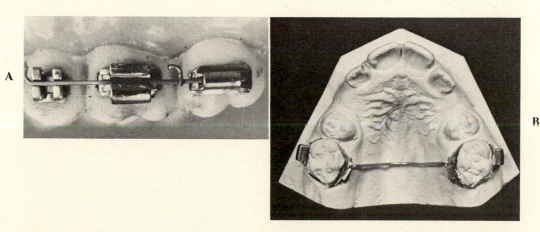

Fig. 16-22 ■ Stabilization of the posterior segments in Burstone's segmented arch technique. **A,** .021 × .025 wire in the bracket slots on tubes of the posterior teeth (courtesy Dr. C.J. Burstone); **B,** transpalatal lingual arch tying the right and left posterior segments together. A similar approach is used in the lower arch, except that the stabilizing lingual arch must curve forward (see Fig. 15-31).

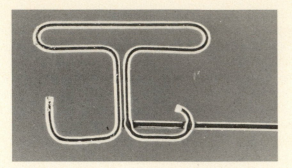

Fig. 16-23 ■ Composite retraction spring designed by Burstone for use with the segmented arch technique, consisting of .018 TMA wire (the loop) welded to .017 × .025 TMA. This spring can be used for either en masse retraction of incisors or canine retraction.

on the first molar tooth. With TMA wire, the design of the retraction spring can be greatly simplified over the design necessary with steel wire (Fig. 16-23).[2] These springs are very effective, and with careful initial activation, an impressive range of movement can be produced before reactivation is necessary.

The greatest disadvantage with segmented arch space closure is not its increased complexity, but that it does not fail safe. Without a rigid connection between the anterior and posterior segments, there is nothing to maintain arch form and proper vertical relationships if a retraction spring is distorted or activated incorrectly. For this reason, despite the excellent results usually obtained with segmented arches and retraction springs, it is important to monitor these patients especially carefully and to avoid long intervals without observation.

■ Maximum Incisor Retraction (Maximum Anchorage)

It is not always desirable to retract the anterior teeth as far as possible after premolars have been extracted. In fact, overretraction of incisors is as much of a potential problem as leaving them too prominent by not maintaining adequate posterior anchorage. When maximum retraction is needed, however, it is vital that the orthodontic mechanotherapy be structured to provide this. Techniques to produce maximum retraction combine two possible approaches. The first is reinforcement of posterior anchorage by appropriate means, including extraoral force, stabilizing lingual arches, and interarch elastics. The second approach involves reduction of strain on the posterior anchorage, which includes any combination of eliminating friction from the retraction system, tipping the incisors before uprighting them, or retracting the canines separately.

Maximum retraction with the .018 appliance. With the .018 appliance, friction from sliding is usually avoided and tipping/uprighting is rarely part of the anchorage control strategy. If maximum retraction of the anterior teeth is required with the .018 appliance and closing loops are normally used, a sequence of steps to augment anchorage and

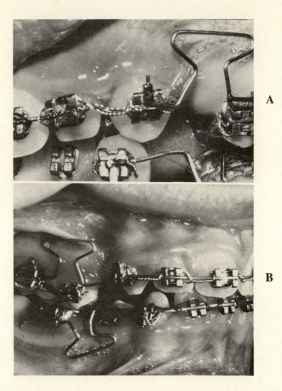

Fig. 16-24 ■ Space closure with the segmented arch technique. **A,** En masse retraction of the anterior maxillary segment and canine retraction in the mandibular arch. Note that the retraction springs fit into a vertical tube on the canine bracket. Braided wire in the maxillary anterior area will be replaced by a stabilizing anterior segment. **B,** Upper and lower en masse space closure using TMA T-loops. (Courtesy Dr. C.J. Burstone.)

reduce anchorage strain could be as follows:

1. Add stabilizing lingual arches and proceed with en masse space closure. The resulting increase in posterior anchorage, though modest, will change the ratio of anterior retraction to posterior protraction to approximately 2:1.

2. Reinforce maxillary posterior anchorage with extraoral force and (if needed) use Class III elastics from the high-pull headgear to supplement retraction force in the lower arch, while continuing the basic en masse closure approach. Depending on how efficiently the patient cooperates, additional improvement of retraction, perhaps to a 3:1 or 4:1 ratio, can be achieved.

3. Retract the canines independently, preferably using a segmental closing loop, and then retract the incisors with a second closing loop archwire. Used with stabilizing lingual arches (which are needed to control the posterior segments in most patients), this technique will produce a 3:1 retraction ratio. When this procedure is reinforced with headgear, even better ratios are possible.

Discussing each of these approaches in more detail:

Reinforcement with stabilizing lingual arches. Stabilizing lingual arches must be rigid and should be made from .036 steel wire for use with either the .018 or .022 appliance. These can be soldered to the molar bands, but it is convenient to be able to remove them, and Burstone's horizontal

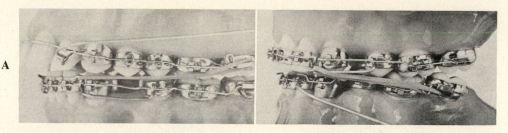

A B

Fig. 16-25 ■ Anchorage preparation in Tweed technique. Class III elastics from a stabilized upper arch reinforced with headgear are being used to tip back the lower posterior teeth. Note the second order bends in the lower archwire. **A,** Sliding jig is being used to transfer the Class III elastic force to the posterior segment; **B,** anchorage preparation completed in the lingual arch. Note the distally tipped position of the lower posterior teeth and the use of Class II elastics to accomplish similar distal tipping of the upper posterior teeth. (From Tweed, C.H.: Clinical orthodontics, St. Louis, 1966, The C.V. Mosby Co.)

insertion design (see Figs. 16-22 and 15-31) is preferred.

The stabilizing lingual arch for the lower arch is more conveniently inserted from the distal than from the mesial of the molar tube. It is important that the lower lingual arch lie behind and below the lower incisors, so that it does not interfere with their retraction. The maxillary stabilizing lingual arch is a straight transpalatal design. Because maximum rigidity is desired for anchorage reinforcement, an expansion loop in the palatal section of this wire is not recommended unless a specific indication exists for including it.

If lingual arches are needed for anchorage control, they should be present during the first and second stages of treatment, but can be removed after space closure is complete. Their presence during the finishing stage of treatment, after extraction spaces have been closed, is usually not helpful and may interfere with final settling of the occlusion.

Reinforcement with headgear and interarch elastics. Extraoral force against the maxillary posterior segments is an obvious and direct method for anchorage reinforcement. It is also possible to place extraoral force against the mandibular posterior segments, but usually more practical to use Class III elastics to transfer the extraoral force from the upper to the lower arch.

Interarch elastics for anchorage reinforcement were a prominent part of the original Tweed method for maximum retraction of protruding anterior teeth. In the Tweed approach to bimaxillary protrusion, lower but not upper premolars were extracted initially, so that an intact upper arch was available to resist the pull of Class III elastics. This step was the first component of the anchorage reinforcement: pitting an intact upper arch against a segmented lower arch (and later, the reverse).

The second part of Tweed anchorage reinforcement was ''anchorage preparation,'' achieved by tipping the molars and premolars distally (Fig. 16-25). Class III elastics were used to maintain lower incisor position while this was done. The distally tipped molars then allowed the incisors to be retracted further than otherwise would have occurred. Only after the lower incisors had been retracted, sliding the canine initially and then using a closing loop, were the upper pre-

molars extracted. At that point, the lower arch was stabilized and Class II elastics were used to prepare anchorage by tipping back the upper molars, before the upper incisors were retracted (Fig. 16-25, *B*).

Although the original Tweed approach can be used with the contemporary .018 appliance, it is rarely indicated. Prolonged use of Class II and III elastics is extrusive and requires good vertical growth for acceptable results. Distally tipping the molars augments their anchorage value primarily by first moving these teeth distally, then mesially.

Segmented retraction of the canines. Segmented retraction of the canines with frictionless springs is an attractive method for reducing the strain on posterior anchorage and is a readily available approach with the modern .018 appliance. It is also possible to retract the canines by sliding them on the archwire, but the narrow brackets usually used with the .018 appliance and the small clearance of the archwire produce friction problems.

For frictionless retraction of the canines, as in Ricketts' bioprogressive technique, an auxillary tube on the molar is needed. An auxiliary tube on the canine is unnecessary, because the retraction spring can fit directly into the canine bracket. Instead of stabilizing lingual arches, a base or utility arch from the first molar to the incisors is normally used (Fig. 16-26). Handled correctly, this technique provides efficient space closure with excellent force characteristics.

Segmented canine retraction springs used in bioprogressive technique are shown in Fig. 16-26. These flexible springs require a root-paralleling gable bend of approximately 60 degrees and an antirotation bend of approximately 20 degrees. Closing loops are then used for the second stage of retraction of the incisors (Fig. 16-27).

Segmented canine retraction presents two problems. The first is that it is difficult to control the position of the canine in all three planes of space as it is retracted. If the canine is pulled distally from an attachment on its buccal surface, the point of attachment is not only some distance occlusal but is also buccal to the center of resistance. This means that without appropriate moments, the tooth will tip distally and rotate mesiobuccally. Both a root-paralleling moment

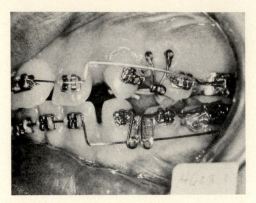

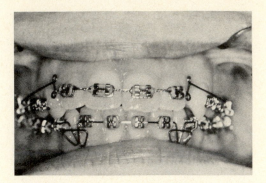

Fig. 16-26 ■ Utility arches from the first molars to the incisor segment used in conjunction with segmented canine retraction springs. This frictionless retraction of the canines reduces the strain on posterior anchorage and produces greater total retraction of the anterior teeth compared to en masse space closure.

Fig. 16-27 ■ Alternative archwires for retraction of the anterior segment after segmented retraction of the canines in .018 edgewise using Rickett's bioprogressive technique. In the upper arch, a contraction utility arch with helical loops to increase its anteroposterior flexibility is being used for anterior retraction. In the lower arch, double-delta loops are being used.

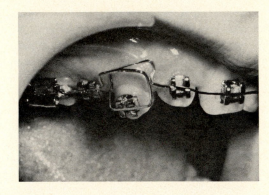

Fig. 16-28 ■ Vertical control of this canine was lost during retraction with a segmented retraction spring. A box-loop in .016 × .016 wire is being used to regain the correct vertical level. The greatest problem with segmented retraction springs is that they have no fail safe component, allowing displacements of this type to occur if a spring is distorted and the patient misses scheduled appointments.

and an antirotation moment must be obtained by placing gable bends in the spring. Control of the vertical position of the canine, particularly after the gable bends in two planes of space have been placed, can be a significant problem.

Second, much more than with en masse retraction using segmented mechanics, segmental retraction of canines does not fail safe. The canine is free to move in three dimensional space, and there are no stops to prevent excessive movement in the wrong direction if a spring is distorted or improperly adjusted. A missed appointment can lead to the development of a considerable problem (Fig. 16-28), and patients must be monitored carefully.

Maximum retraction with the .022 appliance. The same basic approaches are available with the .022 as with the .018 appliance: to increase the amount of incisor retraction, a combination of increased reinforcement of posterior anchorage and decreased strain on that anchorage is needed. All the possible strategies for anchorage control can be used. With a .022 appliance in which sliding retraction of canines is the approach to moderate anchorage, the following sequence of steps to increase incisor retraction might be logical:

Reinforcement of posterior anchorage with extraoral force. Stabilizing the posterior segments with extraoral force while sliding the canine along an archwire sifnificantly increases posterior anchorage. This approach can be especially helpful in the upper arch, where headgear attached to the molars is easily placed, but the same approach can be used in the lower arch. Wearing two facebows to apply force to upper and lower molar teeth at the same time is difficult but not impossible. Reinforcing the upper arch with headgear, with Class III elastics off the headgear to reinforce anchorage for retraction of the lower canines, is a more typical arrangement.

Application of extraoral force directly against the canines to slide them posteriorly. With this approach, a headgear using four hooks (Fig. 16-29) is normally used.[4] The hooks

fit over a base arch wire, typically .019 × .025, and approximately a 200 gm force is supplied at each point of attachment to slide the canines posteriorly. It is easier to attach extraoral force to the mandibular anterior than posterior region, and this arrangement is tolerated well by patients, much better than two facebows.

Retracting the canines in this way totally avoids strain on posterior anchorage during the first retraction step. The disadvantages are the same as when protruding maxillary incisors are retracted with headgear: friction may cause asymmetric space closure. Moreover, this approach requires excellent headgear cooperation by the patient, who should wear the headgear essentially full time to achieve effective tooth movement. For cooperative patients, however, this method is quite effective.

The second step, after retraction of the canines, is done with a closing loop as described previously.

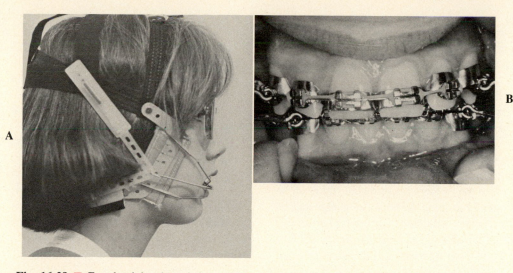

Fig. 16-29 ■ Four-hook headgear being used for retraction of the canines (in a patient who is also wearing a facebow to the molars). **A,** The hooks extend forward from a head cap and, **B,** attach over the upper and lower archwires mesial to the canines.

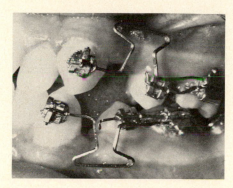

Fig. 16-30 ■ Retraction of upper and lower canines with T-loops in TMA wire, in segmented arch techniques with the .022 edgewise appliance. (Courtesy Dr. C.J. Burstone.)

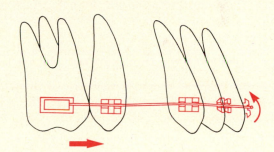

Fig. 16-31 ■ Torque forces against the incisors create a crown-forward as well as a root-backward tendency. Preventing the incisors crowns from tipping forward creates a strain on posterior anchorage, which can be advantageous if it is desired to close space by bringing the posterior teeth forward.

Use of segmented arch mechanics for canine retraction. As discussed earlier, use of a segmented arch system to retract the canines independently, followed by retraction of the four incisors, is a practical method for conserving anchorage and equally adaptable to .022 and .018 appliances (Fig. 16-30). It produces a result approximately equivalent to retracting the canines with headgear, provided that at least a stabilizing lingual arch is used to reinforce posterior anchorage. The problems are also the same as with the .018 slot: the canine can become displaced during its retraction and may become spectacularly malpositioned if something goes wrong, because no fail safe mechanism is in place.

Segmented arch mechanics for tipping/uprighting. Rather than independent retraction of the canines, Burstone[2] now recommends two-step space closure in maximum anchorage cases by en masse distal tipping of the anterior teeth, followed by uprighting. The segmented arch technique is used, but with a differently activated spring assembly from the

one needed for space closure in moderate retraction cases. Compared to independent retraction of the canines with loops, the fail-safe characteristics of this approach are much improved (though still not as good as with continuous arch wires). Excellent control of anchorage for maximum retraction, without the use of headgear, can be obtained. The segmented arch approach is particularly valuable in treatment of adults (see Chapter 20) but can be used very effectively in adolescents.

■ Minimum Incisor Retraction

As with any problem requiring anchorage control, the approaches to reducing the amount of incisor retraction involve reinforcement of anchorage (the anterior teeth in this situation) and reduction of strain on that anchorage. An obvious strategy, implemented at the treatment planning stage, is to incorporate as many teeth in the anterior anchor unit as possible. Therefore, if extraction of teeth is necessary at all, extracting a second premolar or molar, not a first premolar, is desirable. All other factors being equal, the amount of incisor retraction will be less the further posteriorly in the arch an extraction space is located (see Chapter 8).

A second possibility for reinforcing incisor anchorage is to place active lingual root torque in the incisor section of the archwires, maintaining a more mesial position of the incisor crowns at the expense of somewhat greater retraction of the root apices (Fig. 16-31). When the incisors protrude, some degree of forward tipping of these teeth is usually present, so that when the incisors are retracted, they can be allowed to tip lingually at least slightly. Advantage can be taken of this when incisor retraction is desired. Conversely, in patients in whom it is desired to close extraction sites by moving the posterior teeth forward, the incisors are often already upright, and lingual root torque is likely to be desired for both esthetic reasons and control of anchorage. Burstone's segmented arch technique can be used to particular advantage when this strategy for producing differential forward movement of posterior teeth is used.[2]

A third possibility for maximizing forward movement of posterior teeth is to break down the posterior anchorage, moving the posterior teeth forward one tooth at a time. After extraction of a second premolar, for example, it may be desired to stabilize the eight anterior teeth and to bring the first molars forward independently, creating a space between them and the second molars before bringing the second molars anteriorly.

A final possibility for maximizing protraction of posterior teeth is the use of extraoral force, pulling the teeth forward from a facemask or equivalent device (see Chapter 14). This provides the same opportunities and limitations as any other use of extraoral force for tooth movement. If the patient can be persuaded to wear this reverse headgear essentially full time, excellent tooth movement can be obtained. With only 10 to 14 hours per day, the results are often disappointing. Since a reverse headgear inevitably crosses the face, it is difficult to obtain the same level of cooperation as with a conventional posteriorly placed headgear.

It should rarely be necessary to use involved mechanotherapy to protract posterior teeth. The need for this approach arises from an effort to close spaces from congenitally missing teeth, teeth that were lost to decay, or perhaps teeth that should not have been extracted for orthodontic purposes. If the temptation to use first premolars as a routine extraction is avoided, most of the need for minimum retraction mechanotherapy is also avoided.

■ *References*

1. Booth, F.A.: Optimum forces with orthodontic loops. Houston, 1971, M.S. Thesis, University of Texas Dental Branch.
2. Burstone, C.J.: The segmented arch approach to space closure. Am. J. Orthod. **82:**361, 1982.
3. Ricketts, R.M., et al.: Bioprogressive Therapy. Denver, 1979, Rocky Mountain Orthodontics.
4. Hickham, J.H.: Direct edgewise orthodontic approach. J. Clin. Orthod. **8:**617, 1974.

Chapter 17

The Third Stage of Comprehensive Treatment: Finishing

Root paralleling at extraction sites
Torque of incisors
Correction of vertical relationships
   Excessive overbite
   Anterior open bite
Midline discrepancies
Tooth size discrepancies
Final "settling" of teeth
Removal of bands and bonded attachments
Positioners for finishing
Special finishing procedures to avoid relapse
   Control of unfavorable growth
   Control of soft tissue rebound

By the end of the second stage of treatment, the teeth should be well aligned, extraction spaces should be closed, and the teeth in the buccal segments should be in a normal Class I relationship. In the Begg technique, major root movements of both anterior and posterior teeth still remain, to obtain root paralleling at extraction sites and proper axial inclination of tipped incisors. With contemporary edgewise techniques, relatively little finishing is required, but minor versions of these same movements are likely to be required. In addition, most techniques require some adjustment of the vertical relationship of incisors as a finishing procedure, either correcting moderately excessive overbite or closing a mild anterior open bite.

■ *Root Paralleling at Extraction Sites*

In the Begg technique, extraction spaces are closed by initially tipping the teeth together, and then uprighting them (Fig. 17-1). In the finishing stage, the moments necessary for root uprighting are generated by adding auxiliary springs that fit into the vertical slot of the Begg (ribbon arch) bracket. In most instances, a heavier (.020) archwire replaces the .016 archwire used as a base arch up to that point, to provide greater stability. Root paralleling is accomplished by placing an uprighting spring in the vertical slot, and hooking it beneath the archwire. Since the root uprighting forces are also crown separating forces, the crowns must be tied together across the extraction site. The Begg uprighting

springs extend only a short distance from the point of insertion into the bracket to the point where they are hooked to the archwire. Therefore, it is necessary both to make the uprighting springs from small diameter wire (usually .014) and to increase their length by bending a double helix at the base of the spring.

During space closure with the edgewise appliance, it is usually a goal of treatment to produce bodily tooth movement during space closure, preventing the crowns from tipping together. If proper moment-to-force ratios have been used, little if any root paralleling will be necessary as a finishing procedure. On the other hand, it is likely that at least a small amount of tipping will occur in some patients, and some degree of root paralleling is often necessary.

Exactly the same approach used in Begg technique can be employed with the edgewise appliance if it includes a vertical slot behind the edgewise bracket (Fig. 17-2). This allows an uprighting spring to be inserted and hooked beneath a base archwire, in the same way as in Begg technique. This approach is reasonably effective with narrow edgewise brackets and an undersized round wire (typically .018) in the .022 edgewise appliance. In contemporary edgewise technique, this method has been almost totally abandoned in favor of angulated bracket slots that produce proper root paralleling when a full-dimension edgewise arch is placed as a finishing archwire.

With the .018 appliance, the typical finishing archwire is either .017 × .022 or .017 × .025 steel. These wires are flexible enough to engage narrow brackets even if a moderate degree of tipping has occurred, and the archwire will generate the necesary root paralleling moments. If a greater degree of tipping has occurred, a more flexible full dimension rectangular archwire is needed. To correct more severe tipping, a beta-titanium or even a nickel-titanium .017 × .025 wire might be needed initially, with a steel archwire to obtain final positioning.

With wider .022 brackets on the canines and premolars and with the use of sliding rather than loop mechanics, there is usually even less need for root paralleling as a finishing procedure than with narrow brackets and closing loop archwires. If teeth do tip even slightly into the extraction space, however, a full-dimension steel archwire in an .022 bracket is much too stiff to produce the needed root up-

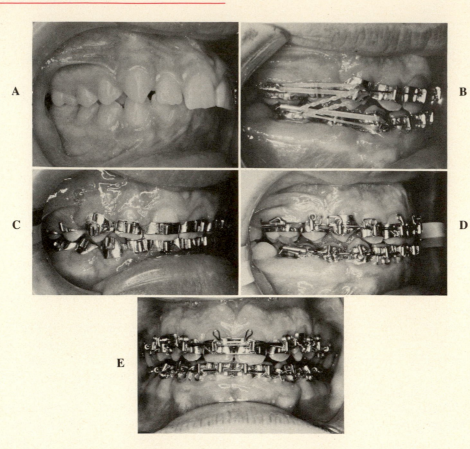

Fig. 17-1 ■ Stages in Begg technique. **A,** The original Class II division I malocclusion; **B,** space closure during stage 2; **C,** tooth positions at the end of stage 2. Note the lingual tipping of incisors and mesiodistal tipping of canines and premolars; **D,** lateral view of the Begg appliance, during stage 3, showing auxiliary root uprighting springs on second premolars, canines, and lateral incisors. These springs extend into the vertical slot of the Begg bracket and hook beneath the archwire adjacent to the tooth. **E,** Anterior view showing a torquing auxiliary to the maxillary central incisors. This auxiliary archwire is "piggy backed" over the base arch and hooks beneath the base arch posteriorly.

righting moment. Even an .019 × .025 steel wire is undesirably stiff. A rectangular beta-titanium wire is an excellent choice if root paralleling is needed.

A root-paralleling moment is a crown-separating moment in edgewise just as it is in Begg, and this effect is important to remember. Either the teeth must be tied together at the extraction site, or the entire archwire tied back against the molars (Fig. 17-3), to prevent the extraction site from reopening during finishing.

Occasionally, a severely tipped canine tooth will be encountered, and a longer range of action is needed than can be delivered by even the most flexible continuous archwire. In this situation, there are two options: (1) bending a loop into a rectangular archwire to provide the desired flexibility (Fig. 17-4), or (2) using an auxiliary root uprighting spring.

With the .018 appliance, the best choice is usually a box

loop in .016 × .022 or .017 × .025 wire. At the same time that the root of the canine tooth is being positioned distally, this loop can also be used to obtain a last bit of space closure. A similar box loop archwire can be used with the .022 appliance, made from .018 × .025 wire (the smallest size that will not twist in an .022 bracket). The alternative is to bypass the tipped canine with a rectangular base arch and use an auxiliary root uprighting spring extending from the auxiliary tube on the first molar and tied into the canine bracket. In .022 edgewise, this is the preferred approach.

■ *Torque of Incisors*

If protruding incisors tipped lingually while they were being retracted, lingual root torque as a finishing procedure may be required. In the Begg technique, the incisors are

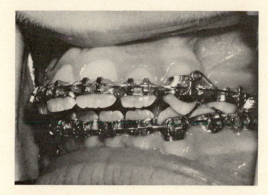

Fig. 17-2 ■ An auxiliary uprighting spring placed in a vertical slot behind an otherwise standard edgewise bracket, for distal root positioning of the canine tooth. This use of auxiliary uprighting springs and edgewise technique has been almost completely abandoned in favor of preangulated brackets and modern resilient archwires.

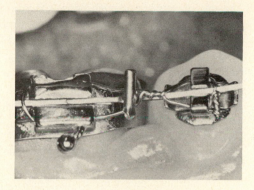

Fig. 17-3 ■ A rectangular archwire that incorporates active root paralleling moments or torque must be tied back against the molar teeth, to prevent space from opening within the arch. If the ligature used to tie back the archwire is cabled forward and also used to tie the second premolar, the tieback is less likely to come loose.

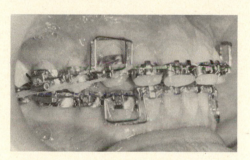

Fig. 17-4 ■ **A,** Box loops in .017 × .025 wire for canine root positioning, in this case after surgical repositioning of the maxillary and mandibular incisor segments. A loop of this type can also serve as a closing loop if it is activated posteriorly, as has been done here in the upper arch.

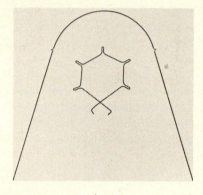

Fig. 17-5 ■ Torquing auxiliary archwires exert their effect when the auxiliary, originally bent into a tight circle as shown, is forced to assume the form of the base archwire over which it will be placed. This tends to distort the base archwire, which therefore should be relatively heavy wire, at least .018 steel.

deliberately tipped back during the second stage of treatment, and lingual root torque is a routine part of the third stage of treatment. Like root paralleling, this is accomplished with an auxiliary appliance that fits over the main or base archwire. The torquing auxiliary is a "piggyback arch" that contacts the labial surface of the incisors near the gingival margin, creating the necessary couple with a moment arm of 4 to 5 mm (see Fig. 17-1). Although these piggyback torquing arches come in a number of designs, the basic principle is the same: the auxiliary arch, bent into a tight circle initially, exerts a force against the roots of the teeth as it is partially straightened out to normal arch form (Fig. 17-5).

A torquing force to move the roots lingually is also, of course, a force to move the crowns labially (see Fig. 16-31). In a typical Class II patient, anchorage is required to

maintain overjet correction while upper incisor roots are torqued lingually. Class II elastics are normally worn during the third stage of Begg treatment to ensure that the maxillary incisor crowns do not become repositioned labially. In addition, the incisors are usually taken to an edge-to-edge relationship during the second stage of Begg treatment, allowing some possibility for the maxillary crowns to move forward during the third stage (see Fig. 17-1). The Class II elastics that reinforce the upper arch, however, further add to the tendency to displace the lower arch mesially, and the inclination of the lower incisors will be improved as much by labial tipping as by lingual root torque.

The torquing auxiliaries normally used in Begg technique not only place lingual force against the incisor roots, they tend to alter the form of the arch itself, because the torquing auxiliary wire tends to constrict the base arch posteriorly.

A major reason for using a heavier base archwire in the third stage of treatment is to resist this potential distortion of arch form. Better results are achieved with an .020 base arch during the third stage than with an .016 wire, as originally used by Dr. Begg.

Precise positioning of individual teeth is difficult to obtain with the Begg appliance. The minimal area of contact between the base archwire and the bracket, though helpful in providing for relatively free tipping and sliding movements, makes it impossible to use the base arch to obtain detailed tooth positioning, and the auxiliaries used for root positioning have no fail safe component at all. They continue to work until disconnected. Tooth positioners (see following) are usually used with the Begg appliance to detail the occlusal relationships, but a positioner is unable to materially affect root position.

For this reason, modifications of the Begg appliance, so that a rectangular archwire in a rectangular slot can be used for finishing purposes, have been proposed repeatedly. This method requires a combination bracket, incorporating an edgewise bracket slot along with the vertically oriented Begg slot. A recent version of such a combination bracket is shown in Fig. 17-6. With this variation, root paralleling and torquing are done with Begg style auxiliary wires, up to a stage of completion approximately equivalent to that at which patients treated with the current edgewise appliances usually enter the finishing stage. Then a rectangular archwire is used in exactly the same way that it would be in edgewise treatment (Fig. 17-7).

In edgewise technique, only moderate additional torque should be necessary during the finishing stage. With the .018 edgewise appliance, an .017 × .025 steel archwire has excellent torsion properties, and active torque with the archwire is entirely feasible. Building torque into the bracket slot initially means that it is unnecessary to place torquing bends in the archwire, making the accomplishment of torque as a finishing procedure relatively straightforward.

With the .022 edgewise appliance, steel full-dimension rectangular wires are far too stiff for effective torquing, and if incisors have been allowed to tip lingually too much, as can happen in the correction of maxillary incisor protrusion, correcting this merely by placing a rectangular steel archwire is not feasible. Torquing auxiliaries similar to those in the Begg appliance were commonly used with .022 standard edgewise technique, and a number of designs have been offered commercially. These piggyback arches are usually used with round rather than rectangular base archwires. Alternatively, an auxiliary torquing spring can be soldered to a rectangular base archwire (see Chapter 10).

One of the great virtues of pretorqued brackets is that, even in the .022 appliance, tipping of incisors can be largely prevented during retraction and space closure. For this reason, torquing auxiliaries for the .022 edgewise appliance have almost disappeared from contemporary use. In addition, full-dimension nickel-titanium or beta-titanium archwires can be used to torque incisors with .022 brackets (provided the brackets have torque built in), further reducing any need for auxiliary arches.

One torquing auxiliary deserves special mention: the Burstone torquing arch (Fig. 17-8). It can be particularly helpful in patients with Class II division 2 malocclusion whose maxillary central incisors are severely tipped lingually and require a long distance of torquing movement, while the lateral incisors need little if any torque. Because of the long lever arm, this is the most effective torquing auxiliary for use with the edgewise appliance. It is equally effective with the .018 or .022 appliance.

Two factors determine the amount of torque that will be expressed by any rectangular archwire in a rectangular slot: the inclination of the bracket slot relative to the archwire, and the tightness of the fit between the archwire and the bracket. The variation in torque prescriptions in contemporary edgewise appliances is shown in Table 12-1. These variations largely reflect different determinations of the average contour of the labial and buccal surfaces of the teeth, but some differences are also related to the expected fit of archwires. With the .018 appliance, it is assumed that the rectangular archwires used for finishing will fit tightly in the bracket slot, i.e., that the finishing archwires will have a minimum dimension of .017 or .018. With the .022 appliance, on the other hand, some brackets may have extra built-in torque to compensate for rectangular finishing archwires that will have more clearance. Torque will not be expressed to the same extent with an .019 wire in an .022 bracket as with an .017 wire in an .018 bracket. The difference amounts to several degrees of torque. Obviously, it is important to know what finishing wires were intended in any given straight arch appliance.

For full expression of the torque built into brackets in the .022 edgewise appliance, it is better to use an .021 × .025 beta-titanium arch wire for finishing, taking advantage of the greater resilience of this modern material. A less effective alternative is .021 × .025 braided rectangular steel wire. A solid .021 × .025 steel wire cannot be recommended because of its stiffness and the resulting extremely high forces and short range of action.

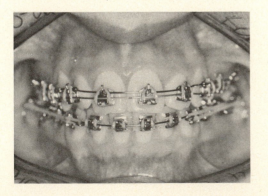

Fig. 17-6 ■ A contemporary combination bracket for use with Begg technique, fabricated so that a rectangular archwire in a rectangular slot can be used in finishing. (Courtesy Dr. W.J. Thompson.)

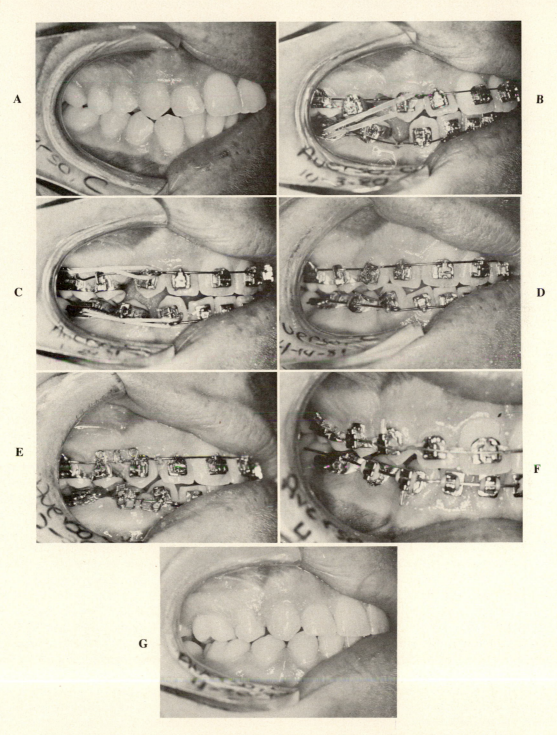

Fig. 17-7 ■ Stages with a combination Begg-edgewise appliance. **A,** The original malocclusion; **B,** stage 1; **C,** beginning stage 2; **D,** end stage 2; **E,** Stage 3 with Begg uprighting springs and a round base arch; **F,** finishing stage continued with a rectangular finishing archwire added; **G,** posttreatment occlusion. (Courtesy Dr. W.J. Thompson.)

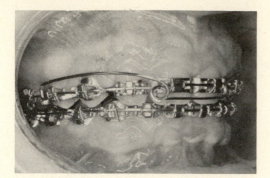

Fig. 17-8 ■ Burstone torquing auxiliary used with .022 standard edgewise appliance. The torquing auxiliary is .021 × .025 steel wire that fits in the brackets only on the central incisors. The base arch extends forward from the molars through the lateral incisor brackets, then steps down and rests against the labial surface of the central incisors. When the torquing auxiliary is passive, its long posterior arms are up in the buccal vestibule. It is activated by pulling the arms down and hooking them beneath the base archwire mesial to the first molar. The segment of the base arch that rests against the labial surface of the central incisors prevents the crowns from going forward, and the result is efficient torque of the central incisor roots.

■ *Correction of Vertical Relationships*

If the first two stages of treatment have gone smoothly, no change in the vertical position of incisors will be needed during the finishing stage of treatment. At this stage, anterior open bite is more likely to be a problem than residual excessive overbite, but either situation may occur.

■ Excessive Overbite

Before attempting to correct excess overbite at the finishing stage of treatment, it is important to carefully assess why the problem exists, and particularly to observe the vertical relationship between the maxillary lip and maxillary incisor. An excessive curve of Spee with relative elongation of the lower incisors may still be the cause of overbite, but by this stage of treatment, the problem is often slight elongation of the maxillary incisors. If so, an auxiliary intrusion arch is the preferred solution.

If a rectangular finishing archwire is already in place, the simplest approach may be to cut this archwire distal to the lateral incisors and install an auxiliary intrusion arch (Fig. 17-9). Alternatively, if the patient is still growing and relative rather than absolute intrusion would be satisfactory (see Chapter 15), a light round continuous archwire with an accentuated curve of Spee (.016 or .018) can be placed, and an auxiliary arch added to it. As a general rule, if an auxiliary depressing arch is added to a continuous base archwire, the base arch should be a relatively small round wire, while if the base arch is segmented, the segments should be rectangular wire.

It is important to remember that when an auxiliary intrusion arch is used, a stabilizing transpalatal lingual arch may

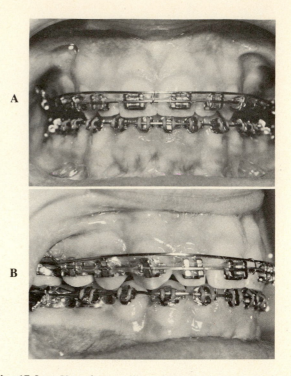

Fig. 17-9 ■ Use of an auxiliary depressing arch at the finishing stage to correct a mildly excessive overbite. **A,** Anterior view; **B,** lateral view. If the intrusion is desired, the base arch must be segmented.

be needed to maintain control of transverse relationships and prevent excessive distal tipping of the maxillary molars. The greater the desired vertical change in incisor position, the more important it will be to have a stabilizing lingual arch in place, and vice versa. Small corrections during finishing usually do not require placing a lingual arch.

■ Anterior Open Bite

As with deep bite, it is important to analyze the source of the difficulty if an anterior open bite persists at the finishing stage of treatment. Only rarely is a persistent open bite caused by lack of eruption of the upper incisors, and elongating these teeth is usually undesirable. If the open bite results from excessive eruption of posterior teeth, whether from a poor growth pattern or improper use of interarch elastics, correcting it at the finishing stage can be extremely difficult. High-pull headgear to the upper molars is the best approach if excessive vertical development of the posterior maxilla is the basic problem, and this treatment will have to be continued until growth is nearly complete, usually well into the retention period.

If no severe problems with the pattern of facial growth exist, however, a mild open bite at the finishing stage of treatment is usually caused by an excessively level lower arch. This condition is managed best by elongating the lower but not the upper incisors, creating a slight curve of Spee. Because of the stiffness of the rectangular archwires used for finishing, particularly with .022 edgewise, it is futile to

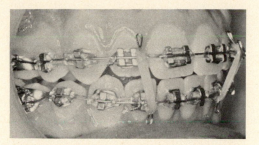

Fig. 17-10 ■ Anterior vertical elastics used to close a mild anterior open bite at the end of the treatment. In this photograph, two small elastics are being used on the right and left sides. An alternative is to use a single larger elastic in a box configuration.

use vertical elastics without altering the form of the archwires to provide a curve of Spee in the lower arch. Moreover, it is preferable to replace a heavy rectangular lower archwire with a lighter round wire before using anterior vertical elastics.

Posterior marginal ridge discrepancies, which may also contribute to the open bite, should be eliminated with small vertical steps in the archwires. The preferred approach is to place a light round wire (.016 or .018) in the lower arch, with a slight curve of Spee and any necessary vertical steps to correct marginal ridge discrepancies, while retaining a full-dimension rectangular archwire in the upper. Light elastic force is then used to elongate the lower incisors and close the open bite (Fig. 17-10). Elongating anterior teeth in this way, of course, is no substitute for controlling posterior vertical development. If carried to an extreme, this will reintroduce overjet and produce an esthetically unacceptable relationship even if proper occlusion is achieved.

■ *Midline Discrepancies*

A relatively common problem at the finishing stage of treatment is a discrepancy in the midlines of the dental arches. This condition can result either from a preexisting midline discrepancy that was not completely resolved at an earlier stage of treatment, or an asymmetric closure of spaces within the arch. Minor midline discrepancies at the finishing stage are no great problem, but it is quite difficult to correct large discrepancies after extraction spaces have been closed and occlusal relationships have been nearly established. As with any discrepancy at the finishing stage, it is important to establish as clearly as possible exactly where the discrepancy arises. Although coincident dental midlines are an important component of functional occlusion—all other things being equal, a midline discrepancy will be reflected in how the posterior teeth fit together—it is undesirable esthetically to displace the maxillary midline, bringing it around to meet a displaced mandibular midline. A correct maxillary midline is important for good facial esthetics, while a small displacement of the mandibular midline creates no esthetic difficulty.

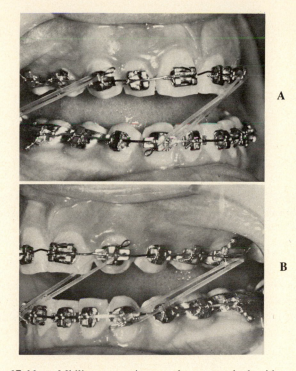

Fig. 17-11 ■ Midline correction can be approached with any combination of asymmetric posterior and anterior diagonal elastics. **A, B,** In this patient, a combination of Class II, Class III, and anterior diagonal elastics are being used, with a rectangular archwire in the lower arch and a round wire in the upper, attempting to shift the maxillary arch to the right.

If a midline discrepancy results from a skeletal asymmetry, it may be impossible to correct it orthodontically, and treatment decisions will have to be made in the light of camouflage versus surgical correction (see discussion in Chapter 8). Fortunately, midline discrepancies in the finishing stage are not usually this severe and are caused only by lateral displacements of maxillary or mandibular teeth. Usually, the midline discrepancy is accompanied by a mild Class II or III relationship on one side.

In this circumstance, the midline can often be corrected by using asymmetric Class II (or Class III) elastic force. As a general rule, it is more effective to use Class II or III elastics bilaterally with heavier force on one side than to place a unilateral elastic. However, if one side is totally corrected while the other is not, a unilateral elastic is usually tolerated reasonably well by the patient. It is also possible to combine a Class II or Class III elastic on one side with a diagonal elastic anteriorly, to bring the midlines together (Fig. 17-11).

An important consideration in dealing with midline discrepancies is the possibility of a mandibular shift contributing to the discrepancy. This can arise easily if a slight discrepancy in the transverse position of posterior teeth is present. For instance, a slightly narrow maxillary right posterior segment can lead to a shift of the mandible to the left on final closure, creating the midline discrepancy. The cor-

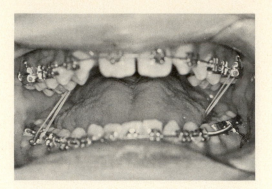

Fig. 17-12 ■ Parallel cross elastics, used to correct a mild transverse discrepancy leading to a lateral mandibular shift late in treatment.

rection in this instance, obviously, must include some force system (usually careful coordination of the maxillary and mandibular archwires, perhaps reinforced by a posterior cross elastic) to alter the transverse arch relationships. Occasionally, the entire maxillary arch is slightly displaced transversely relative to the mandibular arch so that with the teeth in occlusion, relationships are excellent, but there is a lateral shift to reach that position. Correction again would involve posterior cross elastics, but in a parallel pattern as shown in Fig. 17-12.

If a midline discrepancy is more from displacement of mandibular than maxillary teeth, or vice versa, the difference in stability with rectangular versus round wires can be used to help in correcting the situation. If the maxillary midline is correct while the mandibular midline deviates slightly toward one side, and a mild Class II relationship still exists on that side, replacing the rectangular mandibular finishing arch with an .016 or .018 round wire, while retaining a full-dimension rectangular arch in the upper arch, can facilitate correction with a unilateral Class II elastic. This approach should be reserved for small discrepancies, and it is important to carefully observe and control any expansion of the lower molar while a Class II elastic is worn against a light archwire. Prolonged use of Class II or III elastics during the finishing stage of treatment should be avoided, but a brief period of interarch elastic force is often necessary to obtain final positioning of teeth.

■ Tooth Size Discrepancies

Tooth size discrepancy problems must be taken into account when treatment is planned initially (see Chapter 7), but many of the steps to deal with these problems are taken in the finishing stage of treatment. Reduction of interproximal enamel (stripping) is the usual strategy to compensate for discrepancies caused by excess tooth size. When the problem is tooth size-deficiency, it is necessary to leave space between some teeth, which may or may not ultimately be closed by restorations.

One of the advantages of a bonded appliance is that interproximal enamel can be removed at any time. When stripping of enamel is part of the original treatment plan, most of the enamel reduction should be done initially, but final stripping can be deferred until the finishing stage. This procedure allows direct observation of the occlusal relationships before the final tooth size adjustments are made.

Tooth size deficiency problems are often caused by small maxillary lateral incisors. Having a small space distal to the lateral incisor is usually esthetically and functionally acceptable. Addition of composite resins to small teeth is an excellent way to compensate for tooth size problems, and is often the best plan for small incisors (Fig. 17-13). It is better to add small amounts of resin on both sides of a small tooth than a large amount on one side. During finishing, segments of coil spring are usually placed on the finishing archwire to precisely position the small tooth. The composite buildups should be done as soon possible after the patient is in retention, but not until soft tissue inflammation has been resolved.

More generalized small deficiencies can be masked by altering incisor position in any of several ways. To a limited extent, torque of the upper incisors can be used to compensate: leaving the incisors slightly more upright makes them take up less room relative to the lower arch and can be used to mask large upper incisors, while slightly excessive torque can partially compensate for small upper incisors. These adjustments require third order bends in the finishing archwires. It is also possible to compensate by slightly tipping teeth, or by finishing the orthodontic treatment with mildly excessive overbite or overjet, depending on the individual circumstances.[1]

■ Final "Settling" of Teeth

At the conclusion of Class II or III correction, particularly if interarch elastics have been used, the teeth tend to rebound back toward their initial position despite the presence of rectangular archwires. In addition, it is not uncommon for a full-dimension rectangular archwire, no matter how carefully made, to hold some teeth slightly out of occlusion.

Because of the rebound after Class II or III treatment, it is important to slightly overcorrect the occlusal relationships. In a typical Class II, anterior deep bite patient, the teeth should be taken to an end-to-end incisor relationship, with both overjet and overbite totally eliminated, before the headgear or elastic forces are discontinued (Fig. 17-14). Similar overcorrection is needed for other problems, providing some latitude for the teeth to rebound or settle into the proper relationship.

A need for settling can also be seen in Class I cases. A rectangular finishing archwire nearly always requires some first, second, or third order bends to precisely position the teeth. One cannot simply place an ideal rectangular archwire in a straight arch appliance and assume that the ideal position of each tooth will result. For essentially every patient, vari-

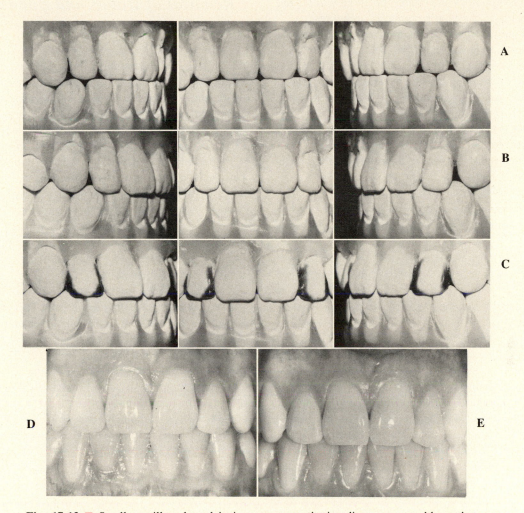

Fig. 17-13 ■ Small maxillary lateral incisors create tooth size discrepancy problems that may become apparent only late in treatment. **A,** Setup showing anterior edge-to-edge relationship with the upper incisors in proximal contact; **B,** spaces distal to the lateral incisors with proper overjet/overbite relationship. This approach can be a satisfactory solution for some patients. **C,** Wax-up showing possible addition of composite restorative material to build up the small laterals and allow space closure; **D,** clinical photograph of same patient immediately after; **E,** 12 months after composite buildups of the laterals. (From Fields, H.W.: Am J. Orthod. **79:**176-183, 1981.)

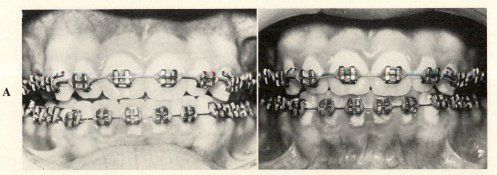

Fig. 17-14 ■ In finishing, overcorrection of Class II or III relationships is necessary to compensate for the rebound that occurs when headgear or elastic force is discontinued. **A,** Occlusion at the time active force in this boy with Class II malocclusion was discontinued; **B,** same patient 8 weeks later.

ations in tooth morphology and bracket positions will require some adjustments in the final rectangular archwires.

The more precisely the archwire fits the brackets and the more bends that it requires, the more likely that some teeth will be almost but not quite in occlusion. This phenomenon was recognized by the pioneers with the edgewise appliance, who coined the term ''arch-bound'' to describe it. They found that with precisely fitting wires, it was almost impossible to get every tooth into solid occlusion, although one could come close.

These considerations lead to the formulation of two rules in finishing treatment:

1. Interarch elastics and headgear should be discontinued, and the rebound from their use should be allowed to express itself, 4 to 8 weeks before the orthodontic appliances are removed.

2. As a final step in treatment, the teeth should be brought into a solid occlusal relationship without heavy archwires present.

The final step of finishing, therefore, is appropriately called ''settling,'' since its purpose is to bring all teeth into a solid occlusal relationship before the patient is placed in retention. There are two ways to settle the occlusion: with the use of a tooth positioner, as discussed following, or by replacing the rectangular archwires at the very end of treatment with light round arches that provide some freedom for movement of the teeth (.016 in the .018 appliance, .016 or .018 in the .022 appliance) and allowing the teeth to find their own occlusal level. These light final arches must include any first or second order bends used in the rectangular finishing arches. It is usually unnecessary for the patient to wear light posterior vertical elastics during this settling, but they can be used if needed (Fig. 17-15). These light arches will quickly settle the teeth into final occlusion and should remain in place for only a few weeks at most.

■ *Removal of Bands and Bonded Attachments*

Removal of bands is accomplished by simply breaking the cement attachment, then lifting the band off the tooth—which sounds simpler than it is in some instances. For upper molar and premolar teeth, a band removing plier is placed so that first the lingual, then the buccal surface is elevated by the plier (Fig. 17-16). A welded lingual bar is needed on these bands to provide a point of attachment for the plier, if lingual hooks or cleats are not a part of the appliance. For the lower posterior teeth, the sequence of force is just the reverse: the band removing plier is applied first on the buccal, then the lingual surface. Maxillary anterior bands are removed from the labial surface with an anterior band removing plier, while tightly fitted mandibular anterior bands usually must be slit with a cutting plier to make it possible to take them off.

Bonded brackets must be removed, insofar as possible, without damaging the enamel surface. This is done by creating a fracture within the resin bonding material or between the bracket and the resin, and then removing the residual resin from the enamel surface (Fig. 17-17). If a shearing stress is applied to the bracket, twisting it away from the tooth surface, the resin usually fractures, but there is some risk of enamel damage. Applying a cutting plier to the base of the bracket so that the bracket bends has the disadvantage of destroying the bracket, which otherwise could be reused, but this is the safest method.[2]

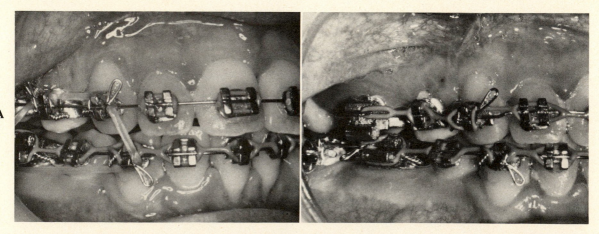

Fig. 17-15 ■ Use of vertical elastics for settling. **A,** Heavy archwires have been replaced by .016 archwires, and ⅜ inch light vertical elastics in a box pattern are being worn to bring the teeth into tight occlusion; **B,** 4 weeks later.

Cement left on the teeth after debanding can be removed easily by scaling, but residual bonding resin is more difficult to remove. The best results are obtained with a 12-fluted carbide bur at moderate speeds in a dental handpiece[3] (Fig. 17-18). This bur cuts resin readily but has little effect on enamel. Topical fluoride should be applied when the cleanup procedure has been completed, however, since some of the fluoride-rich outer enamel layer may be lost with even the most careful approach.

■ *Positioners for Finishing*

An alternative to light round archwires for final settling is a rubber or plastic tooth positioner. A positioner is most effective if it is placed immediately on removal of the fixed orthodontic appliance. Normally, it is fabricated by removing the archwires 4 to 6 weeks before the planned removal of the appliance, taking impressions of the teeth and a registration of occlusal relationships, and then resetting the teeth in the laboratory, incorporating the minor changes in position of each tooth necessary to produce appropriate settling (Fig. 17-19). All erupted teeth should be included in

the positioner, to prevent supereruption. As part of the laboratory procedure, bands and brackets are trimmed away, and any band space can be closed.

This indirect approach allows individual tooth positions to be adjusted with considerable precision, bringing each tooth into the desired final relationship. The positioning device is then fabricated by forming either a hard rubber or soft plastic material around the repositioned and articulated casts, producing a device with the inherent elasticity to move the teeth slightly to their final position (Fig. 17-20).

The use of a tooth positioner rather than final settling archwires has two advantages: (1) it allows the fixed appliance to be removed somewhat more quickly than otherwise would have been the case, and (2) it serves not only to reposition the teeth but also to massage the gingiva, which is almost always at least slightly inflamed and swollen after comprehensive orthodontic treatment. The gingival stimulation provided by a positioner is an excellent way to promote a rapid return to normal gingival contours (Fig. 17-21).

The use of positioners for finishing also has disadvantages. First of all, these appliances require a considerable

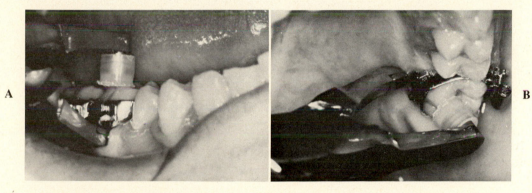

Fig. 17-16 ■ Removal of molar bands with a band removing plier. **A,** Lower posterior bands are removed primarily with pressure from the buccal surface; **B,** upper posterior bands are removed from the lingual surface, using a lingual attachment welded to the band.

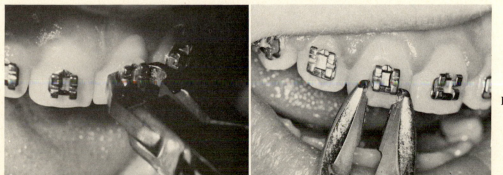

Fig. 17-17 ■ Removal of bonded brackets. **A,** A special plier can be used to grasp the edges of the base and break the attachment with a twisting motion; **B,** a cutter can be used to distort the bracket base, breaking the attachment. The first approach is more compatible with recycling of brackets, but the second is less likely to damage enamel.

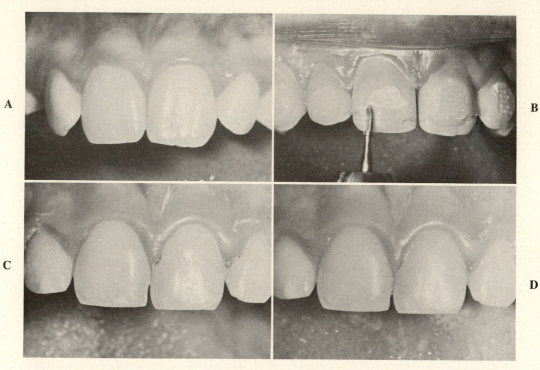

Fig. 17-18 ■ Removing excess bonding resin is best accomplished with a smooth 12-fluted carbide bur, followed by pumicing. **A,** Closeup view of the virgin surface of upper incisors; **B,** excess resin left on the tooth surface after removal of brackets. Upon debonding, the bond failure usually occurs between the base of the bracket and the resin, leaving excess resin on the tooth. The carbide bur is used with a general wiping motion to remove the resin; **C,** tooth surface after the remainder of the resin has been removed with the bur; **D,** tooth surface after final removal of resin (compare to **A**).

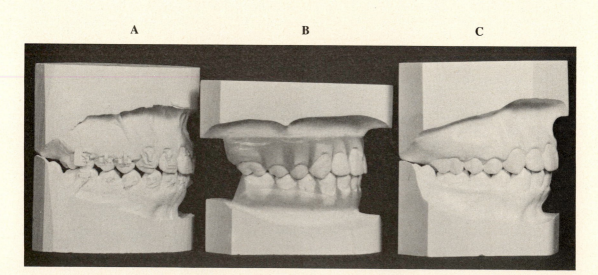

Fig. 17-19 ■ Use of a positioner for finishing. **A,** Casts 1 month before appliance removal, used to fabricate an immediate positioner; **B,** the positioner setup, with bands and brackets carved off the teeth in the laboratory; **C,** casts 2 weeks after appliance removal and placement of the positioner, showing the teeth settled into their finished relationship.

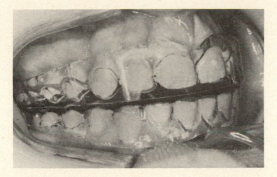

Fig. 17-20 ■ A tooth positioner made from a transparent plastic material, placed in the patient's mouth. The patient bites into the positioner, which creates forces to slightly displace the teeth and also massages the gingiva. A device of this type is most effective in moving teeth if it is placed immediately after the fixed appliance is removed.

amount of laboratory fabrication time, and therefore are expensive. Second, settling with a positioner tends to increase overbite more than the equivalent settling with light archwires. This is a disadvantage in patients who had a deep overbite initially but can be advantageous if the initial problem was an anterior open bite. Third, a positioner does not maintain the correction of rotated teeth well, which means that minor rotations may recur while a positioner is being worn. Finally, good cooperation is essential.

A positioner should be worn by the patient at least 4 hours during the day, and during sleep. Since the amount of tooth movement produced by a positioner tends to decline rapidly after a few days of use, an excellent schedule is to remove the orthodontic appliances, clean the teeth and apply a fluoride treatment, and place the positioner immediately, asking the patient to wear it as nearly full time as possible for the first 2 days. After that, it can be worn on the usual night-plus-4 hours schedule.

As a general rule, a tooth positioner in a cooperative patient will produce any changes it is capable of within 3

weeks. Final (posttreatment) records can be taken 2 or 3 weeks after the positioner is placed. Beyond that time, if the positioner is continued, it is serving as a retainer rather than a finishing device (see Chapter 18).

■ *Special Finishing Procedures to Avoid Relapse*

Relapse after orthodontic treatment has two major causes: (1) continued growth by the patient in an unfavorable pattern, and (2) tissue rebound after the release of orthodontic force.

■ Control of Unfavorable Growth

Changes resulting from continued growth in a Class II, Class III, deep bite, or open bite pattern contribute to a return of the original problem, and so are relapse in that sense. These changes are not attributed to tooth movement alone, however, but to the pattern of skeletal growth. It is more accurate to say that their control requires a continuation of active treatment than to describe this treatment as specific procedures to prevent relapse. For patients with skeletal problem who have undergone orthodontic treatment, this "active retention" takes one of two forms. One possibility is to continue extraoral force in conjunction with orthodontic retainers (high-pull headgear at night, for instance, in a patient with a Class II open bite growth pattern). The other appropriate option is to use a functional appliance rather than a conventional retainer after the completion of fixed appliance therapy. This subject is discussed in more detail in Chapter 18.

■ Control of Soft Tissue Rebound

A major reason for retention is to hold the teeth until soft tissue remodeling can take place. Even with the best remodeling, however, some rebound from the application of orthodontic forces occurs, and indeed the tendency for rebound after interarch elastics are discontinued has already

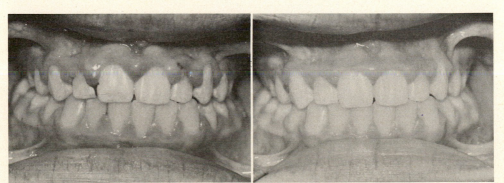

Fig. 17-21 ■ Gingival improvement with positioner wear. **A,** Swollen maxillary papillae immediately after band removal, just before placement of a positioner; **B,** 2 weeks later. This degree of gingival reaction anteriorly is rarely seen, especially with bonded attachments.

been discussed. There are two ways to deal with this phenomenon: (1) overtreatment, so that any rebound will only bring the teeth back to their proper position, and (2) adjunctive periodontal surgery to reduce rebound from elastic fibers in the gingiva. In some cases, permanent retention is required to maintain the desired relationships, but this need not be planned if either of the two approaches described here would make it unnecessary.

Overtreatment. Since it can be anticipated that teeth will rebound slightly toward their previous position after orthodontic correction, it is logical to position them at the end of treatment in a somewhat overtreated position. Only a small degree of overtreatment is compatible with precise finishing of orthodontic cases as described previously, but it is nevertheless possible to apply this principle during the finishing phase of treatment. Considering three specific situations:

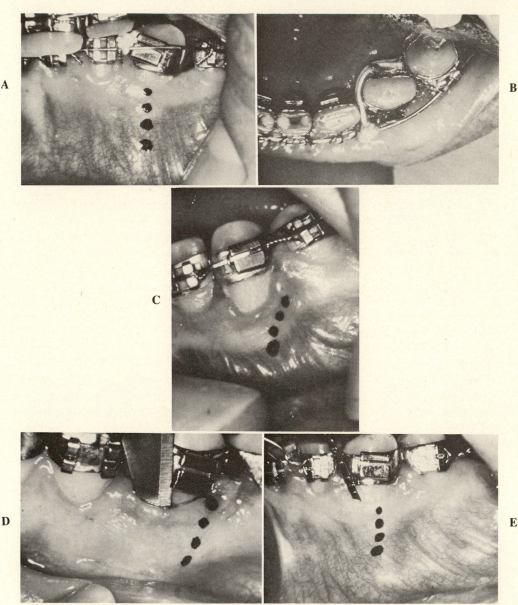

Fig. 17-22 ■ Elastic stretch of the supracrestal gingival fibers and the release of this elastic stretch by fiber section can be demonstrated by placing tattoo marks in the gingiva. **A,** India ink tattoos placed in the vicinity of a rotated maxillary canine before correction of the rotation; **B,** elastic thread used to rotate the tooth into position; **C,** the tooth rotated to its correct position in the arch. Note the displacement of the gingival tissues, as revealed by the deviation of the tattoo marks. **D,** Circumferential incision around the tooth, penetrating to the crest of the alveolar bone; **E,** after the incision, the gingival tissue returns to its original position. Periodontal probing shows a normal sulcus depth after the incision. (From Edwards, J.G.: Am. J. Orthod. 57:35-46, 1970.)

Correction of Class II or III malocclusion. The rebound or settling after Class II or III has already been discussed. After the headgear or elastics correcting the occlusal relationship have been discontinued, it can be expected that the teeth will rebound 1 to 2 mm (see Fig. 17-14), so this degree of overtreatment is required. This rebound is entirely different from relapse tendencies caused by continued growth, which appear long term. The rebound from the forces used for Class II or III correction occurs relatively quickly, within 3 to 4 weeks.

Crossbite correction. Whatever the mechanism used to correct crossbite, it should be overcorrected by at least 1 to 2 mm before the force system is released. If the crossbite is corrected during the first stage of treatment, as should be the case, the overcorrection will gradually be lost during succeeding phases of treatment, but this should improve stability when transverse relationships are established precisely during the finishing phase.

Irregular and rotated teeth. Just as with crossbites, irregularities and rotations can be overcorrected during the first phase of treatment, carrying a tooth that has been lingually positioned slightly too far labial, for instance, and vice versa. Similarly, a tooth being rotated into position in the arch can be overrotated. It is wise to hold the teeth in a slightly overcorrected position for at least for at least a few months, during the end of the first stage of treatment and the second stage. Maintaining an overrotated position can be done by adjusting the wings of single brackets, or by pinching shut one of a pair of twin brackets. Maintaining overcorrected labiolingual positions of incisors is done readily with first order bends in working archwires.

Overcorrection of the position of irregular incisors may be helpful if maintained for a few months, but as a general rule it is not wise to build this into rectangular finishing archwires. Rotated teeth should be maintained in an overcorrected position as long as possible, but even then, these teeth are often candidates for the periodontal procedures described following.

Adjunctive periodontal surgery. The major cause of rebound after orthodontic treatment is the network of elastic supracrestal gingival fibers. As teeth are moved to a new position, these fibers tend to stretch, and they remodel very slowly. If the pull of these elastic fibers could be eliminated, a major cause of relapse of previously irregular and rotated teeth should be eliminated. In fact, if the supracrestal fibers are sectioned and allowed to heal while the teeth are held in the proper position, relapse caused by gingival elasticity is greatly reduced.

Surgery to section the supracrestal elastic fibers is a simple procedure that does not require referral to a periodontist. It can be carried out by either of two approaches. The first method, originally developed by Edwards,[4] is called circumferential supracrestal fibrotomy (CSF) (Fig. 17-22). After infiltration with a local anesthetic, the procedure consists of inserting the sharp point of a fine blade into the gingival sulcus down to the crest of alveolar bone. Cuts are made interproximally on each side of a rotated tooth and along the labial and lingual gingiva margins unless, as is often the case, the labial or lingual gingiva is quite thin, in which case this part of the circumferential cut is omitted. No periodontal pack is necessary, and there is only minor discomfort after the procedure.

An alternative method is to make an incision in the center of each gingival papilla, sparing the margin but separating the papilla from just below the margin to 1 to 2 mm below the height of the bone buccally and lingually[5] (Fig. 17-23). This modification is said to reduce the possibility that height of the gingival attachment will be reduced after the surgery, but there is little if any risk of gingival recession with the circumferential supracrestal fibrotomy unless cuts are made across thin labial or lingual tissues. From the point of view of improved stability after orthodontic treatment, the surgical procedures appear to be equivalent.

Neither the CSF nor the papilla-dividing procedure should be done until malaligned teeth have been corrected and held in their new position for several months, so this surgery is always done toward the end of the finishing phase of treatment. It is important that the teeth continue to be held in good alignment while gingival healing occurs. This means that either the surgery should be done a few weeks before

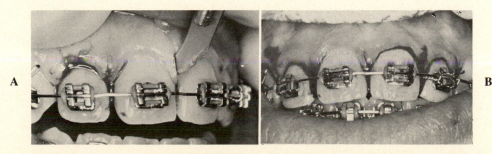

Fig. 17-23 ■ The "papilla split" procedure is an alternative to the CSF approach for sectioning gingival circumferential fibers to improve posttreatment stability. Vertical cuts are made in the gingival papillae without separating the gingival margin at the papilla tip. **A,** The blade inserted to make the vertical cut; **B,** view at completion of the papilla splits. One advantage of this procedure is that it is easier to perform with an orthodonic appliance and archwire in place.

removal of the final orthodontic appliance or, if it is performed at the same time the appliance is removed, a retainer must be inserted almost immediately. It is easier to do the CSF procedure after the orthodontic appliances have been removed, although it can be carried out with appliances in place. An advantage of the papilla-dividing procedure may be that it is easier to perform with the orthodontic appliance still in place. The only problem with placing a retainer immediately after the surgery is that it may be difficult to keep the retainer from contacting soft tissue in a sore area.

■ *References*

1. Fields, H.W.: Orthodontic-restorative for relative mandibular anterior excess tooth size problems. Am. J. Orthod. **79:**176-183, 1981.
2. Bennett, C.G., Shen, C., and Waldron, J.M.: The effects of debonding on the enamel surface. J. Clin. Orthod. **18:**330-334, 1984.
3. Rouleau, B.R., Marshall, G.W., and Cooley, R.D.: Enamel surface evaluation after clinical treatment and removal of orthodontic brackets. Am. J. Orthod. **81:**423-426, 1982.
4. Edwards, J.G.: A surgical procedure to eliminate rotational relapse. Am. J. Orthod. **57:**35-46, 1970.
5. Ahrens, D.G., Shapira, Y., and Kuftinec, M.M.: An approach to rotational relapse. Am. J. Orthod. **80:**83-91, 1981.

Chapter 18

Retention

Why is retention necessary?
  Reorganization of the periodontal tissues
  Occlusal changes related to growth
Removable appliances as retainers
  Hawley retainers
  Other removable retainers
Fixed retainers
Active retainers
  Realignment of irregular incisors: spring retainers
  Correction of occlusal discrepancies: modified functional
    appliances as active retainers

At sporting events, no matter how good things look for one team late in the game, the saying is ''It's not over till it's over.'' In orthodontics, although the patient may feel that treatment is complete when the appliances are removed, an important stage lies ahead. Orthodontic control of tooth position and occlusal relationships must be withdrawn gradually, not abruptly, if excellent long-term results are to be obtained. The type of retention should be included in the original treatment plan.

■ *Why is Retention Necessary?*

Orthodontic treatment results are potentially unstable, and therefore retention is necessary, for three reasons: (1) the gingival and periodontal tissues are affected by orthodontic tooth movement and require time for reorganization when the appliances are removed; (2) changes produced by growth may alter the orthodontic treatment result; (3) the teeth may be in an inherently unstable position after the treatment, so that soft tissue pressures constantly produce a relapse tendency. In the latter situation, gradual withdrawal of orthodontic appliances is of no value. The only possibilities are accepting relapse or using permanent retention. Fortunately, only the first two reasons apply to most orthodontic patients, and maintaining the position of the teeth until remodeling of the supporting tissues is completed and growth has essentially ceased allows a stable orthodontic result without further retention.

■ Reorganization of the Periodontal Tissues

Widening of the periodontal ligament space and disruption of the collagen fiber bundles that support each tooth are normal responses to orthodontic treatment (see Chapter 9). In fact, these changes are necessary to allow orthodontic tooth movement to occur. Even if tooth movement stops before the orthodontic appliance is removed, restoration of the normal periodontal architecture will not occur as long as a tooth is strongly splinted to its neighbors, as when it is attached to a rigid orthodontic archwire. Once the teeth can respond individually to the forces of mastication, i.e., once each tooth can be displaced slightly relative to its neighbor as the patient chews, reorganization of the periodontal ligament occurs over a 3 to 4 month period,[1] and the slight mobility present at appliance removal disappears.

The gingival fiber networks are also disturbed by orthodontic tooth movement and must remodel to accommodate the new tooth positions. Both collagenous and elastic fibers occur in the gingiva, and the reorganization of both occurs more slowly than the periodontal ligament itself.[2] Within 4 to 6 months, the collagenous fiber networks within the gingiva have normally completed their reorganization, but the elastic supracrestal fibers remodel extremely slowly and can still exert forces capable of displacing a tooth at 1 year after removal of an orthodontic appliance. In patients with severe rotations, sectioning the supracrestal fibers around severely malposed or rotated teeth, at or just before the time of appliance removal, is a recommended procedure because it reduces relapse tendencies resulting from this fiber elasticity[3] (see Chapter 17).

This timetable for soft tissue recovery from orthodontic treatment outlines the principles of retention against intraarch instability. These are:

1. The direction of potential relapse can be identified by comparing the position of the teeth at the conclusion of treatment to their original positions. Teeth will tend to move back in the direction from which they came, primarily because of elastic recoil of gingival fibers but also because of occlusal forces immediately after appliance removal (Fig. 18-1).

2. Teeth require essentially full-time retention after comprehensive orthodontic treatment for the first 3 to 4 months after a fixed orthodontic appliance is removed. To promote reorganization of the periodontal ligament, however, the teeth should be free to flex individually during mastication, as the alveolar bone bends in response to the heavy occlusal loads (see Chapter 9). This requirement can be met by a

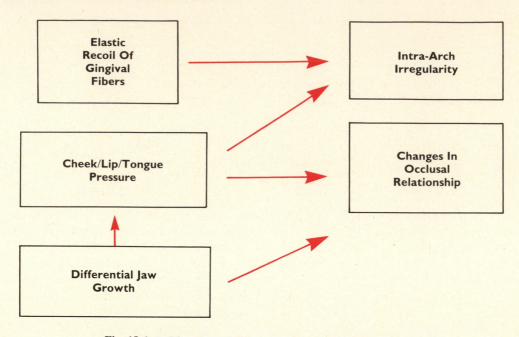

Fig. 18-1 ■ Diagrammatic representation of the causes of relapse.

removable appliance worn full-time except during meals or by a fixed retainer that is not too rigid.

3. Because of the slow response of the gingival fibers, retention should be continued for at least 12 months, but can be reduced to part-time after 3 to 4 months. After approximately 12 months, it should be possible to discontinue retention in nongrowing patients. More precisely, the situation should be stable by that time if it ever will be. Some patients who are not growing will require permanent retention to maintain the teeth in what would otherwise be unstable positions because of lip, cheek, and tongue pressures. Patients who will continue to grow, however, usually need retention until growth has reduced to the low levels that characterize adult life (see Chapter 5 and the discussion following).

■ Occlusal Changes Related to Growth

A continuation of growth is particularly troublesome in patients whose initial malocclusion resulted, largely or in part, from the pattern of skeletal growth. Skeletal problems in all three planes of space tend to recur if growth continues (Fig. 18-2). Because transverse growth is completed first, long-term transverse changes are less troublesome clinically than changes from late anteroposterior and vertical growth.

The tendency for skeletal problems to recur after orthodontic correction results from the fact that most patients continue in their original growth pattern throughout the period of growth. Comprehensive orthodontic treatment is usually carried out in the early permanent dentition, and the duration is typically between 18 and 30 months. This means that active orthodontic treatment is likely to conclude at age 14 to 15, while anteroposterior and particularly vertical growth often do not subside even to the adult level until

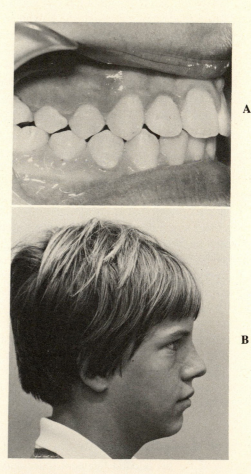

Fig. 18-2 ■ For legend see opposite page.

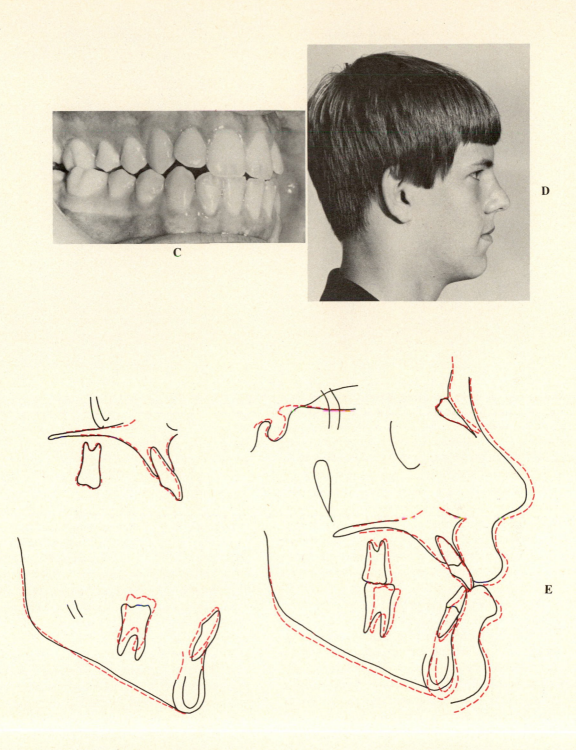

Fig. 18-2 ■ Relapse accompanying a mild Class III growth pattern: **A,** Dental occlusion at the completion of orthodontic treatment; **B,** profile appearance at the conclusion of active treatment; **C,** occlusal relationships 3 years later; **D,** facial appearance 3 years later; **E,** cephalometric superimpositions showing changes resulting from treatment and posttreatment growth (*solid black,* pretreatment; *red,* end of treatment; *dotted red,* 3 years after treatment). Note the mandibular growth, the uprighting of the lower incisors, and the compensatory forward movement of the entire maxillary arch during posttreatment growth.

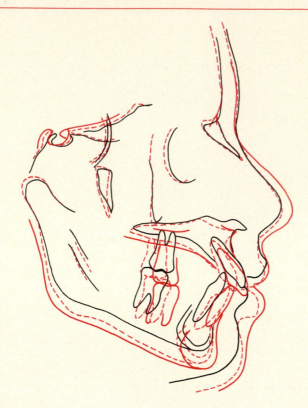

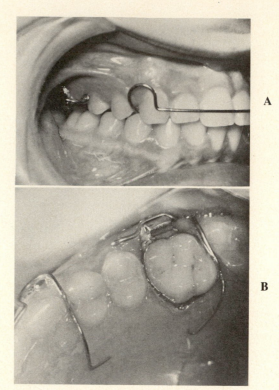

Fig. 18-3 ■ Cephalometric superimposition demonstrating growth-related relapse in a patient treated to correct Class II malocclusion. *Black,* pretreatment, age 11; *dotted red,* immediate posttreatment, age 13; *red,* recall, age 17. After treatment, both jaws grew downward and forward, and the maxillary dentition moved forward relative to the maxilla.

Fig. 18-4 ■ Retention after Class II correction: bands with headgear tubes remain on the upper first molars so that headgear at night can be continued. This is compatible with a removable maxillary retainer using circumferential clasps that fit under the headgear tubes. **A,** Lateral view; **B,** occlusal view.

several years later. Continued growth in the pattern that caused a Class II, Class III, deep bite, or open bite problem in the first place is a major cause of relapse after orthodontic treatment[4] and requires careful management during retention.

Retention after Class II correction. Relapse toward a Class II relationship must result from some combination of tooth movement (forward in the upper arch, backward in the lower, or both) and differential growth of the maxilla relative to the mandible (Fig. 18-3). As might be expected, tooth movement caused by local periodontal and gingival factors can be an important short-term problem, whereas differential jaw growth is more important long-term both because it directly alters jaw position and because it contributes to repositioning of teeth.

Overcorrection of the occlusal relationships as a finishing procedure is an important step in controlling tooth movement that would lead to Class II relapse. Even with good retention, 1 to 2 mm of anteroposterior change caused by adjustments in tooth position is likely to occur after treatment, particularly if Class II elastics were employed. This change occurs relatively quickly after active treatment stops.

The slower, long-term relapse that occurs in some patients results from differential jaw growth. The amount of growth

remaining after orthodontic treatment will obviously depend on the age, sex, and relative maturity of the patient, but after active treatment is completed, more forward growth of the maxilla than the mandible is likely to occur. If maxillary growth has been restrained by either extraoral force or a functional appliance, some posttreatment rebound may occur, accentuating the tendency toward differential growth of the upper jaw.

This relapse tendency can be controlled in one of two ways. The first is to continue headgear to the upper molars on a reduced basis (at night, for instance) in conjunction with a retainer to hold the teeth in alignment (Fig. 18-4). The other method is to use a functional appliance of the activator-bionator type to hold both tooth position and the occlusal relationship. This type of retention is often needed for 12 to 24 months or more in a patient who had a severe skeletal problem initially. The guideline is: the more severe the initial Class II problem and the younger the patient at the end of active treatment, the more likely that either headgear or a functional appliance will be needed as a retainer. It is better to prevent relapse from differential growth than to try to correct it later.

Retention after Class III correction. Retaining a patient after correcting a Class III malocclusion early in the per-

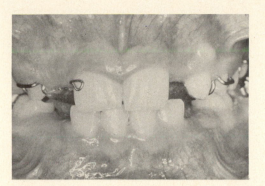

Fig. 18-5 ■ Bite plane on a maxillary retainer used to prevent deepening of the bite. With the posterior teeth in occlusion, the mandibular incisors just touch the baseplate of the retainer lingual to the upper incisors. The baseplate can be seen more clearly than usual because of this patient's missing laterals, but a similar relationship between the lower incisors and the baseplate of the upper retainer is a feature of most retainers.

manent dentition can be frustrating, because relapse from continuing mandibular growth is very likely to occur and such growth is extremely difficult to control. Applying a restraining force to the mandible, as from a chin cap, is not nearly as effective in controlling growth in a Class III patient as applying a restraining force to the maxilla is in Class II problems. As we have noted in previous chapters, a chin cap tends to rotate the mandible downward, causing growth to be expressed more vertically and less horizontally, and Class III functional appliances have the same effect. If face height is normal or excessive after orthodontic treatment, and relapse occurs from mandibular growth, surgical correction after the growth has expressed itself may be the only answer. In mild Class III problems, a functional appliance or a positioner may be enough to maintain the occlusal relationships during posttreatment growth.

Retention after deep bite correction. Correcting excess overbite is an almost routine part of orthodontic treatment, and therefore the majority of patients require control of the vertical overlap of incisors during retention. This is accomplished most readily by using a removable upper retainer made so that the lower incisors will encounter the baseplate of the retainer if they begin to slip vertically behind the upper incisors (Fig. 18-5). The procedure, in other words, is to build a potential bite plane into the retainer, which the lower incisors will contact if the bite begins to deepen. The retainer does not separate the posterior teeth.

Because vertical growth continues into the late teens, control of overbite correction often requires that the patient wear a maxillary removable retainer with a bite plane for several years after completion of the fixed appliance orthodontics. Bite depth can be maintained by wearing the retainer only at night, after stability in other regards has been achieved.

Retention after anterior open bite correction. Relapse into anterior open bite can occur by any combination of depression of the incisors and elongation of the molars. Active habits (of which thumbsucking is the best example) can produce intrusive forces on the incisors, while at the same time leading to an altered posture of the jaw that allows posterior teeth to erupt. If thumbsucking continues after orthodontic treatment, relapse is all but guaranteed. Tongue habits, particularly tongue thrust swallowing, are often blamed for relapse into open bite, but the evidence to support this contention is not convincing (see discussion in Chapter 5). In patients who do not place some object between the front teeth, return of open bite is almost always the result of elongation of the posterior teeth, particularly the upper molars, without any evidence of intrusion of incisors (Fig. 18-6). Controlling eruption of the upper molars, therefore, is the key to retention in open bite patients.

High-pull headgear to the upper molars, in conjunction with a standard removable retainer to maintain tooth position, is the most effective way to control open bite relapse (Fig. 18-7,A). An alternative is an appliance with bite blocks between the posterior teeth (an open bite activator or bionator), which stretches the patient's soft tissues to provide a force opposing eruption (Fig. 18-7,B). Excessive vertical growth and eruption of the posterior teeth often continue until late in the teens or early twenties, making a persistent open bite tendency difficult to control, but this can be accomplished with good patient cooperation over a long enough period of time.

Retention of lower incisor alignment. Not only can continued skeletal growth affect occlusal relationships, it has the potential to alter the position of teeth. If the mandible grows forward or rotates downward, the effect is to carry the lower incisors into the lip, which creates a force tipping them distally. For this reason, continued mandibular growth in normal or Class III patients is strongly associated with crowding of the lower incisors (see Fig. 18-1). Incisor crowding also accompanies the downward and backward rotation of the mandible seen in skeletal open bite problems (see Fig. 18-6). A retainer in the lower incisor region is needed to prevent crowding from developing, until growth has declined to adult levels.

It has often been suggested that orthodontic retention should be continued, at least on a part-time basis, until the third molars have either erupted into normal occlusion or have been removed. The implication of this guideline, that pressure from the developing third molars causes late incisor crowding, is almost surely incorrect (see Chapter 5). On the other hand, because the eruption of third molars or their extraction usually does not take place until the late teen years, the guideline is not a bad one in its emphasis on prolonged retention in patients who are continuing to grow.

Some crowding of lower incisors is present in most adults, including those who had orthodontic treatment and once had perfectly aligned teeth. In a group of patients who had first premolar extraction and treatment with the edgewise appliance, only about 30% had perfect alignment 10 years after retainers were removed and nearly 20% had marked crowd-

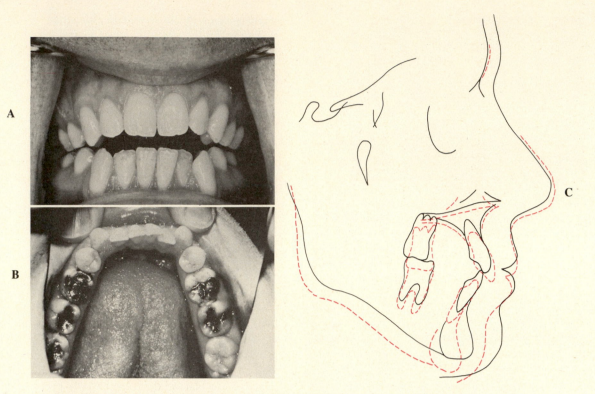

Fig. 18-6 ■ **A, B,** Relapse after comprehensive orthodontic treatment with premolar extraction. Four years after removal of the orthodontic appliances, this 19-year-old has an anterior open bite, 5 mm of overjet with an end-on molar relationship, and severe crowding of the mandibular incisors. Relapse of this type is associated with a downward and backward rotation of the mandible, which is accompanied by excessive eruption of the maxillary posterior teeth. **C,** Cephalometric superimposition showing the pattern of growth associated with this relapse. Note that the increase in both open bite and overjet is related to the downward and backward mandibular rotation, while the incisor crowding is associated with uprighting and lingual repositioning of the incisors as the mandibular rotation thrusts them into the lower lip.

ing. Which individuals would have post-treatment crowding could not be predicted from the characteristics of the original malocclusion or variables associated with treatment.[5] It seems likely that the pattern of late mandibular growth is the major contributor to this crowding tendency.

In summary, retention is needed for all patients who had fixed orthodontic appliances to correct intraarch irregularities. It should be essentially full-time for the first 3 to 4 months, except that the retainer can be removed while eating unless there is a need for permanent splinting. Retention should continue on a part-time basis for at least 12 months, to allow time for remodeling of gingival tissues. In nongrowing patients, retention can often be discontinued at that point, but if significant growth remains, part-time retention is usually needed until completion of growth. For practical purposes, this means that nearly all patients treated in the early permanent dentition will require retention of incisor alignment until the late teens, and in those with skeletal disproportions initially, part-time use of extraoral force or a functional appliance will probably be needed in addition.

Removable appliances can serve effectively for retention

against intraarch instability and are also useful as retainers (in the form of modified functional appliances or part-time headgear) in patients with growth problems. If permanent retention is needed, a fixed retainer should be used in most instances, and fixed retainers (see following) are also indicated for intraarch retention when irregularity in a specific area is likely to be a problem.

■ *Removable Appliances as Retainers*

■ Hawley Retainers

By far the most common removable retainer is the Hawley retainer, designed as an active removable appliance in the 1920s. It incorporates clasps on molar teeth and a characteristic outer bow with adjustment loops, spanning from canine to canine (Fig. 18-8).

The ability of this retainer to provide some tooth movement was a particular asset with fully banded fixed appliances, since one function of the retainer would be to close band spaces between the incisors. With bonded appliances on the anterior teeth or after using a tooth positioner for

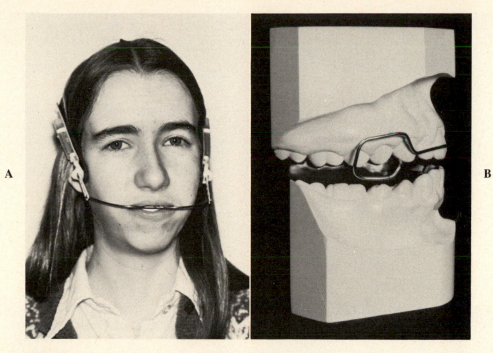

Fig. 18-7 ■ Controlling the eruption of upper molars during late vertical growth is the key to preventing open bite relapse. There are two major approaches to accomplishing this: **A,** high-pull headgear, as worn every night by this 16-year-old patient with a long face pattern of growth, to prevent the recurrence of open bite and overjet, and **B,** a functional appliance with bite blocks to impede eruption, continued as a night time retainer through the late teens.

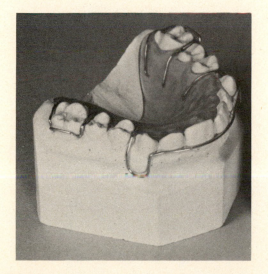

Fig. 18-8 ■ A standard maxillary Hawley retainer. Note the canine-to-canine anterior bow, with clasps on the first molars. The anterior bow is the characteristic feature of this retainer design.

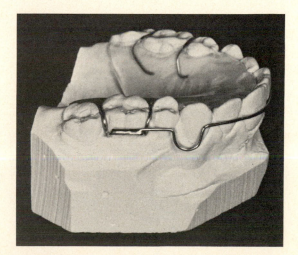

Fig. 18-9 ■ Hawley retainer for premolar extraction patient, with the outer bow soldered to the bridge portion of Adams clasps on the first molars. This design allows the anterior bow to keep the extraction space closed and is usually preferred for extraction cases.

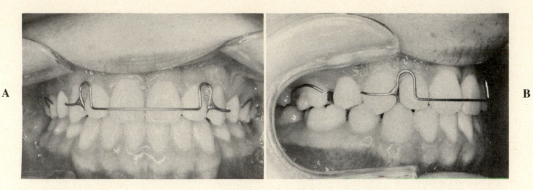

Fig. 18-10 ■ **A, B,** An alternative design for the anterior bow of a retainer, using a distal extension from a short anterior bow to control the maxillary canines.

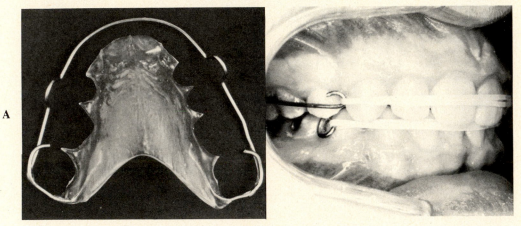

Fig. 18-11 ■ **A,** Maxillary retainer for an individual with very tight occlusal interdigitation. To avoid bringing a wire across the occlusion, the outer bow is soldered to circumferential clasps on the second molar. **B,** Modification of maxillary and mandibular retainers, replacing the Hawley bow with a light elastic across the incisor teeth. This appliance is more esthetic than the standard design, but does not give as good control of tooth positions.

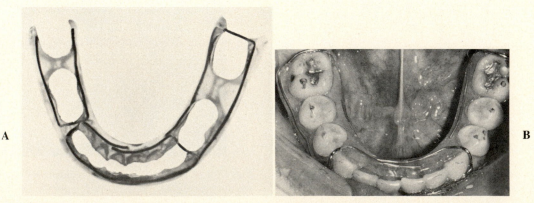

Fig. 18-12 ■ A wraparound retainer for the lower arch. **A,** The retainer out of the mouth, showing the wire reinforcement of the plastic material; **B,** the retainer in the mouth.

finishing, there is no longer any need to close spaces with a retainer. However, the outer bow provides excellent control of the incisors even if it is not adjusted to retract them.

When first premolars have been extracted, one function of a retainer is to keep the extraction space closed, which the standard design of the Hawley retainer cannot do. Even worse, the standard Hawley labial bow extends across a first premolar extraction space, tending to wedge it open. A common modification of the Hawley retainer for use in extraction cases is a bow soldered to the buccal section of Adams clasps on the first molars, so that the action of the bow helps hold the extraction site closed (Fig. 18-9). An alternative design for extraction cases is to bring the labial wire from the baseplate between the lateral incisor and canine and to bend or solder a wire extension distally to control the canines (Fig. 18-10). The latter alternative does not provide an active force to keep an extraction space closed, but at least avoids having the wire cross through the extraction site.

The clasp locations for a Hawley retainer must be selected carefully, since clasp wires crossing the occlusal table can disrupt rather than retain the tooth relationships established during treatment. Circumferential clasps on the terminal molar or lingual extension clasps (see Chapter 11) may be preferred over the more effective Adams clasp if the occlusion is tight (Fig. 18-11).

The palatal coverage of a removable plate like the Hawley retainer makes it possible to incorporate a bite plane lingual to the upper incisors, to control bite depth. As noted previously, this design consideration is important for any patient who once had an excessive overbite. Light contact of the lower incisors against the baseplate of the retainer is desired.

A Hawley retainer can be made for the upper or lower arch. The lower retainer is somewhat fragile and may be difficult to insert because of undercuts in the premolar and molar region. If the major reason for lower retention is maintenance of incisor position, a retainer for that region only is a logical alternative.

■ Other Removable Retainers

A second major type of removable orthodontic retainer is the wraparound or clipon retainer, which consists of a plastic bar (usually wire-reinforced) along the labial and lingual surfaces of the teeth (Fig. 18-12). A full arch wraparound retainer firmly holds each tooth in position. This is not necessarily an advantage, since one object of a retainer should be to allow each tooth to move individually, stimulating reorganization of the periodontal ligament. In addition, a wraparound retainer, though quite esthetic, is often less comfortable than a Hawley retainer and may not be effective in maintaining overbite correction. A full-arch wraparound retainer is indicated primarily when periodontal breakdown requires that the teeth be splinted together.

A variant of the wraparound retainer, the canine-to-canine clip-on retainer, is widely used in the lower anterior region.

This appliance has the great advantage that it can be used to realign irregular incisors, if mild crowding has developed after treatment (see Active Retainers, following) but it is well tolerated as a retainer alone.

A tooth positioner can also be used as a removable retainer, either fabricated for this purpose alone, or more commonly, continued as a retainer after serving initially as a finishing device. Positioners are excellent finishing devices and under special circumstances can be used to an advantage as retainers. For routine use, however, a positioner as a retainer has significant drawbacks. The major problems are:

1. The pattern of wear of a positioner does not match the pattern usually desired for retainers. Because of its bulk, patients often have difficulty wearing a positioner full-time or nearly so. In fact, positioners tend to be worn less than the recommended 4 hours per day after the first few weeks, although they are reasonably well tolerated by most patients during sleep.

2. Positioners do not retain incisor irregularities and rotations as well as standard retainers. This problem follows directly from the first one: a retainer is needed nearly full-time initially to control intraarch alignment. Also, overbite tends to increase while a positioner is being worn, and this effect too probably relates in large part to the fact that it is worn only a small percentage of the time.

A positioner does have one major advantage over a standard removable or wraparound retainer, however—it maintains the occlusal relationships as well as intraarch tooth positions. For a patient with a tendency toward Class III relapse, a positioner made with the jaws rotated somewhat downward and backward may be useful. Although a positioner with the teeth set in a slightly exaggerated ''super-normal'' from the original malocclusion can be used for patients with a skeletal Class II or open bite growth pattern, it is less effective in controlling growth than part-time headgear or a functional appliance.

In fabricating a positioner, it is necessary to separate the teeth by 2 to 4 mm. This means that an articulator mounting

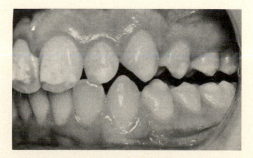

Fig. 18-13 ■ Separation of the posterior teeth after 3 weeks of intensive positioner wear. This unusual complication results from an incorrect hinge axis in constructing the positioner. A patient wearing a positioner long-term should be observed so that no problems of this type occur.

that records the patient's hinge axis is desirable. As a general guideline, the more the patient deviates from the average normal, and the longer the positioner will be worn, the more important it is to obtain an individualized hinge axis mounting on an adjustable articulator for positioner construction. If a positioner is to be used for only 2 to 4 weeks as a finishing device in a patient who will have some vertical growth during later retention, and if the patient has an approximately normal hinge axis, an individualized articulator mounting may be unnecessary. If a positioner is to be worn for many months as a retainer or if no growth can be anticipated, a precisely correct hinge axis becomes more important.

The usual sign of a positioner made to an incorrect hinge axis is some separation of the posterior teeth when the incisors are in contact (Fig. 18-13). Patients wearing a positioner as a retainer should be checked carefully to see that this effect is not occurring.

■*Fixed Retainers*

Fixed orthodontic retainers are normally used in situations where intraarch instability is anticipated and prolonged retention is planned. There are three major indications:

1. Maintenance of lower incisor position during late growth. As has been discussed previously, the major cause of lower incisor crowding in the late teen years, in both patients who have had orthodontic treatment and those who have not, is late growth of the mandible in the normal growth pattern. Especially if the lower incisors have previously been irregular, even a small amount of differential mandibular growth between ages 16 and 20 can cause recrowding of these teeth. Relapse into crowding is almost always accompanied by lingual tipping of the central and lateral incisors in response to the pattern of growth. An excellent retainer to hold these teeth in alignment is a fixed lingual bar, attached only to the canines (or to canines and first premolars) and resting against the flat lingual surface of the lower incisors above the cingulum (Fig. 18-14). This prevents the

incisors from moving lingually and is also reasonably effective in maintaining correction of rotations in the incisor segment.

A fixed lingual canine-to-canine retainer can be fabricated with bands on the canines or can be bonded to the lingual surface. Since the labial part of a band tends to trap plaque against the cervical part of the labial surface, predisposing this area to decalcification, and is also unsightly, a bonded canine-to-canine retainer is preferred.

The fabrication of a bonded canine-to-canine retainer is shown in Fig. 18-15. It is attached only to the canines, resting passively against the central and lateral incisors. If the retainer wire is fitted to a cast of the lower arch, a silicone carrier of the type used for indirect bonding of brackets can be made to assist in placing the retainer. An alternative approach is to tie the retainer wire in place with wire ligatures or dental floss around the contacts, to hold it so that it can be bonded.

It is also possible to bond a fixed lingual retainer to one or more of the incisor teeth. The major indication for this variation is a tooth that had been severely rotated. Whatever the type of retainer, however, it is desirable that teeth not be held rigidly during retention. For this reason, if the span of the retainer wire is reduced by bonding an intermediate tooth or teeth, a more flexible wire should be used. A good choice for a fixed retainer with short spans between the teeth is a braided steel archwire of .0175 diameter (Fig. 18-16).

2. Diastema maintenance. A second indication for a fixed retainer is a situation where teeth must be permanently or semipermanently bonded together to maintain the closure of a space between them. This is encountered most commonly when a diastema between maxillary central incisors has been closed. Even if a frenectomy has been carried out (see Chapters 7 and 17), there is a tendency for a small space to open up between the upper central incisors. Since this is unsightly, prolonged or permanent retention is usually needed.

The best retainer for this purpose is a bonded section of flexible wire, as shown in Fig. 18-17. The wire should be

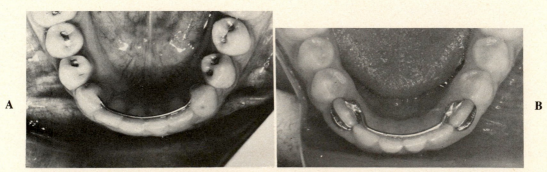

A   **B**

Fig. 18-14 ■ Fixed lingual retainers for the mandibular anterior segment. **A,** Bonded canine-to-canine retainer; **B,** banded canine-to-canine appliance. Although the banded version of this retainer is less likely to be lost, the bonded version avoids labial plaque retention at the band margin and is preferred, especially in patients who had bonded attachments during treatment.

contoured so that it lies near the cingulum to keep it out of occlusal contact. The object of the retainer is to hold the teeth together while allowing them some ability to move independently during function, hence the importance of a flexible wire.

A removable retainer is not a good choice for prolonged retention of a central diastema. In troublesome cases, the diastema is closed when the retainer is removed but opens up quickly. The tooth movement that accompanies this back and forth closure is potentially damaging over a long period of time.

3. Maintenance of pontic space. A fixed retainer is also the best choice to maintain a space where a bridge pontic will eventually be placed. Using a fixed retainer for a few

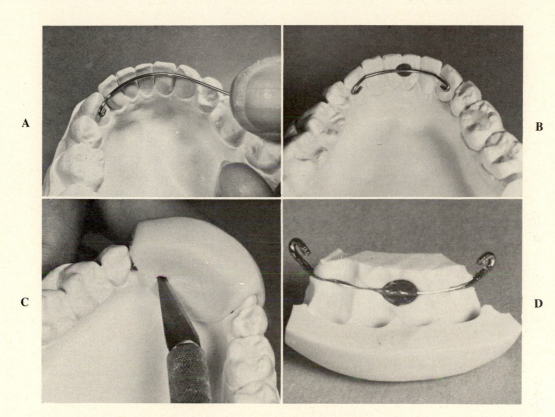

Fig. 18-15 ■ Steps in the fabrication of a canine-to-canine retainer: **A,** .030 wire is bent so that it rests against the flat part of the lingual surface of the incisors, with a loop over the cingulum of the canines; **B,** the wire is held in place with candy adhesive; **C,** a silicone carrier material is mixed, placed over the incisors, and trimmed; **D,** wire in place in the carrier, ready to be carried to the mouth for bonding.

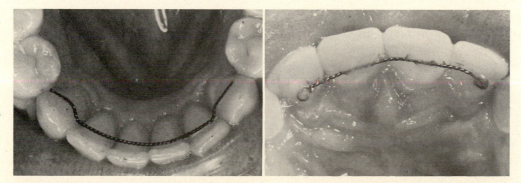

Fig. 18-16 ■ A fixed lingual retainer bonded to several anterior teeth. If multiple teeth are bonded, a lighter wire, such as the .0175 (3 × .008) twist wire shown here, should be used to prevent splinting the teeth too rigidly. **A,** Mandibular incisor retainer, with the wire lightly bonded to the canines, before the incisors are bonded; **B,** completed maxillary retainer, with all four incisors bonded.

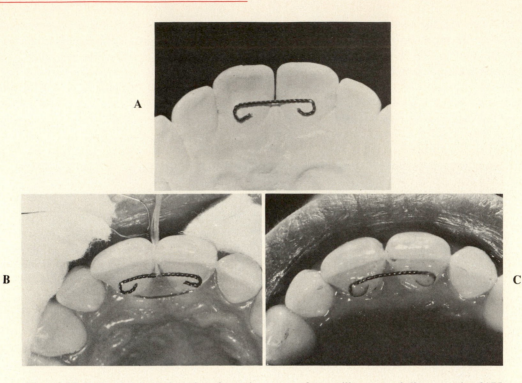

Fig. 18-17 ■ Bonded lingual retainer for maintenance of a maxillary central diastema. **A,** .0175 twist wire contoured to fit passively on the dental cast; **B,** a wire ligature is passed around the necks of the teeth to hold them tightly together while they are bonded. The wire retainer is held in place with dental floss passed around the contact, and composite resin is flowed over it. **C,** The finished retainer. Note that the retainer is up on the cingulum, to avoid occlusal interference with the lower incisors.

months reduces mobility of the teeth and often makes it easier to place the fixed bridge that will serve, among other functions, as a permanent orthodontic retainer. If further periodontal therapy is needed after the teeth have been positioned, several months or even years can pass before a bridge is placed, and a fixed retainer is definitely required.

The preferred orthodontic retainer for maintaining pontic space posteriorly is a heavy intracoronal wire, bonded in shallow preparations in the future abutment teeth (Fig. 18-18). Obviously, the longer the span, the heavier the wire should be. Bringing the wire down out of occlusion decreases the chance that it will be displaced by occlusal forces.

Anterior spaces need a replacement tooth, which can be attached to a removable retainer. This approach guarantees nearly full-time wear and is satisfactory for short periods. An alternative is a fixed retainer in which the replacement tooth is held by twist wires bonded to adjacent teeth, forming a simple acid-etch bridge (Fig. 18-19). If a permanent bridge will be delayed for a long time, it is better to go to a temporary bridge of this type, which is compatible with a removable retainer worn at night.

The major objection to any fixed retainer is that it makes interproximal hygiene procedures more difficult. It is possible to floss between teeth that have a fixed retainer in place by using a floss-threading device. With proper flossing, there

is no reason that fixed retainers, if needed, cannot be left in place indefinitely.

■ *Active Retainers*

"Active retainer" is a contradiction in terms, since a device cannot be actively moving teeth and serving as a retainer at the same time. It does happen, however, that relapse or growth changes after orthodontic treatment will lead to a need for some tooth movement during retention. This is usually accomplished with a removable appliance that continues as a retainer after it has repositioned the teeth, hence the name. A typical Hawley retainer, if used initially to close a small amount of band space, can be considered an active retainer, but the term is usually reserved for two specific situations: realignment of irregular incisors, and functional appliances to manage Class II or III relapse tendencies.

■ Realignment of Irregular Incisors: Spring Retainers

Recrowding of lower incisors is the major indication for an active retainer to correct incisor position. If late crowding has developed, it is often necessary to reduce the interproximal width of lower incisors before realigning them, so that the crowns do not tip labially into an obviously unstable position. Not only does this approach reduce the mesiodistal width of the incisors, decreasing the amount of space required for their alignment, it also flattens the contact areas, increasing the inherent stability of the arch in this region.

Peck and Peck found that the well-aligned lower incisors

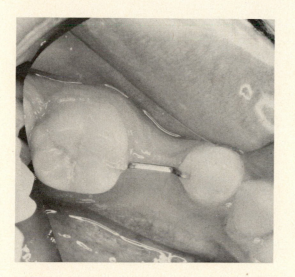

Fig. 18-18 ■ Fixed retainer to maintain space for a missing second premolar. A shallow preparation has been made in the enamel of the marginal ridges adjacent to the extraction site, and a section of .021 × .025 wire is bonded as a retainer.

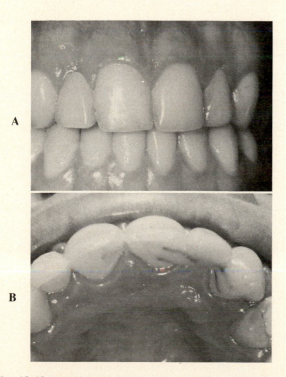

A

B

Fig. 18-19 ■ Acid-etch bridge using segments of braided orthodontic wire to attach the pontic to the abutment tooth. **A,** Frontal view; **B,** occlusal view in mirror showing the bonded attachment. This type of inexpensive fixed retainer is preferred over a removable retainer with a replacement tooth.

tend to have a smaller ratio of width to thickness (the MD-FL ratio) (Fig. 18-20) than irregular incisors.[6] They suggested that stable alignment would be found only when the MD-FL ratio did not exceed 0.92 for the centrals and 0.95 for the laterals. This ratio is smaller than the one for most unmodified incisors, suggesting that some reduction of mesiodistal width would be indicated for the majority of patients. As a general rule, however, removal of interproximal enamel from the lower incisors is indicated only when a tooth size discrepancy has been verified or when a tendency to posttreatment crowding is observed. Studies of long-term stability after orthodontic treatment do not indicate that the MD-FL ratio is an important determinant of incisor crowding.[7,8]

Interproximal enamel can be removed with either abrasive strips or thin discs in a handpiece (Fig. 18-21). Obviously, enamel reduction should not be overdone, but if necessary, the width of each lower incisor can be reduced up to 0.5 mm on each side without going through the interproximal enamel. If an additional 2 mm of space can be gained, reducing each incisor 0.25 mm per side, it is usually possible to realign typically crowded incisors.

A canine-to-canine clip-on is usually the active retainer used to realign crowded incisors. The steps in making such an active retainer are: (1) reduce the interproximal width of the incisors, and apply topical fluoride to the newly exposed enamel surfaces; (2) prepare a laboratory model, on which the teeth can be reset into alignment; (3) fabricate a canine-to-canine clip-on appliance (Fig. 18-22).

Any active removable appliance can be used as an active retainer to recover the position of teeth that have relapsed after orthodontic treatment. Only minor relapse should be observed after correctly planned comprehensive treatment,

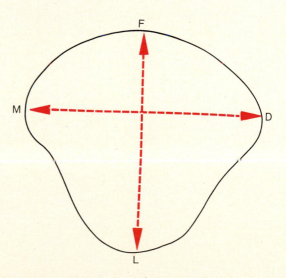

Fig. 18-20 ■ The ratio between the mesiodistal and faciolingual dimensions of the lower incisors (MD/FL ratio) has been suggested as a guideline for stripping lower incisors to control posttreatment crowding.

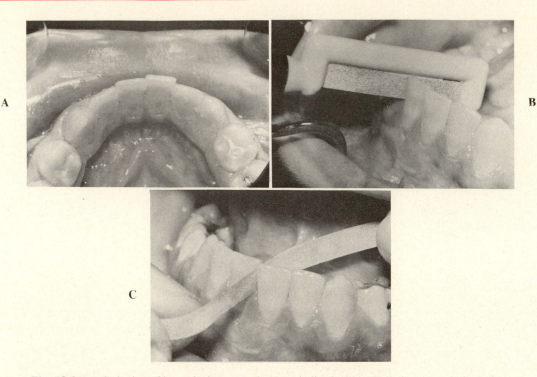

Fig. 18-21 ■ Stripping of lower incisors to reduce mesiodistal width. **A,** Incisor irregularity before realignment; **B,** interproximal enamel being removed with a relatively coarse steel-backed abrasive strip; **C,** enamel surface being polished with a sequence of plastic-backed strips with finer abrasives. Topical fluoride should be applied immediately after stripping procedures.

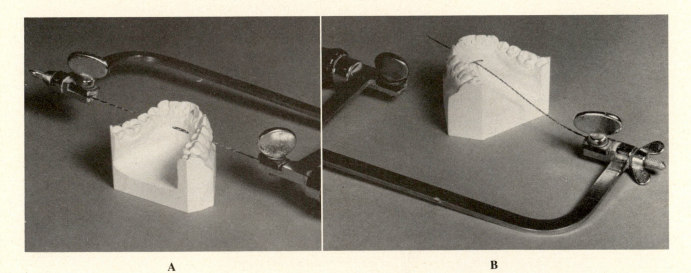

Fig. 18-22 ■ Steps in the fabrication of a canine-to-canine clip-on appliance to realign lower incisors. **A,** After the teeth have been stripped appropriately, an impression is made for a laboratory cast. A saw-cut is made beneath the teeth through the alveolar process to the distal of the lateral incisors; **B,** the saw blade is then passed from front to back beneath the incisors; **C,** cuts are made up to but not through the contact points; **D,** the incisor teeth are broken off the cast and broken apart at the contact points, creating individual dies, and the cast is trimmed to provide space for resetting the teeth; **E,** the teeth are reset in wax in proper alignment; **F,** .028 wire is contoured around the labial and lingual surface of the teeth as shown, with the wire overlapping behind the central incisors; **G,** a covering of acrylic is added over the wire, completing the retainer; **H,** occlusal view of completed retainer; **I,** facial view, showing the upper and lower retainers for this patient who had premolar extraction for correction of crowded and irregular incisors.

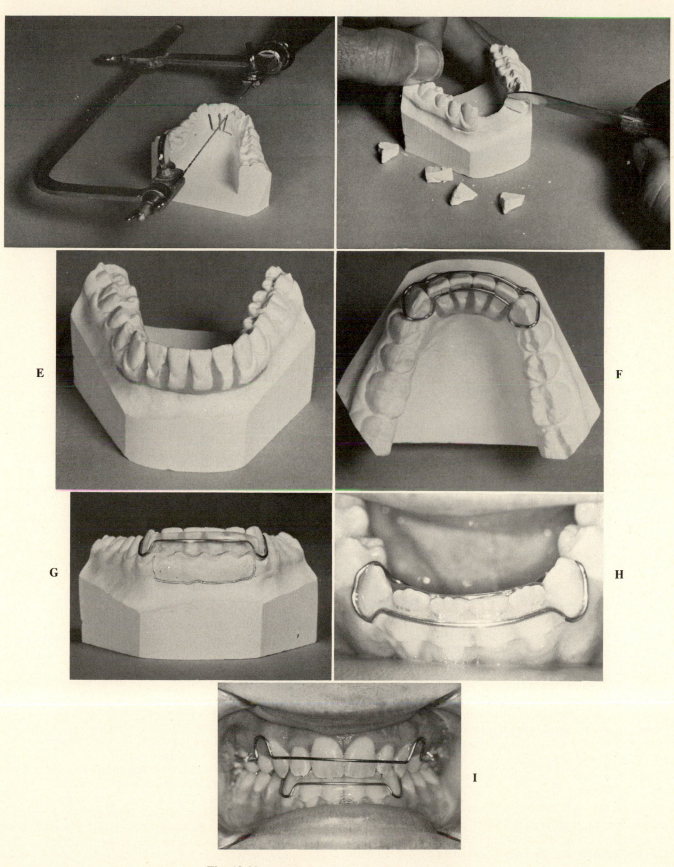

Fig. 18-22, cont'd ■ For legend see opposite page.

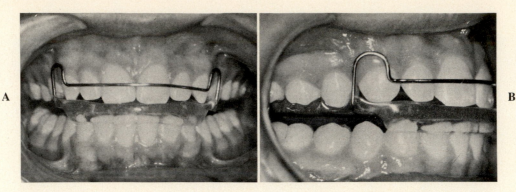

Fig. 18-23 ■ Modified activator being used as an active retainer. The mandible was advanced 3 mm in the construction bite, and the appliance has been trimmed to allow forward eruption of the mandibular posterior teeth to correct the mild Class II relationship that developed after comprehensive treatment. **A,** Anterior view; **B,** lateral view. Vertical growth is necessary with this appliance to prevent downward and backward rotation of the mandible that could make the Class II problem worse.

which means that the inherent limitations of removable appliances should not be exceeded by the demands on them in active retention. If there is more than a modest degree of relapse, however, placing a fixed appliance for comprehensive retreatment must be considered.

■ Correction of occlusal discrepancies: modified functional appliances as active retainers

It is possible to describe an activator as consisting of maxillary and mandibular retainers joined by an interocclusal bite block. Although even the simplest activator is more complex than that (see Chapter 14), the description does illustrate the potential of an activator to simultaneously maintain the position of teeth within the arches while altering, at least minimally, the occlusal relationships.

A typical use for an activator as an active retainer would be a male adolescent who had slipped back 2 to 3 mm toward a Class II relationship after early correction. If he is still growing actively, it may be possible to recover the proper occlusal position of the teeth. Differential anteroposterior growth is not necessary to correct a small occlusal discrepancy—tooth movement is adequate—but some vertical growth is required to prevent downward and backward rotation of the mandible. For all practical purposes, this means that a functional appliance as an active retainer can be used in teenagers but is of no value in adults. Stimulating skeletal growth with a device of this type simply does not happen in adults, at least to a clinically useful extent.

The use of an activator as an active retainer differs somewhat from its use to guide skeletal growth during the mixed dentition or when it is used as a pure retainer. In the latter circumstances, the object is to control growth, and tooth movement is largely an undesirable side effect. In contrast, an activator as an active retainer is expected primarily to move teeth—no significant skeletal change is expected. An activator as an active retainer is not indicated if more than 3 mm of occlusal correction is sought, and over this dis-

tance, tooth movement as a means of correction is a possibility. The correction is achieved by restraining the eruption of maxillary teeth posteriorly and directing the erupting mandibular teeth anteriorly (Fig. 18-23).

The whole family of modified activators designed to produce tooth movement is most useful in this active-retention mode, not in early mixed dentition treatment where tooth movement for the most part is undesirable. On the other hand, the more flexible a removable appliance becomes, the less suited it is for the retention part of active retention, and the more likely it would be to require replacement with another type of retainer when the occlusal relationship had been reestablished. An activator or bionator with an acrylic framework that contacts most teeth, therefore, is usually the best compromise when this type of active retention is needed.

■ References

1. Reitan, K.: Principles of retention and avoidance of post-treatment relapse. Am. J. Orthod. **55:**776-790, 1969.
2. Reitan, K.: Tissue rearrangement during the retention of orthodontically rotated teeth. Angle Orthod. **29:**105-113, 1959.
3. Boese, L.R.: Fiberotomy and reproximation without lower retention: nine years in retrospect. Angle Orthod. **50:**88-97, 1980.
4. Horowitz, S., and Hixon, E.: Physiologic recovery following orthodontic treatment. Am. J. Orthod. **55:**1-4, 1969.
5. Little, R.M., Wallen, T.R., and Riedel, R.A.: Stability and relapse of mandibular incisor alignment—first premolar extraction cases treated by traditional edgewise orthodontics. Am. J. Orthod. **80:**349-365, 1981.
6. Peck, H., and Peck, S.: An index for assessing tooth shape deviations as applied to the mandibular incisors. Am.J. Orthod. **61:**384-401, 1972.
7. Puneky, P.J., Sadowsky, C., and BeGole, E.A.: Tooth morphology and lower incisor alignment many years after orthodontic treatment. Am. J. Orthod. **86:**299-305, 1984.
8. Gilmore, C.A., and Little, R.M.: Mandibular incisor dimensions and crowding. Am. J. Orthod. **86:**493-502, 1984.

TREATMENT FOR ADULTS

Orthodontic treatment for adults has been the fastest growing area in orthodontics in recent years. There appear to be two reasons for this, and therefore two groups of adult patients: (1) many adults with other dental problems are being recognized as candidates for adjunctive orthodontic treatment to make control of dental disease and restoration of missing teeth easier and more effective, and (2) many young adults who desired but did not receive comprehensive orthodontic treatment as youths now seek it as they become financially independent.

Adjunctive treatment procedures are discussed in Chapter 19. Treatment of this type, particularly the simpler procedures, often can and should be carried out within the context of general dental practice, and the chapter is written with that in mind. The discussion in this chapter does not presume a familiarity with the principles of comprehensive orthodontic treatment.

In contrast, the discussion of comprehensive treatment for adults in Chapter 20 builds on Chapters 15 to 18 and focuses on the aspects of comprehensive treatment for adults that are different from treatment for younger patients. Chapter 21, dealing with orthognathic surgery, is written at an intermediate level, emphasizing the possibilities for this type of treatment and the principles that guide the interaction among surgeon, orthodontist, periodontist, and restorative dentist in the treatment of patients with these complex problems.

Chapter 19

Adjunctive Treatment for Adults

■ *The Goals of Adjunctive Treatment*

Adjunctive orthodontic treatment is, by definition, tooth movement carried out to facilitate other dental procedures necessary to control disease and restore function. Although malocclusion as classically described is not necessarily an unhealthy condition, some tooth positions are not conducive to long-term oral health. These differences can perhaps best be understood by reference to Amsterdam's concepts of physiologic versus pathologic occlusion.[1] A physiologic occlusion, although not necessarily an ideal or Class I occlusion, is one that adapts to the stress of function and can be maintained indefinitely, whereas a pathologic occlusion cannot function without contributing to its own destruction. A pathologic occlusion may manifest itself by any combination of (1) excessive wear of the teeth without sufficient compensatory mechanisms, (2) temporomandibular joint problems, (3) pulpal changes ranging from hyperemia to necrosis, and (4) periodontal damage.

If dental treatment to correct or control such problems is impossible because of the existing tooth positions, or if dental treatment itself may produce a pathologic situation unless tooth positions are changed, then orthodontic tooth movement becomes an important step in the overall treatment plan. For example, when a tooth is lost, the adjacent teeth tend to tip, drift, and rotate. Whether or not this requires correction will depend on whether the signs of pathologic occlusion are present. If the patient can still maintain adequate plaque control, if the occlusal forces are within the physiologic tolerance of the support mechanism, and if the patient can function without prematurities or functional

shifts, then the occlusion may be considered physiologic and there is little indication for orthodontic treatment.

If any of the signs of pathologic occlusion exist, however, or if placement of restorations such as overcontoured anterior crowns to close an unattractive space or a posterior bridge to maintain the occlusal table, would prevent adequate plaque clearance or overstress the support apparatus, then tooth movement should become an important part of the overall treatment plan.

Typically, adjunctive orthodontic treatment will involve repositioning teeth that have drifted after extractions or bone loss caused by periodontal disease, forced eruption of badly broken down teeth to expose sound root structure on which to place crowns, correction of crossbites if these compromise jaw function (not all do), and alignment of anterior teeth for more esthetic restorations while maintaining good interproximal bone contour and embrasure form.

Whatever the occlusal status originally, the goals of adjunctive treatment should be to:

- Facilitate restorative treatment by positioning the teeth so that more ideal and conservative techniques can be used.
- Improve the periodontal health by eliminating plaque-harboring areas, improving the alveolar ridge contour adjacent to the teeth, establishing favorable crown-to-root ratios, and positioning the teeth so that occlusal forces are transmitted along the long axes of the teeth.

Adjunctive treatment implies limited orthodontic goals, improving a particular aspect of the occlusion rather than comprehensively altering it. Typically, appliances are required in only a portion of the dental arch and for only a short time. Orthodontic treatment for temporomandibular joint problems should not be considered adjunctive treatment. Admittedly, the boundary between adjunctive and comprehensive treatment is somewhat indistinct. However, treatment that requires a complete fixed appliance or that is complex enough to require more than 6 months for completion should be considered comprehensive, and is discussed in Chapter 20. With the distinction made in this way, most of the adjunctive treatment discussed in this chapter can and should be carried out in the context of general dental practice.

■ *Principles of Adjunctive Treatment*

■ Diagnostic and Treatment Planning Considerations

Just as in planning comprehensive orthodontic treatment, planning for adjunctive treatment requires two steps: (1) collecting an adequate database and (2) developing a comprehensive but clearly stated list of the patient's problems, taking care not to focus unduly on any one aspect of a complex situation. The importance of this stage in planning adjunctive orthodontic treatment cannot be overemphasized, since the solution to the specific problems may involve the synthesis of all branches of dentistry.

The steps outlined in Chapter 6 should be followed when developing the problem list. The patient's motivation for and expectations of treatment, general dental awareness, enthusiasm for and ability to cooperate with the treatment regime, must all be evaluated. A careful clinical examination must determine the patient's dental health status, including any existing destruction or deficiencies of the teeth and their support, and ability to achieve and maintain good overall oral hygiene.

Diagnostic records for adjunctive orthodontic patients differ in several important ways from those for children. For this mainly adult dentally compromised population, these records should include a full series of individual intraoral radiographs (Fig. 19-1). The panoramic radiograph usually does not give sufficient detail of the root morphology, dental disease, or periodontal breakdown. Cephalometric radiographs are not usually required, but it is sound practice to perform a facial form analysis so that the impact of various tooth movements on the face can be anticipated (see Chapter 6).

As with any orthodontic patient, dental casts should be obtained from impressions that have been fully extended so that the crown position, inclination of the teeth, and the contour of the supporting alveolar bone can be clearly identified. The dental casts for adjunctive orthodontic patients should be mounted in centric relation on a semiadjustable articulator if an appreciable functional shift exists, if there are other reasons to suspect pathologic occlusion, or if extensive restorative procedures are contemplated.

Analysis of the records will establish whether a pathologic occlusion is present with evidence of a destructive process.

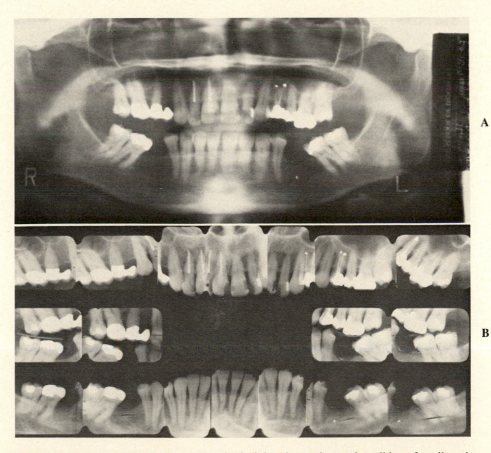

A

B

Fig. 19-1 ■ For the periodontically compromised adults who are the usual candidates for adjunctive orthodontics, periapical as well as panoramic radiographs are usually needed. **A,** The panoramic radiograph gives a good indication of the relative position of the posterior teeth but the anterior teeth are not clearly depicted. **B,** Adequate detail of root morphology, dental disease, and periodontal breakdown is obtained only from carefully taken periapical radiographs.

The key treatment planning question is: Can the occlusion be restored within the existing tooth positions, or must some teeth be moved to achieve a satisfactory, stable, healthy, and esthetic result? The goal of adjunctive treatment is to provide a physiologic occlusion and facilitate other dental treatment and has little to do with Angle's concept of an ideal Class I tooth relationship.

Once all the problems have been identified and categorized, special attention may then be turned to tooth positions that require modification. Possible tooth movements include mesial or distal movement of specific crowns, roots, or both; correction of axial inclination of drifted teeth; correction of the buccolingual position of certain teeth; correction of rotations; and vertical movements of individual teeth. Intrusion of teeth should be avoided as an adjunctive procedure because of the technical difficulties involved and because this approach may complicate long-term periodontal treatment.[2,3] However, intrusion can be an important part of comprehensive treatment for adults (see Chapter 20). As a general rule for adjunctive treatment, teeth that are excessively extruded are best treated by reduction of crown height, which has the added advantage of improving the ultimate crown-to-root ratio of the teeth.

Although certain tooth positions may be considered ideal

for restorative procedures, it may be impossible or impractical to achieve this with adjunctive orthodontics. Factors that should be considered in deciding how ideal the treatment should be, must include the systemic health of the patient, the general dental condition (including existing destruction of teeth and supporting apparatus), and the patient's ability to achieve and maintain good overall oral hygiene. Occlusal considerations such as the space available for tooth movement, the presence or absence and position of antagonist teeth, and the number of teeth to be moved may also modify the treatment goals.

The treatment time depends on the severity of the problem and the amount of tooth movement desired. As a general guideline, adjunctive orthodontic treatment that would take more than 6 months should be avoided. On the other hand, because there is a limit to the amount of possible compromise, the dentist may decide that more comprehensive treatment is needed, perhaps even including orthognathic surgery, than was envisioned originally.

■ Biomechanical Considerations

The design of the appliance to be used for adjunctive orthodontics will depend on the number of teeth to be moved, the availability of other teeth or tissues for anchorage, and the desired direction and amount of crown or root movement. Careful control and judicious balancing of forces between the active and reactive units, using the principles outlined in Chapter 10, are required.

Since patients who need adjunctive orthodontic treatment often have periodontal problems, the amount of bone support of each tooth is an important special consideration when planning force systems. When bone has been lost, the periodontal ligament (PDL) area decreases, and the same force against the crown produces greater pressure in the PDL of a periodontally compromised tooth than a normally supported one. The absolute magnitude of force used to move teeth must be reduced when periodontal support has been lost, to prevent damage to the PDL, bone, cementum, and root.

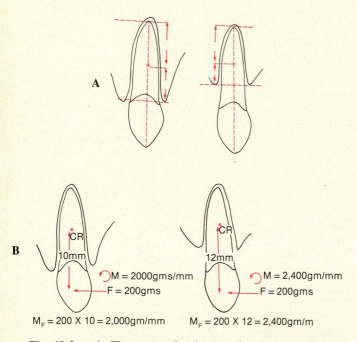

A

B

CR
10mm

$M = 2000gms/mm$
$F = 200gms$

$M_F = 200 \times 10 = 2,000gm/mm$

CR
12mm

$M = 2,400gm/mm$
$F = 200gms$

$M_F = 200 \times 12 = 2,400gm/m$

Fig. 19-2 ■ **A,** The center of resistance of a single rooted tooth lies approximately six-tenths of the distance between the apex of the tooth and crest of the supporting alveolar bone. Loss of alveolar bone height or periodontal attachment, as in the tooth on the right, leads to apical relocation of the center of resistance. **B,** The magnitude of the tipping moment produced by a force is equal to the force times the distance from the point of force application to the center of resistance. Apical relocation of the center of resistance increases the magnitude of the tipping moment (M_F) for a given force and consequently a larger countervailing couple *(M)* would be necessary to effect bodily movement.

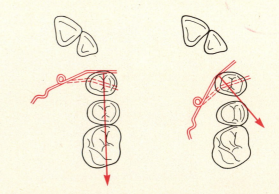

Fig. 19-3 ■ The direction of tooth movement is always at right angles to the initial contact of a fingerspring on a removable appliance, thus control of tooth position and correction of rotations can be extremely difficult. On the right, applying the spring so that the premolar rotation would improve carries the tooth buccally.

In addition, the greater the loss of attachment, the smaller the area of supported root and the further apical the center of resistance will become (Fig. 19-2). Orthodontic forces must be applied to the crown of a tooth, and the further the point of force application is from the center of resistance, the greater will be the tipping moment produced by any given force. Conversely, if bodily movement is required, a countervailing moment must be applied. When bone support has been lost, this will have to be greater to balance the greater tipping moment.

In general, control of anchorage requires that anchor teeth not be allowed to tip. For this reason, adjunctive tooth movement usually requires a fixed appliance. For adjunctive orthodontic treatment, we recommend wide .022 edgewise attachments (no wider than one-half the width of the crown). The rectangular (edgewise) bracket slot permits control of buccolingual axial inclination, and the wide bracket helps control undesirable tipping. The larger slot size allows the use of stabilizing wires that are somewhat stiffer than ordinarily might be used in comprehensive treatment with continuous archwires.

Adult patients traditionally have been somewhat reluctant to wear obvious fixed appliances and frequently indicate their preference for a removable appliance. However, this method is rarely satisfactory for adjunctive (or comprehensive) treatment. Removable appliances by their very nature produce simple tipping movements of teeth, making control of tooth position extremely difficult (Fig. 19-3). In addition, removable appliances are by definition removable, and the adult patient's concept of continuous appliance wear does not always coincide with that of the dentist. Intermittent

forces, though capable of producing tooth movement, are not as efficient as continuous forces, particularly in the presence of occlusal interferences.

Removable appliances, however, may have an advantage over fixed appliances for some patients with multiple missing teeth. They permit the reaction forces from tooth movement to be spread over adjacent supporting tissues such as the palatal vault and alveolar mucosa as well as the anchor teeth. If many teeth are missing, this approach may be the only way to generate sufficient anchorage. In nearly all cases, however, provided the patient can be convinced of the importance of treatment, resistance to fixed appliances is minimal. Discomfort and interference with speech and mastication are far less with a carefully designed and placed fixed appliance than with most removable appliances.

No matter what the type of orthodontic appliance, it must meet certain basic design criteria: it (1) should not interfere with function; (2) should cause no harm to the oral tissues or interfere with the maintenance of good oral hygiene; (3) should be as light and inconspicuous as possible, yet sufficiently strong to withstand masticatory forces and a reasonable amount of abuse; (4) must be firmly retained in position; (5) must be capable of exerting an appropriately controlled force in the correct direction and delivering this force for as long as possible between adjustment visits; and (6) should allow control of anchorage, so that tooth movements other than those intended are minimized.

Modern edgewise brackets of the straight-arch type (see Chapter 12) are designed for a specific location on an individual tooth. With the brackets in this position, a rectangular wire bent to ideal arch form, if deflected and fully engaged into the bracket slot, would produce a force system to move the teeth into an ideal relationship with correct tip, torque, and rotations. For an ideal patient, it would not be necessary to include first, second, and third order bends in the wire, thus the "straight-arch" name. If the teeth were severely malposed, of course, a large rectangular wire could not be used initially, and a series of progressively stiffer archwires would be required.

Placing the bracket in its ideal position on each tooth implies that the position of every tooth will be changed during treatment. Since adjunctive treatment is concerned with only limited tooth movements, it is usually neither necessary nor desirable to alter the position of every tooth in the arch. For this reason, when placing a partial fixed appliance for adjunctive treatment, the brackets are placed in an ideal position only on teeth to be moved, and the remaining teeth to be incorporated in the anchor system are bracketed or banded in the most convenient way possible, with the archwire slots closely aligned (Fig. 19-4). This allows the anchorage segments of the wire to be engaged passively in the brackets with little bending. Passive engagement of wires to anchor teeth produces minimal disturbance of teeth that are in a physiologically satisfactory position. This important point is illustrated in more detail in the section on specific treatment procedures following.

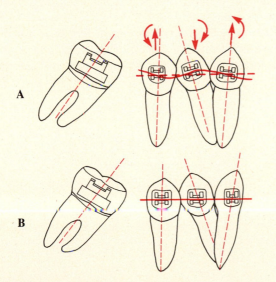

Fig. 19-4 ■ **A,** Brackets placed in the "ideal" position on the anchor teeth. Placement of a straight length of wire will cause uprighting of the anterior teeth as the brackets are brought into alignment. For adjunctive orthodontic treatment, movement of the anchor teeth is often undesirable. **B,** Brackets placed in the position of maximum convenience. Placement of a straight length of wire will maintain the existing bracket and hence tooth alignment.

Timing and Sequence of Treatment

The timing and sequence of treatment are critically important in adjunctive orthodontic treatment (Fig. 19-5). After the development of a comprehensive treatment plan, the first step is the control of any active dental disease. Before any orthodontic treatment, gingival inflammation must be controlled since orthodontic tooth movement in the presence of inflammation can lead to rapid and irreversible breakdown of the periodontal support apparatus.[4,5] Scaling, curettage (by open flap procedures, if necessary), and gingival grafts should be undertaken as appropriate before any tooth movement. In addition, periodontal therapy should be continued once orthodontic treatment is under way, since it has been shown that regular professional cleaning and repeat curettage may halt or even reverse the destruction of the attachment apparatus.[6] Osseous surgery should be delayed until completion of the orthodontic phase of treatment, because a significant amount of bone recontouring occurs during orthodontic tooth movement. Active caries and pulpal pathology should be eliminated, using extractions, restorative procedures, and pulpal or apical treatment as necessary. Teeth should be restored with well-placed amalgams or composite resins. Crowns, bridges, and other restorations requiring detailed occlusal anatomy should not be placed until any adjunctive orthodontic treatment has been completed,

since the occlusal relationships will inevitably be changed by orthodontic tooth movement, and these occlusal changes may be far more widespread than simply repositioning an individual tooth.

During this preparatory phase, the patient's enthusiasm for treatment and ability to achieve and maintain good overall oral hygiene should be carefully monitored. Because attempts to reposition the teeth and restore the occlusion of patients who are insufficiently motivated to maintain good oral hygiene are doomed to failure, less time-consuming and costly treatment alternatives should be adopted. However, if the disease process can be controlled and the patient has demonstrated that he or she is prepared to undergo the necessary treatment, adjunctive orthodontic tooth movement can significantly improve the final restorative and periodontal procedures.

Adjunctive Treatment Procedures

Uprighting Posterior Teeth

Treatment planning considerations. Loss of posterior teeth, usually first permanent molars, is a frequent problem in adults. The sequel to this will depend on the position and number of teeth lost, the age at which this occurs, the time elapsed since the loss, and the occlusion.

When a posterior tooth is lost, the adjacent teeth usually tip, drift, and rotate. As the teeth move, the adjacent gingival tissue becomes folded and distorted, forming a plaque-harboring pseudopocket that may be virtually impossible for the patient to clean. The accumulation of bacterial plaque can cause direct damage to the periodontium from toxic and antigenic bacterial substances,[7] and indirect damage by stimulating an immune response.[8]

Additional periodontal damage can also occur as a result of misdirected occlusal forces.[9] The precise effects of occlusal forces depend on how they are distributed and on the

---

Collection and Analysis of Data

Problem List

Tentative Treatment Plan

Phase I   Treatment: Control of Active Disease
   oral hygiene: scaling; curettage;
   extractions; endodontic treatment;
   caries control; amalgams; composite resins.

Patient Evaluation

Phase II Treatment:
   orthodontic tooth movement;
   continued periodontal control.

Stabilization of Tooth Position

Perio Surgery: osseous and/or soft tissue
                recontouring as necessary

Crowns

Fixed and/or Removable Partial Dentures

Continued Maintenance

Fig. 19-5 ■ Suggested sequence of steps in treatment of patients requiring adjunctive orthodontic treatment.

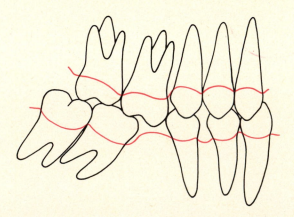

Fig. 19-6 ■ Loss of a lower molar can lead to tipping and drifting of adjacent teeth, poor interproximal contacts, poor gingival contour, reduced interradicular bone, and supraeruption of unopposed teeth. Since the bone contour follows the cementoenamel junction, pseudopockets form adjacent to the tipped teeth.

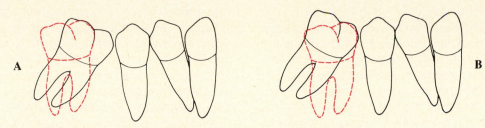

Fig. 19-7 ■ **A,** Uprighting a tipped molar by distal crown movement leads to increased pontic space, whereas (**B**) uprighting the molar by mesial root movement reduces pontic space and might eliminate the need for a prosthesis.

patient's resistance. Most of the fibers of the periodontal ligament of posterior teeth run obliquely from the cementum to a more coronal insertion in the bone and are thus best designed to resist axial loadings.[10] Any tilt of the teeth will alter the way occlusal stresses are transmitted to the supporting structures.

In general, the effect of any injury depends on the frequency of the irritation. In the case of a tipped tooth, bacterial plaque retention will provide a constant irritation, while occlusal stress is only an intermittent factor. Thus, prophylactic control of bacterial plaque is more important than prophylactic occlusal adjustment or tooth repositioning. This fact, together with variations in the immune response, explains why some teeth in an abnormal position exhibit little loss of attachment as long as the patient maintains adequate oral hygiene in the area. Notwithstanding, the elimination of potentially pathologic conditions associated with tipped molars is probably the most important procedure in adjunctive orthodontic treatment and has the added advantage of simplifying the ultimate restorative procedures.

Since the first molar is so frequently lost, one often sees the second and third molar tipped mesially, rotated, and in a position that is neither conducive to long-term health nor to simple restorative procedures (Fig. 19-6). In addition, the premolars may have drifted distally and rotated, resulting in open contacts and poor marginal ridge relationships. The opposing teeth may supererupt into the edentulous spaces, further complicating restorative procedures and frequently contributing to occlusal interferences, especially in protrusive and excursive movements. The treatment objectives should be to restore the normal tooth positions.

When planning molar uprighting, a number of interrelated questions must be answered. The first is, if the third molar is present, whether one molar or two should be uprighted. For many patients, distal positioning of the third molar would move it into a position where good hygiene could not be maintained, or the uprighted third molar would not be in functional occlusion after being uprighted. In these circumstances, it is more appropriate to extract the third molar and simply upright the remaining second molar tooth.

The second question is whether to upright the tipped teeth by distal crown movement (tipping), which would increase the space available for a later pontic, or by mesial root movement, which would reduce the edentulous span and occasionally close the extraction space, thereby eliminating the need for a bridge (Fig. 19-7). The choice will depend on the ultimate occlusion desired, the anchorage available for such movement, and perhaps most importantly, the contour of the bone in the edentulous ridge area. If extensive ridge resorption has occurred, particularly in the buccolingual dimension (Fig. 19-8), mesial movement of a wide molar root into such an area will proceed very slowly. It will also probably result in a dehiscence of bone from the mesial, buccal, and lingual root surfaces, which is not conducive to long-term physiologic health. In general, distal tipping for uprighting molars is preferred over mesial root movement.

The third question is whether there should be slight extrusion, maintenance of the existing occlusal height, or intrusion as the teeth are uprighted. Extrusion of a tipped molar has the merit of reducing the depth of the pseudopocket found on the mesial surface, and since the attached gingiva follows the cementoenamel junction while the mucogingival junction remains stable, it also increases the width of the keratinized tissue in that area. In addition, if the height of the clinical crown is systematically reduced,

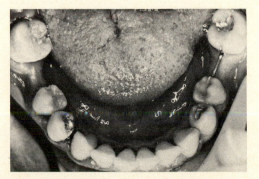

Fig. 19-8 ■ Loss of the first molar has led to resorption of the alveolar ridge in the edentulous space. The second molars have been uprighted by distal crown tipping since attempts to move the roots mesially would almost certainly have resulted in a dehiscence of bone on the mesiolingual root. Note the teeth on the right side prepared for a stabilizing splint, which has been bonded in place on the left side.

the ultimate crown–root length ratio will be improved (Fig. 19-9). On the other hand, maintaining the occlusal ridge height requires intrusion, which carries with it as least the theoretic possibility of increasing the pocket depth (see Chapter 20) and of relocating infected crevicular tissue further subgingivally. Moreover, intrusion of molars is technically difficult, requiring precisely directed and gentle long-acting forces. Unless slight extrusion is acceptable, which it usually is, the patient should be considered to have problems that require comprehensive treatment and should be treated accordingly.

The final question is whether the premolars should be

repositioned as part of the treatment. This decision will depend on the position of these teeth, the existing contacts, and the opposing intercuspation. It is desirable to close spaces between premolars when uprighting molars.

A variety of appliances have been proposed to upright tipped molars. Although the design and application may vary slightly, the principles are the same. Each appliance can be separated into an active and a reactive (stabilizing or anchor) unit. To provide appropriate anchorage, all teeth as far forward as the canine in the treatment quadrant should be included. The canine on the contralateral side should also be linked to the anchor teeth by the use of a heavy stabilizing lingual arch (Fig. 19-10). This approach is mandatory in

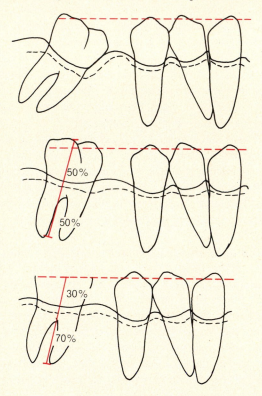

Fig. 19-9 ■ Uprighting a tipped molar increases the crown height while it reduces the depth of the mesial pocket. Subsequent crown reduction improves the ratio of crown height to supported root length of the molar.

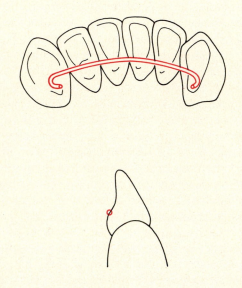

Fig. 19-10 ■ Canine-to-canine stabilizing lingual arch of .030 wire is needed in most patients who require molar uprighting to increase the anterior anchorage and prevent buccal displacement of the anchor premolars. The archwire should be placed at the cingula for maximum mechanical efficiency and so the patient can maintain good oral hygiene.

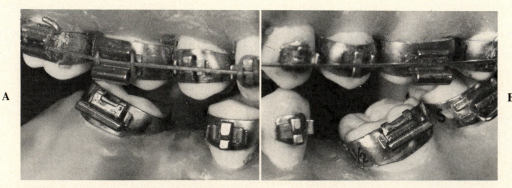

Fig. 19-11 ■ **A,** If a single molar is to be uprighted, it should carry a wide twin bracket with a convertible cap and gingivally placed auxiliary tube as shown here on the lower second molar. **B,** If two adjacent molars are to be uprighted, the convertible cap on the mesial molar bracket should be removed before cementing the band, and the terminal molar should carry a single tube.

the mandibular arch and advisable in the maxillary arch, particularly if a premolar also is missing. This canine-to-canine stabilizing arch not only increases the anterior anchorage but also resists buccal displacement of the anchor teeth.

Although directly bonded brackets are suitable for the premolars and canine teeth, it is advisable to band the molars because of the difficulty in maintaining the necessary moisture control in that area and because the occlusal forces may be heavy. The second molar should carry a combination attachment consisting of a wide twin bracket with a convertible cap and a gingivally placed auxiliary tube. This attachment is listed in most orthodontic catalogs as being for first molars. In molar uprighting, of course, the first molar is missing. If two molars are being uprighted simultaneously, the convertible cap should be removed before cementing the second molar band, and the third molar should carry a second molar band with a single molar tube (Fig. 19-11). Lingual buttons or cleats may be helpful if rotations or crossbites are to be corrected (Fig. 19-12).

The placement of the premolar brackets depends on the intended tooth movement. If these teeth are to be repositioned, the brackets should be placed in the ideal position at the center of the facial surface of each tooth. However, if the teeth are merely serving as anchor units and no repositioning is planned, then the brackets should be placed in the position of maximum convenience where minimum wire bending will be required to engage a passive archwire (see Fig. 19-5).

Orthodontic technique: single molar uprighting. Initial alignment of the brackets can be achieved using a light flexible wire, such as .017 × .025 braided stainless steel, nickel-titanium, or beta-titanium wire (Fig. 19-13). Provided such a wire can be placed in the brackets without permanent distortion, it will provide some initial gentle leveling of the teeth. However, it is unlikely that this wire will provide sufficient force to upright the molar against the forces of occlusion. The molar uprighting is done with a helical uprighting auxiliary spring of .017 × .025 stainless

steel wire placed in the auxiliary tube on the molar. The mesial arm of the helical spring should be adjusted to lie passively in the vestibule and upon activation should hook over the archwire in the stabilizing segment. It is important that the hook be positioned so that it is free to slide distally as the molar uprights. A slight lingual bend placed in the uprighting spring is needed to counteract the forces that tend to tip the anchor teeth buccally and the molar lingually (Fig. 19-14).

Since a helical uprighting spring causes considerable occlusal as well as distal crown movement, it should be used only when the terminal molar has an occlusal antagonist. Frequent occlusal adjustments are necessary to reduce developing interferences, making the helical uprighting spring

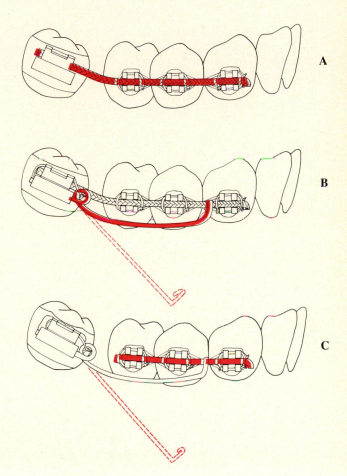

Fig. 19-13 ■ Fixed appliance technique for uprighting a single molar. **A,** Initial bracket alignment is achieved by placing a light flexible wire such as .017 × .025 braided stainless steel wire, from molar to canine; **B,** subsequently, a helical uprighting spring of stiffer wire, .017 × .025 stainless steel, is placed in the auxiliary molar tube and activated by engaging the mesial hook over the stabilizing wire. **C,** If the relative alignment of the molar precludes extending the stabilizing segment into the molar bracket, then a rigid stabilizing wire, .019 × .025 stainless steel, is placed in the premolars and canine only. The mesial arm of the uprighting spring should be adjusted to lie passively in the vestibule before engagement.

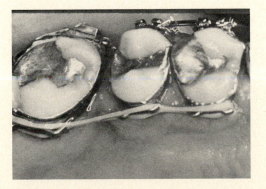

Fig. 19-12 ■ Lingual buttons or cleats (shown here) permit the use of auxiliary elastics that help in correction of rotations or crossbites. Here, lingual attachments and an elastomeric chain are being used for rotation of the molar.

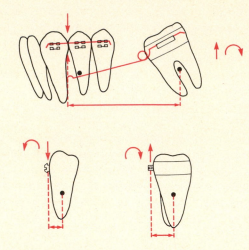

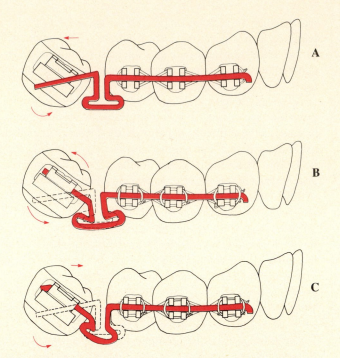

Fig. 19-14 ■ Because the spring is attached to the facial surface of the teeth, a helical uprighting spring tends not only to extrude the molar but also to roll it lingually, while intruding the premolars and flaring them buccally. The uprighting spring should be curved buccolingually so that when it is placed into the molar tube, the hook lies lingual to the archwire to counteract this side effect.

Fig. 19-15 ■ **A,** T-loop spring in .017 × .025 showing the degree of gabling necessary to upright a single tipped molar; **B,** T-loop spring active to upright the tooth by distal crown tipping; **C,** pulling the distal of the wire through the molar tube and opening the T-loop generate a mesial force that results in molar uprighting by mesial root movement with space closure.

most useful when a fixed partial denture is planned or the terminal molar is to be crowned. A helical uprighting spring should never be used to upright an unopposed terminal molar because it will rapidly extrude such a tooth.

If the anchor teeth show a tendency to move, the light stabilizing wire should be replaced by a stiffer wire. Whether this wire can be placed into the premolar brackets and molar tube without permanent distortion will depend on the relative axial inclination of the tipped molar and distal premolar, and the distance between the molar and premolar brackets. Extending the stabilizing wire distally through the molar bracket has the advantage of increasing the buccolingual and vertical control of the molar during uprighting.

However, the degree of molar tipping frequently prevents placement of all but the most flexible wires that may not have sufficient stiffness to control the anchor segments adequately. If this is so, it is advisable to replace the initial stabilizing wire with a rigid wire segment of .019 × .025 stainless steel, extending from the canine to the distal premolar only (see Fig. 19-13c). In this case, the lingual contour of the helical uprighting spring should be increased to counteract the forces that tend to roll the premolars bucally and the molar lingually (Fig. 19-14).

If the molar to be uprighted has no occlusal antagonist, if extrusion is considered undesirable, or if the crown is to be maintained in position while the roots are brought mesially, then an alternative uprighting spring should be used. After the initial alignment with a light flexible wire, a single "T-loop" sectional archwire of .017 × .025 stainless steel should be adapted to fit passively into the brackets on the anchor teeth and gabled at the T to exert an uprighting force

on the molar (Fig. 19-15). When engaged in the molar bracket, this wire will deliver a couple or anticlockwise rotation to the molar, thrusting the roots mesially while the crown tips back.

If the treatment plan calls for space closure rather than increasing the pontic space, the distal end of the archwire should be pulled distally through the molar tube opening the T-loop by 1 to 2 mm. The end of the wire is then bent sharply gingivally to maintain this opening. This provides a mesial force on the molar that prevents the crown from moving distally while the tooth uprights. The fit of the rectangular wire into the rectangular molar tube controls the position of the tooth in all three planes of space.

Since the extrusive forces generated with this appliance are small, it is ideally suited for those patients in whom the opposing tooth has been lost. Severely rotated teeth may also be treated using this appliance, but in this case, the design of the T-loop is modified so that the end of the archwire is inserted from the posterior aspect of the molar tube (Fig. 19-16).

Once the molar uprighting has been almost accomplished, it may be desirable to increase the available pontic space and close any open contacts in the anterior segment. A round wire of .018 diameter should be bent to engage the anchor teeth passively and extended through the molar tube, projecting about 1 mm beyond the distal. An open coil spring compressed between the molar and distal premolar to exert

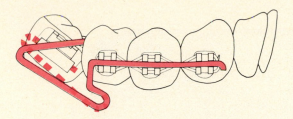

Fig. 19-16 ■ Modification of a T-loop that may be used to upright a severely tipped or rotated molar. The terminal part of the spring is inserted from the distal opening of the molar bracket.

a force of approximately 100 gm will move the premolars mesially while continuing to tip the molar distally (Fig. 19-17). The coil spring may be reactivated by compressing it and adding a split tube spacer over the wire between the coil and the bracket. However, continued use of a compressed coil spring once the premolar spaces are closed may result in anterior displacement of the anchor teeth and incisors. Therefore, the occlusion should be checked carefully against the original study casts at each visit.

These appliances may be used in the maxilla or the mandible (Fig. 19-18), unilaterally or bilaterally (Fig. 19-19). However, it must be remembered that during bilateral molar uprighting, the strain on the anterior anchorage is increased. Very light forces should be used and the anterior occlusion carefully monitored. If it appears that the anchor teeth are moving, then it is probably advisable to deactivate one segment, complete molar uprighting in one quadrant, stabilize those teeth, and then upright the contralateral quadrant.

Orthodontic technique: uprighting two molars in the same quadrant by either mesial root movement or distal crown tipping. When both the second and third molar are to be uprighted, the third molar should carry a single rectangular tube and the cap should be removed from the convertible bracket on the second molar. The initial archwire should be .017 × .025 braided steel wire, which will level the brackets in the anchor segment. After this, a segmental uprighting arch is placed.

Since the second molar is usually more severely tipped than the third molar, increased flexibility of the wire mesial and distal to the second molar is required. This effect may be achieved by using paired T-loops mesial and distal to the second molar (Fig. 19-20), or a box-type loop (Fig. 19-21). Because the resistance offered when uprighting two molars is considerable, careful attention must be paid to the anchorage. As with the single T-loop, distal crown movement may be controlled by opening the loops 1 to 2 mm. However, because of the unfavorable anchorage balance between two molars and the premolars and canines, only small amounts of space closure should be attempted. It is inadvisable to attempt to upright both the second and third molars bilaterally at the same time. Such extensive treatment would require additional augmentation of the anchorage of the anterior teeth and would fall into the category of comprehensive treatment.

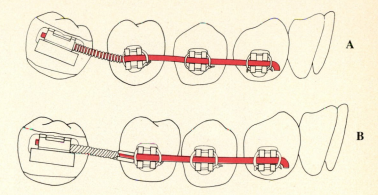

Fig. 19-17 ■ **A,** Compressed coil spring on a round wire (usually .018 steel) may be used to complete molar uprighting while closing remaining spaces in the premolar region. **B,** The coil spring may be reactivated by addition of a split spacer over the archwire.

Clinical management. The most frequent problem encountered with molar uprighting appliances is soft tissue irritation from the loops. Great care must be taken to ensure that the loops lie parallel to but about 1 mm buccal from the dentoalveolar contour, when the wire is engaged in the brackets. Modification of loop design may be required, particularly when uprighting a third molar, since the vestibule in that region is frequently shallow and the buccal mucosa against the dentoalveolar units.

Excessive mobility of the teeth being uprighted can result from either overactivation of the springs or failure to reduce the occlusal interferences. As the teeth upright, the intercuspal contacts will change. To avoid excessive crown reduction, it may be helpful to use a bite splint on the opposing arch so that what may be only transient occlusal interferences can be handled without excessive destruction of tooth material. However, the vertical position of the teeth should be carefully considered when planning treatment and, if extensive crown reduction will be necessary, endodontic treatment should be planned as part of therapy from the beginning rather than provided as an afterthought.

In general, the springs are sufficiently active on placement to complete the molar uprighting, and failure to upright the teeth usually results from occlusal interferences rather than insufficient force. However, T-loop and box-loop springs may have to be removed during treatment to check whether sufficient activation is still present. Unwanted movement of the anchor teeth can be minimized by careful planning and sequencing of treatment, using light forces, and incorporating a cross arch stabilizing splint where appropriate.

Careful attention to oral hygiene must be maintained throughout treatment because the stresses induced by orthodontic force may cause irreversible tissue damage if inflammation is not controlled. However, for many patients the reason for adjunctive tooth movement is the elimination of plaque-harboring periodontal pockets that the patient is unable to clean. Thus, during treatment, it is advisable to see the patient every 2 or 3 weeks for professional cleaning

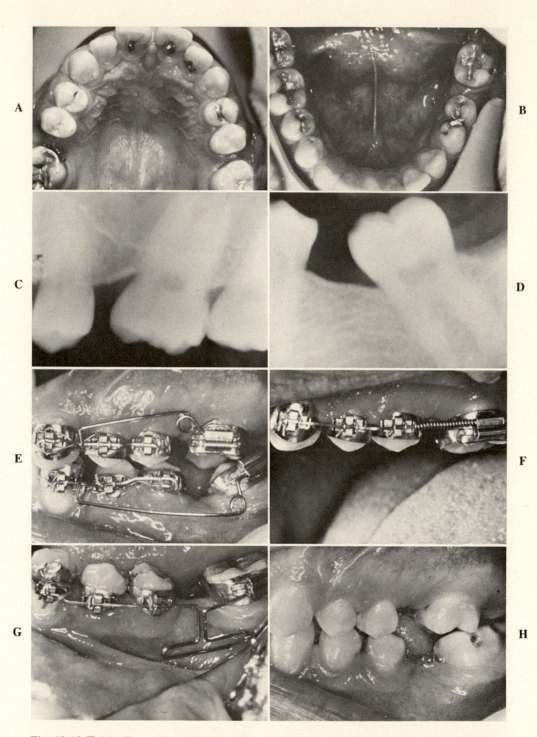

Fig. 19-18 ■ Maxillary and mandibular unilateral uprighting. **A** and **B,** Maxillary and mandibular first molars have been lost and the molars on the left side have tipped so far mesially that molar uprighting is necessary before a pontic can be placed; **C** and **D,** radiographs showing mesial tilt and poor alveolar bone contour. It is necessary to remove the upper third molar to reposition the second molar. **E,** Helical uprighting springs in place; **F,** a compressed coil spring is placed on an .018 round wire in the maxilla to increase the pontic space while continuing to upright the molar. **G,** .017 × .025 T-loop sectional arch placed in the lower arch to continue uprighting the tooth. Since the distal of this archwire has been pulled through the molar tube and bent gingivally, the crown cannot move distally so the roots translate mesially; **H,** both molars uprighted and stabilized; **I,** bridges in place. **J** and **K,** Radiographs showing improved root inclinations and bone contour.

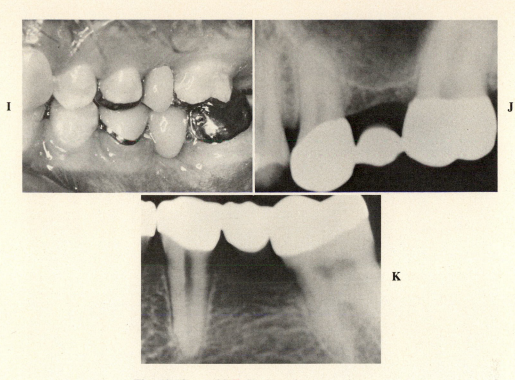

Fig. 19-18, cont'd ■ For legend see opposite page.

of the pockets on the mesial and mesiolingual of the teeth being uprighted. Root planing, curettage, and polishing should be performed gently but thoroughly at each appointment, but care should be taken not to destroy the epithelial attachment since this may result in irreversible crestal bone loss.

The treatment time will vary with the type and extent of the tooth movement required. Uprighting a tooth by distal crown tipping proceeds more rapidly than mesial root movement. Failure to eliminate occlusal interferences will also prolong treatment. The simplest cases should be completed in 8 to 10 weeks, but uprighting two molars with mesial root movement could easily take 20 to 24 weeks.

Retention. Once the teeth have been repositioned, they must be retained while the periodontal ligament reorganizes. A fixed or removable prosthesis placed on teeth that have been uprighted will obviously provide the long-term retention. However, before placement of a prosthesis, an intermediate form of splinting is necessary to maintain the position of abutment teeth. Recently moved teeth are often quite mobile and may change position easily during prosthesis construction. There are two methods of intermediate splinting (Fig. 19-22).

Extracoronal splinting. An .019 × .025 wire designed to fit the brackets passively will prevent any tooth movement. Such a splint must be free of any occlusal interferences. This type of retention, however, should not be used for prolonged periods because orthodontic appliances themselves make effective oral hygiene maintenance difficult.

Intracoronal splinting. Shallow cavities may be prepared in the abutment teeth and a splint of .019 × .025 or heavier wire is secured intracoronally with either amalgam or composite resins (see Figs. 19-22 and 19-8). This type of splint causes very little gingival irritation and can be left in place for considerable time. The adjacent teeth are then free to adjust to a stable position before prosthetic treatment.

■ Forced Eruption

Indications. A second major type of adjunctive orthodontic treatment is the forced eruption of teeth. Teeth with defects in the cervical third of the root pose a complex dental problem (Fig. 19-23). These problems can arise after horizontal or oblique fracture, internal or external resorption, decay, or pathologic perforation. To obtain good access for endodontic and restorative procedures, it is frequently necessary to perform extensive crown lengthening. However, this surgery causes sacrifice of surrounding bone and may result in root sensitivity, long clinical crowns, poor esthetics, and open embrasures.

Controlled vertical extrusion is an excellent way of retaining such teeth in what might otherwise be a hopeless situation. Extrusion of a tooth improves endodontic access and can allow isolation under rubber dam when it would not be possible otherwise. This technique allows the placement of crown margins on sound tooth structure while maintaining a uniform gingival contour that produces improved esthetics. In addition, the alveolar bone height is not compromised, the apparent crown length is maintained, and the

Text continued on p. 488.

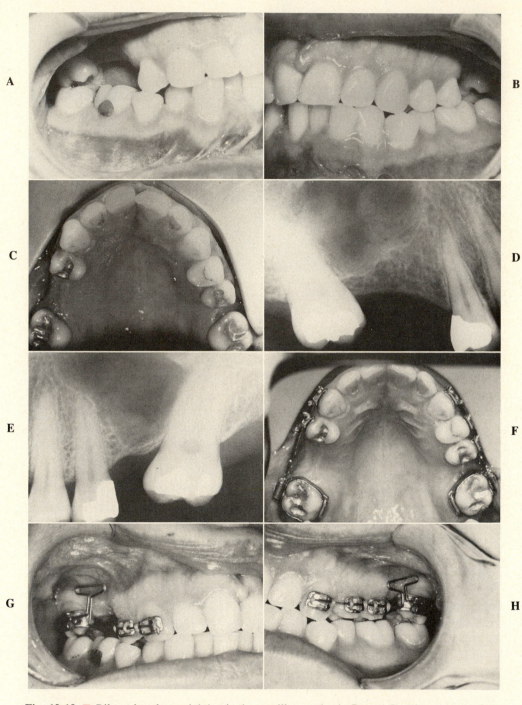

Fig. 19-19 ■ Bilateral molar uprighting in the maxillary arch. **A, B,** and **C,** After the loss of the maxillary teeth, the second molars have tipped and rotated mesially, resulting in poor mesial gingival contour; **D** and **E,** radiographs show the poor bone contour and degree of tipping. **F** to **H,** T-loop uprighting springs active on the right to bring the root mesially and on the left to tip the crown distally.

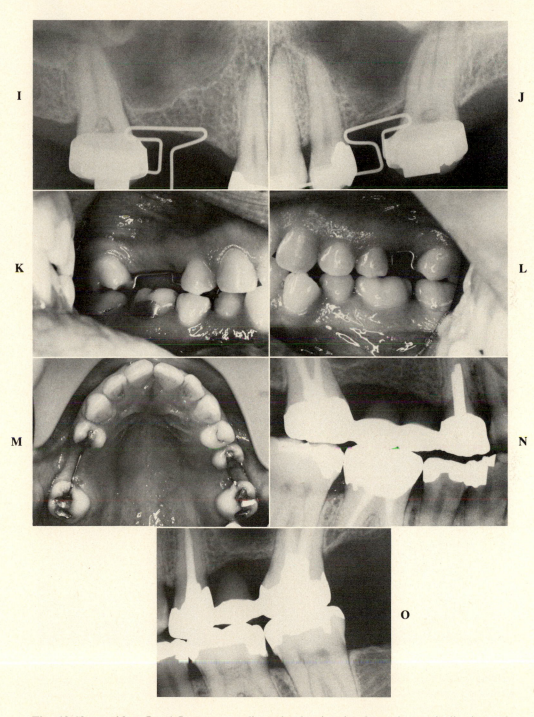

Fig. 19-19, cont'd ■ **I** and **J**, progress radiographs showing the change in root inclination and alveolar bone contour; **K** to **M**, intracoronal splints stabilizing the uprighted teeth for about 6 weeks before bridge construction; **N** to **O**, radiographs showing restorative procedures completed. Note the improved root paralleling and alveolar ridge contour.

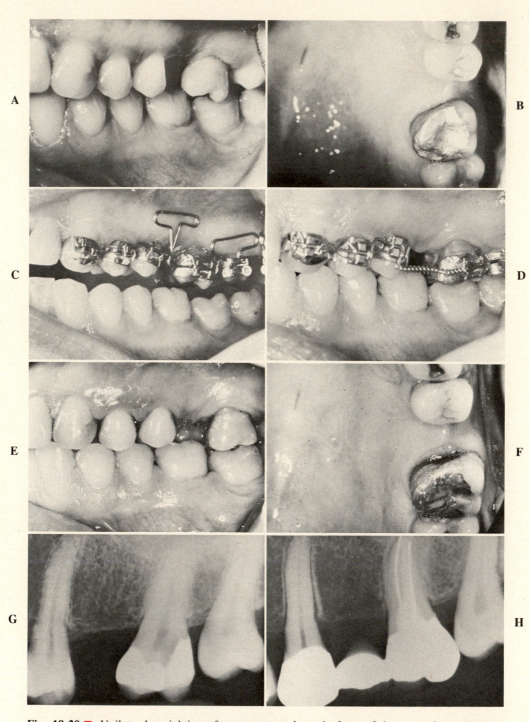

Fig. 19-20 ■ Unilateral uprighting of two upper molars. **A,** Loss of the upper first molar has resulted in tipping of the second molar with extrusion of the distal cusp. **B,** The second molar has rotated around the palatal root, and the mesial gingival tissue has produced a soft tissue pocket. **C,** Initial alignment is achieved with a double T-loop in .017 × .025 wire. It is important that the wire, when not engaged in the mesial molar bracket, should lie obliquely across the bracket from the mesioocclusal to the distogingival tie wing. When the wire is engaged in the bracket, an uprighting couple is generated. **D,** Once initial alignment has been achieved, the pontic space is increased with a compressed coil spring on a round wire. **E,** The molar has been uprighted and the pontic space increased. **F,** The gingival tissue has followed the crown movement reducing the soft tissue pocket. **G,** Pretreatment radiograph of the tipped molar (note the recurrent caries). **H,** Post-treatment radiograph showing that the roots of the abutment are parallel, the bone contour is good, and the endodontic treatment has permitted adequate reduction in crown height.

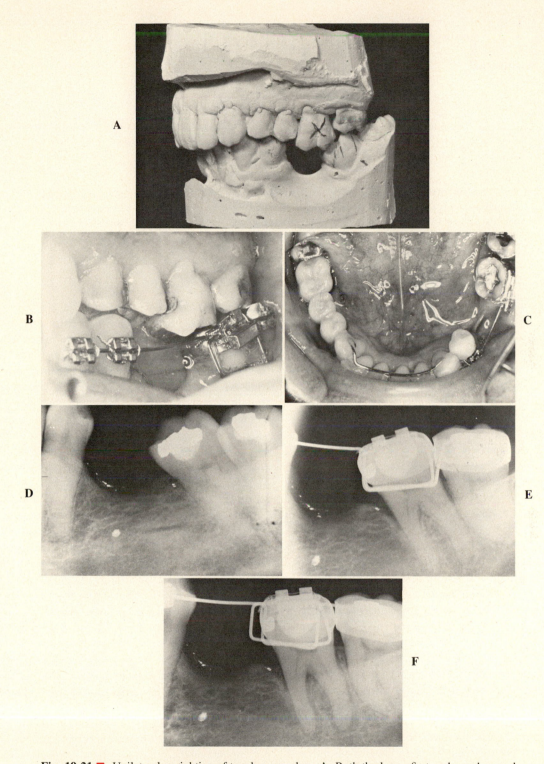

Fig. 19-21 ■ Unilateral uprighting of two lower molars. **A,** Both the lower first molar and second premolar have been lost. Both molars must be uprighted, though the loss of alveolar ridge necessitates doing this by distal crown tipping. **B,** Box loop uprighting spring in place. The spring is bent to lie passively from the mesioocclusal to distogingival tie wing and is activated for molar uprighting upon engagement in the bracket. **C,** A canine-to-canine lingual arch is mandatory to increase the anterior anchorage. **D,** Radiograph of the pretreatment tooth position showing molar tipping, poor alveolar ridge contour, and root approximation of the molars. **E and F,** Radiographs showing progress in uprighting the molars at 12 and 18 weeks, improved bone contour at the mesial of the anterior molar, and generation of good interradicular bone.

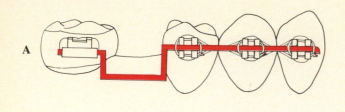

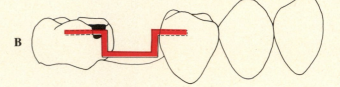

Fig. 19-22 ■ Stabilization after tooth movement should continue until the prostheses are placed. A minimum of 6 weeks is suggested. **A,** An extracoronal splint using an .019 × .025 wire engaging the brackets passively; **B,** an intracoronal splint when bonded in place with composite resin causes minimal tissue disturbance. The intracoronal splint is preferred, particularly if retention is to be continued for more than a few weeks.

procedure does not involve removing bony support from adjacent teeth. As the tooth is extruded, the attached gingiva should follow the cementoenamel junction, thereby increasing the width of the keratinized tissue as the mucogingival junction remains stable. However, it may be necessary to recontour the gingiva to produce an even gingival contour in the adjacent teeth, returning the width of attached gingiva to its original level.

Treatment planning. Before beginning treatment, it is essential to have good periapical radiographs to examine the vertical extent of the defect, the periodontal support, and the root morphology and position. The ideal morphology is a single tapering root. Flared or divergent roots will result in increasing root proximity with extrusion and the possibility of exposing the root furcation area. In rare instances, hypercementosis or dilaceration of the root may make forced eruption complicated or impossible.

The occlusion should also be examined to make sure that sufficient space still exists within the arch and the opposing teeth will permit the placement of a satisfactory esthetic restoration. The crown-to-root ratio at the end of treatment should be 1:1 or better, though the possibility of stabilizing a tooth with an endodontic implant does exist.

The orthodontic movement must often be completed before definitive endodontic procedures since one purpose of the orthodontic movement is to provide better access for endodontic and restorative procedures. However, preliminary endodontic treatment should be performed to relieve symptoms of pulp damage and death. Pulpless teeth move as readily as vital teeth, and root resorption is unlikely to be a problem if treatment time is short.

The length of time required for forced eruption will vary with the age of the patient, the distance the tooth has to be moved, and the viability of the periodontal ligament. In general, 3 to 6 weeks is sufficient. As the tooth erupts, the alveolar bone crest will move with the tooth, particularly if the tooth is moved slowly. Thus, some recontouring of bone may be required around the erupted tooth, but this is usually a relatively minor procedure.

Orthodontic technique. Since extrusion is the tooth movement that occurs most readily and intrusion the movement that occurs least readily, ample anchorage is usually available from adjacent teeth. It has been suggested that the teeth on either side should be used as anchorage with a straight orthodontic wire.[11] Activating such a wire apically will undoubtedly generate an extrusive force, but it also tips adjacent teeth toward the tooth being extruded, reducing the space for subsequent restorations and disturbing the interproximal contacts within the arch. For this reason, a modification of the T-loop used to upright tipped molars is preferred (Fig. 19-24).[12]

If the buccal surface of the tooth to be extruded is intact, a bracket should be bonded as far gingivally as possible (Fig. 19-25). If the crown is hopelessly destroyed, an orthodontic band with a welded bracket can usually be placed over the remaining crown (Fig. 19-26). Two or three additional teeth should be sufficient to provide anchorage. On the anchor teeth, brackets can be placed somewhat more occlusally than the ideal position. A T-loop archwire segment is fabricated from .017 × .025 stainless steel wire, with the height of the loops being determined by the depth of the vestibule. The rectangular wire gives positive control of tooth position in three planes of space. The part of the wire engaging the tooth to be extruded should be somewhat occlusal to the anchor unit (Fig. 19-27). The wire must fit the brackets of the anchor teeth passively and the loops must not impinge on the gingival or buccal tissues when engaged in the bracket. As the tooth is extruded, its occlusal surface may have to be reduced to create space in which to continue forced eruption. The patient should be seen every week or two to reduce the occlusion, control any inflammation, and monitor progress. The objective of treatment is to extrude the tooth sufficiently to produce a level alveolar bone contour and permit placement of a satisfactory esthetic restoration on the exposed root margin.

After active tooth movement has been completed, the

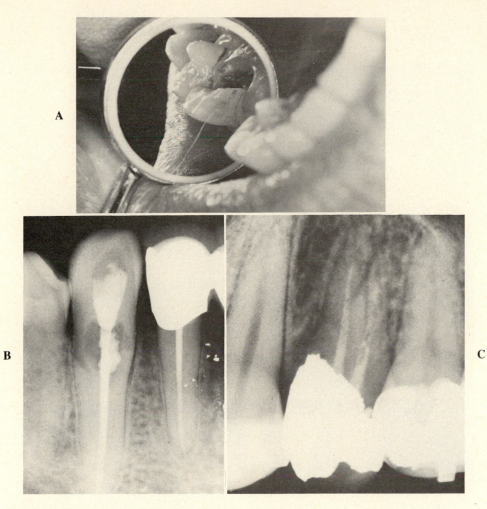

Fig. 19-23 ■ Situations in which forced eruption of teeth will improve restorative procedures. **A,** Crown fracture at the alveolar crest; **B,** internal root resorption; **C,** extensive deep decay at the mesial margin of the first premolar.

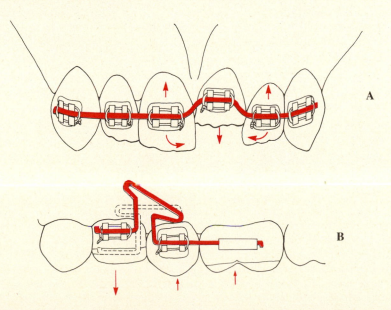

Fig. 19-24 ■ **A,** Although a straight orthodontic wire activated apically will produce an extrusive force on a tooth, it will also cause the teeth on either side to tip toward each other, reducing the space available for the extruding tooth; **B,** a modified T-loop in .017 × .025 will extrude a tooth while controlling mesiodistal tipping.

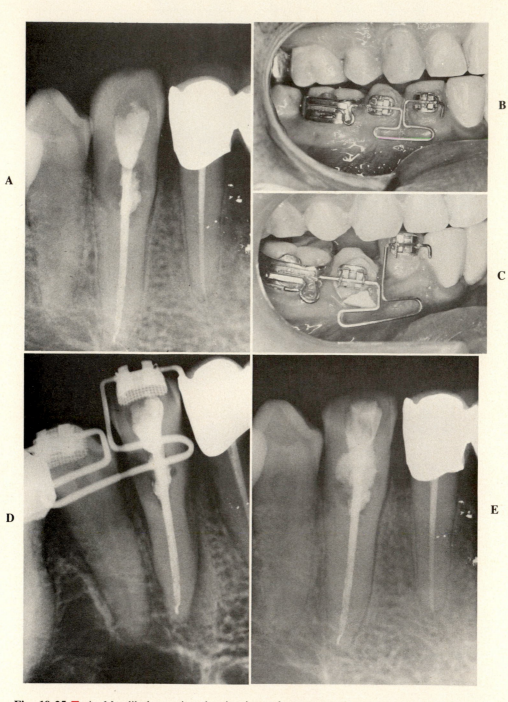

Fig. 19-25 ■ **A,** Mandibular canine showing internal root resorption and suspected lateral perforation. Access is poor and surgical crown lengthening may jeopardize the periodontal integrity of adjacent teeth. **B,** Segmental T-loop appliance active to extrude the canine. The bracket has been placed as far gingival as possible and the crown must be reduced vertically to permit extrusion. **C,** The canine has been extruded. Note the relationship of the bracket to the gingival margin. **D,** Extrusion has moved the lateral perforation to the alveolar margin, where it is accessible for endodontic treatment. **E,** Two-year followup showing stable condition. Note the excellent bone height on the adjacent teeth. (From Tuncay, O.C. J. Prosthet. Dent. **46:**41-47, 1981.)

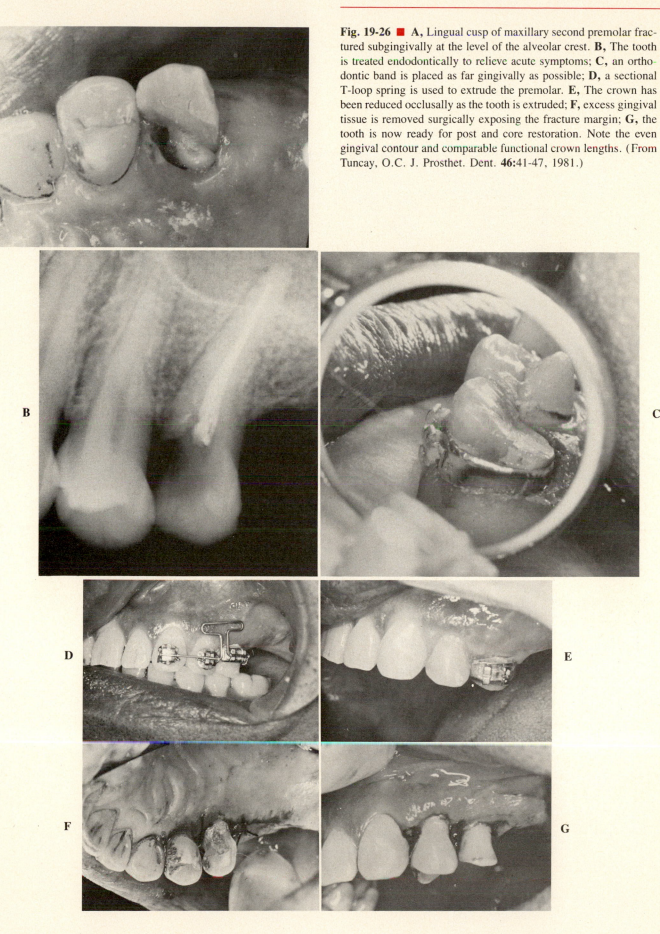

Fig. 19-26 ■ **A,** Lingual cusp of maxillary second premolar fractured subgingivally at the level of the alveolar crest. **B,** The tooth is treated endodontically to relieve acute symptoms; **C,** an orthodontic band is placed as far gingivally as possible; **D,** a sectional T-loop spring is used to extrude the premolar. **E,** The crown has been reduced occlusally as the tooth is extruded; **F,** excess gingival tissue is removed surgically exposing the fracture margin; **G,** the tooth is now ready for post and core restoration. Note the even gingival contour and comparable functional crown lengths. (From Tuncay, O.C. J. Prosthet. Dent. **46:**41-47, 1981.)

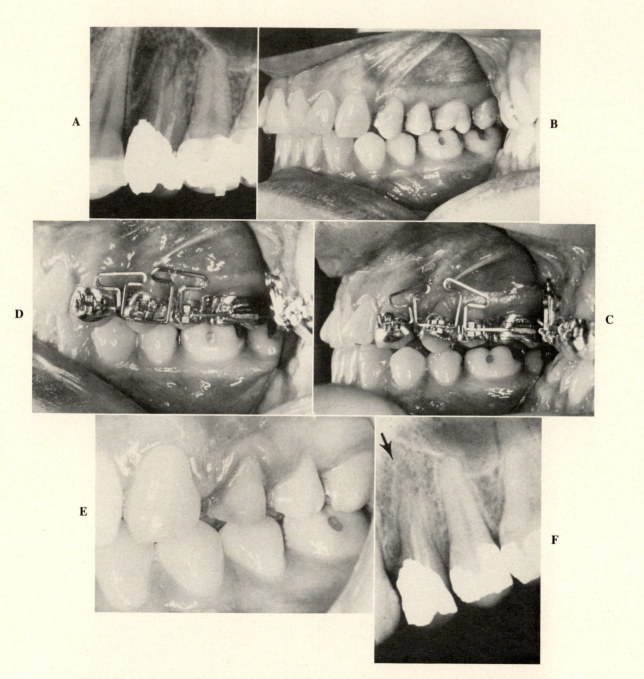

Fig. 19-27 ■ **A,** Gross decay on the mesial of the first premolar with poorly placed amalgam restoration has resulted in periodontal damage. **B,** The first premolar is in occlusion but shows gingival damage and a long clinical crown. **C,** T-loop wire engaging only the anchor teeth to show the degree of activation necessary to extrude the premolar; **D,** T-loop ligated into the premolar. Note the deflection of the loops. These must be carefully checked for soft tissue irritation. **E,** The tooth has been extruded. Crown reduction has maintained the length of the clinical crown and the gingival contour is level. **F,** The gingival margin is now above the alveolar crest. The arrow indicates the former position of the root apex.

tooth should be stabilized by bending a rectangular wire to fit passively into all the brackets. Stabilization allows for proper reorganization of the periodontal ligament fibers and allows the bone to remodel, which discourages relapse. In general, 3 to 6 weeks of stabilization should be sufficient after extrusion.

■ Alignment of Teeth

Indications. Rotations, crowding, spacing, crossbites, and tipped teeth all pose problems for restorative and periodontal procedures. Orthodontic alignment of malpositioned teeth can greatly improve access and permit placement of well adapted and contoured restorations with minimal sacrifice of sound tooth material. Repositioning closely approximated roots improves the embrasure form and increases the amount of interradicular bone, which in turn increases the chance that periodontal disease can be controlled. Eliminating crossbites and uprighting tipped teeth establish good interproximal contacts, provide better directed occlusal loadings, and minimize the possibility of occlusal interferences. Space closure or redistribution permits placement of crowns and pontics without overcontoured crowns that produce poor embrasure form.

Most alignment problems are reflections of crowding or spacing within the dental arch. As such, it is first necessary to assess how much space would be required or created during arch alignment. Moving teeth lingually and correcting rotations of anterior teeth require additional space within the arch. Derotating posterior teeth and uprighting tipped teeth usually cause them to occupy less space within the arch, while moving teeth facially increases arch length. Space may also be created by removing interproximal enamel to reduce the mesiodistal width of selected teeth. This does not seem to increase the risk of caries, providing that at least one-half of the enamel structure remains and the exposed surface is protected by topical application of fluoride.

Treatment planning. A "diagnostic setup" can be very helpful in planning treatment for alignment problems, particularly if crowding or spacing must be corrected. For this procedure, the study casts are duplicated and the malaligned teeth are carefully cut from the model, crown dimensions are modified if appropriate, and the teeth are then waxed back onto the cast in a new position (Fig. 19-28). This allows one to assess what tooth movements, crown reshaping, or pontic replacement would be necessary to produce an esthetically satisfying and functional occlusion. Alternative tooth positions may be tried to determine the optimum for each patient. Once the most satisfactory occlusion has been established, the feasibility of the orthodontic treatment can be evaluated in light of the crown and root movements required, the anchorage available, the periodontal support for each tooth, and the possible occlusal interferences.

Teeth that can be arranged satisfactorily in a diagnostic setup may not always be as easy to adjust clinically. On the other hand, an orthodontic appliance certainly cannot ac-

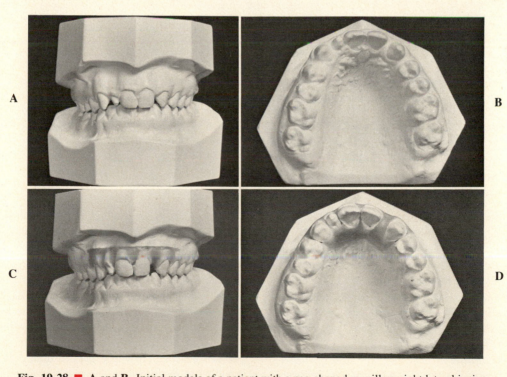

Fig. 19-28 ■ **A** and **B,** Initial models of a patient with a peg-shaped maxillary right lateral incisor, congenital absence of the maxillary left lateral, and one mandibular incisor; **C** and **D,** the diagnostic setup suggests that both canines be retracted, the peg-shaped lateral moved to the right and built up, and space for the replacement of the left lateral be increased.   *Continued.*

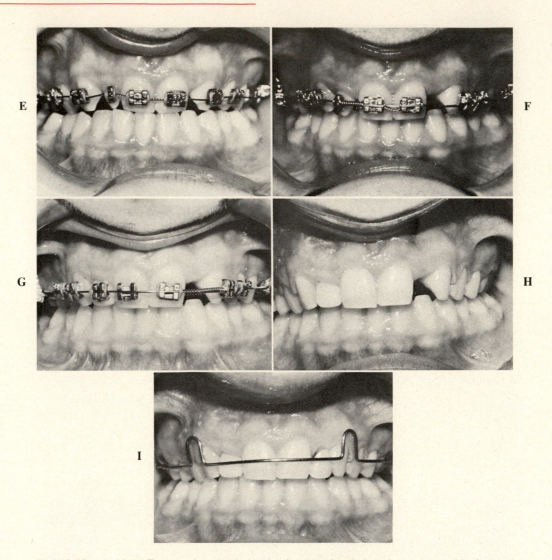

Fig. 19-28, cont'd ■ **E,** A sectioned twin bracket has been bonded on the peg-shaped incisor and an .0175 multistranded wire is used for initial alignment. **F** and **G,** Mesial and distal movement of teeth with elastomeric modules or coil spring requires a stiffer wire (.018 stainless steel) to control tipping. Rectangular wire (0.018 × .025) is used only if the buccolingual inclination must be adjusted. **H,** The teeth are repositioned, the peg-shaped lateral built up with resin. **I,** Retainer with a replacement lateral incisor can be used before definitive restorative procedures.

complish in the mouth what cannot be done on the laboratory bench. The length of time required to align teeth will vary with the age of the patient, the distance the teeth have to be moved, and the cellular activity within the periodontal ligament. As a general guideline, adjunctive tooth movement that would take longer than 6 months should be avoided, since such patients almost certainly have a complicated malocclusion that would be better handled with comprehensive orthodontic treatment.

Orthodontic technique

Alignment of crowded, rotated, and displaced incisors. Anterior teeth that require alignment should be brought into their proper position before definitive restorative procedures (Fig. 19-29). Progressive interproximal stripping can be used to create space, within limits established by the mesiodistal diameter of the crowns at the gingival margin in the maxillary arch. Approximately ½ mm of enamel may be removed from the mesial and distal surface of each maxillary anterior tooth, giving a maximum 4 to 5 mm additional space in the anterior part of the arch. In the mandibular arch, the smaller mesiodistal width of the incisor teeth reduces the amount of interproximal stripping that can be undertaken without producing unacceptable root proximity. For this reason, crowding greater than 3 to 4 mm in the mandibular anterior arch nearly always requires the extraction of a lower incisor. While stripping anterior teeth may be an excellent way of gaining a small amount of space, such treatment should be undertaken with caution since it

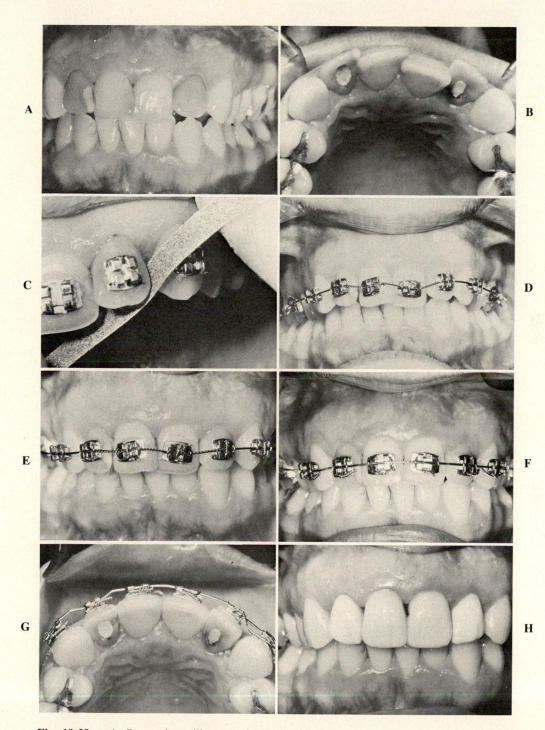

Fig. 19-29 ■ **A,** Decayed maxillary anterior teeth with discoloration after endodontic treatment; **B,** the occlusal view shows the degree of crowding and rotation; **C,** although the lateral incisor has been treated endodontically, the mesiodistal width of the crown at the gingival margin limits the amount of interproximal stripping possible; **D,** initial alignment is achieved with a highly flexible archwire, .0175 multistranded steel, **E,** which is retied or replaced after 3 to 4 weeks; **F,** final alignment is achieved with a stiffer wire (.016 or .018 steel). **G,** If anterior crowns are to be placed, minor rotations need not be corrected orthodontically since they can be masked restoratively. This procedure is easier on endodontically treated teeth since there is no danger of accidental pulp exposure during crown preparation. **H,** Anterior crowns in place. Unless the crowns are fused together, retention must be continued to prevent rotational relapse.

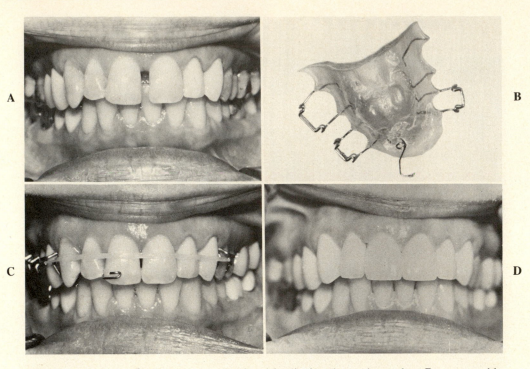

Fig. 19-30 ■ **A,** Small diastema may be closed by tipping the teeth together; **B,** a removable appliance with fingersprings in place. **C,** Any labial flaring can be controlled with an anterior elastic or a labial bow; **D,** space redistribution has permitted placement of more equal sized anterior crowns.

may have an undesirable effect on the esthetics, overbite and overjet relationship, and posterior intercuspation.

Alignment nearly always requires a fixed appliance. The first molars should be banded to serve as anchorage, augmented if necessary with a rigid lingual arch (see Chapters 9 and 12). Edgewise brackets are bonded on the anterior teeth, usually canine-to-canine, and an initial ideal archwire is placed. This wire must be light and flexible enough to be tied to all the brackets (but not necessarily completely into them) without either becoming permanently distorted or exerting excessive forces on the teeth. A braided .0175 stainless steel or .016 NiTi wire is usually suitable (see Chapter 15). Unless the wire is turned gingivally at the distal of the molar tubes, the teeth will flare labially while they align, which is usually undesirable. Crown reduction should be started the day the appliances are placed and continued at subsequent appointments.

The initial wire can be tied more tightly at 4-week intervals and can generally be replaced by an .016 or .018 steel wire about 4 weeks after it has been fully engaged in the bracket slots. This second wire will exert sufficient force to complete alignment of the teeth. Although round wires can correct rotations and tip teeth into alignment, precise positioning of roots requires the use of an additional rectangular wire. However, rectangular wires should not be used for preliminary alignment since they may cause undesirable back and forth root movement at that stage (see Chapter 15).

Once the ideal crown and root positions have been achieved, the teeth must be stabilized. Their tendency to relapse after correction of rotation may be reduced by severing the distorted supracrestal gingival fibers (see Chapter 18). A carefully constructed retainer with a closely adapted labial bow must be placed immediately upon removal of the fixed appliance. If a fiber section has been performed, retention should be continued for 6 months. If fibers are not sectioned, then retention should be continued at night for an indefinite period. It is probably advisable to delay any crown construction for 6 to 8 weeks after alignment of incisors to allow bone remodeling to be completed. The retention schedule outlined previously should then be followed unless the crowns are fused together to form a permanent retainer.

Anterior diastema closure and space redistribution. Loss of posterior teeth, abnormally small teeth, or loss of bone support may all result in drifting and spacing of incisors. Space closure or redistribution will greatly simplify restorative procedures and improve the esthetics. Closure of anterior spaces is usually relatively simple but often requires permanent retention with a bonded lingual retainer, overcontoured crowns, fused crowns, or a fixed partial denture.

If the diastema is small or results from adjacent teeth being tipped in opposite directions, a removable appliance with fingerspring may be used to close the space by simple tipping (Fig. 19-30). However, if the teeth are bodily dis-

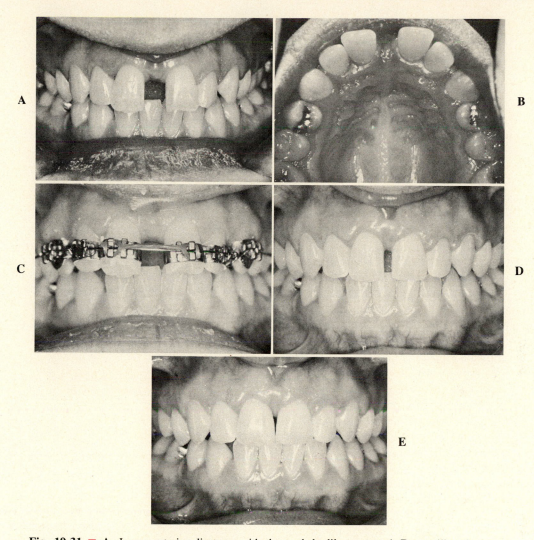

Fig. 19-31 ■ **A,** Large anterior diastema with the teeth bodily separated; **B,** maxillary incisors are flared labially with generalized spacing. **C,** Fixed appliances on the teeth prevent tipping as the incisors are approximated and retracted with elastomeric chain. The mesial bracket wings of the central incisors also must be tied to prevent rotation. **D,** Overjet reduction complete but residual anterior spacing still present. **E,** Anterior spaces closed with small composite buildups that have produced good embrasure form and esthetics.

placed or widely separated, a fixed appliance must be used to control both crown and root position (Fig. 19-31). Once again, a wire bent to ideal arch form is used, which may be continuous from molar to molar if several teeth are to be moved, or involve just the anterior segment of the arch if only two or three teeth are to be moved.

Brackets are placed on the teeth to be moved and on appropriate anchor teeth. Initial alignment is carried out using a light wire such as .0175 braided steel or .016 NiTi. This wire is replaced 3 to 4 weeks after bracket engagement is achieved, with an .016 or .018 round steel wire along which the teeth are repositioned, using elastomeric modules or coil springs. Initially the teeth tip but the stiffness of the wire in the wide bracket counteracts this effect and results in bodily movement. If the spacing is the result of abnormally small teeth in one arch (i.e., a tooth size discrepancy

exists), it will be impossible to close all the space while maintaining the posterior intercuspation. In such a case, the teeth must be moved into an ideally separated position and the crowns built up either with composite resins (see Chapter 17) or castings.

Crossbite correction. Crossbites may occur in any part of the arch and often cause functional problems such as occlusal interferences, occlusal trauma, and improper occlusal loading. Anterior crossbites are an esthetic problem as well. If only one or two teeth are involved, the crossbite usually results from displacement of crowded teeth or ectopic eruption. If a group of teeth are involved, it is more likely that the crossbite is a skeletal problem and will not respond to limited orthodontic treatment. In this case, if successful restorative or periodontal treatment cannot be done with the teeth in the crossbite position, the patient

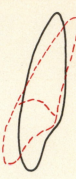

Fig. 19-32 ■ A labially directed force from a removable appliance will tip the tooth and cause an apparent intrusion of the crown, which reduces the overbite.

should be referred for comprehensive orthodontic treatment that may include orthognathic surgery.

If a crossbite is due only to displaced teeth and if the tooth correction requires only tipping movements, then a removable appliance may be used to tip the teeth into a normal position. However, since removable appliances only tip teeth, as a tooth rotates labially or buccally into its new position, there is an apparent intrusion that reduces the overbite (Fig. 19-32). This effect is particularly noticeable on anterior teeth. Alternatively, "through the bite elastics" may be used from the tooth in crossbite to a conveniently placed tooth in the opposing arch. This approach also tips the teeth but tends to extrude them (Fig. 19-33).

If bodily movement is required in crossbite correction and vertical control is critical, an ideal arch system should be used, incorporating the first molars and two or three teeth on either side of the tooth to be moved (Fig. 19-34). Progressively stiffer round wires are placed to align the crown, but the final correction of root position can be achieved only by placing a rectangular wire that will almost fill the bracket slot. The reciprocal force will tend to move the anchor teeth into crossbite. This may be resisted by the use of a soldered transpalatal arch on the molars or the addition of a removable acrylic plate that closely contacts the palatal surface of the adjacent anchor teeth. The rectangular wire can be adjusted to control the tooth in three planes of space.

Establishing a good overbite relationship is the key to maintaining crossbite correction. Alternatively, crown reconstruction can provide the same positive occlusal indexing, while eliminating any balancing interferences from the lingual cusps of posterior teeth. If a deep overbite exists on the teeth in crossbite, correction will be much easier if a temporary bite plane that frees the occlusion is added. This bite plane should be carefully constructed to contact the occlusal surfaces of all teeth to prevent any supraeruption during treatment.

Separation of approximated teeth. Occasionally two teeth may exhibit close root proximity. The lack of interradicular space at the gingival margin is the critical factor since this will not only prevent satisfactory restorative procedures but also predispose both teeth to periodontal disease. If the roots

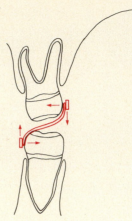

Fig. 19-33 ■ "Through the bite" or cross elastics have both horizontal and vertical forces and will extrude the teeth while moving them buccolingually. These elastics are used frequently to correct posterior crossbites but are rarely indicated for an anterior crossbite.

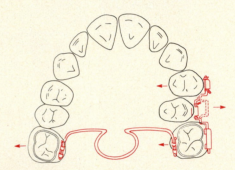

Fig. 19-34 ■ Tipping and extrusion of a tooth during crossbite correction may be controlled by using a fixed appliance. Anchorage is obtained from adjacent teeth and the contralateral molar if necessary, which can be included via a lingual arch as shown here. A flexible wire engaged in the brackets generates the necessary controlled forces.

of such teeth must be separated, the necessary tooth movement can be achieved only with a fixed appliance, since a force system that applies a moment effective in moving roots must be used (see Chapter 10). The anchorage for such movement may be gained from the adjacent teeth or from a removable appliance (Fig. 19-35). Root movement proceeds more slowly than crown tipping, and 8 to 10 weeks should be allowed for such procedures. Periapical radiographs will confirm that adequate root separation has been achieved.

In summary, adjunctive orthodontic treatment should be considered as a means of eliminating pathologic occlusion, permitting placement of more ideal restorations by more conservative techniques, and positioning teeth where periodontal health can be maintained. Providing that a correct diagnosis has been established and careful control of three dimensional tooth position is maintained, such limited tooth movement can greatly enhance general dental treatment.

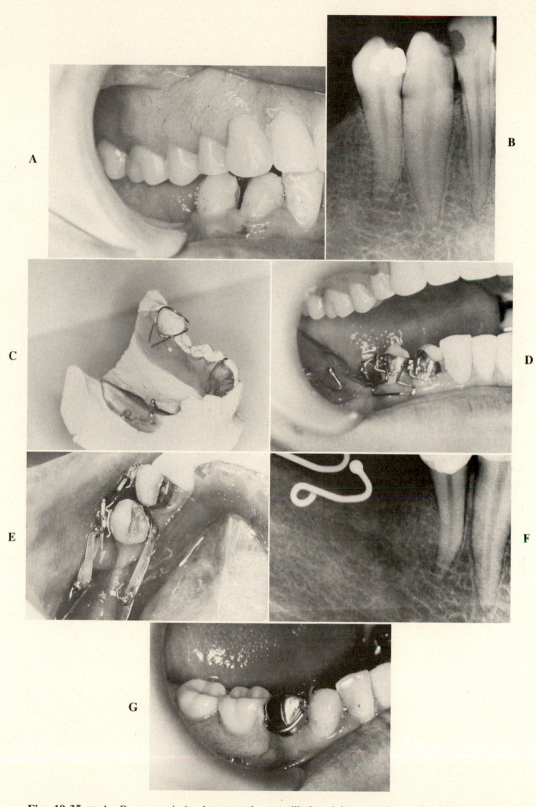

Fig. 19-35 ■ **A,** Root proximity between the mandibular right premolar and canine poses a prosthetic and periodontal problem. **B,** Radiograph showing the difficulty of restoring the premolar and lack of interradicular bone. The premolar must be moved distally without tipping if damage to the root surfaces of the adjacent teeth is to be avoided. This requires the combination of a translational force and a root-uprighting moment. **C,** Removable appliance used to augment anchorage. **D,** T-loop spring active to provide the moment that moves the premolar root distally. **E,** Rubberbands hooked to removable appliance provide distal translational force to the premolar. **F,** Radiographs showing the resultant distal bodily movement of the premolar and formation of new interradicular bone. **G,** Partial denture in place with rests on the crown of the premolar. (From Tuncay, O.C. J. Prosthet. Dent. **46:**41-47, 1981.)

■ *References*

1. Amsterdam, M.: Periodontal prosthesis, twenty-five years in retrospect. Alpha Omegan Sci. Issue **67:**8-52, 1974.
2. Muhlemann, H., and Herzog, H.: Tooth mobility and microscopic tissue changes produced by experimental occlusal trauma. Helv. Odontologica Acta **5:**33-39, 1961.
3. Polson, A.M., Neitner, S.W., and Zander, H.A.: Trauma and progression of marginal periodontitis in squirrel monkeys. IV. Reversibility of bone loss due to trauma alone and trauma superimposed upon periodontitis. J. Periodontal. Res. **11:**290-298, 1976.
4. Nisengard, R.J.: The role of immunology in periodontal disease. J. Periodontol. **48:**505-516, 1977.
5. Lindhe, J., and Svanberg, G.: Influence of trauma from occlusion on progression of experimental periodontitis in the Beagle dog. J. Clin. Periodontol. **1:**3-14, 1974.
6. Ericsson, I., Thilander, B., Lindhe, J., et al.: The effect of orthodontic tilting movements on the periodontal tissues of infected and non-infected dentition in dogs. J. Clin. Periodontol. **4:**278-293, 1977.
7. Ericsson, I., Thilander, B., and Lindhe, J.: Periodontal condition after orthodontic tooth movements in the dog. Angle Orthod. **48:**210-218, 1978.
8. Lindhe, J., and Nyman, S.: The effect of plaque control and surgical pocket elimination on the establishment and maintenance of periodontal health: a longitudinal study of periodontal therapy in cases of advanced disease. J. Clin. Periodontol. **2:**67-79, 1975.
9. Page, R.C., and Schroeder, H.E.: Pathogenesis of inflammatory periodontal disease: a summary of current work. Lab. Invest. **34:**235-249, 1976.
10. Zander, H.A., and Polson, A.M.: Present status of occlusion and occlusal therapy in periodontics. J. Periodontol. **48:**540-544, 1977.
11. Ten Cate, A.R.: Oral Histology: Development, Structure and Function. St. Louis, 1980, The C.V. Mosby Co.
12. Guildford, J.H., and Grubb, T.A.: Vertical extrusion: a standardized technique. Compendium Continuing Educ. **5:**562-567, 1984.

Chapter 20

Special Considerations in Comprehensive Treatment of Adults

Since the 1960s, there has been a dramatic increase in the number of adults receiving comprehensive orthodontic treatment. Although no precise data are available, informal practice surveys indicate that the number of adults seeking orthodontic treatment in the United States has increased nearly fivefold in recent years. Adults represented approximately 5% of all orthodontic patients before 1970, but are estimated to be 20% to 25% in the 1980s[1] (Fig. 20-1).

The response to orthodontic force may be somewhat slower in an adult than in a child, but tooth movement occurs in a very similar way at all ages, and comprehensive treatment can be divided into the same stages discussed in Chapters 15 to 18. Despite this fact, comprehensive treatment for adults brings with it a set of problems that simply do not exist with younger patients. Special considerations for adults fall into three major categories: (1) their different motivations for seeking orthodontic treatment and different psychologic reactions to it, (2) their heightened susceptibility to periodontal disease and the possibility that active periodontal disease is one reason for seeking treatment in the first place, and (3) their lack of growth, even the small amounts of vertical growth on which orthodontists can rely for patients in late adolescence.

■ *Motivation for Adult Treatment*

■ Psychologic Considerations

A major motivation for orthodontic treatment of children and adolescents is the parents' desire for treatment. The typical child accepts orthodontics in about the same way that he accepts going to school, summer camp, and the inevitable junior high school dance—just another in the series of events that one must endure while growing up. Occasionally, of course, an adolescent actively resists orthodontic treatment, and the result can be unfortunate for all concerned if the treatment become the focus of an adolescent rebellion. In most instances, however, adolescents tend not to become emotionally involved in their treatment.

Adults, in contrast, seek comprehensive orthodontic treatment because they themselves want something. That something, however, is not always clearly expressed, and in fact some adults have a remarkably elaborate hidden set of motivations. It is important to explore why the patient wants treatment, and why now, to avoid setting up a situation in which the patient's expectations from treatment cannot possibly be met. Sometimes orthodontic treatment is sought as a last-ditch effort to improve personal appearance to deal with a series of complicated social problems. An extreme example might be an individual whose marriage is failing and who thinks that perhaps this would not happen if his or her protruding front teeth were corrected. Orthodontic treatment obviously cannot be relied on to repair personal relationships, save jobs, or overcome a series of financial disasters, and if the prospective patient has unrealistic expectations of that sort, it is much better to deal with them sooner rather than later.

Most adult patients, fortunately, understand why they are seeking orthodontic treatment and are realistic about what they can obtain from it. One might expect those who seek treatment to be less secure and less well adjusted than the average adult, but for most part, those who seek treatment tend to have a more positive self-image than average.[2] It apparently takes a good deal of ego strength to seek orthodontic treatment as an adult, and ego strength rather than weakness characterizes most potential adult patients. A patient who seek treatment primarily because he or she wants to improve the appearance or function of the teeth (internal motivation) is more likely to respond well psychologically

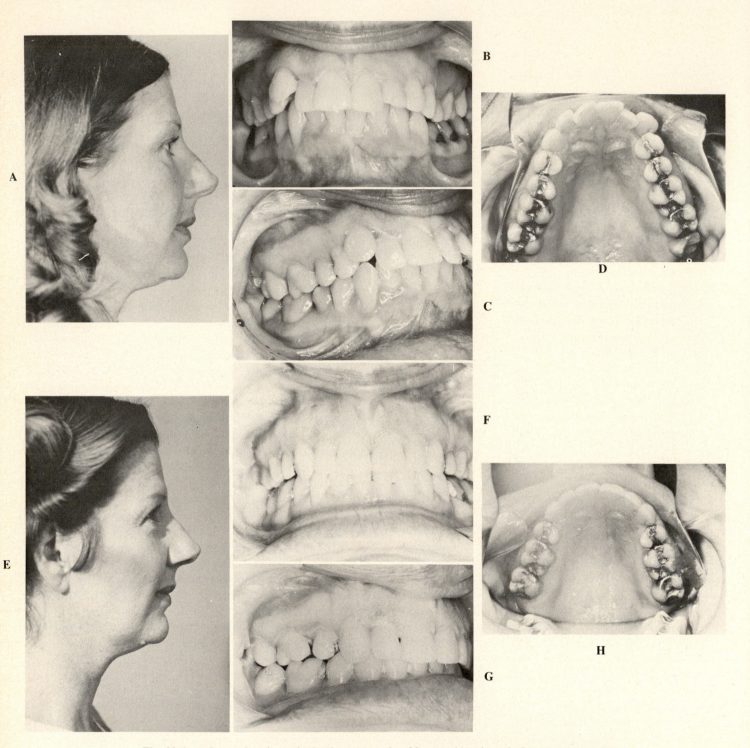

Fig. 20-1 ■ Comprehensive orthodontic treatment in a 38-year-old patient. **A,** Pretreatment profile, showing reasonably good facial proportions despite moderate mandibular deficiency. Her chief complaint was of irregular and protruding incisors. **B,** Frontal view of the dental occlusion; note the midline discrepancy; **C,** lateral view, demonstrating the Class II molar and canine relationships; **D,** occlusal view, showing the crowded maxillary arch; **E,** posttreatment facial profile after 22 months of active treatment and extraction of upper first and lower second premolars; **F,** frontal view of occlusion after treatment; **G,** lateral occlusal view after treatment; **H,** posttreatment occlusal view of maxillary arch; **I,** cephalometric superimposition, demonstrating that correction of occlusal relationships was obtained largely by retracting the upper incisors, using the mandibular posterior segments as anchorage. Note that slight downward rotation of the mandible did occur as a consequence of the extrusive components of the orthodontic force systems.

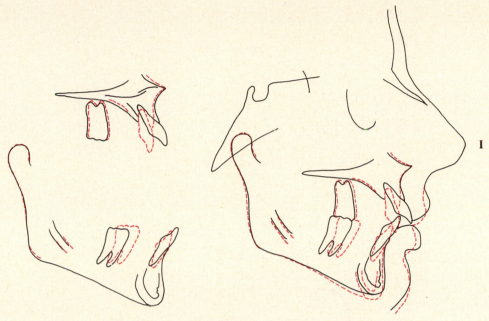

Fig. 20-1, cont'd ■ For legend see opposite page.

than a patient whose motivation is the urging of others or the expected impact of treatment on others (external motivation). External motivation is often accompanied by an increasing impact of the orthodontic problem or personality (Fig. 20-2). The same type of patient is most likely to have a complex set of unrecognized expectations for treatment, the proverbial hidden agenda.

One way to identify the minority of individuals who may be problems because of their unrealistic expectations is to compare the patient's perception of his or her orthodontic condition with the doctor's evaluation. If the patient thinks that the appearance or function of the teeth is creating a

severe problem, while an objective assessment simply does not corroborate that, orthodontic treatment should be approached with caution.

Even highly motivated adults express some concern about the appearance of orthodontic appliances. The demand for an invisible orthodontic appliance comes almost entirely from adults who are concerned about the reaction of others to obvious orthodontic treatment. In an earlier era, this was a major reason for using removable appliances in adults, particularly the Crozat appliance in the United States. However, it is simply impossible to do effective comprehensive treatment with a removable appliance, particularly one that

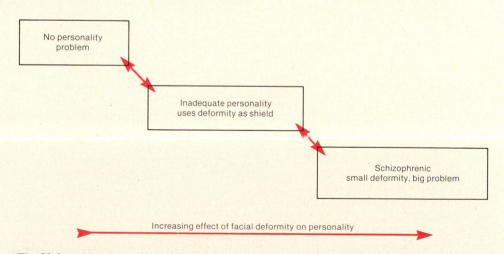

Fig. 20-2 ■ Most potential orthodontic patients do not have personality problems, but it is important to recognize that for some individuals, the orthodontic condition can become the focus for a wide-ranging set of social adjustment problems. An important aspect of orthodontic diagnosis for adults is understanding where a patient fits along this spectrum.

is not worn constantly. In recent years, the search for less visible appliances has led to clear or tooth-colored labial brackets (Fig. 20-3), and most recently to fixed lingual appliances.

At present, it is not possible to produce an invisible or minimally visible appliance that does not compromise the orthodontic treatment. Plastic brackets create problems in controlling root position and closing spaces. Lingual appliances, primarily because of the small interbracket span, also make control of complex tooth movements difficult. Although there is nothing wrong with using the most esthetic possible appliance for an adult patient, the compromises associated with this approach should be thoroughly discussed in advance. It is unrealistic for a patient to expect that orthodontic treatment can be carried out without other people knowing about it.

The whole issue of the visibility of the orthodontic appliances is much less important, at least in the United States at present, than many patients fear. Orthodontic treatment for adults is certainly socially acceptable, and one does not become a victim of discrimination because of visible orthodontic appliances. In a sense, the patient's expectations become a self-fulfilling prophecy. If the patient faces others confidently, a visible orthodontic appliance causes no problems. Only if the patient acts ashamed is there likely to be any negative reaction from others.

The question of whether the treatment area for adult patients should be separated from the adolescents who still constitute the bulk of most orthodontic practices is related to the same set of attitudes. Most comprehensive orthodontic treatment for adolescents is carried out in open treatment areas, not only because the open area is efficient but also because the learning effect from having patients observe what is happening to others is a positive influence in adapting to treatment (Fig. 20-4). Should adults be segregated into private rooms, rather than joining the group in the open treatment area? This arrangement is logical only if the adult is vaguely ashamed of being an orthodontic patient. Sometimes, for some adults, treatment in a private area may be preferable, but for most adults, learning from interacting with other patients is extremely beneficial. There are positive advantages in having patients at various stages of treat-

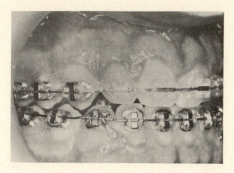

Fig. 20-3 ■ Small bonded metal brackets have less esthetic impact than bands, and plastic brackets on the maxillary incisors as shown here further reduce visibility of the appliance. Lingual appliances (see Chapter 12) are almost totally invisible. Whether a less visible appliance is worth the additional cost, effort, and treatment time is a judgment to be made individually with each patient.

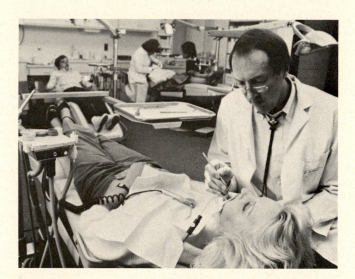

Fig. 20-4 ■ For most adults, there is a positive advantage in carrying out orthodontic treatment in an open treatment area that allows interaction with other patients, just as there is with adolescents. The interplay between doctor, assistants, and other patients enhances the patient's learning about orthodontic treatment.

Fig. 20-5 ■ Comprehensive treatment for a patient with advanced periodontal disease. **A,** Periapical radiograph of the mandibular incisor region before treatment, showing severe bone loss and subgingival calculus; **B,** frontal view of occlusal relationships after initial scaling. One lower incisor had been lost previously. **C,** Lateral occlusal view initially. The horizontal and vertical discrepancies in the lower incisor region made splinting almost impossible, and the necessity for splints in the future was one of the reasons for orthodontic treatment; **D,** Loop arches used for initial alignment; **E,** progress in leveling the mandibular arch; **F,** occlusal relationships after 16 months of comprehensive treatment, showing resolution of the occlusal discrepancies; **G,** lateral view of occlusal relationships; **H,** periapical radiograph of the lower incisor region. It is unrealistic to expect that bone will regenerate as a consequence of orthodontic treatment, but further bone loss can be avoided with careful periodontal management during the active orthodontic treatment, and the overall periodontal situation often improves.

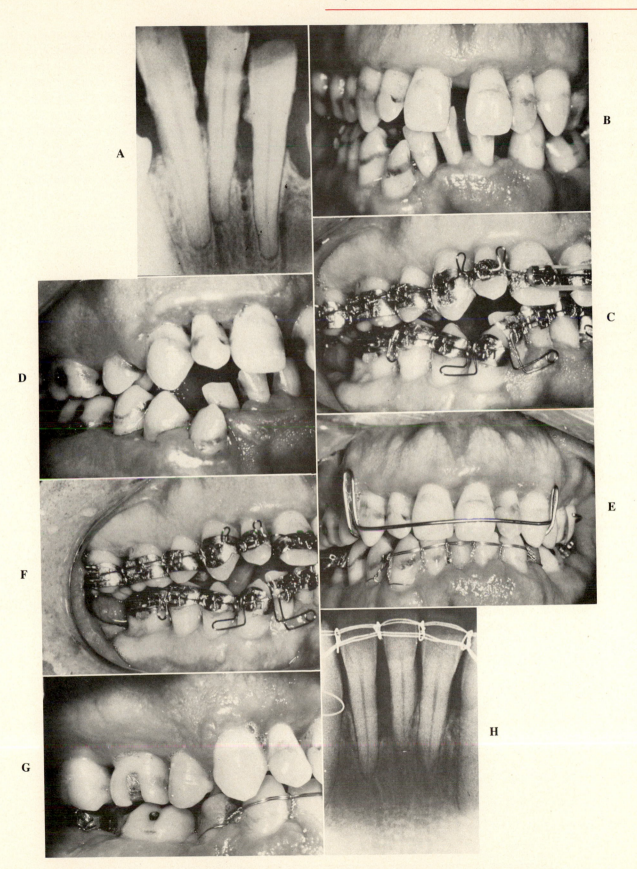

Fig. 20-5 ■ For legend see opposite page.

ment compare their experiences, and this is at least as beneficial to adults as to children, perhaps more so.

Despite the fact that adult patients can be treated in the same area as adolescents, they cannot be handled in exactly the same way. The typical adolescent's passive acceptance of what is being done is rarely found in adult patients, who want and expect a considerable degree of explanation of what is happening and why. The fact that an adult can be counted on to be interested in the treatment does not automatically translate into compliance with instructions. Unless adult patients understand why they have been asked to do various things, they may choose not to do them, not in the passive way an adolescent might just shrug it off, but from an active decision not to cooperate. In addition, adults, as a rule, are less tolerant of discomfort and more likely to complain about pain after adjustments and about difficulties in speech, eating, and tissue adaptation. Additional chair time to meet these demands should be anticipated.

These characteristics might make adults sound like less desirable orthodontic patients than adolescents, which is not necessarily so. Working with individuals who are intensely interested in their own treatment can be a pleasant and stimulating alternative to the less involved adolescents. If the expectations of both the doctor and the patient are realistic, comprehensive treatment for adults can be a rewarding experience for both.

■ Periodontal and Restorative Needs as Motivating Factors

Although comprehensive orthodontic treatment cannot preclude the possibility of periodontal disease developing later, it can be a useful part of the overall treatment plan for a patient who already has periodontal involvement (Fig. 20-5). It may be necessary, for instance, to align teeth and improve occlusal relationships after initial therapy has brought periodontal disease under control, to make definitive periodontal and restorative treatment possible. In a sense, this is adjunctive orthodontic treatment, but even if the major focus of treatment is the periodontal situation, when the orthodontic therapy involves changing the entire occlusal scheme it can be considered comprehensive. Not more than 10% of adult patients have comprehensive orthodontic treatment primarily because of periodontal problems, but periodontal considerations are important for all adults who undergo orthodontic treatment (see following).

■ Temporomandibular Joint Symptoms as a Reason for Orthodontic Treatment

Temporomandibular joint (TMJ) pain and dysfunction are rarely encountered in children seeking orthodontic treatment, but this condition is a significant motivating factor in approximately 15% of adults who consider orthodontic treatment. The relationship between dental occlusion and TMJ symptoms is highly controversial, and it is important to view this situation reasonably objectively. Orthodontic treatment can sometimes help patients with TMJ problems, but it cannot be relied on to correct them, and it is important for patients to understand what may happen to their symptoms during and after orthodontics.

Patients with TMJ symptoms can be divided into two large groups: those with internal joint pathology, including displacement or destruction of the intraarticular disc; and those with symptoms primarily of muscle origin, caused by spasm and fatigue of the muscles that position the jaw and head

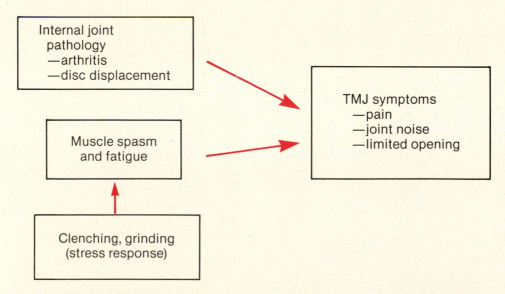

Fig. 20-6 ■ Temporomandibular joint symptoms arise from two major causes: internal joint pathology, and muscle spasm and fatigue. As a general guideline, patients with symptoms of muscle spasm and fatigue may be helped by orthodontic treatment, but orthodontics alone is rarely useful for patients with internal joint pathology.

(Fig. 20-6). The distinction in many patients is difficult diagnostically and is oversimplified in the sense that often other causes are possible and that muscle spasm and joint pathology can coexist. Nevertheless, the distinction is important when orthodontic treatment is considered. It is unlikely that orthodontic treatment alone will be of significant benefit to the patient who has internal joint problems or other nonmuscular sources of pain. Those who have myofascial pain, on the other hand, may benefit from improved occlusal relationships.

Most of us develop some symptoms of degenerative joint disease as we grow older, and it is not surprising that the jaw joints sometimes show internal degenerative changes (Fig. 20-7). Arthritic involvement of the temporomandibular joints is most likely to be the cause of TMJ symptoms in patients who have arthritic changes in other joints of the body. A component of muscle spasm and muscle pain should be suspected in individuals whose only symptoms are in the TMJ area, even if radiographs show moderate arthritic degeneration of the joint.

Displacement of the disc (Fig. 20-8) can arise from a number of causes. One possibility is trauma to the joint, so that the ligaments that oppose the action of the lateral pterygoid muscle are stretched or torn. In this circumstance, muscle contraction moves the disc forward as the mandibular condyles translate forward on wide opening, but the ligaments do not restore the disc to its proper position when the jaw is closed. The result is a click upon opening and closing, as the disc pops into place over the condylar head as the patient opens, but is displaced anteriorly on closure.

The click and symptoms associated with it can be corrected if an occlusal splint is used to prevent the patient from closing beyond the point at which displacement occurs. The resulting relief of pain influences patients and dentists to seek either restorative or orthodontic treatment to increase facial vertical dimension. However, orthodontic elongation of all posterior teeth to control disc displacement is not a treatment procedure that should be undertaken lightly. Often the patient whose symptoms have been controlled by a splint can tolerate its reduction or removal, without requiring major occlusal changes. As a general rule, there are better ways of handling disc displacement problems than orthodontic treatment.

Myofascial pain develops when muscles are overly fatigued and tend to go into spasm. It is all but impossible to overwork the jaw muscles to this extent during normal occlusal function. To produce myofascial pain, the patient must be clenching or grinding the teeth for many hours per day, presumably as a response to stress. Great variations are seen in the way different individuals respond to stress, both in the organ system that feels the strain (those who develop stomach ulcers rarely have TMJ symptoms also) and in the amount of stress that can be tolerated before symptoms appear (tense individuals develop stress-related

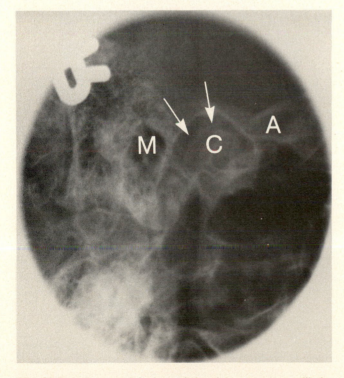

Fig. 20-7 ■ Transcranial view of the right temporomandibular joint in a patient with arthritis. Note the obvious destruction and remodeling of the head of the condyle. (Courtesy Dr. M. Tucker.)

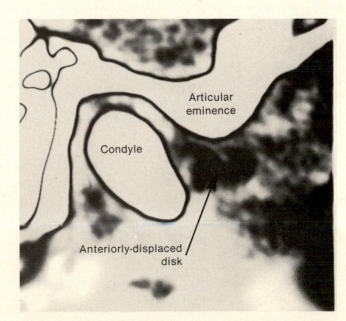

Fig. 20-8 ■ Computerized tomographic view of a displaced mandibular disc, which can be visualized clearly in front of the head of the condyle. Computerized tomography is rapidly becoming the preferred radiographic method for demonstration of disc position, replacing joint arthrography.

Table 20-1 ■ Periodontal problems as a function of age in patients with severe orthodontic problems

Age	No. of patients	% with pocketing >5 mm	% with inadequate attached gingiva	% with any mucogingival problem
Under 10	15	6	7	47
10-19	267	17	27	60
20-26	180	32	38	69
27-32	144	48	27	62
33-39	59	64	25	54
40 and over	35*	66	17	49

From Moriarty, J.D., and Simpson, D.M.: J. Dent. Res. **63**:IADR abstract 1249, 1984.
*Three had previous periodontal surgery.

symptoms before their relaxed colleagues do). For this reason, it is impossible to say that occlusal discrepancies of any given degree will lead to TMJ symptoms.

It is possible to demonstrate that some types of occlusal discrepancies predispose patients who clench or grind their teeth to the development of TMJ symptoms, and to construct a rational case for helping to control those problems by altering the occlusion.[3] It must be kept in mind, however, that it takes two factors to produce TMJ symptoms from myofascial pain: an occlusal discrepancy *and* a patient who clenches or grinds the teeth. The dictum "let your teeth alone" would solve myofasical pain problems if it could be followed by the patient.

From this perspective, it is apparent that three broad approaches to myofascial pain symptoms can be considered: reducing the amount of stress; reducing the patient's reaction to the stress; or improving the occlusal relationships, thereby making it harder for the patient to hurt himself or herself. Drastic alteration of the occlusion, by either restorative dental procedures or orthodontic treatment, is logical only if the less invasive stress-control and stress-adaptation approaches have failed. In that circumstance, orthodontic treatment to alter the occlusion, so that potentially damaging occlusal characteristics are eliminated, may be the treatment of choice.

■ *Periodontal Aspects of Adult Treatment*

Periodontal problems are rarely a major concern during orthodontic treatment of children and adolescents, both because periodontal disease usually does not arise at an early age and because tissue resistance to the irritation produced by orthodontic appliances is higher in younger patients. For the same reasons, periodontal considerations are increasingly important as patients become older, regardless of whether periodontal problems were a motivating factor for orthodontic treatment.

The prevalence of periodontal disease as a function of age in one group of potential orthodontic patients is shown in Table 20-1. These data are from individuals with severe

problems who were candidates for possible surgical and orthodontic correction of dentofacial deformity. Note that there is nearly a straight-line relationship between periodontal pocketing (defined here as the presence of pockets greater than 5 mm) and age. In contrast, the prevalence of mucogingival problems is maximal in the twenties.[4] The odds are that any patient over the age of 35 has some periodontal problems that could affect orthodontic treatment. There is no contraindication to treating adult patients who have periodontal disease, as long as the disease has been brought under control, but the periodontal situation must

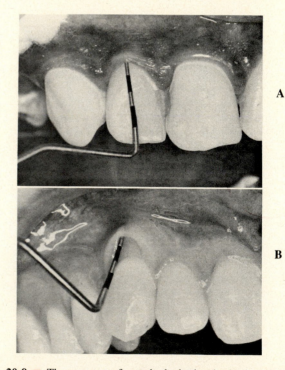

Fig. 20-9 ■ The amount of attached gingiva is the keratinized tissue between the depth of periodontal probing and the beginning of alveolar mucosa. **A,** In this young and healthy patient, 2-3 mm of attached gingiva are apparent; **B,** in this older patient with gingival recession over the canine, the probe penetrates to the mucosal margin, indicating essentially no attached tissue.

receive major attention in planning and executing orthodontic treatment for all adults.

■ Minimal Periodontal Involvement

In adults with no other periodontal problems, the factor most likely to be significant in planning orthodontic treatment is the condition of the attached gingiva. Wherever the amount of attached gingiva is inadequate, there is a risk that the soft tissue attachment will strip away from the tooth. Orthodontic treatment accentuates this tendency, particularly when irregular teeth are aligned by expanding the dental arch.

There is a difference, of course, between the amount of keratinized gingiva and the amount of attached gingiva. The distinction can be made most readily by inserting a periodontal probe and observing the distance between the point at which the gingival attachment is encountered and the point at which the alveolar mucosa begins (Fig. 20-9). A minimal area of attached gingiva, which might be adequate in the absence of orthodontic treatment, can be inadequate to withstand the stresses of labial or buccal tooth movement. It is much better to prevent stripping of tissue before orthodontic treatment than to correct it later. A gingival graft to create additional attachment must be considered in many patients (Fig. 20-10), particularly those for whom moderate arch expansion will be used to align incisors and those who

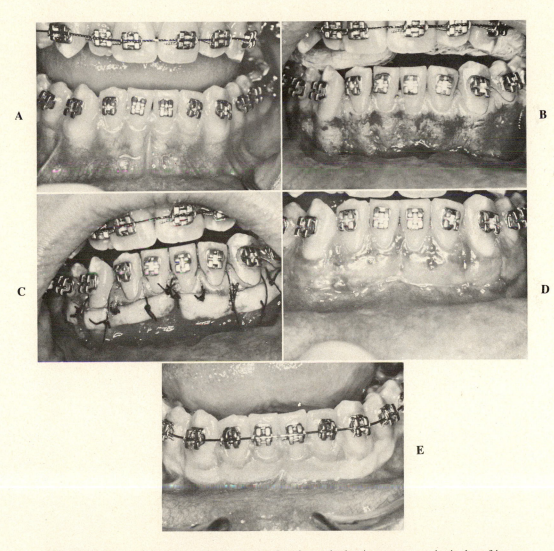

Fig. 20-10 ■ In adults who will have comprehensive orthodontic treatment, gingival grafting to create adequate attached gingiva before beginning orthodontic tooth movement is important. **A,** Lack of attached gingiva in the mandibular anterior region in a patient whose lower incisors must be advanced to align them. Note the alveolar mucosa extending almost to the gingival margin on all anterior teeth; **B,** surgical preparation of a bed for grafting; **C,** grafts sutured in place; **D,** healing 10 days later, showing incorporation of the grafts; **E,** orthodontic alignment nearly completed 5 months later, with the gingival grafts creating a generous band of attached tissue. (Courtesy Dr. J. Moriarty.)

will have surgical mandibular advancement or genioplasty (see Chapter 21).

Any patient undergoing orthodontic treatment must take extra care to clean the teeth, but this is even more important for adults. Orthodontic appliances simultaneously make maintenance of oral hygiene more difficult and more important. In children and adolescents, even if gingivitis develops in response to the presence of orthodontic appliances, it almost never extends into periodontitis. This cannot be taken for granted in adults, no matter how good their initial periodontal condition.

The difficult area for orthodontic patients to clean is the area of each tooth between the brackets and the gingival margin, and because of the greater length of the clinical crown in adults, it is at least easier for adult patients to approach these areas. Hygiene aids such as rubber interdental stimulators and proximal brushes to reach between teeth are often needed.

■ Moderate Periodontal Involvement

Before orthodontic treatment is attempted for patients who have moderate preexisting periodontal problems, it is important that dental and periodontal disease be brought under control. Unless a patient can maintain periodontal health after initial therapy, orthodontic treatment is potentially damaging rather than beneficial. A period of observation following the preliminary treatment, to make sure that the patient is adequately controlled, should precede comprehensive orthodontics.

Preliminary periodontal therapy can include all aspects of periodontal treatment except osseous surgery. It is important to remove all calculus and other irritants from periodontal pockets before any tooth movement is attempted, and it is often wise to use surgical flaps to expose these areas to ensure the best possible scaling. Treatment procedures to facilitate the patient's long-term maintenance, like osseous recontouring, are best deferred until the final occlusal relationships have been established.

Disease control also requires that any pulpally involved teeth be treated endodontically, and that immediate restorative needs should be met. There is no contraindication to the orthodontic movement of an endodontically treated tooth, so root canal therapy before orthodontics will cause no problems (Fig. 20-11). Movement of a pulpally involved tooth is likely to cause a flareup of the periapical condition.

The general guideline for preliminary restorative treatment is that temporary restorations should be placed to control caries, with the definitive restorative dentistry delayed until after the orthodontic phase of treatment. Temporary restoration, however, often implies the use of a cement that will last only a few months, and short-lived temporaries of this type are incompatible with orthodontic treatment. Amal-

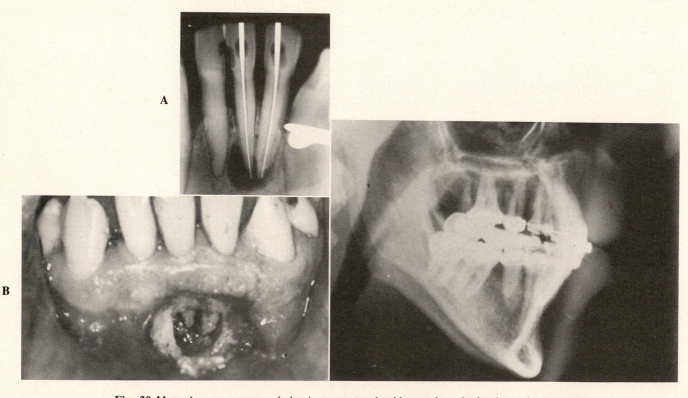

Fig. 20-11 ■ Any necessary endodontic treatment should precede orthodontic tooth movement. **A,** Periapical lesion around two nonvital mandibular incisors; **B,** apicoectomy and retrograde amalgam seal in connection with endodontic treatment of these teeth; **C,** cephalometric radiograph during orthodontic treatment, with the apical amalgam on the lower incisors clearly visible. In this patient, the lower incisors were successfully intruded despite the previous endodontic treatment.

gam is the preferred temporary restorative material while orthodontics is being carried out. Cast restorations should be delayed until after the final occlusal relationships have been established by orthodontic treatment.

During comprehensive orthodontic treatment, a patient with moderate periodontal problems must be on a periodontal maintenance schedule, with the frequency of cleaning and scaling depending on the severity of the periodontal disease. For a typical patient with moderate involvement, periodontal maintenance therapy at 2- to 4-month intervals is the usual plan.

■ Severe Periodontal Involvement

The general approach to treatment for patients with severe periodontal involvement is the same as that outlined earlier, but the treatment itself must be modified in two ways. (1) Periodontal maintenance should be scheduled at more frequent intervals, with the patient being seen as frequently for periodontal maintenance as for orthodontic appliance adjustments in many instances, i.e., every 3 or 4 weeks. (2) Orthodontic treatment goals and mechanics must be modified to keep orthodontic forces to an absolute minimum, because of the reduced area of the periodontal ligament after significant bone loss. Modifications in treatment mechanics for these patients are discussed in more detail following.

■ *Orthodontic Appliance Therapy*

Both the goals and the stages of comprehensive orthodontic treatment for adults are the same as those in the treatment of adolescents (see Chapters 15 to 18). The orthodontic mechanotherapy, however, must often be modified. Because of the lack of growth, particularly the small amounts of vertical growth that allow some extrusion of the posterior teeth in adolescents without leading to mandibular rotation, segmented arch mechanics for intrusion are often required. If the patient has lost some periodontal support,

it is especially important to keep forces light. Orthodontic space closure may be contraindicated if teeth have been lost because of periodontal disease, and previous treatment of TMJ problems can be a factor in later orthodontic treatment.

For orthodontic patients with jaw discrepancies, there are always three broad categories of possible treatment: (1) correction through growth; (2) correction through orthodontic camouflage, i.e., bringing the teeth into proper occlusion without correcting the jaw discrepancy; and (3) surgical correction of the jaw discrepancy. In adults, because the first option is no longer available, an important treatment planning criterion is the extent to which a jaw discrepancy can be camouflaged successfully rather than requiring surgical correction (see Chapters 6 and 21). In the following discussion, it is assumed that an appropriate and feasible treatment plan has been prepared.

■ Segmented Arch Procedures for Intrusion

Growth is important in normal orthodontic treatment even for patients who have Class I problems and excellent jaw relationships, because most mechanotherapy has an extrusive component and tends to elongate the teeth (see Fig. 20-1). In young patients, the choice between intrusion or extrusion to correct a deep overbite and level an excessive curve of Spee can often be resolved in favor of extrusion, because vertical growth will compensate for it. In adults, the choice must often be intrusion, which can be achieved only by segmented arch mechanics. The practical effect is to make segmented arch treatment more important in adults than it is in younger patients.

The principles of segmented arch treatment have been discussed in Chapter 10, and more specific indications for leveling and space closure are presented in Chapters 15 and 16. The basic idea in segmented arch treatment is to create a stable anchor unit, consisting of several teeth rigidly connected to create the functional equivalent of a single large multirooted anchor tooth, and to use this anchorage to provide precisely controlled force against the teeth whose

Fig. 20-12 ■ Segmented arch treatment for intrusion of the maxillary incisors. **A,** Maxillary transpalatal arch for anchorage control, which is essential with intrusion mechanics; **B,** buccal view showing the maxillary intrusion arch with stabilized segments. Note that the intrusion arch is tied between the lateral incisors and canines, moving the point of force application nearer the center of resistance of the anterior segment to prevent labial tipping during the intrusion.

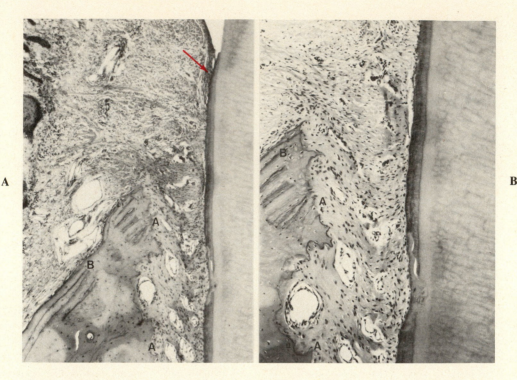

Fig. 20-13 ■ **A,** Histologic preparation from a dog's lower first premolar that was extruded and slightly tipped buccally for 12 weeks, then intruded for 16 weeks, and finally had 3 days without orthodontic force immediately before sacrifice. Oral hygiene was maintained during the treatment. **A,** Tight epithelial cuff is seen where epithelium penetrates apically in consequence of the intrusion. **B,** Higher magnification view of the alveolar crest area. Note the formation of new bone **(B)** on the alveolar crest, which occurred during extrusion, and resorption of bone from intrusion only on the periodontal ligament side of the alveolar crest **(A)**, without loss of alveolar crest height. (Courtesy Dr. B. Melsen.)

movement is desired (Fig. 20-12). In addition to its use for intrusion, the segmented arch approach can also be helpful in controlling the magnitude of force in space closure. This is even more important in periodontally involved patients than in those with an intact periodontium, because the periodontal ligament area over which the force is distributed is smaller.

One potential problem with intrusive tooth movement in periodontally involved adults is the prospect that a deepening of periodontal pockets might be produced by this treatment. Ideally, of course, intruding a tooth would lead to a reattachment of the periodontal fibers, but there is no basis for expecting true reattachment in response to orthodontic treatment. What seems to happen instead is the formation of a tight epithelial cuff, so that the position of the gingiva relative to the crown improves clinically, while periodontal probing depths do not increase. Histologic slides from experimental animals show a relative invagination of the epithelium, but with a tight area of contact that cannot be probed (Fig. 20-13). It can be argued that this leaves the patient at risk for rapid periodontal breakdown if inflammation is allowed to recur. Certainly intrusion should never be attempted without excellent control of inflammation. On the other hand, if good hygiene is maintained, clinical experience has shown that it is possible to maintain

teeth that have been treated in this way, and both dental esthetics and function improve after the intrusion.

The mechanotherapy needed to produce intrusion in an adult is not different from the methods for younger patients described in Chapter 15. Burstone-type depressing arches (see Fig. 20-12) or (less commonly) Ricketts utility arches, both using a long span from the stabilized posterior sgments to the anterior area where intrusion is desired, are normally selected for adults. The use of extremely light forces is very important, since excessive force will lead to posterior extrusion rather than the desired anterior intrusion. The point at which the intrusion arch attaches to the anterior segment is important, because it influences the extent to which the anterior segment tips buccally or lingually, as intrusion occurs (see Chapter 15).

■ **Space Closure**

In contrast to leveling of vertical arch discrepancies, continuous arch treatment can be used with adults to correct anteroposterior discrepancies, but segmented arch treatment does have special advantages. The same comments apply to space closure in adults as to adolescents (see Chapter 16), with two exceptions:

1. It is unrealistic to expect an adult to wear a headgear on the nearly continuous basis necessary to produce efficient

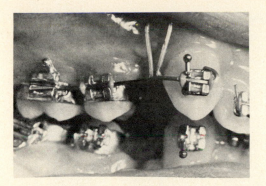

Fig. 20-14 ■ Segmental closing loop in .019 × .025 TMA wire, for initial retraction of the canine in a patient being treated with first premolar extraction. Retracting the canines separately without friction can be particularly advantageous in adults with reduced periodontal support, because it allows the application of minimal and precisely controlled forces.

tooth movement, so direct extraoral force to slide teeth along an archwire during closure of extraction spaces is impractical. For the same reason, headgear to control anchorage is probably less reliable than it might be in a younger patient and other methods of anchorage control must be sought. The most effective of these is the creation of posterior stabilizing segments with lingual arches and buccal stabilizing wires, the same setup needed for leveling by intrusion. In addition, it is often wise to use segmental closing loops for retraction of the canines as a first stage in space closure (Fig. 20-14), followed by a second stage of retraction of the incisors, to minimize the strain on posterior anchorage

and keep forces as light as possible. This approach has inherent problems in vertical control of the canines (see Chapter 16), and therefore it is important to see the patient on a regular schedule for close supervision. Fortunately, compliance with appointments is less likely to be a problem with adults than with many adolescents.

2. Old extraction sites in adults pose a mechanical and biologic challenge in orthodontic treatment. In a young patient, any extraction site is recent and can usually be closed without any particular problems. In an adult, closure of an extraction site many years after the tooth is lost is neither straightforward nor predictable. It may be good judgment not to attempt space closure, but rather to plan for prosthetic replacement of the missing tooth.

The problem in closing an old extraction site arises because of resorption and remodeling of alveolar bone. After several years, resorption results in a decrease in the vertical height of the bone, but more importantly, remodeling produces a buccolingual narrowing of the alveolar process as well (see Fig. 19-8). When this has happened, closing the extraction space requires a reshaping of the cortical bone that comprises the buccal and lingual plates of the alveolar process. Cortical bone will respond to orthodontic force in most instances, but the response is significantly slower. Typically, an old extraction site can be closed part way, but it is difficult to close it completely and keep it closed.[5] It is also difficult to close a space of this type by differential forward movement of the posterior teeth or backward movement of the anterior teeth, no matter what the apparent anchorage situation is (Fig. 20-15). The involvement of cortical bone tends to produce a reciprocal space closure,

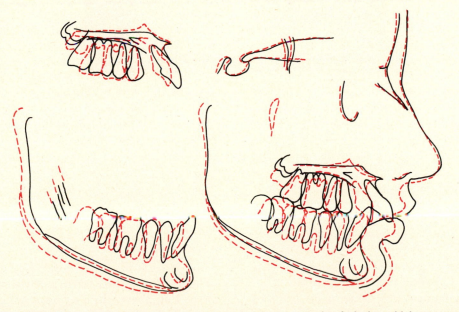

Fig. 20-15 ■ Cephalometric superimpositions showing the result of closing old lower second premolar extraction sites in an adolescent. Despite the use of Class II elastics and space closing techniques designed to slip the lower molars forward, reciprocal space closure resulted. This effect is often observed in the closure of old extraction sites and probably arises because of the narrowed buccal and lingual cortical plates.

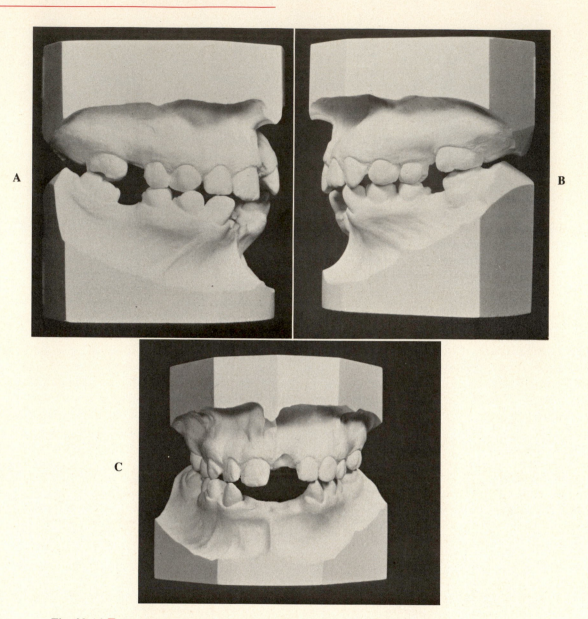

Fig. 20-16 ■ Pretreatment records of a girl with juvenile periodontitis. **A,** to **C,** Dental casts after the periodontitis had been brought under control, which required extraction of all first molars, the mandibular incisors, and one maxillary incisor; **D,** periapical radiographs at the time of initial periodontal treatment; **E,** periapical radiographs at the beginning of orthodontic treatment.

which means that anterior teeth may be retracted more than anticipated in the closure of an old extraction site.

A space closure problem is also posed by the loss of a tooth to periodontal disease. As a general rule, it is unwise to move a tooth into an area where bone has been destroyed by periodontal disease, because of the risk that normal bone formation will not occur as the tooth moves into the defect. It is better to move teeth away from such an area, in preparation for prosthetic replacement.

However, there is an exception. First molars and incisors are lost in some adolescents to juvenile periodontitis, which differentially attacks these teeth and has a characteristic and unique bacterial flora. Once the disease process has been brought under control, the causative agent seems to disappear. Although bone around the first molars is often totally destroyed, neither the second molar nor the second premolar is significantly affected in most patients (Fig. 20-16). Orthodontic closure of the incisor spaces is rarely feasible, but

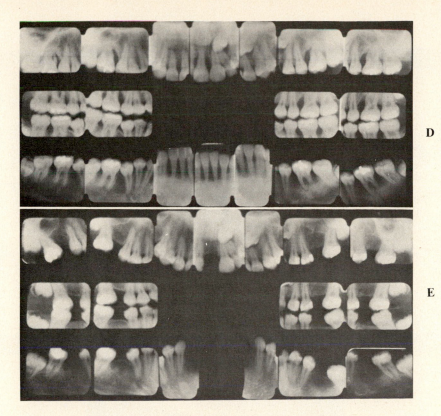

Fig. 20-16, cont'd ■ For legend see opposite page.

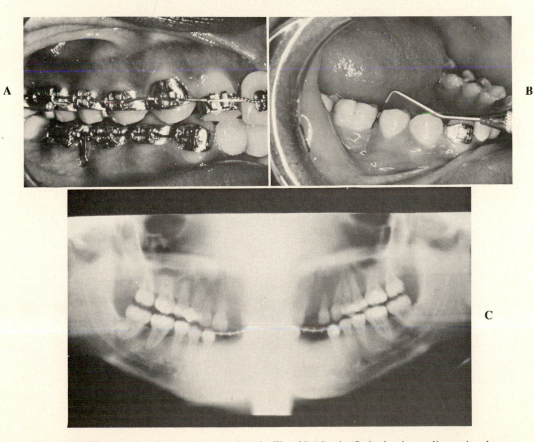

Fig. 20-17 ■ Orthodontic treatment (patient in Fig. 20-16). **A,** Orthodontic appliance in place, showing closure of the first molar extraction space. Note that a replacement maxillary central incisor is tied to the archwire, while replacement mandibular incisors are attached to a heavy lingual wire from canine to canine; **B,** at the completion of space closure, pocket depths are normal at the first molar extraction site; **C,** panoramic radiograph at the completion of orthodontic treatment.

Continued.

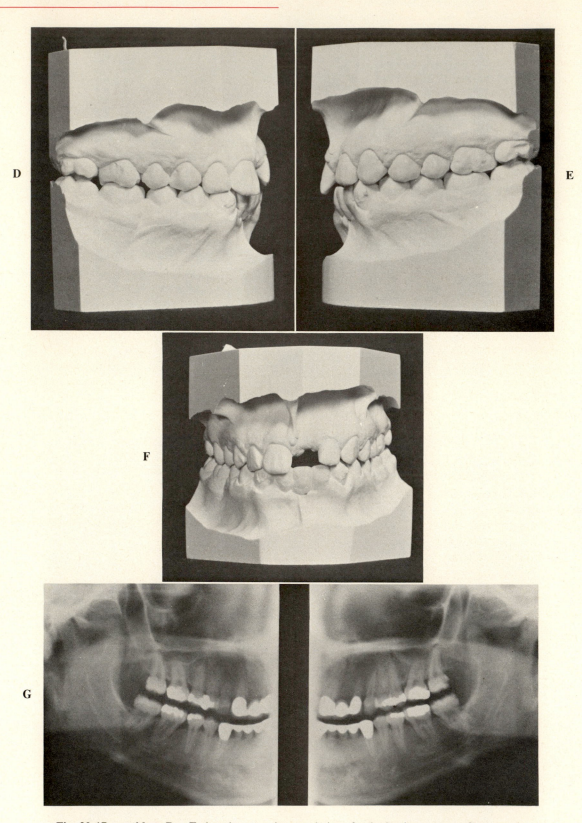

Fig. 20-17, cont'd ■ **D** to **F,** dental casts at the completion of orthodontic treatment; **G,** panoramic radiograph on 4-year recall.

in these adolescent or young adult patients, it is often possible to orthodontically close the first molar extraction sites,[6] bringing the second permanent molar forward into the area where the first molar was lost (Fig. 20-17). The second molar brings its own investing bone with it, and the large bony defect disappears.

This favorable response is attributed to some combination of three factors: the relatively young age of the juvenile periodontitis patients, the fact that the original attack was almost entirely on the first molars, and the disappearance of the specific bacterial flora. In an older patient who has lost a first molar to periodontal disease, it is unlikely that the other teeth have been totally spared or that the bacterial flora have changed, and it would not be good judgment to attempt to close the space.

■ Finishing and Retention Procedures

Orthodontic finishing with archwires does not differ significantly in adults from the finishing procedures for younger patients, except for those who have had a combination of surgical and orthodontic treatment. This special circumstance is discussed in Chapter 21. Positioners are indicated less often as finishing devices for older patients, however. Without any vertical growth to compensate for slight vertical repositioning of the teeth, a positioner can contribute to rotational repositioning of the mandible. This problem can be overcome by fabricating the positioner from casts mounted with an accurate hinge axis mounting. Even with this technique, it is unwise to use a positioner for finishing in a patient with moderate to severe periodontal bone loss. These patients should be brought to their final orthodontic relationship with archwires, and then stabilized with immediately placed retainers before eventual detailing of occlusal relationships by equilibration.

Part of the purpose of a traditional orthodontic retainer is to allow each tooth to move during function, independently of its neighbors, to produce a restoration of the normal periodontal architecture. This clearly does not apply to patients who have had a significant degree of periodontal bone loss and who have mobile teeth. In these patients, splinting of the teeth is necessary both short- and long-term. A rigid removable splint often serves as the best short-term retainer. This can be either an occlusal wafer, providing a positive indexing of the teeth and extending buccally and lingually to maintain tooth position (Fig. 20-18), or a wrap-around retainer as illustrated in Chapter 18. Long-term splinting usually involves cast restorations.

■ Special Treatment Considerations in Patients with Temporomandibular Joint Syndrome

The extent to which temporomandibular joint symptoms in many adults diminish and disappear when comprehensive orthodontic treatment begins, can be surprising and overly gratifying to those who do not understand the etiology of myofascial pain. Orthodontic intervention can appear almost magical in the way that TMJ symptoms disappear long before the occlusal relationships have been corrected. The explanation is simple—orthodontic treatment makes the teeth sore, and grinding or clenching sensitive teeth as a means of handling stress does not produce the same subconscious gratification as previously. The changing occlusal relationships also contribute to breaking up the habit patterns

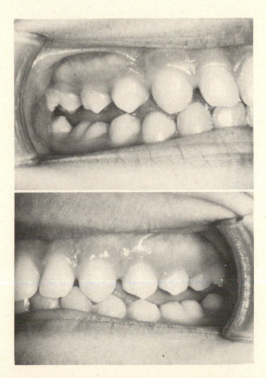

Fig. 20-19 ■ Occlusal relationships in a 16-year-old girl who had worn a splint covering only the posterior teeth for the previous 8 months. The posterior open bite is created, not by intrusion of the posterior teeth, but by further eruption of the anteriors. Discarding the splint had become impossible.

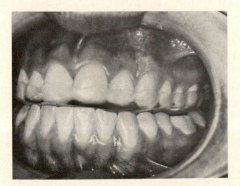

Fig. 20-18 ■ An occlusal splint, of the same type often used for initial treatment of patients with TMJ problems, can serve as an orthodontic retainer for one arch for patients with periodontal involvement. These individuals require permanent retention, so the usual orthodontic retention procedures based on gradual withdrawal of the retainer do not apply. A rigid retainer is needed immediately upon the removal of the orthodontic appliance.

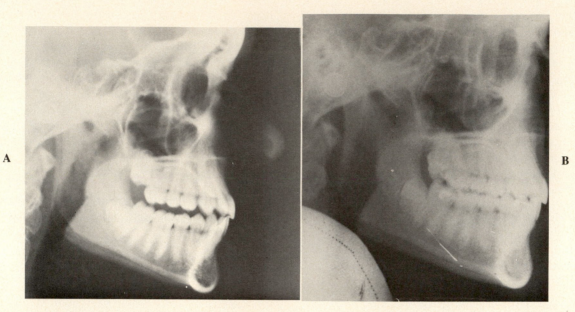

Fig. 20-20 ■ Cephalometric films for the patient shown in Fig. 20-19, **A,** before, and **B,** after orthodontic treatment to extrude the posterior teeth back into occlusion.

that contributed to the muscle fatigue and pain. No matter what the type of orthodontic treatment, symptoms are unlikely to be present while movement of a significant number of teeth is occurring, as long as treatment that produces strongly deflective contracts is avoided. Prolonged use of Class II or III elastics should be avoided in adults who have had TMJ problems (and for that matter, in most other patients as well).

The moment of truth for TMJ symptoms comes some time after orthodontic treatment is completed, when the clenching and grinding that originally caused the problem tend to recur. At that point, even if the occlusal relationships have been significantly improved, it may be impossible to keep the patient from moving into extreme jaw positions and engaging in parafunctional activity that produces pain. The use of interocclusal splints in this situation may be the only way to keep symptoms from recurring. In short, the miraculous cure that orthodontic treatment often provides for myofascial pain tends to disappear with the appliance. Those who have had TMJ symptoms in the past are always at risk of having them recur.

Occasionally, orthodontic treatment is made more complicated by previous splint therapy for TMJ problems. If an occlusal splint for TMJ symptoms covers the posterior but not the anterior teeth, the anterior teeth that have been taken out of occlusion begin to erupt again and may come back into occlusion even though the posterior teeth are still separated (Fig. 20-19). Clinically, it may appear that the posterior teeth are being intruded, but rarely if ever occurs. Significant incisor eruption can occur in only a few months, and the patient may end up in a situation in which discarding the splint has become impossible. The only treatment possibilities are elongation of the posterior teeth, either prosthetically or orthodontically, or intrusion of the anterior teeth orthodontically.

Orthodontic intervention at this stage is difficult, because TMJ symptoms are likely to develop immediately if the splint is removed, and it is not possible to elongate the posterior teeth orthodontically without discarding or cutting down the splint. Placing orthodontic attachments on the posterior teeth and using light vertical elastics to the posterior segments (Fig. 20-20) can be used to bring the posterior teeth back into occlusion, if the patient can tolerate this treatment. Some reintrusion of the elongated anterior teeth is likely to occur, but a significant increase in face height is often maintained. Permanently increasing the vertical dimension to control disc displacement can be accomplished in this way, but this treatment plan should be used with extreme caution.

■ References

1. Gottlieb, E.L., and Vogel, D.S.: 1983 JCO Orthodontic practice survey. J. Clin. Orthod. **18:**167-173, 1984.
2. Kiyak, H.A., Hohl, T., West, R.A., et al.: The psychological impact of orthognathic surgery. Am. J. Orthod. **81:**404-412, 1982.
3. Sadowsky, C., and Polson, A.M.: Temporomandibular disorders and functional occlusion after orthodontic treatment: results of two long-term studies. Am. J. Orthod. **86:**386-390, 1984.
4. Moriarty, J.D., and Simpson, D.M.: Incidence of periodontal problems to patients with dentofacial deformities. J. Dent. Res. **63:**IADR abstract 1249, 1984.
5. Hom, B.M., and Turley, P.K.: The effects of space closure of the mandibular first molar area in adults. Am. J. Orthod. **85:**457-469, 1984.
6. McLain, J.B., Proffit, W.R., and Davenport, R.H.: Adjunctive orthodontic therapy in the treatment of juvenile periodontitis. Am. J. Orthod. **83:**290-298, 1983.

Combined Surgical and Orthodontic Treatment

For patients whose orthodontic problems are so severe that neither growth modification nor camouflage offers a solution, surgical realignment of the jaws or repositioning of dentoalveolar segments is the only possible treatment. Surgery is not a substitute for orthodontics in these patients. Instead, it must be properly coordinated with orthodontics and other dental treatment to achieve good overall results. Dramatic progress in the past decade has made it possible for combined treatment to correct many severe problems that simply were untreatable only a few years ago.

Surgical treatment for mandibular prognathism began early in the twentieth century. Edward Angle, commenting on a patient who had treatment of this type, described how the result could have been improved if orthodontic appliances and occlusal splints had been used.[1] Although there was gradual progress in techniques for setting back a prominent mandible throughout the first half of this century, Trauner and Obwegeser's introduction of the sagittal split ramus osteotomy in 1959 marked the beginning of a new era in orthognathic surgery.[2] This technique used an intraoral ap-

proach, which avoided the necessity of a potentially disfiguring skin incision. The sagittal split design also offered a biologically sound method for lengthening or shortening the lower law with the same bone cuts, thus allowing treatment of mandibular deficiency or excess (Fig. 21-1). During the 1960s, American surgeons began to use and modify techniques for maxillary surgery that had been developed in Europe,[3,4] and a decade of rapid progress in maxillary surgery culminated in the development by Bell, Epker, and associates of the LeFort I downfracture technique that allowed repositioning of the maxilla in all three planes of space (Fig. 21-2).[5,6] With this came the realization that skeletal open bite, a historically difficult problem for surgeons and orthodontists, could be successfully treated by maxillary impaction, sometimes coupled with mandibular surgery.

By the 1980s, progress in oral and maxillofacial surgery made it possible to reposition either or both jaws, to move the chin in all three planes of space, and to reposition dentoalveolar segments surgically as desired. Combined orthodontic-surgical treatment can now be planned for patients with a severe dentofacial problem of any type. This is an incredible contrast to the situation not long ago, when the only surgical treatment was for mandibular prognathism.

■ Types of Orthodontic-Surgical Treatment

To review the changes that can be achieved by contemporary surgical techniques, it is helpful to consider how the jaws can be repositioned in three planes of space.

■ Problems in Transverse Relationships

It is possible to move the maxillary segments both away from and toward the midline with relative ease and stability (Fig. 21-3). The same movements, however, are more difficult to perform in the mandible because of the temporomandibular joint articulation and problems with soft tissue management. The mandible can be narrowed anteriorly, but for all practical purposes, it cannot be widened.

Maxilla. Maxillary constriction or expansion can be easily accomplished in the course of LeFort I downfracture surgery. Parasagittal osteotomies in the lateral floor of the

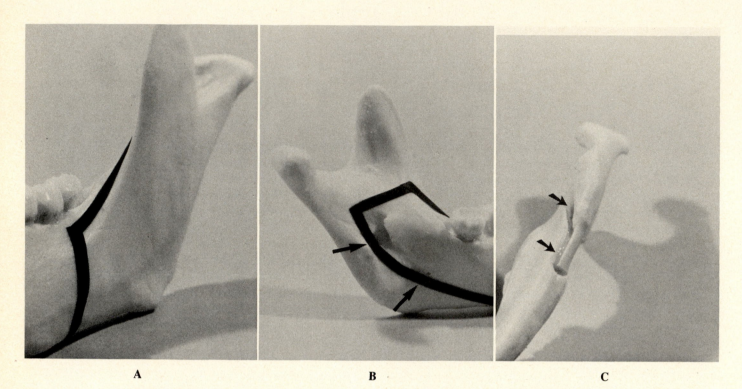

A   B   C

Fig. 21-1 ■ **A,** The black lines on this model of the mandible as viewed from the lateral aspect indicate the path of osteotomy cuts for the sagittal splitting technique. The vertical cut is placed distal to the second molar and extended posteriorly along the superior and anterior aspect of the ascending ramus. **B,** The horizontal extension of this cut is seen on this medial view of the mandible. This cut is placed midway between the entrance of the inferior alveolar nerve and the depth of the sigmoid notch. In the modified technique diagrammed here, the posterior aspect of this cut extends just beyond the foramen. The inferior and posterior portion of the osteotomy *(arrows)* is not actually cut by instrumentation but occurs along natural cleavage lines during the splitting technique. **C,** This photograph shows the inferior border and a portion of the medial aspect of a model of the mandible that has actually been sectioned. The area splitting along natural cleavage lines is indicated by arrows and connects the lateral and medial cuts.

nose or medial floor of the sinus are connected anteriorly by a transverse cut, with an extension being made between the central incisors (Fig. 21-4). If constriction is desired, bone is removed with the parasagittal osteotomies according to presurgical planning. In expansion, either bone harvested in the downfracture or bank bone is used to fill the void created by lateral movement of the posterior segments.

The parasagittal design has several advantages over a single midline approach. The osteotomies are placed through an area of the palate where the soft tissue is thicker and glandular in nature. The loose underlying connective tissue is more compliant than midline palatal mucosa and produces less relapse tendency. Spreading the amount of

movement over two cuts further decreases the tissue adaptation necessary. Clinical experience has shown that the blood supply to the three segments can be maintained with careful attention to detail, and this procedure affords extraordinary flexibility in movement.

Rapid palatal expansion of the type used in adolescents is not stable in adults because of the increasing resistance of the midpalatal and lateral maxillary sutures. Surgically assisted palatal expansion, using bone cuts to reduce the resistance without totally freeing the maxillary segments, is another possible treatment approach for the adult patient with skeletal maxillary constriction. A midpalatal corticotomy can recreate the suture, which is then opened with an

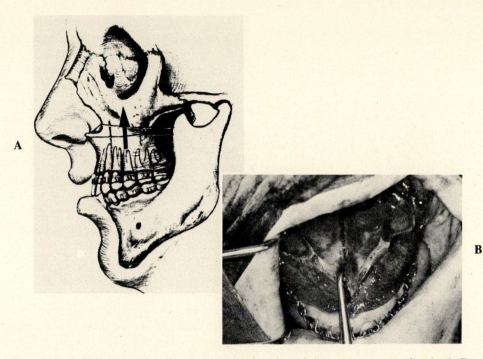

Fig. 21-2 ■ This illustration demonstrates the location of the osteotomy cuts for the LeFort I downfracture technique. In patients whose mandible is normal in size, the retrognathic appearance results from downward and backward rotation of the chin. **A,** Superior repositioning of the maxilla as indicated by the arrow allows the mandible to rotate upward and forward, hinging at the temporomandibular joint, which simultaneously shortens facial height and provides more chin prominence. **B,** This intraoperative photograph shows the maxilla in its downfractured position. The osteotomy locations are exposed through an intraoral incision in the vestibule and by careful elevation of the mucosa lining the nose. The nasal and antral floors are seen in this illustration. (**A** and **B** from Bell, W.H., Proffit, W.R., and White, R.P.: Surgical Correction of Dentofacial Deformity. Philadelphia, 1980, W.B. Saunders Co.)

expansion device; however, this approach violates sound surgical principles. Since the incision must heal over a void, dehiscence and development of an oronasal fistula may occur. Corticotomies of the lateral antral wall also reduce resistance enough for jackscrew expansion,[7] but this approach involves more morbidity and requires deep sedation or general anesthesia.

In either case, maxillary separation is still impaired by articulation at the nasal septum, vomer, medial nasal walls, and pterygomaxillary suture. There are few indications for surgically assisted expansion of either type.

Constriction of the maxilla without some coexisting vertical or sagittal problem rarely occurs. If downfracture surgery is indicated for correction of other problems, the transverse dimension can be addressed easily, accurately, and efficiently at that time. It would be particularly inefficient to plan surgically assisted expansion in a patient who would require another operation later to reposition the maxilla in the anteroposterior or vertical planes of space.

Mandible. The range of expansion or constriction possible in the mandible is more limited. Movements in the posterior region are limited by the architecture of the glenoid fossa. Expansion anteriorly is limited by the necessity to cover the defect with soft tissue. Although regional flaps could be used, these are rarely indicated except in secondary reconstructive surgery. Constriction by a body osteotomy is possible anteriorly, but removal of teeth is necessary unless adequate interdental spacing exists. Improved techniques and instrumentation have made surgical repositioning of the dentoalveolar process possible but only to the limit allowed by the underlying bone support.

■ Problems in Anteroposterior Relationships

Both the maxilla and mandible can be moved forward or backward (Fig. 21-5). The mandible can be moved anteriorly or posteriorly in the sagittal plane with relative ease. Extreme advancement may create stability problems associated with neuromuscular adaptation and stretch of the investing soft tissues. The maxilla can be moved forward if bone grafts are interposed posteriorly to help stabilize the new position. Posterior movement of the entire maxilla is not easily achieved because other skeletal components that normally support

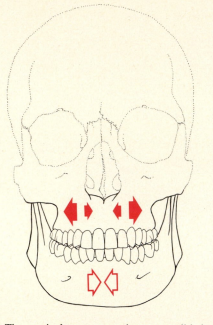

Fig. 21-3 ■ The surgical movements that are possible in the transverse dimension are shown on this posteroanterior illustration of the skull. The solid red arrows indicate that the maxilla can be expanded laterally or constricted with reasonable stability. The smaller size of the arrows pointing to the midline represents the fact that the amount of constriction possible is somewhat less than the range of expansion. The only transverse movement easily achieved in the mandible is constriction, and this is limited to the chin area.

the maxilla interfere with moving it back. As shown in Fig. 21-5, however, this difficulty is overcome by segmenting the maxilla so that only the anterior portion is retracted.

Maxillary surgery. Considerable maxillary advancement is possible with the downfracture technique, with the limiting factors being the vascular pedicle and soft tissue compliance. A graft in the retromolar area or at a step created in the lateral wall is usually required. Various materials, including autogenous and freeze-dried bone and alloplastic substances, can be used.

Maxillary retraction is limited by the anatomic structures immediately distal to the pterygomaxillary fissure. Although some movement can be accomplished by removal of bone in the tuberosity area, access is difficult and close to areas of increased vascularity. More commonly, retraction of the anterior segment is achieved by removal of a premolar, segmentation, and movement of the anterior segment into the space created (Fig. 21-5). Rarely does this technique fail to provide adequate room for the correction needed.

Mandibular advancement. Several techniques can advance the mandible. The inverted L osteotomy can be accomplished intraorally but has never been widely popular. Stabilization is difficult without a graft since the bony interface is limited (Fig. 21-6, *A*).

The C osteotomy and its variants are most frequently performed extraorally (Fig. 21-6, *B*). If significant advancement is planned, grafting is suggested to help stability and prevent the formation of a "window" defect in the void created by the advancement. Today this approach is gen-

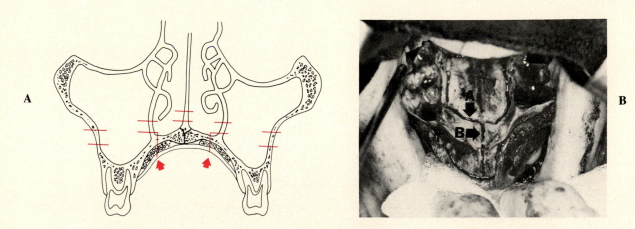

A   B

Fig. 21-4 ■ **A,** The osteotomy cuts necessary to surgically reposition the maxilla using the LeFort I downfracture approach are indicated in red. The arrows point to the vertical cuts that are placed immediately medial or lateral to the nasal wall to allow changes in transverse dimensions. The vertical cuts are placed in this location because there is more loose connective tissue underlying the mucosa in this area than at the midpalatal suture. This technique allows repositioning with less soft tissue tension than would be experienced if a midline approach were used. **B,** This photograph is the surgeon's view of a downfractured maxilla in which the osteotomy cuts for parasagittal expansion have been completed. The anterior-posterior cuts in the lateral nasal floor are connected by transverse osteotomy *(arrow A)*. An extension *(arrow B)* passes between the roots of the central incisors and completes the separation of the maxillary halves.

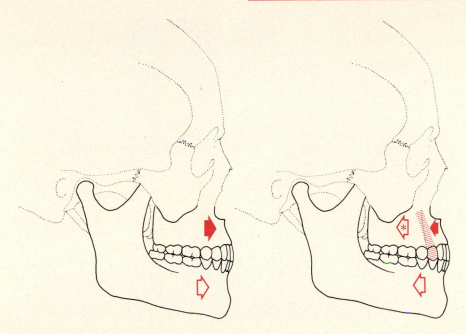

Fig. 21-5 ■ The maxilla and mandible can be moved anteriorly and posteriorly as indicated by the red arrows in these line drawings. Anterior movements of the mandible greater than 10 to 12 mm create considerable tension in the investing soft tissues and tend to be unstable. Posterior movement of the entire maxilla, though possible, is difficult and usually unnecessary. Instead, posterior movement of protruding incisors up to the width of a premolar is accomplished by removal of a premolar tooth on each side *(cross-hatched area)*, followed by segmentation of the maxilla. Although the maxilla can be advanced more than it can be retracted, the possibility of relapse or speech alteration from nasopharyngeal incompetence increases with larger movements.

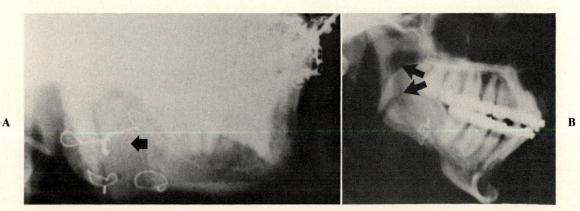

A   B

Fig. 21-6 ■ **A,** This lateral oblique radiograph demonstrates mandibular advancement by an inverted L osteotomy. The interpositional bone graft is indicated by the arrow. Contact of the distal and proximal segments can be maintained only at the superior osteotomy site with this design. **B,** Mandibular advancement using the C osteotomy is shown on this lateral cephalometric film. The proximal and distal segments remain in contact at both the superior and inferior osteotomy cuts, an advantage in providing stability. The arrow indicates the "window defect."

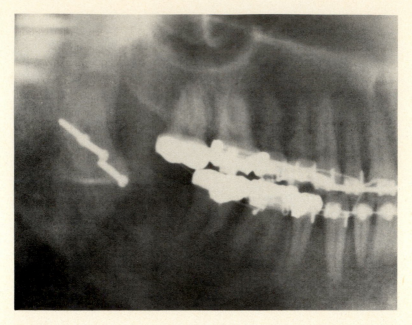

Fig. 21-7 ■ Osteosynthesis screws placed transorally are seen at the superior border of this sagittal split osteotomy site. The excellent stability provided by this rigid fixation system permits jaw mobilization soon after surgery and allows the resumption of a normal diet as well as orthodontic finishing.

erally reserved for patients in whom an intraoral procedure would be difficult because of limited access or preexisting pathology.

Currently, the intraoral sagittal split ramus osteotomy (see Fig. 21-1) is most frequently used for mandibular advancement. Since its introduction, the technique has undergone various modifications to reduce stripping of the muscular attachments that provide the vascular pedicle. These changes have resulted in increased stability and decreased morbidity. The osteotomy design provides a broad interface of medullary bone for rapid healing. The overlapping of the two segments allows easy fixation by intraosseous wiring or placement of osteosynthesis screws (Fig. 21-7), and problems with postoperative instability are rare.

The greatest drawbacks of the sagittal split are altered sensation and a reduced interincisal opening postoperatively. Although the long buccal nerve is frequently cut in the access incision, patients rarely complain of parasthesia in the tissues that it supplies. Altered sensation in the lingual nerve distribution is generally transient. Inferior alveolar nerve involvement, which may be caused by the reflection and retraction of the soft tissues in gaining access to place the medial osteotomy cut, creates an area of altered sensation on the lower lip and chin that occasionally persists but usually disappears in 2 to 6 months. Unless the nerve is actually torn or cut, it is difficult to determine at what point the insult occurs.

Modifications in surgical design have decreased the need

for medial dissection, but some stretching and retraction are still necessary to place the osteotomy cut. If malleting is used to complete the sagittal split, this may compress the nerve where it passes through the medullary bone. Injury may occur during the direct manipulation of the neurovascular bundle, which is frequently needed to gently tease it away from the proximal osteotomy segment and place it with the portion of mandible that will be moved. The incidence of prolonged paresthesia varies widely with operator expertise, but 20% to 25% of patients commonly experience this complication. This adverse effect is less of a problem if the patient has received adequate explanation and understands that the involvement has no relationship to motor function.

Although some limitation in opening can be expected after any ramus surgery, recent reports indicate that the decrease with the sagittal split osteotomy is greater than with other procedures.[8] This effect may be related to the additional dissection done on the medial aspect of the mandible. Postoperative physical therapy may help in reestablishing a normal range of motion.

Advancement of only the teeth and alveolar process is also possible, using subapical surgery. This approach is indicated for individuals who have adequate chin projection but distal placement of the dentoalveolus on the mandibular corpus (Fig. 21-8). A component of vertical deficiency is often associated with this sagittal problem and can be corrected with a bone graft beneath the alveolar segment. Ad-

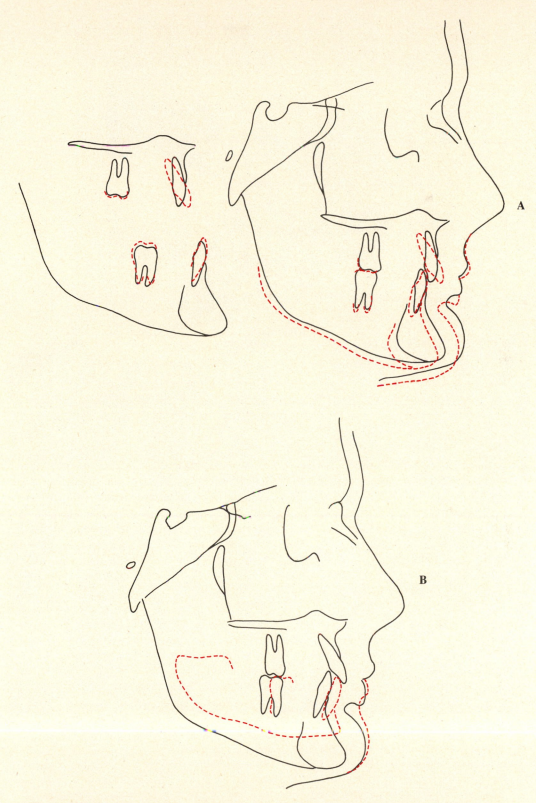

Fig. 21-8 ■ **A,** Cephalometric superimposition showing presurgical orthodontic preparation *(red)* in a patient having mandibular dentoalveolar retrusion. Proclination of the upper anterior teeth has established the overjet necessary for surgical alveolar advancement. Bite opening by extensive leveling mechanics has helped to increase lower facial height. **B,** Superimposition of cephalometric tracings from films taken immediately before and after surgery (same patient). The broken red outline shows the amount of alveolar advancement. The overjet has been corrected and better lip to chin balance established.

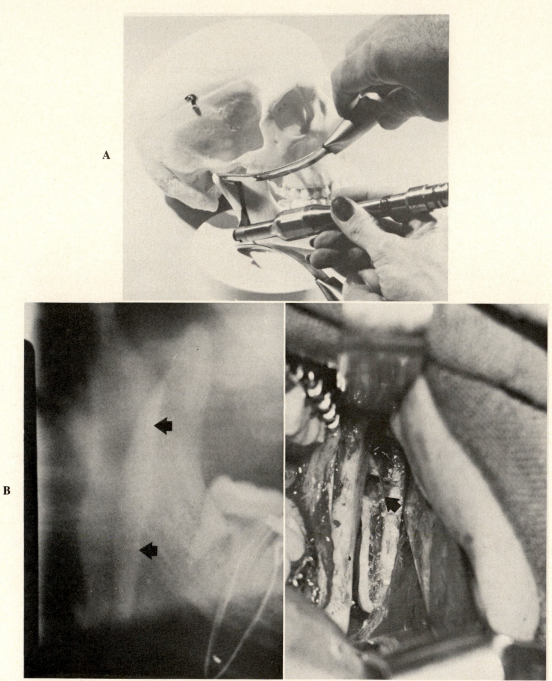

Fig. 21-9 ■ Illustration of the intraoral transoral vertical oblique osteotomy, used for correction of mandibular prognathism. **A,** Typical instrumentation for completing the transoral vertical oblique osteotomy of the mandibular ramus. The bone cut is made with a nitrogen driven oscillating saw. **B,** This radiograph of the right mandibular ramus shows the postoperative position of the surgical segments. This technique is limited to posterior movement of the mandible because good contact of the bony segments can only be achieved by overlapping them. (The area of overlap is indicated by the arrows.) **C,** Photograph of the surgery site as viewed by the surgeon. The proximal (condyle containing) segment can be seen overlapping the larger portion of the mandible on the lateral surface. This osteotomy cut passed just distal to the interior alveolar nerve since the posterior part of the mandibular foramen is visible *(arrow)*.

vancement is limited to the dimensions of the underlying bony base.

Mandibular setback. Reduction of the mandibular skeletal base usually is accomplished by one of two techniques performed in the ramus, each having advantages and disadvantages. The sagittal split osteotomy discussed previously can be used to move the mandible posteriorly as well as anteriorly. In addition to the pros and cons already mentioned, it has the advantage of producing less lateral rotation of the mandibular condyle when the mandible is set back.

The transoral vertical oblique ramus osteotomy incorporates cuts from the sigmoid notch to the mandibular angle (Fig. 21-9). The vertical oblique design is limited to the reduction of mandibular prognathism and necessitates full-thickness overlapping of the segments, which makes internal fixation difficult. This technique was done originally from an extraoral approach, but with improved instrumentation can now be performed intraorally. Limited visibility is a major difficulty with the intraoral version of this technique. Although this concern has been addressed with better instrumentation, it still requires a somewhat "blind" approach. Because fixation is minimal and dissection is limited to the lateral aspect of the ramus, the procedure can generally be accomplished in less time than the sagittal split.

Studies indicate little or no difference in sagittal stability between the two techniques but significantly greater neurologic morbidity with the sagittal split approach.[9] This design has increased tendency for postsurgical opening of the gonial angle, which may be related to superior rotation of the proximal segment, resorption caused by the amount of muscle stripping necessary, or both. Although this result has no effect on surgical stability, it is a cosmetic concern to some individuals.

Occasionally, the original operation for mandibular prognathism, a body ostectomy, is still indicated. Sagittal reduction performed by removing a segment of bone from the mandibular body, allows closure of bilateral edentulous spaces and produces a slight narrowing of the mandible. In some instances, the anterior alveolus is so thin that orthodontic treatment risks the periodontal health of the associated teeth. The compensatory lingual angulation of the teeth can be corrected by designing the ostectomy to allow clockwise rotation of the anterior segment. Rigid fixation techniques have solved previous problems with postsurgical stability.

Segmental surgery to retract the anterior dentoalveolus after extraction of premolars can be helpful in the rare cases of mandibular excess with associated chin deficiency, since tooth-lip-chin balance is then enhanced by the surgery. Since similar results could be achieved by premolar extraction and maximum anchorage orthodontics, the primary indication for surgery would be a narrow anterior alveolar configuration in which orthodontic treatment would risk the periodontal health of the associated teeth.

■ Problems in Vertical Relationships

Problems of excessive and deficient face height, which are usually accompanied by severe anterior open bite and deep bite respectively, were not treated in a reliable manner until the 1970s. At present, as diagrammed in Fig. 21-10, the maxilla can be moved up quite successfully but can be positioned downward with less predictability. The mandible can be moved up or down anteriorly but cannot be moved down at the gonial angle with stability. As a general guideline, this means that long face problems are treated best by intrusion of the maxilla. This method allows the mandible to rotate around the condyle, thereby reducing the mandibular plane angle and shortening the face.

Short face problems, in contrast, are treated most predictably by mandibular ramus surgery that allows the mandible to move downward only at the chin, increasing the mandibular plane angle by shortening the ramus and opening the gonial angle rather than by rotating at the condyle. When vertical positions of the jaws are changed, it is often necessary to change anteroposterior positions as well.

Maxillary surgery. Historically, the skeletal open bite deformity has been one of the most difficult problems to treat by any means. The contemporary surgical approach involves maxillary intrusion after removal of bone from the lateral walls of the nose, sinus, and nasal septum. It is important to shorten the nasal septum or free its base so that the septum is not bent when the maxilla is elevated. The inferior turbinate can be partially resected if needed to allow the intrusion, although this procedure is rarely necessary. The overall facial height is shortened as the mandible responds by rotating upward and forward, altering both its occlusal and postural positions (Fig. 21-11). Further surgery for correction of the anteroposterior mandibular position may not always be necessary after this rotation, depending on functional and esthetic concerns. Longitudinal study has shown that this type of maxillary intrusion provides stable correction of long face problems because the maxilla does not tend to move back down postsurgically.[10]

In contrast, when the maxilla is moved downward surgically to increase face height, it tends to relapse back up postsurgically. Slow adaptation of the facial soft tissues that are stretched when the mandible rotates down may be partly responsible. Inability to stabilize the graft material in the osteotomy site against contraction of the mandibular elevator muscles may also contribute to the instability. Both problems have been addressed with mechanical approaches to increase fixation stability, but at this time, data are insufficient to draw conclusions about long-term results of the modified fixation techniques. Where the deformity allows an equally satisfactory alternative approach, moving the maxilla down should be avoided.

Mandibular surgery. Patients with a long face, skeletal open bite, and an anteroposterior mandibular deficiency often have a short mandibular ramus. As Fig. 21-10 suggests,

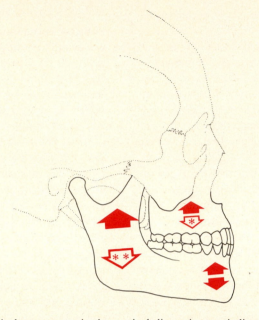

Fig. 21-10 ■ The surgical movements in the vertical dimension are indicated by the red arrows on this diagram of the skull. The maxilla, mandibular angles, and chin can be moved upward reliably, while downward movement of the maxilla by bone grafting is less predictable *(arrow with single asterisk)*. Downward movement of the chin is possible in combination with slight advancement. Lengthening the ramus *(arrow with double asterisks)* stretches the muscular sling and usually results in relapse.

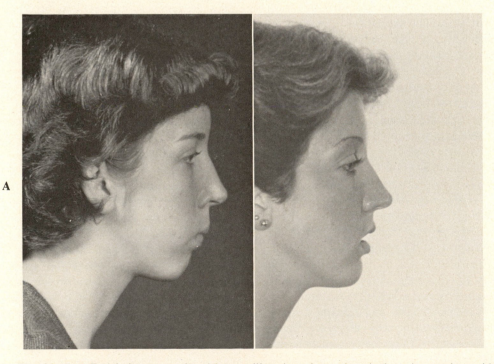

A   B

Fig. 21-11 ■ Facial changes produced by maxillary intrusion and genioplasty in a patient with increased facial height caused by a skeletal open bite. **A,** The poor chin projection and steep mandibular plane seen in this pretreatment photograph are caused by downward and backward rotation of the mandible. **B,** The improved facial balance on this postoperative photograph has been achieved by upward and forward rotation of the mandible, which closed the open bite and provided better chin projection. Genioplasty further augmented the chin.

surgery to reduce the mandibular plane angle and close the open bite by rotating the mandible down posteriorly and up anteriorly, has been found to be highly unstable. Because the fulcrum for rotation is the posterior teeth, this rotation lengthens the ramus and stretches the muscles of the pterygomandibular sling. The instability is attributed primarily to lack of neuromuscular adaptation in these powerful muscles, which can produce relapse to presurgical or even worse mandibular positions (Fig. 21-12). Mandibular ramus surgery in open bite patients should be avoided for this reason, unless it is combined with maxillary intrusion so that lengthening of the ramus does not occur.

Long-face patients often have excessive eruption of mandibular anterior teeth, indicated cephalometrically by an abnormally long distance from the incisal edge to the base of the chin. This vertical tooth-chin problem can be corrected by orthodontic intrusion or by anterior segmental surgery to depress the elongated incisor segment. Often, however, the preferred treatment is genioplasty to reduce the vertical height of the chin at the same time it is augmented horizontally (see Fig. 21-11). Many long face patients are treated best with a combination of maxillary intrusion and genioplasty.

Occasionally, anterior or posterior open bite occurs in a patient who does not have vertical maxillary excess. Kolë[11] devised a procedure for treating anterior open bite problems by elevation of the mandibular alveolar segments and interposition of a graft taken from the lower border of the chin, thus shortening face height (Fig. 21-13). Clinical experience has shown that this is an extremely successful alternative method for closure of anterior open bite when maxillary impaction surgery is not indicated. Rarely, posterior open bite results from deficient eruption and lack of dentoalveolar development. This condition can be treated by elevation of a dentoalveolar segment or even the entire mandibular dentition, with a graft placed beneath to hold the teeth in position. Stable results are obtained.

Patients with a short face (skeletal deep bite) problem are characterized by a long mandibular ramus, square gonial angle, and short nose-chin distance. Despite the deep overbite, excessive eruption of the lower incisors often has not occurred, as demonstrated by a normal distance from the chin to the incisal edge. These patients often have an associated mild mandibular deficiency and are treated best by sagittal split mandibular ramus surgery, to rotate the mandible slightly forward and down and the gonial angle area up (Fig. 21-14). Orthodontic leveling of the lower arch can be done before or after surgery (see following).

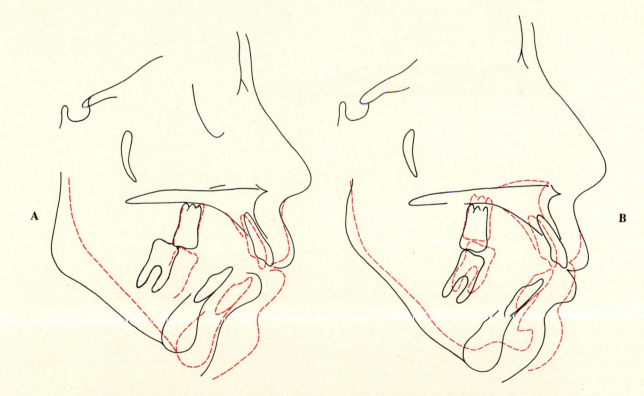

Fig. 21-12 ■ Cephalometric superimpositions for a patient who had two different operations for correction of mandibular deficiency and skeletal open bite. **A,** Pretreatment (black) and 3-month postsurgical (red) tracings. The first operation, mandibular advancement only, produced an unstable increase in posterior face height. Note the opening and shortening of the gonial angle. Although some advancement has been maintained, the patient experienced relapse of the open bite and lingual compensation of the upper incisors. **B,** The broken red outline shows the postoperative result of surgical retreatment with a three-segment maxillary osteotomy and genioplasty. Maxillary intrusion and protraction have allowed upward rotation of the mandible and decrease in face height. Advancement genioplasty was necessary in this instance for improved chin projection.

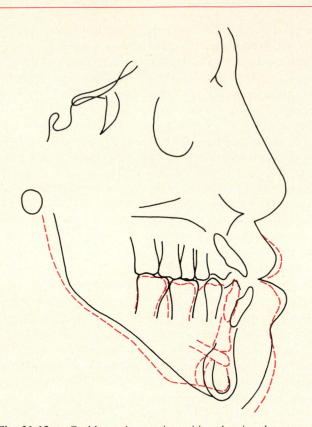

Fig. 21-13 ■ Cephlometric superimposition showing the correction of Class III open bite malocclusion by elevation of the mandibular anterior segment, using a modified Kolë procedure. The postsurgical result is indicated by the red outline. After the removal of two premolar teeth, the anterior mandibular segment was retracted, positioned superiorly, and supported by a section removed from the inferior symphysis.

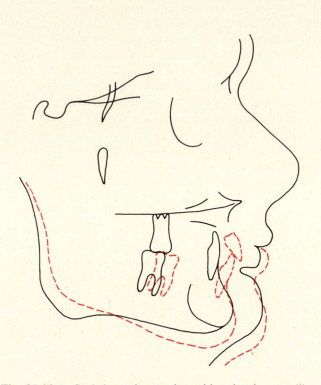

Fig. 21-14 ■ Cephalometric superimposition showing mandibular advancement in a short face patient, which often results in as much vertical as horizontal movement. The black tracing illustrates the parallelism of anatomic planes and deep overbite of the anterior teeth in this patient with skeletal deep bite. The result of surgical mandibular advancement is shown in red. The anterior mandible has rotated downward while maintaining anteroposterior position, producing increased facial height and decreased overbite. Superior rotation in the ramus has resulted in overall normalization of the mandibular plane angle.

■ Role of Genioplasty

Lack of surrounding anatomic structures gives the surgeon considerable latitude in alteration of chin morphology, and movement of the chin in all three planes of space is possible (Fig. 21-15). The chin can be moved in virtually every direction, but esthetic results are unquestionably better and more predictable if the movement increases or the soft tissue support rather than diminishes it. Although the surgical movement of basal bone and dentoalveolar segments clearly has functional benefits in addition to changes in appearance, alteration of the chin is primarily cosmetic. However, there is in theory some potential impact on stability of the lower incisors. Protrusion of the lower incisors relative to the chin is widely considered to be related to incisor stability,[12] though long-term studies of posttreatment orthodontic patients suggest that the relationship is a weak one.[13] Advancing the chin in patients whose lower incisors have been proclined during treatment may contribute to stability. Long-term studies of genioplasty patients, however, are not yet available to support this contention.

The chin can be augmented either by adding an implant material or by using an osteotomy to reposition the symphysis. Addition of a bone graft taken from another area is a possible implant approach but is rarely used because absence of a vascular pedicle results in loss of viability and significant resorption. Silicone implants were commonly placed at one time, but are now used infrequently because of problems with bone resorption and migration of the implant into the symphysis. If an alloplastic material must be used, Proplast is currently considered a better choice, but the sponge-like porosity that helps secure this implant material with fibrous tissue ingrowth also increases the likelihood of contamination, infection, and rejection. Histologic studies have shown giant cell reactions around both implants. This is thought by some researchers to be an osteoclastic response. Regardless of the nature of the reaction, the material cannot be considered inert.

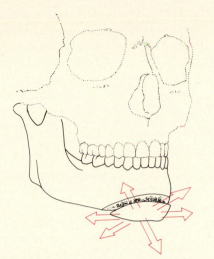

Fig. 21-15 ■ The chin can be sectioned anterior to the mental foramen and repositioned in three dimensions depending on the orientation of the osteotomy. The lingual surface remains attached to muscles in the floor of the mouth, which provide the blood supply. The overlying soft tissues favorably reflect the correction of asymmetry or chin deficiency. The morphology after the reduction of chin prominence is less predictable and may result in a boxy appearance.

For most patients, the preferred approach to genioplasty involves an osteotomy to free a wedge-shaped portion of the symphysis and inferior border that remains pedicled on the genioglossus and geniohyoid muscles. This segment can be advanced to augment chin contour, shifted sideways to correct asymmetry, or downgrafted to increase lower face height. By splitting the segment vertically, the distal aspects of the wedge can be flared or compressed. If narrowing of the anterior portion is needed, bone is removed in that area. When reduction is desired in the distance from the incisal edge to the inferior aspect of the symphysis, a wedge of bone can be removed above the chin as diagrammed in Fig. 21-15.

Less satisfactory results are achieved in the reduction of a prominent symphysis by genioplasty. Reduction by degloving the symphysis and cutting away bone produces an undesirable boxy or blunted appearance. Posterior movement of a pedicled wedge gives results that are better but still less predictable and esthetic than augmentation. If possible, most surgeons attempt to decrease the chin prominence by rotating the body of the mandible in the course of other maxillary or mandibular surgery.

■ Overview of Contemporary Orthognathic Surgery

Today, the vast majority of dentofacial problems are treated with variations of four operations: the LeFort I maxillary downfracture, the bilateral sagittal split ramus osteotomy, the transoral vertical oblique ramus osteotomy, and the horizontal sliding genioplasty. The few remaining prob-

lems can be dealt with using segmental dentoalveolar surgery and mandibular body procedures. Craniofacial abnormalities require more complicated midface and intracranial surgery, but individuals with these problems comprise a small percentage of the total patient population.

Three factors have been important in the selection of these operations as the usual orthognathic surgical procedures: stability of results, predictability of hard and soft tissue changes, and patient response. Ideally, a surgical technique would provide perfectly stable and predictable results, with minimal risk to the patient or untoward responses. The procedures presently used in orthognathic surgery, though not ideal, can be evaluated quite highly against this standard.

It is difficult to perfectly quantify the stability of various surgical procedures because of such variables as the surgeon's expertise, fixation techniques, magnitude of change, and patient compliance with postsurgical instructions. In general, however, when the preferred operation is used, minimal bony changes (less than 2 mm) can be expected postsurgically in the great majority of patients. The changes are almost always in the relapse direction, i.e., a mandible that has been brought forward tends to slip back slightly, while one that has been moved back surgically tends to slip forward a small distance.

Generally speaking, mandibular setback tends to relapse less than mandibular advancement. Both the transoral vertical oblique and sagittal split osteotomies can be used to set the mandible back, and predictable results are obtained with both, but the vertical oblique procedure produces less nerve damage and also seems to give slightly better stability. For mandibular advancement, the sagittal split is the only feasible approach and is quite satisfactory, but about 2 mm of relapse at the chin during the healing phase immediately after surgery must be expected. Maxillary intrusion with the downfracture approach is highly stable, but if the maxilla is moved down, there is an unpredictable but sometimes marked relapse tendency, which is why this movement is recommended only if there is no alternative. Both forward and backward movements of the maxilla give stable results.

It is also difficult to precisely predict the response of facial soft tissues to surgical movement of the supporting bony framework. Existing guidelines for soft tissue changes allow reasonable predictability of chin and lip profile changes when the jaws are moved forward or back. When face height is decreased by moving the maxilla up, the base of the nose becomes wider, the cheeks fill out so that the face looks wider, and the lips become thinner (see Fig. 21-35). These changes usually are pleasing because long faced individuals often have narrow nasal bases and angular cheekbones, but they could be objectionable in a patient with a long but otherwise normally proportioned face. The thickness and tone of the facial soft tissue also affect the response. For example, clinical experience has shown that aging skin that is losing elasticity does not respond well to procedures that decrease soft tissue support. In older patients, double chins become bigger and skin creases and folds deepen when mandibular or maxillary protrusion is reduced.

The patient response to modern orthognathic surgery also is quite good. The surgery typically requires a hospital stay of 3 to 5 days. A well-qualified and experienced nursing team is important in providing the postsurgical care. Patients require surprisingly little pain medication, particularly following maxillary surgery. The discomfort associated with prolonged intermaxillary fixation is being reduced by the rigid fixation techniques that reduce or eliminate wiring the jaws together during healing. Changes in sensation in the lower lip after mandibular ramus osteotomies are the major complications of the current orthognathic surgical procedures.

Although surgical techniques have become more sophisticated with better diagnosis, instrumentation, and knowledge of their biologic basis, they are but one part of the overall treatment picture in surgical orthodontics. The surgery itself tends to receive more attention because of the rapid and major morphologic changes possible, but the other components are equally important in the overall treatment sequence.

■ *Timing of Treatment*

As noted previously, growth modification is the preferred approach to severe dentofacial problems, whereas surgery is reserved for patients who do not respond to growth modification and whose problems are too severe to camouflage. As a general guideline, orthognathic surgery should be delayed until growth is essentially completed in patients who have problems of excessive growth, especially mandibular prognathism. For patients with growth deficiencies, surgery can be considered earlier, but rarely before the adolescent growth spurt.

■ Early Surgery and Growth Excess

There is reasonable agreement that early jaw surgery has little if any effect of preventing further excessive growth. Actively growing patients with mandibular prognathism can be expected to outgrow their correction and require retreatment if operated too early (Fig. 21-16). Problems with psychosocial adjustment may justify early surgery to correct prognathism, but the assessment should be made by a qualified professional and documented carefully. The patient's parents must be informed of the chances that retreatment will be required in these cases. If the decision is to delay surgery until growth is completed, indirect methods of assessing growth status, such as hand-wrist films to determine bone age, are not accurate enough to use for planning the time of surgery. The best method is serial cephalometric tracings, with surgery delayed until good superimposition documents that the adult deceleration of growth has occurred.

The situation is not so clearcut for patients with the long

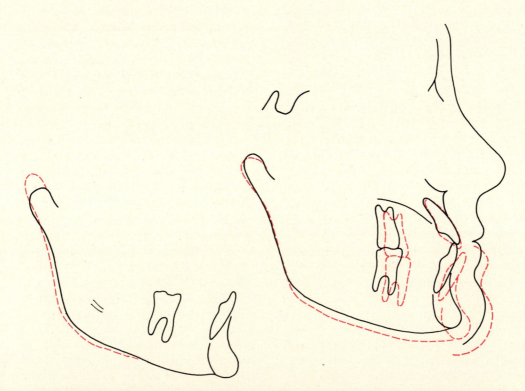

Fig. 21-16 ■ Cephalometric superimposition showing continued mandibular growth after surgical correction at age 15 *(black tracing, completion of initial phase of treatment).* The red outline, from a film 5 years later, demonstrates the increment of mandibular growth and resulting relapse.

face (skeletal open bite) pattern that can be characterized as vertical maxillary excess. Washburn et al.[14] studied 12 patients who had surgery to correct vertical maxillary excess between the ages of 10 and 16, following them for 2 to 3 years after surgery. They reported continued vertical development of the maxilla, most of which was above the dentoalveolar level. Only one patient, who had an increasing mandibular plane angle, was considered to have unfavorable growth postoperatively. In a series of patients treated at the University of North Carolina, skeletal stability of the vertically repositioned maxilla was similar in patients above and below the age of 19, but the maxillary posterior teeth tended to erupt after surgery in the younger patients.[10] There appears to be a reasonable chance for stable surgical correction of this problem before growth is totally completed, but the difference in clinical stability between treatment at, for example, ages 14 and 18, remains incompletely understood.

Long-term followup of these patients will be of interest in light of Behrents' findings of continued slow growth in the original pattern throughout life with the vertical component predominating in later years[15] (see Chapter 4).

■ Early Surgery and Growth Deficiency

Surgery in infancy and early childhood is required for some congenital problems that involve growth deficiency; craniosynostosis and severe hemifacial microsomia are two examples. The major indication for orthognathic surgery before puberty, however, is a progressive deformity caused by restriction of growth. A common cause is ankylosis of the mandible, unilaterally or occasionally bilaterally, after a condylar injury or severe infection (see Chapters 2 and 4). Surgery to release the ankylosis, followed by functional appliance therapy to guide subsequent growth, is needed in these unusual problems.

A child with a severely progressive deficiency should be distinguished from one with a severe but stable deficiency, for example, a child with a small mandible whose facial proportions are not changing appreciably with growth. Although a progressive deficiency is an indication for early surgery, a severe but stable deficiency may not be. In keeping with the general principle that orthognathic surgery has surprisingly little impact on growth, early surgery does not improve the growth prognosis unless it relieves a specific restriction on growth, nor does it produce a subsequent normal growth pattern.

Early mandibular advancement. Wolford, Schendel, and Epker have reported the results of early mandibular advancement surgery.[16] In their sample of 15 patients, the average advancement measured at the mandibular incisal edge was 5.4 mm, a discrepancy that many orthodontists would consider to be within the realm of more conservative treatment. They commented that results were stable and postsurgical growth was harmonious, but their illustrations of computer generated graphics suggest that growth after surgery was primarily vertical (Fig. 21-17).

A retrospective study by Huang and Ross[17] on young mandibular advancement patients suggests that stability is related both to the amount of correction and to age at the time of surgery. Children with advancement of more than 10 mm appeared to have considerably more relapse than those with smaller advancements. There was no further growth after advancement in 68% of the patients studied. In those who had continued growth, there was a 1 year lag period before growth resumed, and in all cases, the individual's preoperative pattern was reestablished.

In our view, mandibular advancement before the adolescent growth spurt is of questionable utility for patients who do not have extremely severe and progressive deformities. On the other hand, there is no reason to delay mandibular advancement after sexual maturity. Minimal facial growth can be expected in patients with severe deficiency during late adolescence and relapse from that cause is unlikely.

Early maxillary advancement. Early surgical advancement of a sagittally deficient maxilla or midface remains relatively stable if there is careful attention to detail and grafts are used to combat relapse. There is no evidence, however, to suggest that normal forward development of midfacial structures is initiated after surgery. Subsequent growth of the mandible is likely to result in reestablishment of the abnormal relationships. If early advancement is needed (for psychological reasons or to control compensatory changes in the mandible), a second stage of surgical treatment should be planned to follow the adolescent growth acceleration.

Problems of this type are most common in patients with cleft lip and palate. Maxillary advancement may be performed soon after puberty, along with bone grafting and fistula closure. If the skeletal discrepancy recurs during subsequent growth, surgical mandibular setback can be done at a later date to reestablish jaw relationships.

In summary, when planning early surgery for dentofacial problems, one must consider psychosocial implications as well as which skeletal components are at fault and whether the problem is one of excessive or deficient growth. Psychologic consultation and objective documentation should be obtained in cases where circumstances would otherwise indicate delaying surgery. The pattern of additional postsurgical growth and its effect on treatment stability should be estimated. It is best to delay, if possible, surgical treatment of problems that involve growth excess and unfavorable (vertical) growth pattern until late adolescence. Patients with a progressive deformity are candidates for surgery at an early age, whereas those with a stable deficiency can have surgery soon after puberty.

■ Special Considerations in Orthodontic-Surgical Planning

■ Team Approach to Evaluation

The approach to treatment planning for orthognathic surgery patients has continued to be refined with increasing

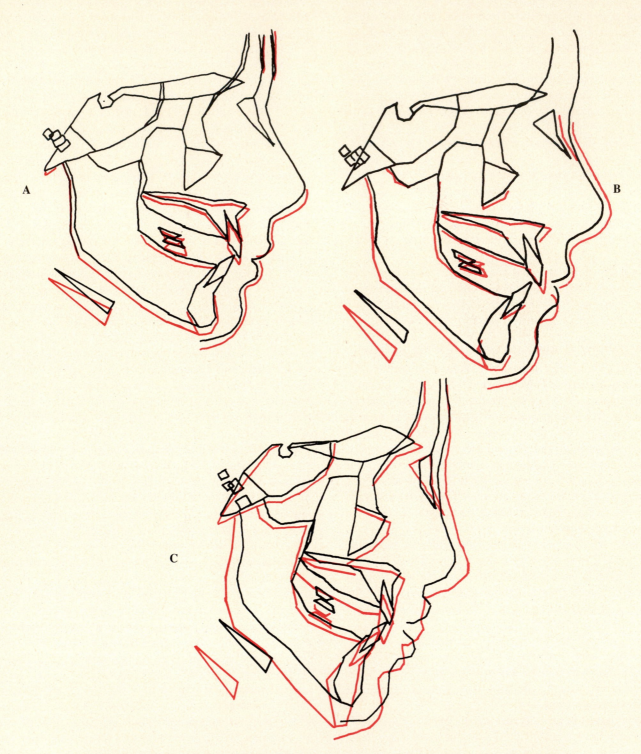

Fig. 21-17 ■ Computer generated average cephalometric tracings showing growth after surgical advancement of the mandible in young patients (black, postsurgical; red, follow-up). **A,** The response in patients with low mandibular plane angle. Note that the increment is primarily in a vertical direction with little if any horizontal projection of the chin. **B,** Postsurgical growth in patients with an average mandibular plane angle was primarily vertical with a small component of clockwise or backward chin rotation. **C,** Growth after surgery in patients with high mandibular plane angle was clearly in a vertical direction with a definite component of clockwise or posterior rotation of the mandible. (From Wolford, L.M., et al.: J. Maxillofac. Surg. **7:**61-72, 1979.)

clinical experience. In the past, practitioners would often proceed unilaterally with diagnosis and treatment, consulting with colleagues in "other" disciplines only when it seemed unavoidable.

The contemporary approach involves a team to ensure close cooperation of those involved in all phases of treatment. In almost all cases, an oral and maxillofacial surgeon and an orthodontist are involved as primary team members. Because of the largely adult patient population and the impact of surgery and orthodontics on tissue support, a periodontist is needed for regular consultation. In instances where extensive prosthetic rehabilitation is required, it may be advantageous to involve a team member with this expertise at an early stage (Fig. 21-18). Although the rela-

tionship of various skeletal malocclusions and temporomandibular joint disorders remains unclear, the problems coexist with sufficient frequency to warrant having at least one team member who is knowledgeable in this area. A person qualified to do psychologic evaluation and counseling should be identified for consultation if the need arises.

Coordination of a treatment team is obviously easier in an institutional setting but can be accomplished by small group practices or solo practitioners with adequate planning. Regular communication and intellectual honesty are perhaps the most important factors in team treatment and should be observed whether the team members are in close proximity to one another or spread over a larger geographic area.

Although problems of scheduling, time constraints, and

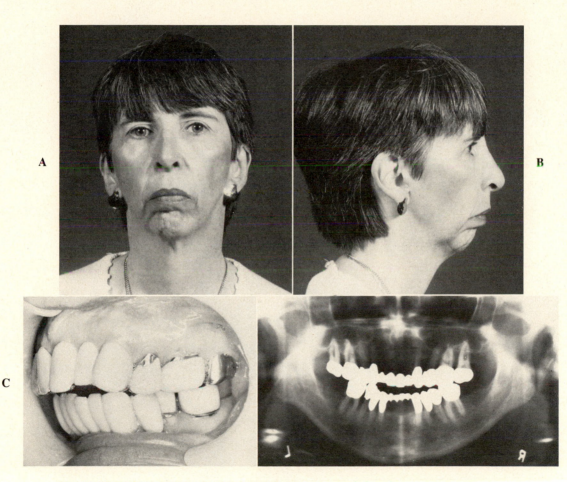

Fig. 21-18 ■ Pretreatment records of a patient requiring periodontal and prosthodontic as well as surgical-orthodontic treatment planning. **A, B,** The frontal and profile photographs demonstrate this woman's severe mandibular retrognathia. This results from a combination of absolute deficiency in overall size and relative deficiency caused by excessive vertical maxillary development and backward rotation of the mandible. **C,** Treatment is complicated by extensive fixed restorations that were fabricated in an attempt to dentally compensate for her skeletal malocclusion. Presurgical orthodontic treatment ordinarily would remove these dental compensations, but in this instance, the bridges must be sectioned and remade after treatment. **D,** This panoramic film shows the generalized periodontal involvement that further complicates treatment in this patient. Generalized bone loss and furcation involvement are evident in all quadrants. Note the flattened condylar heads and decreased posterior ramus height often associated with patients having skeletal open bite malocclusion.

geographic location may cause difficulties, it is helpful to undertake the initial interview and examination as a team. This avoids the problem of the patient varying his or her story when talking with different interviewers. Team members are "kept honest" by the group, and there is less tendency to view the patient in the context of one's particular interest. If nothing else, it is a courtesy to patients to avoid their having to travel to a variety of offices to repeat their story and have records taken. A practitioner who will be involved in treating patients with complex problems should be willing to make the allowances necessary to participate as a member of the team.

The patient interview should be as relaxed as possible. The team member particularly adept at interviewing techniques may be the prime speaker, with others asking for clarification when indicated. The patient's concerns

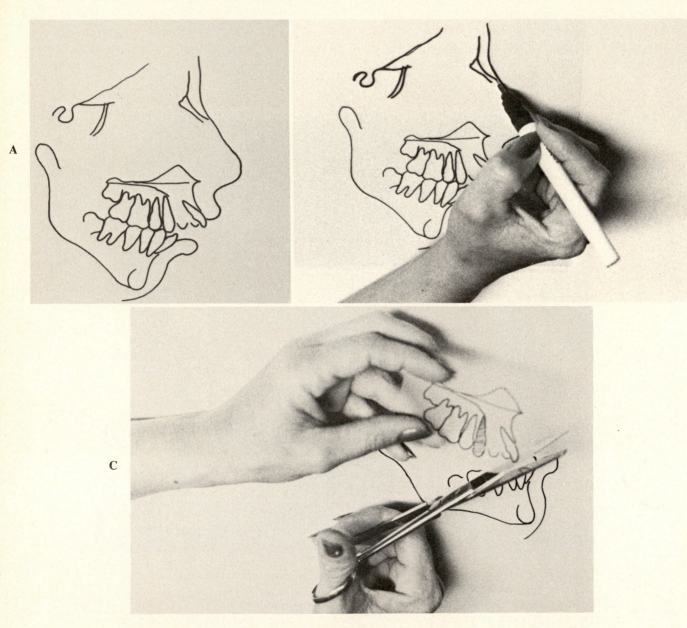

Fig. 21-19 ■ Photographic series demonstrating the technique of cephalometric surgical prediction, in this case for a patient who will have both upper and lower jaws repositioned. **A,** The cephalometric tracing of the pretreatment relationships is prepared; the occlusal outlines of all teeth should be carefully drawn to assist in establishing the new occlusion; **B,** a second sheet of acetate is placed over the surgical tracing and the structures that will not be changed by surgery are traced; **C,** note the maxillary dental and skeletal structures are traced on acetate and cut out in preparation for simulated surgical repositioning. The first premolar, which is to be removed, is indicated by cross hatching. Since the maxilla is to be segmented at this location, the tracing is cut into two pieces.

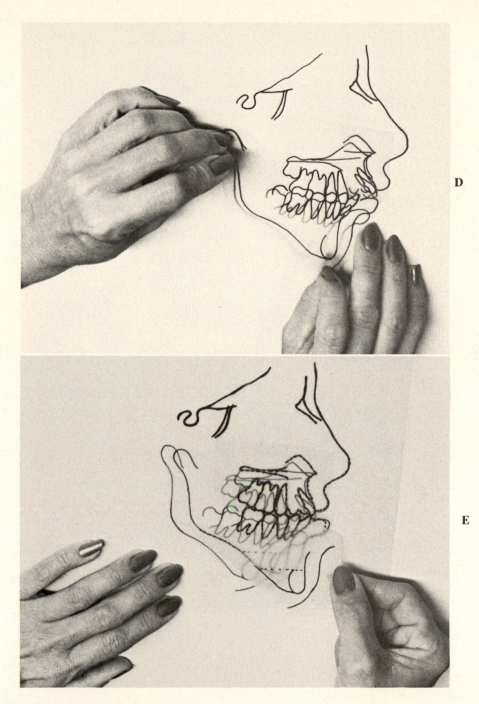

Fig. 21-19, cont'd ■ **D,** Maxillary impaction is needed for this patient, and the anterior segment of the maxilla has been positioned superiorly to provide optimal lip support and esthetic display of incisal edge with lips at rest. (The cephalometric film used in this technique must be taken with the soft tissues at rest if an accurate prediction is to be made.) When the position of the anterior segment is established, the mandibular cutout can be rotated around the center of the condylar head to determine whether rotation alone will provide adequate occlusion or whether surgical advancement of the mandible is necessary. In this patient, it can be seen that the mandible will need to be surgically advanced. **E,** The cutout of the mandible and overlying soft tissue has been advanced into ideal overjet/overbite relationships and the posterior segment of the maxilla placed into Class II molar relationship (a first premolar has been removed). The amount of mandibular advancement can be seen by the discrepancy in the outline of the condyles. Since maxillary impaction and mandibular advancement have still failed to provide adequate chin projection, a tracing of the inferior aspect of the symphysis is prepared and advanced to simulate a sliding genioplasty.

Continued.

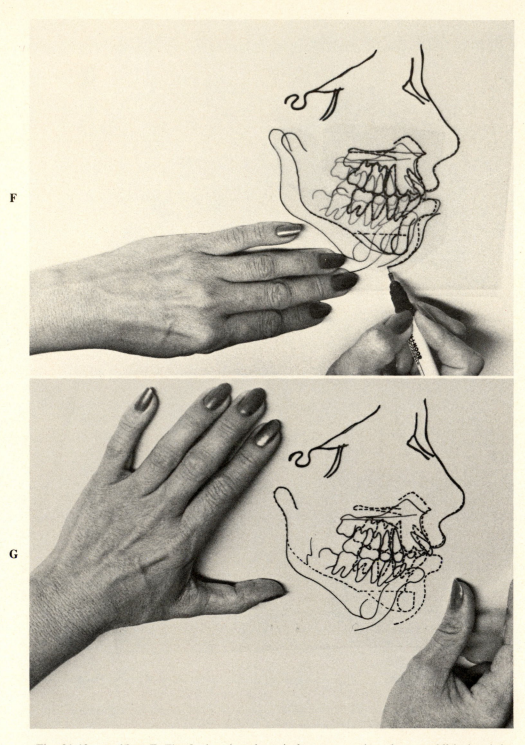

F

G

Fig. 21-19, cont'd ■ **F,** The final projected surgical movements have been established and the acetate cutouts are taped in place. The projected soft tissue changes are sketched in with a dashed line. Published ratios of soft tissue change in response to movement of the underlying skeletal components are used in drawing the projected final soft tissue outlines. **G,** The final prediction for this patient is indicated by the dashed line that has been superimposed on the original tracing shown by the solid line. The maxilla has been impacted using a segmented LeFort I approach to close the open bite and the extraction space left by the removal of the first premolar. The mandible has been surgically advanced and rotated upward into a good occlusal relationship with the maxilla. An advancement genioplasty has been done to provide a more pleasing facial balance.

should be carefully elicited and prioritized. Since the second opinion has become more commonplace, one must determine whether the concerns voiced are really the patient's chief complaint or are secondary issues suggested during a previous consultation. If a hidden agenda is uncovered in the course of gathering psychosocial data, referral for psychologic evaluation and counseling may be indicated. It is helpful to begin the evaluation of facial proportions during the interview to detect any subconscious posturing habits and observe component relationships when the patient is not posed for a clinical examination.

Minimum diagnostic records for potential surgical patients are the same as for any other comprehensive orthodontic treatment (see Chapter 6). To assist in accurate planning, an effort should be made to obtain records with the patient's head normally positioned. If records are being taken in more than one office, the data collection protocol must ensure uniformity to allow longitudinal comparison. In an ideal situation, master records could be kept in one file with duplicates available for the various team members to take back to their offices for individual study.

■ Cephalometric Prediction

In addition to cephalometric analysis, cephalometric tracings are used to evaluate the feasibility of various possible solutions to the patient's problems. The step-by-step approach to diagnosis outlined in Chapter 6 culminates in a prioritized list of the patient's problems. Setting priorities is essential in dealing with individuals who have several problems, which is nearly always the case when surgical-orthodontic treatment is required. An *x-y* coordinate millimeter measurement system is helpful in evaluating skeletal spatial relationships because it is difficult to plan surgical movements with angular measures. Vertical relationships must be assessed to determine the impact that facial geometry will have on orthodontic mechanics and treatment sequence. The changes planned for these relationships must be considered in the context of existing facial width to achieve overall esthetic balance when planning the surgical movements.

Cephalometric prediction of possible surgical results is done by repositioning tracings of the various bony and dental segments over the original tracing, simulating the movements that would occur if possible treatment procedures were used (Fig. 21-19). The probable posttreatment soft tissue outline is established by using published guidelines for the ratio of soft tissue to hard tissue change. The variables of soft tissue thickness and tonicity introduce uncertainties that make prediction of soft tissue change somewhat of an art form. Nevertheless, the predictions are an invaluable guide to planning treatment for maximum benefit to the patient.

When adequate time has elapsed for records analysis, the team members should reconvene to discuss treatment options and sequencing in the context of the patient's concerns. If there is more than one viable option, it is highly desirable to have cephalometric predictions of each approach to facilitate discussion of the pros and cons of each alternative.

■ The Borderline Patient: Possibilities and Limitations

One of the most difficult decisions facing the orthodontist and surgeon is whether the patient with a borderline skeletal discrepancy can be successfully treated with orthodontics alone. The decision must be made from the very beginning, however, because orthodontic preparation for surgery differs significantly from orthodontic treatment for camouflage. Ill-advised attempts to camouflage problems that are too severe extend treatment time and compromise the final result; on the other hand, unnecessary surgery should be avoided. The problem facing the practitioners, therefore, is how to decide which patients have the potential to be successfully camouflaged and which would be better surgical candidates.

Since the information needed to make this judgment has been collected in a thorough diagnostic database, finding the solution is a matter of integrating the data with one's clinical experience. Some guidelines can be offered, depending on the nature of the patient's problems.

Patients with a long face or skeletal open bite pattern are difficult to treat, regardless of growth status. Most orthodontic mechanotherapy extrudes teeth somewhat, and in these patients orthodontic treatment is particularly likely to result in clockwise mandibular rotation and further lengthening of the face (Fig. 21-20, *A*). If an open bite is not present initially, it will frequently develop in the course of leveling the arches. The features that usually add to the efficiency of the contemporary edgewise appliances create further problems. Since these systems were designed to produce ideal dental relationships on normally positioned jaws, one may see varying degrees of anteroposterior, vertical and transverse discrepancy develop as dental compensations for the skeletal problem are removed by the prescription. All these factors complicate camouflage treatment for this type of patient, tipping the balance toward surgery in apparently borderline situations.

The same type of extrusive tooth movement occurs when patients with a short face or skeletal deep bite facial pattern are treated, but generally the results are desirable, since extrusion of the posterior teeth and lengthening of the face improve the situation (Fig. 21-20, B). Clockwise rotation of the mandible still occurs, but because of the geometric arrangement of the skeletal planes, it is often expressed by the mandible dropping inferiorly more than back, facilitating the possibility of camouflage.

As with any orthodontic patient, the amount of arch length discrepancy must be kept in mind when camouflage of a Class II or III problem is considered. Anteroposterior tooth movement to compensate for a jaw discrepancy is limited to the width of an extraction space or by the amount of expansion that will be tolerated by the periodontium and remain stable. If considerable space is required for the relief

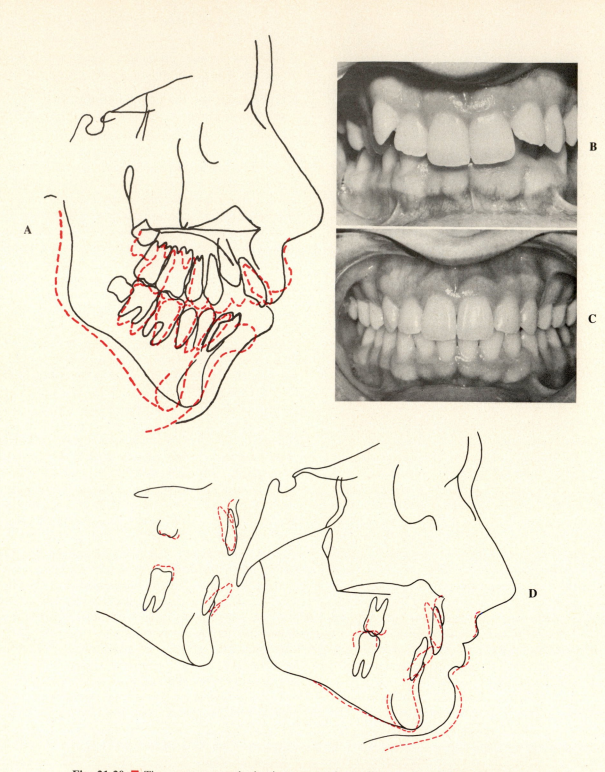

Fig. 21-20 ■ The response to orthodontic treatment is usually more favorable in short face than long face patients. **A,** cephalometric superimposition (black, pretreatment; red, progress) of treatment response in a 15-year-old girl with a long face pattern. Extrusion of posterior teeth during attempted orthodontic treatment made both the open bite and mandibular deficiency worse, as the mandible rotated down and back. Maxillary surgery was eventually necessary. **B** and **C,** pretreatment and post-treatment intraoral photographs of an adult with a short face pattern and a Class II division 2 malocclusion, showing a satisfactory response to orthodontic treatment alone. **D,** cephalometric superimposition for this short face patient. In this case also, extrusion of posterior teeth caused an increase in face height, but for this individual the increase aided in correcting the deep overbite. The chin moved more down and less back for this short face individual than it did in the long face patient shown in **A.** Note the forward movement of the lower incisors, which will require indefinite retention.

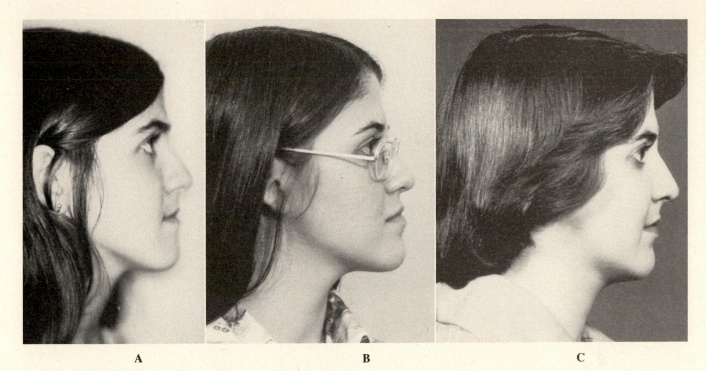

A   B   C

Fig. 21-21 ■ **A,** Dental compensation by extraction of lower premolars was planned for this patient with average facial height and moderate mandibular prognathism; **B,** Continued mandibular growth and the retraction/compensation of the lower anterior dentition has produced a postorthodontic result in which the teeth occlude nicely but overall facial esthetics are compromised by the strong appearance of the chin. At this stage, the patient sought surgical treatment despite her orthodontist's opinion that everything was fine. **C,** Orthognathic surgery has improved the overall facial balance. Treatment was complicated, however, by the dental compensation that had been "built in" to mask the skeletal malocclusion. Patients to be treated with orthodontic camouflage must be carefully selected, since the mechanotherapy and treatment objectives are the opposite of those desired in orthodontic preparation for surgical correction.

of crowding and for leveling, little may be left for the camouflage of a skeletal discrepancy.

The evaluation of soft tissue relationships is an important factor in the decision. A skeketal problem is truly camouflaged only if orthodontic treatment will produce satisfactory facial esthetics as well as good occlusion. If a patient with a skeletal Class II relationship has poor lip support and a large nose, the situation will not be improved by retracting the upper incisors. Likewise, the chin will not become smaller on a Class III patient who has lower premolars removed. If the teeth have been brought into good occlusion orthodontically but the overall facial appearance has been compromised, one must question whether the treatment was appropriate (Fig. 21-21).

Problems in the transverse dimension can be addressed orthodontically if they result mainly from buccal or lingual tipping of the dentition. A jackscrew to open the midpalatal suture is not applicable in adults, and attempts to use this technique may result in subsequent periodontal problems. Skeletal asymmetry can be camouflaged orthodontically only if the chin and external bony contours are not involved.

If they are, dental midline correction alone is unlikely to satisfy the patient. Orthodontic treatment is best confined to problems existing on skeletal bases that are well aligned in the transverse dimension.

The characteristics that can make the difference between satisfactory camouflage treatment and failure are summarized in Table 21-1.

Table 21-1 ■ Orthodontic camouflage of skeletal malocclusion

Acceptable results likely	*Poor results likely*
Average or short facial pattern	Long vertical facial pattern
Mild anteroposterior jaw discrepancy	Moderate or severe anteroposterior jaw discrepancy
Crowding >4-6 mm	Crowding >4-6 mm
Normal soft tissue features (nose, lips, chin)	Exaggerated features
No transverse skeletal problem	Transverse skeletal component of problem

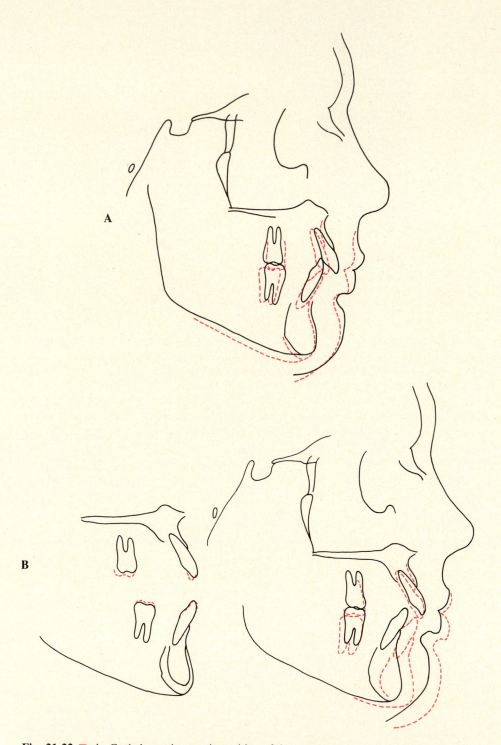

Fig. 21-22 ■ A, Cephalometric superimposition of the pretreatment tracing *(black)* and projected outcome *(red)* of orthodontic camouflage for mild mandibular deficiency. The broken red line shows the anticipated soft tissue profile resulting from maxillary anterior retraction after the extraction of upper first premolars. **B,** Cephalometric superimposition of the same patient's immediate presurgical and postsurgical tracings. This individual was dissatisfied with the projected result of orthodontic camouflage and opted for mandibular advancement surgery. The dashed red line shows the amount of mandibular advancement and increase in facial height. Lower first premolars were extracted to provide room for leveling, alignment, and decompensation of the lower anterior teeth, but there were no extractions in the upper arch.

■ Extraction Patterns in Orthodontic Preparation for Surgery

The importance of deciding on surgery or camouflage from the beginning is further illustrated by the difference in extractions needed with the two approaches. In camouflage, extraction spaces are used to produce dental compensations and the extractions are planned accordingly. For example, a patient with mandibular deficiency and a Class II malocclusion might have upper first premolars removed to allow the retraction of the maxillary anterior teeth (Fig. 21-22). Extraction in the lower arch would be avoided, or if it was necessary because of leveling or alignment requirements, the second premolars might be chosen to provide needed arch length while avoiding retraction of the lower anterior teeth.

The extraction pattern for this same patient would be quite different if mandibular advancement were planned. Removal of lower first premolars would allow leveling of the arch and correction of the lower anterior proclination often associated with this malocclusion. Since retraction of the upper incisors would now be undesirable, the upper arch would be treated without extraction, or if some space were needed because of arch length discrepancy, extractions would be planned to avoid compromising the mandibular advancement by overretraction of the anterior teeth.

A similar but reversed situation would be seen in a patient with a skeletal Class III problem. If camouflage were planned, typical extractions might be lower first premolars alone, or lower first and upper second premolars. Surgical preparation of the same patient often involves the extraction of only upper first premolars to correct the proclination of upper incisors that is usually present. If space were needed in the lower arch, second premolar extraction would be a logical choice so that the lower incisors were not retracted.

Because the treatment objectives of surgical preparation are quite different from those of camouflage, the mechanics seem paradoxical. The Class II interarch forces normally used in a mandibular deficient patient to help close maxillary extraction space and reduce overjet, are often replaced in a patient being prepared for surgery by Class III elastics to retract lower incisors. In the preparation of skeletal Class III patients for surgery, Class II elastics may be needed to increase the reverse overjet. Arch coordination is still necessary in the surgery patient, but each arch must be aligned over individual skeletal base, so that the teeth will be coordinated in their postsurgical, not their presurgical position. The orthodontist and the patient must accept the fact that if proper preparation is to be achieved, the occlusion and cosmetic appearance will temporarily become worse in the preoperative period.

If satisfactory esthetics and functional occlusion can be achieved by either orthodontic camouflage or integrated orthodontic and surgical treatment, the pros and cons of each approach must be carefully explained so that an informed decision can be reached. Returning to a discussion of the patient's concerns often helps clarify the treatment expectations and suggests the appropriate treatment alternative.

■ *Integration of Orthodontics and Surgery*

■ Timing and Sequence of Treatment

Successful management of combined orthodontic and surgical treatment requires the integration of presurgical orthodontic, surgical, and postsurgical orthodontic phases of treatment. In contemporary treatment, dental compensations are removed before surgery and the teeth are properly located in relationship to the individual skeletal components. At this point, heavy archwires are placed and the appliance is used for stability and fixation during surgical reorientation of the bony segments. When satisfactory healing has taken place, active orthodontics is reinitiated to refine the occlusion and complete treatment.

Attempts have been made to separate the surgical and orthodontic treatment, either completing the orthodontics first and then performing the surgery, or vice versa. Aligning the teeth and then terminating the orthodontic phase, by debanding before surgery, make sense only if the orthodontic appliance cannot be used for surgical stabilization. In fact, the contemporary edgewise appliance provides excellent stabilization, better than can be obtained with arch bars or fracture splints. More importantly, appliance removal precludes postoperative orthodontic finishing. Although orthognathic surgery can be performed with reasonable precision, it is always desirable to refine the occlusal relationships after jaw discrepancies have been corrected.

The other possible approach would be to defer any orthodontics until after surgical treatment. It is difficult or impossible to properly position and secure the jaws if the dental arches are incompatible, and the stability of the surgical result may be jeopardized by active orthodontic treatment on recently healed skeletal bases with poor occlusal relationships. Therefore, some orthodontic preparation is nearly always required.

As with any orthodontic patient, dental and periodontal disease must be brought under control before combined surgical-orthodontic treatment is begun. The principles discussed in Chapter 20 are entirely applicable. Three special points should be considered when orthognathic surgery is involved:

1. Incision lines contract somewhat as they heal, and this contracture of vestibular incisions can stress the gingival attachment, leading to stripping or recession in compromised areas. This recession is most likely to be a problem in the lower anterior area in relation to the vestibular incision for a genioplasty (Fig. 21-23). Gingival grafting should be completed before genioplasty if the attached gingiva is inadequate.

2. Many young adults being prepared for orthognathic surgery have unerupted or impacted third molars (Fig. 21-

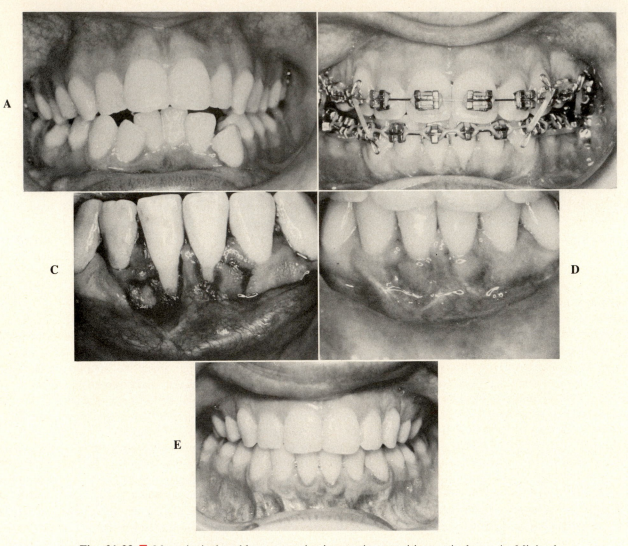

Fig. 21-23 ■ Mucogingival problems can arise in a patient requiring genioplasty. **A,** Minimal amount of attached keratinized gingiva can be seen overlying the lower anterior teeth in this pretreatment photo. Note the inflammation of the marginal gingiva resulting from inadequate hygiene. **B,** After orthodontic alignment and genioplasty, the stresses placed on the periodontium by orthodontic tooth movement and the contracture of the vestibular incision used in advancement genioplasty have resulted in loss of attachment and dehiscence over the lower central incisors. **C,** Periodontal surgery is indicated to prevent further dehiscence and reestablish gingival attachment over the involved teeth. **D,** Early healing of the laterally positioned flaps as seen at the surgical margins of the central incisors. **E,** Excellent contour and reattachment have been established in this patient. Since early grafting procedures are generally more successful than those to reestablish attachment once dehiscence has occurred, it is better to anticipate problems and plan gingival grafts in questionable areas before initiating treatment.

24), but there is no apparent consensus regarding the optimal time to remove them. If the surgeon anticipates using bone screws or other rigid fixation systems that are placed in the third molar area, it is desirable to have the teeth removed far enough in advance of the orthognathic procedure to allow good bone healing. The morbidity associated with removing impacted teeth may be greater than that of orthognathic surgery. This factor, plus greater efficiency and limited anesthetic exposure, is an argument for removal at the time of the major procedure. However, there are legitimate con-

cerns about increasing the surgical morbidity and risking the postoperative complications associated with the removal of impacted teeth. Waiting until the completion of all other treatment to remove the third molars is probably the least desirable option, because patient compliance seems to be better before this stage of treatment.

3. If the patient's prime motivation for treatment is a temporomandibular joint (TMJ) problem, the unpredictable impact of orthognathic surgery must be carefully discussed to avoid unreasonable treatment expectations. The accuracy

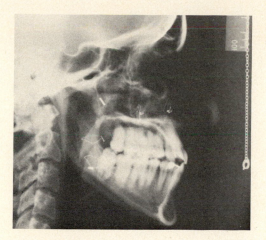

Fig. 21-24 ■ Maxillary and mandibular third molars remain in this patient who underwent LeFort I maxillary impaction and sagittal split osteotomies for mandibular setback. The lower third molars can often be easily removed through the osteotomy site. However, if further bone removal is required, the surgeons may elect to delay extraction rather than jeopardize the integrity of the bony segments.

of diagnostic records may be affected by mandibular posturing if there is acute capsule or muscle involvement. In these instances, it is best to delay the records appointment until initial TMJ therapy alleviates the symptoms and allows the patient to assume an unstrained relationship.

Because of the complex interaction between situational stress and malocclusion, long-term changes are unlikely in patients having muscular hyperactivity disorders. As discussed in Chapter 20, TMJ symptoms usually improve during active treatment, probably because the soreness associated with tooth movement interferes with parafunctional activity, but this improvement may be transient.

If surgical treatment of intracapsular pathology will be required, delaying this treatment until after the orthognathic surgery risks further occlusal impairment from condylar head and meniscal alteration. On the other hand, since condylar rotation accompanies most orthognathic surgical procedures, the joint surgery is more predictable if done after the new jaw positions and occlusal relationships are established, not before. Some surgeons deal with this dilemma by correcting the capsular and orthognathic problems at the same surgery, but the efficacy of such an approach has yet to stand the test of time. An orderly approach to sequencing TMJ and orthognathic treatment may become apparent as more is learned about the relationship between the two.

It is wise to delay definitive restorative and prosthetic treatment until the skeletal relationships are normalized and the finishing orthodontics completed. The patient should be cautioned that existing castings may occlude poorly after surgery because of the change in functional pathways. Fixed bridgework or splinted castings may have to be cut to allow individual tooth alignment. The initial restorative treatment,

then, should stabilize or temporize the existing dentition with restorations that will be serviceable and provide patient comfort during the orthodontic and surgery phases. When the final skeletal and dental relationships have been achieved, it is possible to obtain accurate articulator mountings and complete the final occlusal rehabilitation.

■ Presurgical Orthodontic Treatment

Appliance systems. In contemporary treatment, the fixed orthodontic appliance is used to stabilize the teeth and basal bone at the time of surgery and during healing. For this reason, the appliance system must permit the use of rectangular archwires for strength and stability. Any of the variations of the edgewise appliance and the combination Begg-edgewise appliance (''Stage IV'' or equivalent) are acceptable. The standard Begg appliance does not provide the control needed, even though a ribbon archwire and special retaining pins can provide some additional rigidity. Since most lingual appliances are a variation of the edgewise design, they will accept a rectangular wire, but the lingual location makes using the appliance for surgical stabilization very difficult.

Goals of presurgical treatment. The objective of presurgical treatment is to prepare the patient for surgery, not to make occlusal relationships as ideal as possible.

Since some postsurgical orthodontics will be required in any case, it is inefficient to do presurgical tooth movement that could have been accomplished more easily and quickly during or after surgery. For example, if LeFort downfracture surgery is planned for correction of a vertical or anteroposterior problem, a coexisting transverse skeletal deficiency can be corrected with parasagittal surgical expansion rather than struggling with jackscrews on a fused palatal suture. Likewise, if segmented surgery is planned in an area having residual extraction space, treatment can be shortened by closing the space with judicious osteoplasty.

As previously stated, most orthodontic movement has some component of extrusion, the results of which are exaggerated in the patient with the long face pattern because of the geometric orientation of the anatomic planes. The postoperative functional geometry is generally improved, but posterior dental extrusion still produces undesirable anterior bite opening. Simply stated, this means that the treatment sequence for the patient with a long face pattern should be planned so that postoperative tooth movement involves minor settling only.

The essential steps, then, in orthodontic preparation are to align the arches or arch segments and make them compatible, and to establish the anteroposterior and vertical position of the incisors. Both are necessary so that tooth positions will not interfere with placing the jaws in the desired position. Incisor rotations that may appear minor can markedly alter anteroposterior skeletal movement at the time of surgery.

General guidelines for tooth movement that should be done presurgically and postsurgically are given in Table 21-

Fig. 21-25 ■ Leveling by orthodontic intrusion before mandibular advancement, as compared to leveling by extrusion after surgery. **A,** Superimposition showing intrusion of the lower incisors before surgery; **B,** Superimposition showing mandibular advancement and maxillary intrusion in this patient. Presurgical intrusion was necessary to control lower face height when the mandible was brought forward. **C,** Superimposition of pretreatment and immediate presurgical tracings of a different patient, showing the posterior extrusion, increased facial height, and incisor proclination that occurred in the course of leveling. The slight retraction of the upper incisor occurred in the course of space consolidation. **D,** Superimposition of the immediate postsurgical and 2-year posttreatment cephalometric tracings in the same patient as **C.** The amount of postsurgical extrusion of posterior teeth is shown by the broken red molar outline on the mandibular superimposition. Lower anterior retraction occurred in the course of closing extraction space and has allowed some relapse in bite depth. Although the chin has moved upward and forward slightly, there has been little impact on the soft tissue appearance. For this patient, the increased anterior face height needed as part of the surgical result required that the leveling be done postsurgically by extrusion rather than presurgically by intrusion.

2. Note the implication of the guidelines that the amount of presurgical orthodontics can be quite variable, ranging from only appliance placement in a few patients to 12 months or so in others with severe crowding and incisor malpositions. The presurgical phase should almost never require more than a year, however. In contrast, the postsurgical phase is more constant in duration—not more than 6 months should be needed, and 3 to 4 months is the usual time from resumption of orthodontics to retention.

Special considerations in leveling. As Table 21-2 indicates, extrusive movement of the teeth is generally done more easily postsurgically, whereas intrusion must be accomplished presurgically or handled surgically. Two frequent questions require special consideration: how to level an accentuated curve of Spee in the lower arch of a patient with deep overbite, and how to level the upper arch in an open bite patient who has a large vertical discrepancy between anterior and posterior teeth.

Mandible. When an accentuated curve of Spee is present in the lower arch, the decision to level by intrusion of in-

Table 21-2 ■ Types of tooth movement related to timing of surgery

Must be accomplished before surgery	*Can be delayed until after surgery*
General alignment and arch coordination unless established at surgery	Detailed tooth positioning
Intrusion	Extrusion
Closure of extraction space*	Root paralleling at extraction sites
Major crossbites	Minor crossbites (½ cusp or less)

*Unless the surgery will involve an osteotomy through the extraction site, in which case at least one-half the extraction space should remain at the time of surgery.

cisors or extrusion of premolars should be based on the initial vertical position of the lower incisors. If they are elongated, i.e., if the distance from the incisal edge to the chin is excessive, they should be intruded to allow counterclockwise rotation and projection of the mandible as well as improved lower face height balance (Fig. 21-25). On the other hand, if the distance is normal, leveling by extrusion of posterior teeth, not intrusion of incisors, is needed. It is important to remember that in either case, additional arch length is needed for leveling. The required space results from expansion or extraction, so mechanotherapy decisions must be made while considering the desired final incisor position, crowding, and periodontal support.

Most short face–deep bite patients can benefit from posterior extrusion. It has been considered advantageous to stage the treatment of short face mandibular deficient patients so that much of the leveling of the lower arch is finished after surgery. A curve of Spee is left in the lower archwire, which causes the surgical splint for these patients

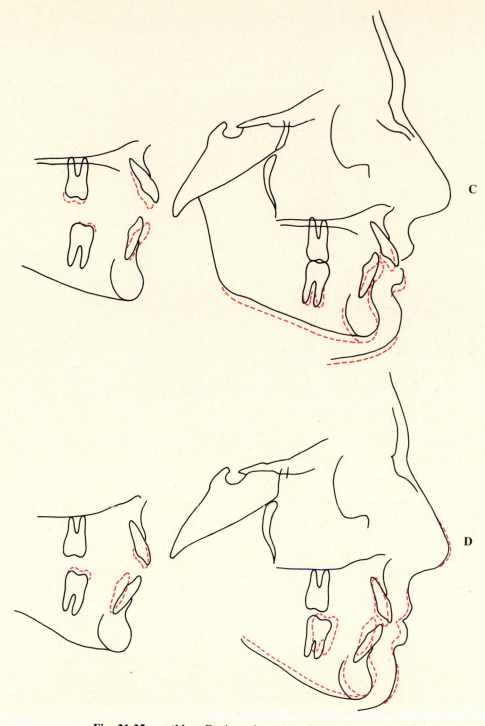

Fig. 21-25, cont'd ■ For legend see opposite page.

to be relatively thick in the premolar region. The incisors are brought into a proper position at surgery, and the leveling is accomplished by postsurgical extrusion (Fig. 21-26). In theory, treatment proceeds more rapidly and with greater increase in total facial height since the space between the teeth after surgery allows teeth in the lower buccal segments to be extruded without having to overcome occlusal force. In practice, extreme care must be taken in controlling the

torque, overbite, and overjet relationships established at surgery, because immediately after the splint is removed, only the terminal molars and the anterior teeth are in occlusal contact. This technique requires more time than the desired 3 to 4 months of postsurgical orthodontics and taxes patients' compliance at a time when they are interested in the rapid completion of treatment.

An alternative in these patients is to use an auxiliary wire

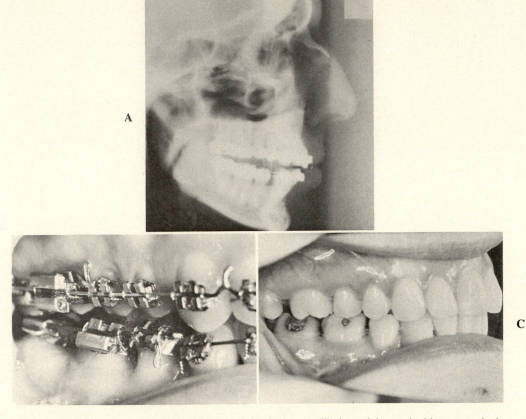

Fig. 21-26 ■ **A,** The amount of leveling remaining in the mandibular arch is seen in this postsurgical cephalometric film of a deep bite patient who had mandibular advancement. Maxillary leveling, alignment, and space consolidation were completed before surgery. Postsurgical leveling of the lower arch is often necessary to obtain the desired increase in face height and can be accomplished without problem. **B,** The mandibular archwire has been segmented between canine and premolars postsurgically. Buccal elastics and segmental mechanics are used to extrude the premolar and molar teeth into occlusion. **C,** The final occlusion after postsurgical leveling by extrusion.

to assist in more rapid preoperative leveling. A Burstone style auxiliary or utility arch (see Chapter 10) can be tied over the continuous reverse curve base archwire to increase its action. Tiebacks and concern for the point of force application aid in controlling final incisor position.

If intrusion is required, a segmented arch approach is usually indicated (see Chapters 15 and 20) but two surgical alternatives may be considered, depending on the treatment proposed. If a genioplasty has been suggested as part of the surgical treatment plan, osteotomy cuts can be designed to decrease the distance from the incisal edge to the chin point in addition to providing better mandibular projection. If large occlusal discrepancies exist, anterior intrusion can be accomplished surgically after each arch component is leveled with segmented wires.

If it appears that there will be no difference in the end treatment result, the decision regarding which technique to use may be one of treatment efficiency. If intrusion can be accomplished orthodontically while other presurgical movement is in progress, there is no reason to consider surgical approaches. When orthodontic intrusion would add an ad-

ditional 6 months to treatment, however, surgical alternatives become more reasonable.

Maxilla. In a patient with open bite, severe vertical discrepancies within the maxillary arch are an indication for multiple segment surgery. When this is planned, the upper arch should *not* be leveled conventionally. Leveling should be done only within each segment (Fig. 21-27) since the surgery allows differential vertical movement of the anterior and posterior segments. If a one-piece osteomy is planned, however, orthodontic leveling is required, but extrusion of anterior teeth before surgery must be avoided since even mild orthodontic relapse could cause a problem with postsurgical bite opening.

Establishment of incisor position and space closure. The anteroposterior position of the incisors determines where the mandible will be placed relative to the maxilla at surgery and therefore is a critical element in planning treatment. This is often the major factor in planning anchorage in the closure of extraction sites.

When several surgical segments are planned for the maxilla, a different consideration arises: the axial inclination of

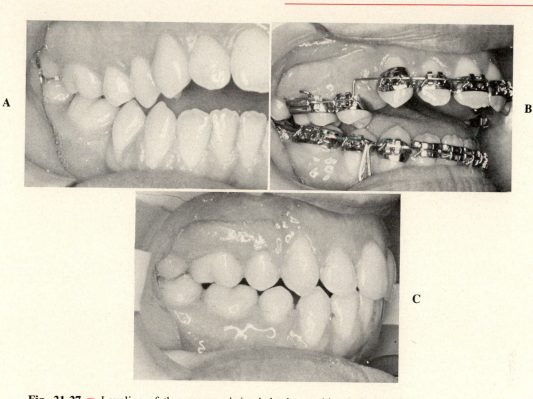

Fig. 21-27 ■ Leveling of the upper arch in skeletal open bite patients with a severe maxillary curve of Spee should be accomplished surgically, not orthodontically. **A,** Pretreatment relationship; **B,** orthodontic preparation for surgery. The stability of the open bite correction is improved if the preoperative leveling within the segments is done by stepped or segmented archwires. The final leveling is then accomplished in the course of segmented LeFort surgery. **C,** Posttreatment result.

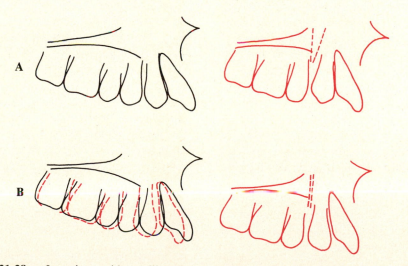

Fig. 21-28 ■ In patients with maxillary incisor protrusion, it usually is necessary to upright the incisors as they are retracted. **A,** The situation when uprighting is accomplished by rotation of the anterior maxillary segment at surgery (black, pretreatment; red, postsurgical). Note that the rotation has elevated the canines and brought their roots forward. **B,** This complication can be avoided by extracting the first premolars before jaw surgery and obtaining the correct incisor inclination (dashed red) by partially closing the extraction space. This technique allows the anterior segment to be retracted at surgery without rotation.

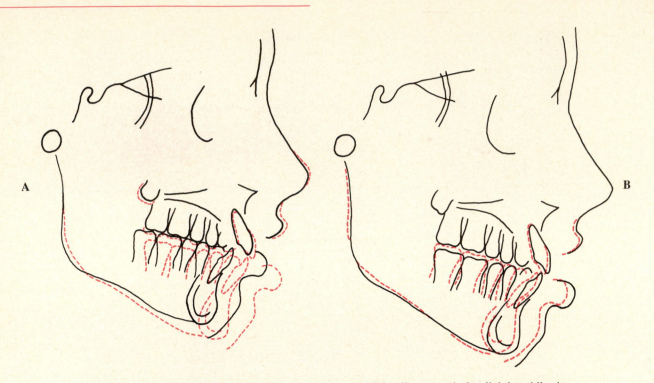

Fig. 21-29 ■ After mandibular advancement, the mandible slips posteriorly slightly while the patient is in intermaxillary fixation, even though the teeth are wired together and the occlusal relationships are preserved. In this instance, orthodontic tooth movement allows the mandible to slip back while the teeth stay in the same position as they were immediately after surgery. **A,** Superimposition showing the changes produced at surgery; **B,** superimposition showing changes during the next 6 months, almost all of which occurred in the 6 weeks of intermaxillary fixation. Note that the mandible has slipped back 2 mm, while the upper incisor has tipped back and the lower incisor has tipped forward, maintaining the occlusal relationships.

the upper incisors and canines should be established presurgically so that rotation of the anterior segment at surgery can be avoided (Fig. 21-28). Unless the arch components have been properly prepared with stepped archwires or segmented mechanics, establishing correct torque of the incisors surgically will elevate the canines above the occlusal plane. In these cases, proper postoperative repositioning of the canines has often been difficult if not impossible. An extraction site that will be the location of an osteotomy cut should not be completely closed before surgery, but up to one-half the extraction space can be used in the course of adjusting incisor inclination without creating difficulty for the surgeon.

Incisor positioning before mandibular advancement poses a special problem, because tooth movement can be anticipated in these patients during intermaxillary fixation.[18] The elastic recoil of the soft tissues that are stretched as the mandible is moved forward causes a Class II elastics effect during intermaxillary fixation (Fig. 21-29). Although the occlusal relationships are maintained by fixation and the acrylic splint, this soft tissue force causes tooth movement, and as a result, the lower jaw slips back, while the lower incisors are tipped forward and the upper incisors are retracted. The amount of this movement is probably related

to a combination of tooth mobility from presurgical orthodontics, tolerances in the fit of the archwire in the brackets and the mobility inherent to the intraosseous wiring technique. These changes stop when bony union occurs at about 6 weeks after surgery.

Overcorrection of the mandibular advancement so that the patient is placed in anterior crossbite at the time of surgery is an error, because the patient will still be in crossbite when he or she returns for postsurgical orthodontics. The proper compensation is to prepare the patient so that ust before surgery, the lower incisors are slightly overretracted and the upper incisors slightly prominent. Rigid fixation techniques appear to combat the forces producing relapse by preventing postoperative movement at the osteotomy site and the resultant changes in incisor regulation.

■ Patient Management at Surgery

As the patient is approaching the end of orthodontic preparation for surgery, it is helpful to take impressions and examine the hand-articulated models for occlusal compatibility. Minor interferences that can be easily corrected with minor archwire adjustment can significantly limit surgical movement. Upper second molars are sometimes elongated

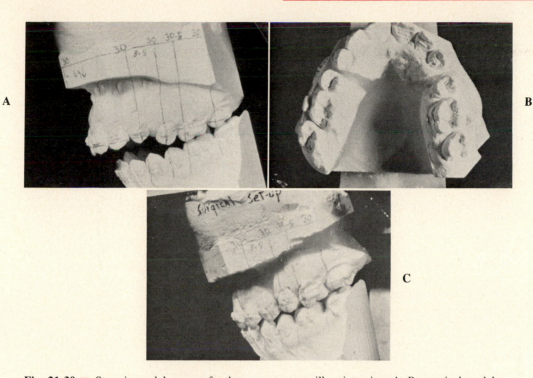

Fig. 21-30 ■ Steps in model surgery for three-segment maxillary intrusion. **A,** Presurgical models are mounted on an anatomic articulator using a facebow transfer and jaw relation records. Measurements from cusp tips to the osteotomy are marked above index lines that indicate the amount of anteroposterior and vertical movement needed at surgery. **B,** The maxillary segments are waxed into position, using the cephalometric prediction as a guide. Extraction space has been closed surgically. **C,** The final occlusion is established and a record is made of segment movement in three dimensions. These models are duplicated and used in the fabrication of the acrylic surgical splint.

by archwires that include no curve of Spee, compounding the potential interference problem.

When any final orthodontic adjustments have been made, the stabilizing archwires should be placed. These are full-dimension edgewise wires, i.e., .017 × .025 steel in the .018 appliance, .021 × .025 TMA or steel in the .022 appliance. Filling the bracket slot minimizes tolerance in the appliance system and provides the strength needed to withstand the forces resulting from intermaxillary fixation. Unless the brackets incorporate ball-hooks, brass lugs should be soldered to the archwire as attachments for the fixation wiring. Prefabricated ball-hooks may also be used if welded, soldered, or carefully crimped in place on the archwire. Crimping these in place without removing the archwire may cause distortion that could go unrecognized and result in unwanted tooth movement. Sliding them over the wire without securing them is equally undesirable, since they frequently will rotate during ligation, making intermaxillary fixation difficult.

Final surgical planning. When the orthodontist considers surgical preparation completed, presurgical records should be secured. These consist of panoramic and lateral cephalometric films, periapical films of interdental osteotomy sites, and dental casts. Casts should be mounted on a

semiadjustable articulator if maxillary vertical repositioning is planned. To avoid distortion, impressions are best made with the stabilizing archwires removed. The archwires should be passive by the time these final presurgical impressions for model surgery and splints are taken.

The orthodontist and surgeon should work closely in the final planning of surgery. The cephalometric film is used to prepare a final tracing, and acetate cutouts are again used to simulate surgical movements and predict the resultant soft tissue profile. When satisfactory functional and esthetic balance is achieved, the surgical movements are duplicated in the model surgery. It is better for the surgeon to perform this phase, since much insight into the final surgical design can be gained. The movements planned on the acetate tracings should closely match those recorded from the model surgery. If there is a significant discrepancy, one should suspect that the patient altered his mandibular position when the radiograph was taken or an error was made in recording jaw relationships. It is important to retake the record in error, since it may affect the final plan.

Splints and stabilization. We recommend the routine use of an interocclusal wafer splint, made from the casts as repositioned by the model surgery. Since this splint will define the postsurgical result, the orthodontist and surgeon

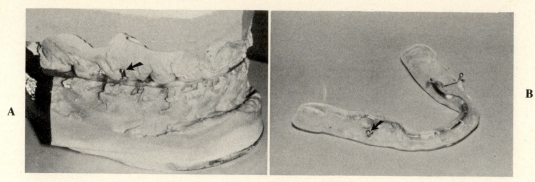

Fig. 21-31 ■ A removable surgical splint for a patient undergoing rigid fixation and early mobilization. **A,** The surgical splint should be trimmed on the buccal aspect to allow adequate visualization of occlusal interdigitation as well as hygiene during the fixation process. A ball clasp *(arrow)* has been incorporated to provide retention during function, but also to allow the patient to remove the splint while eating and for hygiene purposes. **B,** An .040 wire is molded into the lingual aspect of this splint to provide strength and maintain the splint's integrity if the acrylic is fractured during surgery or in postoperative function.

should review the model surgery together (Fig. 21-30). In patients requiring postoperative prosthetic rehabilitation, the dentist responsible for this phase of treatment should provide input regarding the acceptability of abutment and ridge relationships. Minor changes in model orientation that will facilitate subsequent treatment without compromising the surgery can be made at this time.

When the model orientation is deemed acceptable by those involved in treatment, the occlusal wafer splint can be prepared (Fig. 21-31). Plaster mounting of the models on an articulator avoids the possibility of relationships changing during the laboratory procedures. The splint is made with autopolymerizing acrylic and cured in a pressure pot to prevent distortion. It should be as thin as is consistent with adequate strength, and in most patients, some teeth should contact through the splint. It should be trimmed on

the buccal surfaces to allow good hygiene and permit visual verification of proper seating at the time of surgery. The lingual aspect of the splint can be thicker and, if needed for strength, reinforced with a large gauge wire incorporated in the acrylic.

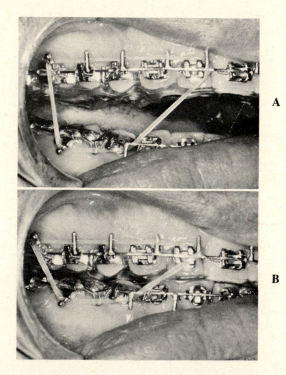

Fig. 21-33 ■ **A, B,** Light elastic traction and the occlusal wafer splint are used to guide jaw closure after the release of intermaxillary fixation. During this time, the patient begins a program of progressively increased function and physiotherapy to reestablish normal range of motion. At this stage, the splint is tied to the upper archwire or held in place by a ball clasp.

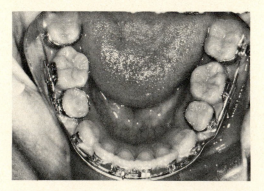

Fig. 21-32 ■ Prefabricated auxiliary wires are now used to stabilize segmented surgery by bridging the gaps between segmented base arches. A wire like this one, which is contoured to fit the model surgery casts and fits into the auxiliary tubes on first molars, can be placed quickly in the operating room and eliminates the need for the orthodontist to bend a passive stabilizing archwire at the time of surgery.

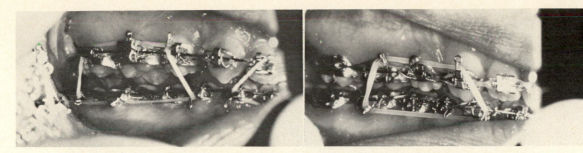

Fig. 21-34 ■ When adequate stability has been achieved, the splint is removed and light flexible archwires are placed to allow final settling. Light elastics placed in the buccal segments guide the occlusal pathway and assist in the final interdigitation that occurs rapidly over a 6- to-8-week period. **A,** Occlusal relationships at the beginning of postsurgical orthodontics; **B,** 8 weeks later.

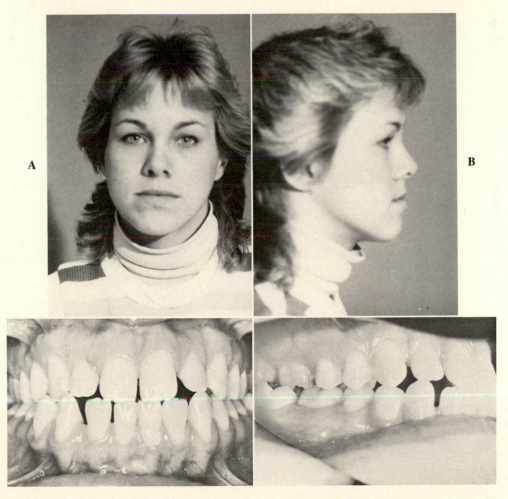

Fig. 21-35 ■ Treatment records for a patient having integrated orthodontic-surgical correction of mandibular prognathism combined with a mild skeletal open bite. **A** and **B,** Frontal and profile photographs show the protrusion and increased height of the lower third of the face. **C,** Dental compensation has resulted in a pretreatment end-to-end incisor relationship with minimum overbite. **D,** Class III canine and molar relationships are seen on the lateral view.

Continued.

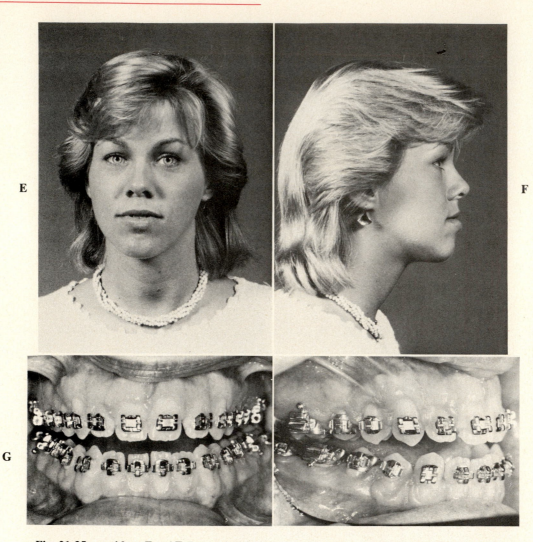

Fig. 21-35, cont'd ■ **E** and **F,** Presurgical frontal and profile photographs taken after the correction of dental compensations show slightly more lip protrusion than the pretreatment photos. **G** and **H,** Orthodontic leveling has resulted in bite opening that will necessitate maxillary as well as mandibular surgery. Presurgical predictions of treatment by mandibular setback alone showed an increase in posterior ramus height, a movement known to be unstable.

Prefabricated auxiliary archwires are useful if segmental surgery is planned. The auxiliary is fitted into headgear tubes and lies lateral to the segmented main archwire (Fig. 21-32). When ligated to the main archwire, the auxiliary, coupled with the wafer splint, provides good stability for the surgical segments. The auxiliary *must* be adjusted to lie passively since this large a wire can exert a considerable amount of force. If the surgeon is not comfortable making these adjustments, they should be done by the orthodontist at the time of surgery or immediately postoperatively. Failure to do so can result in distraction of the segments or undesired tooth movement during fixation.

■ Postsurgical Orthodontics

When there has been adequate bony healing, the patient is allowed to resume limited function under the observation of the surgeon. The acrylic splint is ligated to one of the arches to key the occlusion, and light elastics are used to guide jaw function (Fig. 21-33).

Once satisfactory range of motion and stability are achieved, the finishing stages of orthodontics can be started. It is critically important that when the splint is removed, the stabilizing archwires are also removed and working wires are placed to allow final tooth movement. Light vertical elastics are continued at this time to override proprioceptive impulses from the teeth that otherwise would cause the patient to seek a new position of maximum intercuspation (Fig. 21-34). Removal of the splint without allowing the teeth to settle into better interdigitation can result in the patient adopting an undesirable convenience bite, which in turn complicates orthodontic finishing and could stress recent surgery sites. To prevent this reaction, it is usually

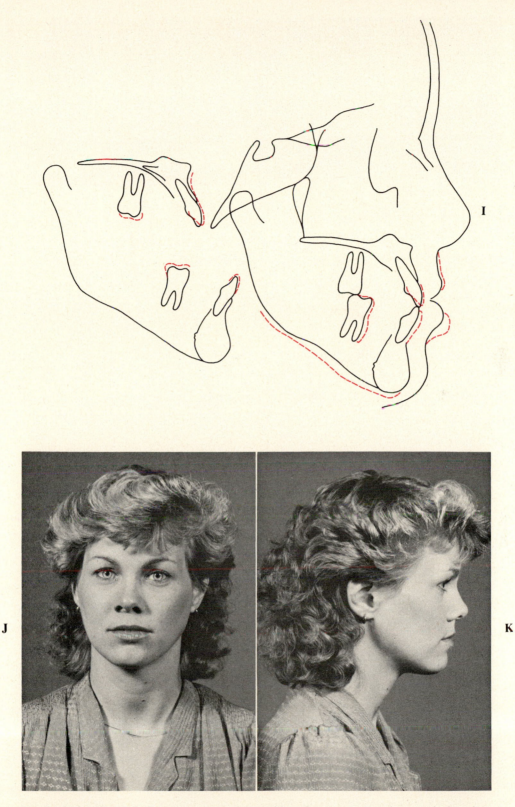

Fig. 21-35, cont'd ▪ **I,** Cephalometric superimposition of pretreatment and presurgical tracings. The red outline shows the bite opening and downward movement of the chin that has occurred during leveling. **J** and **K,** Frontal and profile photographs taken at the completion of treatment show improved vertical facial balance and correction of the prognathism. Surgery consisted of LeFort I osteotomy with posterior intrusion combined with bilateral sagittal split ramus osteotomies and mandibular setback. Rigid fixation with osteosynthesis plates and lag screws allowed mobilization 2 weeks after surgery.

Continued.

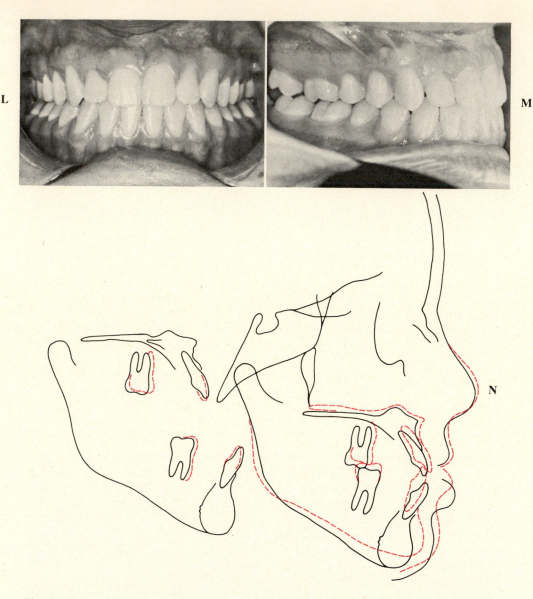

Fig. 21-35, cont'd ■ **L** and **M,** Intraoral photographs taken after appliance removal show correction of the open bite, spacing, and reverse overjet. Postoperative settling and detailing of the occlusion was completed within 3 months after surgery and has remained stable. **N,** Cephalometric superimposition of the presurgical and posttreatment tracings. The final treatment result is shown by the broken red line. Tooth movement has primarily been consolidation and leveling. The maxilla is repositioned upward and forward and the mandible placed backward and upward. The elevation of the nasal tip is typically found after LeFort I procedures.

preferable for the orthodontist, not the surgeon, to remove the splint.

The type of archwire used for final settling is determined by the amount of movement needed. Minor movement can be achieved rapidly using light round wires (typically .016 steel) and buccal box elastics with an anterior vector that supports the sagittal correction. More anterior torque control may be desired if a moderate amount of settling is needed. In these cases, braided rectangular wire preserves the anterior relationships established preoperatively but provides adequate flexibility in the vertical plane to permit interdigitation. If circumstances require a considerable amount of

settling in the buccal segments, precautions must be taken to prevent alteration of the anterior relationships. It may be desirable to segment the archwire and work independently with the posterior occlusion in these instances. An alternative approach is to use wire that is rectangular in the anterior portion and changes to light round posteriorly. In any case, the settling process proceeds rapidly and rarely takes longer than 2 months (Fig. 21-35).

Retention after surgical orthodontics is no different than for other adult patients (see Chapter 20), and definitive periodontal and prosthetic treatment can follow the establishment of the final occlusal relationships.

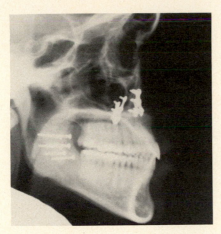

Fig. 21-36 ■ This posttreatment cephalometric film of the patient shown in Fig. 21-35 demonstrates the rigid fixation system used to secure the osseous segments. Four osteosynthesis plates hold the maxilla and three lag screws were used on each side of the mandibular surgery site. There is rarely any indication to remove these devices after healing since patients seldom perceive their presence.

■ Future Directions

In recent years, the growth of knowledge regarding the etiology, diagnosis, and treatment of patients with dentofacial deformities has been almost logarithmic. There is no reason to suspect that activity in this area will diminish in the future.

The full impact of the computer era has yet to be felt in diagnosis and treatment planning. Presently, computers are being used to rapidly retrieve information and compare individual patient data with existing norms. Computed imaging techniques are just beginning to be explored by those interested in dentofacial deformities. Continued development will allow preoperative surgical simulation on three-dimensional images of the patient, thus allowing more detailed analysis of the projected result.

Surgery techniques will continue to undergo refinement, which will enhance stability and minimize morbidity. Procedures will become less invasive and recovery will be faster as smaller and more sophisticated instrumentation is developed. Presently, there is a growing interest in rigid fixation systems that enhance stability and allow earlier mobilization (Fig. 21-36). Research in the area of biomaterials will undoubtedly result in a biocompatible bone adhesive that will eliminate the need for metallic systems.

Much is still to be learned regarding the mechanisms controlling craniofacial growth and the degree to which they can be manipulated. Currently, one sees great interest in neuromuscular physiology and its impact on determining facial morphology. Little is known, however, about the biochemical and mechanical role played by other investing tissues such as fascia and periosteum. All of these factors must be considered in the context of the role played by genetic coding.

At present, treatment is being successfully provided by practitioners at institutions throughout the world. Continued research will surely allow treatment to become directed at the cause of aberrant growth rather than the effect.

■ References

1. Angle, E.H.: Double resection of the lower maxilla. Dental Cosmos **40**:July-Dec., 1898.
2. Trauner, R., and Obwegeser, H.: The surgical correction of mandibular prognathism and retrognathia with consideration of genioplasty. Oral Surg. Oral Med. Oral Pathol. **10**:671-692, 1957.
3. Epker, B.N.: Modifications in the sagittal osteotomy of the mandible. J. Oral Surg. **34**:157-159, 1977.
4. Bell, W.H., and Schendel, S.A.: Biologic basis for modifications of the sagittal split ramus osteotomy. J. Oral Surg. **35**:362-369, 1977.
5. Bell, W.H.: LeFort I osteotomy for correction of maxillary deformities. J. Oral Surg. **33**:412-426, 1975.
6. Epker, B.N., and Wolford, L.M.: Middle third facial osteotomies: their use in the correction of acquired and developmental dentofacial and craniofacial deformities. J. Oral Surg. **33**:491-514, 1975.
7. Glassman, A.S., Nahigian, S.J., Medway, J.M., et al.: Conservative surgical adult rapid palatal expansion. Am. J. Orthod. **86**:207-213, 1984.
8. Aragon, S.B., and Van Sickles, J.E.: Effects of early physiotherapy on opening following orthognathic surgery. J. Dent. Res. **64**:216, 1985.
9. Zaytoun, H., Jr., Phillips, C., and Terry, B.C.: Skeletal alterations following TOVRO or BSSO procedures. J. Dent. Res. **64**:215, 1985.
10. Phillips, C., Schellhase, D.J., Proffit, W.R., et al.: Skeletal stability following surgical maxillary intrusion. J. Dent. Res. **64**:349, 1985.
11. Kolë, H.: Surgical operations on the alveolar ridge to correct occlusal abnormalities. Oral Surg. Oral Med. Oral Pathol. **12**:515-524, 1959.
12. Ricketts, R.M., et al.: Book I. Bioprogressive Therapy. Parts 7 and 8. Denver, 1980, Rocky Mountain Orthodontics.
13. Gilmore, C.A., and Little, R.M.: Mandibular incisor dimension and crowding. Am. J. Orthod. **86**:493, 1984.
14. Washburn, M.C., Schendel, S.A., and Epker, B.N.: Superior repositioning of the maxilla during growth. Oral Surg. Oral Med. Oral Pathol. **53**:142-149, 1982.
15. Behrents, R.G.: A treatise on the continuum of growth in the aging craniofacial skeleton. Ann Arbor, 1984, University of Michigan, Ph.D. dissertation.
16. Wolford, L.M., Schendel, S.A., and Epker, B.N.: Surgical orthodontic correction of mandibular deficiency in growing children: long-term treatment results. J. Maxillofac. Surg. **7**:61-72, 1979.
17. Huang, C.S., and Ross, R.B.: Surgical advancement of the retrognathic mandible in growing children. Am. J. Orthod. **82**:89-103, 1982.
18. Lake, S.L., McNeil, R.W., Little, R.M., et al.: Surgical mandibular advancement: a cephalometric analysis of treatment response. Am. J. Orthod. **80**:376-393, 1981.

INDEX